DIMENSIONS
OF
PROFESSIONAL
NURSING

Lucie Young Kelly, R.N., Ph.D.

DIMENSIONS OF PROFESSIONAL NURSING

FOURTH EDITION

Macmillan Publishing Co., Inc.
New York
Collier Macmillan Publishers
London

Macmillan Publishing Co., Inc.
866 Third Avenue, New York, New York 10022

Collier Macmillan Canada, Ltd.

Library of Congress Cataloging in Publication Data

Kelly, Lucie Young.
    Dimensions of professional nursing.

    Bibliography: p.
    Includes index.
    1. Nursing.   2. Nursing—United States.   I. Title.
[DNLM: 1. Nursing.   WY16 K33d]
RT82.K4   1981   610.73   80-17353
ISBN 0-02-362270-9

Printing: 45678   Year: 34567

ISBN   0-02-362270-9

Preface

In this fourth edition of *Dimensions of Professional Nursing,* the changes in nursing—new and emerging concerns and commitments, opportunities and omens, progress and problems—are evident. More than ever, it is critical that nurses become informed about the broad range of issues that include but go beyond clinical practice. Without such knowledge, we cannot deal with the present, much less the future.

Therefore, once more, this book intends to present what Cordelia Kelly, the author of the first two editions, called, "an overview of the nonclinical aspects of nursing in sufficient detail to be adaptable for use at all stages in all types of preservice programs in professional nursing." To this I add once more, "and in the continuing education of nurses at all levels." The book is directed particularly toward educational programs whose philosophy includes the belief that if nurses are to be professional practitioners, they must not only be knowledgeable and skilled in the clinical aspects of nursing, but also understand what the profession is and work toward making it what it could be.

In this revision, there have been a number of changes. Increasingly, I am convinced that not only can many lessons be learned from the past, but that the understanding of our nursing history and nursing leaders can renew a professional sense of pride in nursing's accomplishments. Therefore, Part I of this book concentrates on the historical background of nursing.

The chapter on Florence Nightingale has been developed more fully, and the following two new chapters on the history of American nursing pinpoint the landmarks of nursing progress with emphasis on the people who made them so. The section ends with an updated overview of major nursing studies.

Part II has five sections that describe contemporary professional nursing. Most are new or greatly expanded to focus on emerging concerns. Section 1 comprehensively delineates how, where, and by whom health care is given. Students are introduced to both the health care setting (people and places) and to major health care issues and trends. Also given attention are the societal changes that affect every aspect of nursing, such as the consumer movement, women's movement, changes in education, and scientific/technological developments. In the next section, the issue of professionalism and the multiple meanings of nursing are explored, with a brief look at the nursing process and some of the theories of nursing. Professional ethics is given considerable attention, with comparisons of varying concepts, as well as presentation of the major codes of ethics. The first American nursing code which few people are aware of presents a fascinating glimpse into the past. In "The Profile of the Modern Nurse," new information on ethnic minorities and men has been added as well as a synthesis of the many new surveys on nursing attitudes and characteristics.

The section on Education and Research is even more comprehensive than before. Besides being updated, it gives particular attention to the serious issues that must be faced, presenting the various points of view about the future of nursing that have caused such divisiveness among nurses.

v

The longest chapter in the book is "Areas of Practice." Never have nurses had so many career opportunities. For instance, the hows and whats of private or independent practice, as well as new data on nurse practitioners merit attention. At the same time, full information is given on the types of positions beginning nurses will be seeking. Immediately following the practice opportunities are the problems and challenges—the struggle for autonomy and influence. The issues and suggested strategies are explored. Nurse power and leadership is discussed, as is the importance of inter- and intraprofessional relationships.

Section 5 on the law has been completely reorganized, updated, and enriched. This section should provide a solid base of knowledge about the many-faceted legal aspects of nursing and includes additional informational resources. Chapter 19 should be particularly useful as a permanent reference; it includes most of the major federal legislation affecting nursing, which, to the best of my knowledge, does not appear elsewhere. At a time when consumerism is reaching a peak, "rights" issues are particularly significant, including the rights of students and RNs.

Section 1 of Part III, besides the expected updating, has added dimensions in Chapter 23, which includes a discussion of the problems and conflicts in professional nursing organizations, and in Chapter 29, which presents a guide to literature search and guidelines for writing and publication.

Finally, the last section assists the new, or not so new, graduate in the critical process of identifying and getting the "right" job. The last chapter focuses on the conflicts that arise on the job, how to deal with reality shock, "burnout," stress, and suggestions to help meet the challenges of professionalism.

Because *Dimensions of Professional Nursing* is intended for and used by a diverse readership and is often used for reference, the references and bibliography are once more broad-based so that students, RNs and others can further research what is of interest and importance to them. References giving more than one point of view on a controversial issue are included wherever possible. Besides the standard nursing journals, references from other professional journals and books give a different flavor to familiar issues.

In using the book, it will be noted that cross references are frequent. For instance, different aspects of collective bargaining are discussed in Chapter 19 (components of the various labor laws); in Chapter 22 (the right of the nurse to organize and engage in collective bargaining and the process used) and in Chapter 25 (the role of the ANA in collective bargaining.) Another major issue, continuing education, is referred to in Chapter 2 (Nightingale's concept), Chapter 6 (the consumer movement and educational trends), Chapter 10 (accountability for competent practice), Chapter 12 (issues), Chapter 13 (types), Chapter 20 (mandatory continuing education), and Chapter 31 (where and how to get it).

I thank the many users—teachers and students—of the book whom I have met as I travel around the country and who have shared with me their concerns and interests in nursing "trends and issues." Equally appreciated are the efforts of those who answered a questionnaire seeking input into the new edition.

I have many others to thank: the staff and officers of the various professional organizations and the AJN Company, the Armed Services and VA nursing services, who all sent much descriptive material and often took time to discuss their programs and organizations with me; the staff of the AJN Company Library and the Columbia University Health Science Library who were always pleasant and helpful; Susan Canfield, then a graduate student in the nurse administrator program in the School of Public Health at Columbia University, who put together Chapters 27 and 28. Special appreciation goes to Carol Cruz, who efficiently typed the major portion of this manuscript.

My deep involvement in nursing has made

the writing of this fourth edition more meaningful than ever. I was constantly reminded of the excitement of being part of our profession in this critical period, having the opportunity to participate in the decisions that will affect the future of nursing and health care. There are serious challenges to be met, but nursing's accomplishments and advances, along with our new sense of accountability, should be a source of continued pride. It is my hope that this book will in some way help nurses to understand and care about the continually new dimensions of professional nursing.

LUCIE YOUNG KELLY

Contents

ix

Part
III
PROFESSIONAL COMPONENTS AND CAREER DEVELOPMENT

DEVELOPMENT OF MODERN NURSING

SECTION

1

EARLY HISTORICAL INFLUENCES

CHAPTER 1

Care of the Sick:
An Historical Overview

The clinical practice of nursing is quite rightly the major focus of most of its practitioners and the prime concern of students. Therefore, there is a tendency to greet nursing history with a "What good is it to me?" attitude. Undoubtedly, nurses can give good nursing care even if they have never heard of Florence Nightingale, Isabel Hampton Robb, Lavinia Dock, or Lillian Wald. But one of the major differences between an occupation and a profession is its practitioners' long-term commitment to the profession, which includes working toward its development. To do so without some understanding of its past is possibly to repeat errors.

Nursing today was formed by its historical antecedents. Its development since ancient times, within the social contexts of those times, explains many things: its power or lack of power, its educational confusion, and the makeup of its practitioners. The changing relationships between nursing and other health care professions, nursing and other disciplines, nursing and the public can be traced and better understood with the knowledge of past history. The impact of social and scientific changes on nursing and nursing's impact on society are ongoing proc-

esses that need to be studied; nursing does not exist in a vacuum. Sometimes there is a repetition of history, with the answer to the problems apparently not much clearer now than a hundred years ago. For instance, a 1901 editorial in the *Journal of the American Medical Association* said, "The usefulness of the nurse is and always will be gauged by her faithfulness as a subordinate intelligently carrying out the directions of the physician. . . ."[1] In 1977, a major medical organization noted, "An independent, autonomous nurse practitioner is inconsistent with (the organization's position that nurses and other health care personnel work under the physician's direction) and must lead to second-class medical care."[2] A hundred years ago, there was objection from within and without nursing to nurses having more education; the scenario is repeated today. Seventy-five years ago, the question of nursing licensure was hotly debated; today, it is again a major concern. These issues affect the practice of every nurse; in some cases, they are a factor in whether the nurse even chooses to stay in the profession. An understanding of the past can bring additional clarity to the decisions that shape the future.

This chapter and those that follow in Part I are not intended in any way as a substitute for the many fine texts that are available on nursing history. Instead, they provide an overview to set the stage for the more detailed study of nursing history an individual may undertake for professional reasons or personal satisfaction. As an additional resource, Appendix A presents vignettes of distinguished nurses of the past.

PRIMITIVE SOCIETIES

Although historians sometimes advance theories and cite an occasional archaeological discovery to prove that prehistoric civilization practiced crude medicine and nursing, the supporting evidence about nursing is somewhat inconclusive. It must be assumed, however, that in most tribes there were some individuals who were more adept than others at caring for the sick and injured and helping the medicine men or witch doctors. It seems reasonable to assume further that some of these men and women taught their sons and daughters and certain members of the tribes to give this care, for these people were able to communicate; they wanted to survive; they were human beings with some ability to think, to recall, and to teach by example, if not by coherent explanation.

Indirect evidence of some of the beliefs and practices of ancient man concerning illness has evolved from recent studies of primitive cultures. Apparently, many concepts of health and illness were related to belief in the supernatural. Everything in nature was seen as being alive with invisible forces and supernatural power. There were good spirits and evil spirits that must be placated. Primitive man believed that a person became sick (1) when an evil spirit entered the body; (2) when a good spirit within the body that was ordinarily able to fend off diseases left, either because someone or something had taken it away or of its own accord; and (3) because witchcraft had been performed upon the affected part of the body, either directly or through some object that had been given to the person.

Thus, although it was probably recognized how heat, cold, certain foods, wounds, and strains were related to health and empirical treatments developed for them, serious illness called for the services of a medicine man (witch doctor, shaman, root doctor). This mysterious figure, sometimes a woman, but usually a man, functioned through a ritualistic mystique, frequently a shock or fright technique that was intended to induce evil spirits to leave the body. Included were the use of frightening masks and noises, incantations, vile odors, charms, spells, sacrifices, and fetishes. In a primitive version of modern trephining, the medicine man cut a hole in the skull to let the evil spirit out. Purgatives, emetics, deodorants, applied hot and cold substances, cauterization, massage, cupping, and blistering were frequently used.

A woman in abnormal labor was treated by similarly drastic measures, such as placing a lighted fire between her outstretched legs to hasten delivery. Needless to say, patients did not always survive this treatment, and if they did, there is no evidence that any daily ongoing care was given by the shaman. Probably a relative gave this "nursing" care. Women generally assisted other women in childbearing. But whether treatment of illness and injury by use of herbs and other "natural" means was carried out by all men, and/or women, or specially designated individuals is not known.

EARLY CIVILIZATIONS

In the written records of the early civilizations (5000 B.C. to A.D. 476), there is very little reference to nursing as such. However, if there is evidence of a high standard of living, a good sanitation system, architectural achievement, interest in education and culture and scientific medicine, or even two or three of these, it is reasonably certain that the health of the inhabitants was of paramount importance and that nurses were not only present but were trained in some fashion to prepare them for the work they did.

The Babylonians

Babylonia was the center of ancient Mesopotamian culture, which was in ruins by the time the Christian era began. Located between the eastern Mediterranean Sea and the Persian Gulf and nourished by the Tigris and Euphrates rivers, this land was very fertile, offering a good life to its settlers. Coveted by many peoples, it was for thousands of years first under the rule of one master and then another who took possession by force. Each influenced the others' development intellectually, socially, and scientifically. Their many wars brought misery and suffering, and, even in that abundant country, there must have been many illnesses and injuries in the normal course of life.

There is evidence that a legalized medical service was instituted and that some type of lay nurse cared for patients. They may have been men, but if they were women, their status was probably quite low, and they must have been subservient to physicians because the women of Babylonia were dominated by men who controlled their every action.

Herodotus, a Greek historian called the "Father of History," recorded that it was customary in Babylon for the sick to go to the marketplace where passersby could see them and stop and inquire into the "nature of their distemper." Those who had knowledge of how to treat a condition (knowledge acquired principally through experience) advised the ill on therapy that had helped them. This was hardly a scientific method of treatment, but it no doubt was effective in many instances.

Excavations made in 1849 of 700 medical tablets show that the Babylonian physician-priest allowed his patient to choose whether he wanted to be treated with medicine or charms. If he selected medicine, the physician had many vegetable and mineral preparations to employ. If he selected charms, the doctor told him which ones to wear for his particular illness and probably uttered a few incantations to accompany them, for they still believed that disease was caused by sin and displeasure of the gods.

However, some of the treatments indicate a realistic attitude toward illness, for they included diet, rest, enemas, bandaging, and massaging plus emphasis on the importance of good personal hygiene. This care might be given by family or a "nurse."

The first Babylonian Empire was founded by King Hammurabi, who developed a code of laws for the whole empire. The code is engraved on a huge stone, unearthed in 1902, and shows Hammurabi worshipping a sun god from whom he is receiving instructions about the laws. Included are laws concerned with the fees that a physician was allowed to charge for his services and also punishment for the physician who committed "malpractice." Payments were to be made in *shekels* of silver—usually two, five, or ten, depending upon whether the patient was a master or a slave. Punishment for causing a patient to lose his life or an eye was to "cut off the physician's hands if the patient was a nobleman." (This kind of punishment was reserved for surgeons, not physician-priests.) Wet nurses were also regulated as to renumeration and responsibility.

The Ancient Hebrews

Much of the story of the ancient Hebrews is told in the *Talmud* and the Old Testament. The Hebrews, alone of their contemporaries, believed in one God, Yahweh, not many.

Their misfortunes and illnesses they attributed to God's wrath, and they depended upon Him more than on man to restore them to health when they were sick. One facet of their religion was that it was their duty to be hospitable to strangers as well as to their own people, and they were obliged to give a tithe to augment their personal service in visiting the sick and needy.

The Hebrews brought many hygienic practices from Babylonia where they had been in captivity, but under the leadership of Moses they also developed principles and practices of hygiene and sanitation. Moses decreed that all meat must be inspected, the selection and preparation of all foods must be carefully supervised, and cleanliness in all areas of living was absolutely essential. This has been called the first sanitary legislation. It represented one of the first public health movements on record.

Their people were taught to help prevent the spread of communicable diseases by burning an infected person's garments and sometimes even his house, and by scrubbing the room in which he was ill and the utensils he used. They were often able to diagnose and control the spread of leprosy and gonorrhea. They performed trephining operations skillfully and humanely, giving the patient a sleeping potion before surgery to dull the pain. They also did Caesarian sections, splenectomies, amputations, circumcisions, and set fractures. They dressed wounds with oil, wine, and balsam and used sutures and bandages.

From these operations and careful examination of animals made primarily for sanitary purposes, they developed a body of knowledge about anatomy and physiology, although we know now that some of their information was understandably superficial and inaccurate.

The nurse is mentioned occasionally in the Old Testament and the *talmud*, but in what capacity she served, except as wet nurse, is not entirely clear. It does appear that the "nurse" visited and possibly cared for the sick in their homes. She probably also had a role in health teaching.

The Persian Contribution

Between c. 550 and 500 B.C., Cyrus the Great, King of Persia, and his son, Cambyses, acquired a vast empire in the Near East. They adopted many of the medical practices and much of the culture from the great lands they conquered—Asia Minor, Babylonia, Syria, Mesopotamia, Egypt, and several others.

In Egypt, the Emperor Darius, successor of Cambyses, restored a school for training priest-physicians and, in effect, established a government-controlled medical center, the first of its kind recorded in history. It is also known that there were practitioners who healed with holy words, with herbs, and with the knife—in decreasing order of practice.

The Art of Medicine in Egypt

There are references to nurses in accounts of Egyptian medicine as it was practiced in the pre-Christian era. The medical *papyri* discovered during excavations contain descriptions of such nursing procedures as feeding a tetanus patient and dressing wounds. The extent of the nurse's duties is not clear, however.

Egyptian medicine, on the other hand, is revealed by graven inscriptions, the *papyri*, and other literature as having been rather far advanced. In spite of the Egyptians' ideas about the origins of life, the journey that man took after death, the causes of disease, and the catastrophic effects of incurring the wrath of the gods, they also practiced some very good medicine, although it may not have been based on scientific principles. Priests and physicians were identical in early Egyptian civilization, and in healing temples, rest, rituals and prayer were part of the treatment. Later there emerged physicians who were concerned only with matters of health and hygiene.

Medical specialization became so common that a physician usually spent his entire career in caring for diseases of one particular part of the body. Members of the profession were organized to protect their medical secrets.

It was in ancient Egypt that the great physician Imhotep lived in about 2980 B.C. Skilled in architecture, magic, and priestcraft as well as medicine, he became so famous that he was never forgotten. More than two and a half centuries after his death, he became the god of medicine, identified by the Greeks with their famous god of healing, Asclepios (Latin, Aesculapius).

In Egypt, as in most countries, one of the important areas of concern was the health of the people.

The Egyptians formulated regulations about diet, baths, purgatives, and other matters of personal hygiene. They initiated laws of health suited to Egypt's climate and terrain. They developed diagnostic procedures (which differed in some respects from those of other ancient civilizations) for the common illnesses of their people. Examinations of mummies indicate that the Egyptians suffered many bone diseases and injuries. Osteoarthritis was apparently very common and there must also have been ailments all humans are subject to such as abdominal, gynecological, and genitourinary conditions.

There were medical schools and at least one school of midwifery for women, the graduates of which taught physicians about "women's conditions." They became quite well informed about some aspects of anatomy and physiology. For example, the *papyri* reveal that Egyptian physicians may have had reasonably accurate knowledge of the circulatory system, which was not described accurately and completely by modern man until the sixteenth century A.D., when William Harvey studied it. Taking the pulse was a common practice, and the quality of both the heart beat and the pulse was considered important in understanding a patient's condition. Treatments included the use of a kind of adhesive plaster for closing small wounds, swabs, bandages, and tampons made from linen ravelings, sutures, and molded splints. The *papyri* also contains records of the preparation of pills, ointments, snuffs, gargles, and emmolients that have continued, at least in name, until modern times. Drugs included opium, castor oil, hemlock, salts of copper, and many others.

Dentistry was practiced skillfully, if the gold-filled teeth of mummies of wealthy citizens are to be accepted as evidence. Egyptians developed the art of embalming the body to provide a home for the soul as it went on its journey after death.

The Ancient Hindus

The history of pre-Christian India reports the establishment of hospitals, probably the first in the world, and also the first special nursing group of which we have accurate information. These male attendants (perhaps more accurately called physician's assistants instead of nurses) staffed the hospitals to which surgeons with remarkable skills sent their patients for care. The Indian philosophy which assigned women to an inferior role in society would not allow them to work outside the home environment. The "nurses'" qualifications were stated as follows in the *Charaka Samhita*, a medical manuscript:

> . . . there should be secured a body of attendants of good behavior, distinguished for purity or cleanliness of habits, attached to the person for whose services they are engaged, possessed of cleverness and skill, endowed with kindness, skilled in every kind of service that a patient may require . . . clever in bathing or washing a patient . . . well skilled in making or cleaning beds . . . and skillful in waiting upon one that is ailing, and never unwilling to do any act that they be commanded to do.

One does not know who did the "commanding" of these workers—patients or doctors, or both. The nurse's status is also unclear (it appears that he might have become a physician after training), but we at least know that he performed some nursing functions.

The knowledge about Indian medicine derives principally from several of their books and writings (in contrast to the reliance on archeological discoveries for data about the Mesopotamian and Egyptian civilizations and others). Of these, the sacred writings called the *Vedas*, a compendium of surgical works *(Susruta Samhita)*, and another of medical works *(Charaka Samhita)* are most informative.

From the *Vedas*, which were the oldest scriptures of Hinduism, it is learned that the Indian people of ancient times were highly religious and believed in divine control of health and disease. They worshipped many gods, and especially the sun god Brahma, until Buddhism originated in the sixth century B.C. They used charms and invocations and other primitive methods to quell the wrath of the gods, but from about 800 B.C. to A.D. 1000, all India flourished and progressed, and medicine advanced also. It was during this period that the hospitals mentioned earlier were built.

The two outstanding physicians of ancient times were Susruta and Charaka who in their writings revealed that physicians were members of the upper castes and were required to be pure of mind and body and ethical in every respect. Their knowledge of anatomy and physiology was often inaccurate, but they evolved some theories that persisted for centuries. Among these was the belief that disease might be caused by impurities in the body fluids or humors. They used blood-letting procedures to rid the body of the impure fluids. This theory of humoral pathology was accepted subsequently by Greek physicians and became a basic concept of European medicine. The Indian physician had a great many drugs and other pharmaceutical preparations to help him in his work.

The surgery practiced in India was particularly outstanding for the time. With instruments they designed themselves, under the cleanest conditions possible, without the aid of effective antiseptics or the benefits of anesthesia, the surgeons performed tonsillectomies, herniorrhaphies, tumor excisions, cataract operations, and other surgery.

To help prevent disease, the Hindus formulated religious laws covering particularly matters of hygiene and diet suitable to the tropical climate.

Scientific medicine in India eventually lost its momentum and during the Mohammedan era beginning about A.D. 622, it began to decline and became almost completely extinguished, a genuine loss to world medicine.

Ceylon, an island just off India's southeast coast, also enjoyed an advanced standard of living during the period of India's greatest achievement. History has recorded the establishment of many hospitals in which well-prepared physicians and nurses attended the sick. Hospitals for animals also were founded in India as well as Ceylon.

The Chinese

As in other ancient cultures, magic, demons, and evil spirits were part of Chinese medical beliefs. The beginning of a more modern medicine is credited to the emperor Shen Nung (c. 2700 B.C.), who apparently originated drug therapy and acupuncture. These were incorporated into the theory of Yang and Yin which still exists. Yang, the male principle, is light, positive, full of life; Yin, the female principle, is dark, cold, lifeless. When the two are in harmony, the patient is in good health. Originally, acupuncture consisted of inserting needles into areas called meridians, which controlled the flow of Yang and Yin. (With new interest in acupuncture, American medicine is trying to determine its anatomic and physiological basis.)

Other Chinese contributions include the use of many still pertinent drugs and further refinement of ancient measures of hydrotherapy, massage, cupping (bloodletting) moxa (a form of counterirritation) cautery, and the promotion of systematic exercise to maintain physical and mental well-being.

Sources of information include a book on medicine written by Shen Nung, and later works, notably the classic *Canon of Medicine,* which is a complete discussion of anatomy and physiology with many details about blood circulation and pulse. Another outstanding book was the *Essay on Typhoid* written in the first century A.D. by Chang Chung Ching, often regarded as China's greatest physician.

There is little mention of any type of hospital, perhaps because of strong family traditions that would naturally include giving care to the sick within the family circle. Thus, nursing care was probably given in the home.

The Great Achievements of Greece

Whenever ancient Greece is mentioned, one immediately thinks of education, progress, philosophy, and democracy. But Plato, Aristotle, Socrates, Herodotus, Homer, Sophocles, Pericles, Euripides, and other great names of Greece were not typical of its earliest times, for this country too began under primitive conditions in about 2000 B.C.

The first of the great philosophers, Socrates, was born in 469 B.C.; his pupil Plato was born in 427 B.C.; and Aristotle, Plato's famous pupil, in 384 B.C. Herodotus, the great historian, was born in 484 B.C.; Homer, the epic poet, in c. 1000 B.C.

The ancient Greeks represented many peoples, principally the Achean, Dorian, Aegean, Ionian, Arcadian, and Aeolian, who came from the mountains, from fertile valleys where they had engaged in agriculture, and from the seacoast where seafaring was their occupation. Collectively they called themselves the Hellenes (after their ancestor Hellen, a legendary king of Phthia).

They were barbaric peoples at first with the superstitions and practices of primitive peoples, but gradually there emerged the well-known Grecian character with a thirst for truth and knowledge. Because of their geographical location and the ease of maritime travel, they were able to visit such comparatively advanced countries as Crete and Mesopotamia and borrow or usurp their culture.

They were also eager to expand their geographical borders and were so successful that within a few centuries their culture extended from Greece to India. Gradually they developed their own Hellenic civilization and by 500 B.C., if not before, they displayed the keen intellect, independence of thought, and democratic action for which they are famous. They also enjoyed religious freedom. Their great center of civilization was Athens which was at its peak in the fourth century B.C. Athenian culture spread to other beautiful cities, principally along the Mediterranean coast, some of which eventually surpassed Athens in brilliance.

In such a vital society, the art of medicine naturally kept pace with advancements in other fields. But, like other ancient cultures, it too went through centuries of belief in demons and spirits as causes of human ills, but with an element of greater complexity (not known to some simple primitive peoples) because of its acquisition of other cultures and a divergence of beliefs and practices among them. Here, too, they gradually evolved their own ideas about the relationships of the gods to health and illness. The famous Greek myths told in story and poem show a mixture of common sense and mysticism in their medical attitudes.

Aesculapius, the classical god of medicine, is part of one such myth. Whether he actually lived or not seems uncertain for his origin is obscure, but it is generally conceded that he did exist in person and that the mystery that surrounds him stems largely from his deification. A parallel is seen in the deification of Imhotep by the Egyptians. Hygieia, the goddess of health, is reputed to have been the daughter of Aesculapius.

His contributions, real or imagined, were further recognized by the founding of temples in his honor in localities suitable for rest and restoration to health. Sometimes referred to as hospitals, they were much more like the spas and health resorts of modern times with mineral springs, baths, gymnasiums, athletic fields, and treatment and consultation rooms.

They differed from modern resorts, however, in that they were controlled by priests and were essentially religious institutions. Prayers, sacrifices, rituals, and thank offerings were part of every patient's regimen in one of these sanitoria. (However, pregnant women and individuals with incurable diseases were not admitted.) The therapeutic effects of the earthly facilities were considerable, however, and knowledge of them was significant in later medical practice. Priestesses served as attendants and waited upon the sick, but they could not be considered nurses. The best known of these temples was Epidauros, about 30 miles from Athens, the ruins of which can still be seen.

To Aesculapius can also be traced the origin of the symbol of the medical profession —a serpent entwined on a staff—known as the Caduceus. The staff was the staff of Aesculapius; the serpent since primitive times had represented wisdom and knowledge.

The greatest name in Greek medicine— and possibly in all medicine—is Hippocrates. Born in Cos in 460 B.C., he is frequently seen as the epitome of the ideal physician both personally and professionally. Humane, brilliant, progressive, a great physician, teacher, and leader, he is often known as the Father of Medicine.

Hippocrates' medical achievements can be grouped in four major areas:

1. *Rejection of all beliefs in the supernatural origin of disease.* He divorced medicine from religion, philosophy, and the remaining traces of magic and taught that illness was caused by a breach of natural laws. He did not accept the theories of others who preceded him, but made his diagnoses on the basis of symptoms he observed in his patients. His emphasis was on the whole patient, and he advocated constant and continuous bedside care.

2. *Development of thorough patient assessment and recording.* He thoroughly examined his patients and then made a systematic recording of his findings: general appearance, temperature, pulse, respiration, sputum, excreta, ability to move about, and so on. Never before had physicians prepared good clinical records.

3. *Establishment of the highest ethical standards in medicine.* Hippocrates considered medicine one of the noblest of arts and believed that the conduct of the physician should be above reproach. He must be loyal to his profession and never bring dishonor upon it. He must be equally loyal to his patients and never injure them in any way. The Hippocratic

Oath (probably written after his death) is reproduced in part on pages 171–172 and presumably encompasses some of his convictions.

4. *Author of medical books.* Although it is thought that much of the writing was actually done by contemporaries or possibly his students, the information is supposed to be based on Hippocrates' teachings. The works include his case histories, descriptions of techniques such as bathing and bandaging, treatises on fractures and dislocations, diet in acute diseases, ulcers, epidemic diseases, and others. He reported on treatments that did not work as well as those that did to avoid repetition of errors.

Also attributed to him by some authorities (questioned by others) is a *Book of Decorum* from which this oft-quoted excerpt is taken:

> *Let one of your pupils be left in charge, to carry out instructions without unpleasantness, and to administer the treatment. Choose out one who has already been admitted into the mysteries of the art, so as to add anything that is necessary and to give treatment with safety. He is there also to prevent those things escaping notice that happen in the intervals between visits. Never put a layman in charge of anything, otherwise if a mischance occurs the blame will fall on you, but achievement will bring you pride.*
> *[From a translation by W. H. S. Jones.]*

It is assumed that the author was not referring to nurses but probably to medical students or attendants, who might also have taught and supervised care of the sick in the patient's home. This kind of care was probably done by the women of the family.

Little is known of nursing as an occupation in pre-Christian Greece. However, because the Greeks never established hospitals in spite of nominal advances in surgery, Greek physicians did not need the assistance of nurses to the degree that the surgeons of India did, for example, and that may have been an important factor. Through the ages, the development of nursing seems to have been greatly influenced by the physician's need for assistance, the quality of help that he wanted, and the amount of responsibility he was willing to delegate to others. If there were nurses who worked outside the home in Greece, they must have all been men because women held a very inferior position and were denied education as well as participation in community activities, both civil and humanitarian, except in the few instances in which women became midwives or physicians.

Advances in Alexandria

After Alexander the Great conquered Greece in about 338 B.C., he spread Greek civilization all over the known world. It reached a particularly high point in Alexandria, an Egyptian city on the Mediterranean Sea. Here the arts and sciences, including medicine, flourished for about three hundred years.

In c. 300 B.C., the first great medical school of this period was established in Alexandria with clinics, laboratories, and a huge library of 500,000 volumes. The physicians were supported by the state and did not have to depend on their practice to make a living. Dissections were permitted, and this resulted in tremendous advances in the knowledge of anatomy and physiology. The studies made by the Alexandrian physicians are considered the first medical research worthy of the name. After Cleopatra was defeated by the Romans in 30 B.C., Alexandria's place in the sun dimmed considerably, and the art of, and interest in, research declined.

Roman Hospitals and Sanitation

When the Etruscans conquered Rome in about 750 B.C., they brought new arts to this farming community, particularly the use of bronze, skill in building stone edifices, and a written language. In about 500 B.C., the Romans overthrew the Etruscans and became a powerful master of the Western world. Rome soon became a thriving commercial center and, through later conquests, a vast empire. Much emphasis was placed on government administration and related activities, on pleasures for the well-to-do, sometimes at the expense of the less fortunate, and on beautifully constructed public buildings, aqueducts, and roads.

Gradually Rome assimilated what it wanted of the Greek culture, and in some fields that was considerable. Although a temple of Aesculapius was built, Romans were somewhat wary of the Greek methods of treating disease, believing that their own deities, folklore, and magic were functioning well enough. Moreover, they were reluctant to accept advice and direction from the Greek physicians who, they thought, might poison or assassinate them in the name of medicine. They considered them social inferiors and thought them mercenary because they charged fees for their services.

Nevertheless, Greek medicine gradually replaced or supplemented Roman practices, and medicine was soon considered part of the necessary education of upper-class Roman men. Celsus (c. first century A.D.), in his lay work *De Medicina,* reported on, among other things, dietetics, pharmacy, medical conditions (particularly dermatological), surgical conditions (including cataract surgery and the use of ligatures), and mental illness. It might be added that physicians of ancient times had little interest in the care of childbearing women. Soranus, another Greek of this period, did write some treatises on obstetrics and gynecology, which is the first indication of male physician interest in these matters. Galen later referred to some of the techniques used by the midwives in delivery and care of the newborn, and it can be assumed that midwives were the key figures in the care of women. Galen (A.D. 130–201), considered one of the greatest of Greek physicians, practiced in Rome after education in many cities, including Alexandria. He wrote some 100 treatises on medicine, so comprehensive that for 200 years they remained unchallenged. He is seen as the greatest scientific experimentalist before the seventeenth century and perhaps the originator of scientific medicine.

Major Roman contributions to health were in public health sanitation and law. Their aqueducts, sewage systems, and baths were unequaled for centuries, and their city planning included both the appointment of a water commissioner and a public health official. In addition, they may be credited with the development of hospitals. *Valetudinaria* were detached buildings or just a large room designated for the care of valuable slaves on Roman estates. Apparently attendants watched over the sick, possibly with the attention of a physician. There is some indication that, at a later time, individuals other than slaves might have been cared for in *valetudinaria*. Given even more attention was the care of sick and injured soldiers. Originally, they were billeted with local Roman families, who tried to outdo each other in the quality of care. But as the Roman wars expanded to new frontiers, permanent convalescent camps succeeded temporary mobile hospitals. Modern excavations along the Rhine and Danube show the remains of hospitals that could accommodate 200 patients, with wards, recreation areas, baths, pharmacies, and rooms for attendants. Roman historians report that military discipline prevailed and, although the patients received good care, they were also required to conduct themselves "quietly."

Thus, it appears that the Romans took Greek medicine an additional step to the care of the sick by both male and female attendants.

THE FIRST FIVE CENTURIES OF CHRISTIANITY

After centuries of vilification, Christianity became the official religion of Rome in A.D. 335. The early Christian era brought another dimension to the care of the sick. Christian charity, based to a great extent on the Hebrew model as well as on the teachings of Christ, was reinforced by the persecution suffered by the early followers. Their beliefs included a strong emphasis on the sanctity of human life, and infanticide and abortion were considered murder. In the institutionalization of these ideals, bishops were given responsibility for the sick, the poor, widows, and children, but deacons and deaconesses were designated to carry out the services. (Deaconesses, found almost entirely in the Eastern church until the eighth century and always fewer in number, had almost disappeared in the East by the eleventh century.)

The duties were not the same in all churches, but a deaconess usually assisted with such church services as the baptism of women, visiting sick women of the church in their homes, acting as ushers for women attending church, carrying messages for the clergy, and visiting prisoners when they could be helped through counseling. Not all were ordained by the church fathers, who resisted giving women too much recognition or freedom. Neither were they permitted to form orders with rules until somewhat later in history. The role of women was seen as marriage and the begetting of children. Young widows were encouraged to remarry. Widows over sixty (which in those days of early death must have restricted the number considerably) were designated to, among other things, watch over the sick. Some virgins also chose to take vows of service. It is not certain to what extent the early deaconesses were involved in such care, but it is clear that a group of specially designated women, whether deaconesses, widows, virgins, or matrons, cared for the sick.

Noted Women

Among the fabled women who made noted contributions to the care of the sick were the following:

Phoebe (spelled *Phebe* in the Bible) of Cenchrea in southern Italy, who lived about A.D. 60, was the first deaconess who performed nursing functions that were referred to in records of such early times. St. Paul, in Romans 16:1–2 (King James Version), commends her to authorities in Rome—to which she traveled—as a "succorer of many and of myself, also."

The **Empress Helena,** mother of Constantine the Great of Rome, lived c. 248–328. In c. 312, she converted to Christianity and made a pilgrimage to Jerusalem reportedly to expiate the sins of her son. In the Holy Land, she built two churches and a Christian hospital. An influential personage, she won support for both the Christian church and especially for its humanitarian aspects.

Olympias, an aristocratic and beautiful young woman of Constantinople, was born in 368. Widowed at nineteen, she became a deaconess and devoted the rest of her life to work among the sick and poor. She was an excellent organizer, and the forty deaconesses who worked under her accomplished a great deal in alleviating suffering, caring for orphans and the aged, and converting others to Christianity.

Perhaps unfortunately, Olympias is remembered in history chiefly for her extreme asceticism. She denied herself the luxury of a bath, dressed as the lowliest of beggars, and refused to observe any of the rules of hygienic living. Fabiola, Paula, and others (both men and women) of the early Christian era had ascetic tendencies, but none to the degree that Olympias demonstrated. Largely because of her personal neglect, she contracted many illnesses and thus lessened the effectiveness of her work.

Fabiola, a beautiful and wealthy matron of Rome, founded the first free hospital in that city in c. 390. Twice married and twice divorced, she embraced Christianity and spent her fortune and the rest of her life in service to the poor and sick. She personally nursed the sickest and filthiest people who came to her hospital and was so gentle and kind that she was beloved by all Romans. Following her death, St. Jerome wrote a letter about her, sometimes called "the first literary document in the history of nursing."

Paula, a friend of Fabiola, widowed at twenty-three, learned and wealthy, also became a Christian. In about 385, she sailed from Rome to Palestine, where she built hospitals and inns for pilgrims and travelers along the route to Jerusalem, a monastery in Bethlehem, and a convent for women in Jerusalem. She, like Fabiola, performed nursing duties.

Hospitals

Following the closing of the temples of Aesculapius, in those same early centuries, another form of hospital emerged, the *diakonia*, providing a combination of outpatient and welfare service, managed by the deacons and supervised by the bishop. These were replaced in time by "a house for the sick," as there was a house for the poor and for the old. Generally, only the poor, the destitute, or the traveller, those who could not be cared for in their own homes, chose this alternative, an attitude that persisted to a great extent into the eighteenth and nineteenth centuries. One of these hospitals may have been the Basilias outside Caesarea, built in the third century by St. Basil, one of the Four Fathers of the Greek Church, and his sister Macrina. Huge and apparently magnificent, it had special rooms or areas for patients with different conditions, a separate building for lepers, and a special area where the physically handicapped could learn a new trade. There were homes for physicians and nurses, for convalescent patients, for the elderly, and schools and workshops for foundlings. Presumably, some kind of attendants had to be present. Some of these were the women cited earlier, who probably came from their homes to give care. A brotherhood known as *parabolani*, organized in the third century during a great plague in Alexandria, gave care to the sick and buried the dead.

The most regrettable fact in the history of this period is the attitude of the Christians toward science and education—an attitude that stultified progress in all intellectual pursuits, including medicine, and permeated the so-called Dark Ages, which continued for another 500 years.

THE MIDDLE AGES

The term *Middle Ages* usually is applied to the years from approximately A.D. 500 to 1500, of which roughly the first half has been called the Dark Ages, to distinguish it from the periods of classical civilization preceding and following it. Some historians acknowledge that the Dark Ages may have been more enlightened than was formerly believed. Certainly there were many areas allied to nursing in which the era might have been termed "light gray" rather than "dark," for progress was made that influenced the later development of nursing as a profession for both women and men.

Politically, the world changed greatly during the Middle Ages. The early centuries brought invasions against the Roman Empire by "barbarians" (to the Romans anyone outside the pale of the Empire), which resulted in the formation of many smaller kingdoms within the Empire. By the twelfth century, many kingdoms existed, chief among them England, Scotland, France, Denmark, Poland, Hungary, Sicily, and several in Spain. In the meantime, the Vikings had settled in the Scandinavian areas and in parts of Russia, and expansions developed rapidly. Trade routes were established between principal cities, and new occupations developed to meet the needs of a rapidly increasing population and changing economies and goals.

The barbarians were all pagans, and it took until the thirteenth and fourteenth centuries to convert them to Christianity. Most of the work of conversion was carried out under the direction of the Pope, and Roman Catholicism quite naturally was the principal religion of the world at that time.

Also significant in the general picture of the known world during medieval times was the rise and fall of feudalism in Central Europe with its devastating effects on the welfare of the common man. It was a time of famine and pestilence with accompanying miseries and serious illnesses. Medical and nursing care were needed, but unfortunately were not available in either sufficient quality or quantity. Beginning in the thirteenth century, feudalism gradually disappeared.

During the Middle Ages, the deaconesses, suppressed by the Western churches in particular, gradually declined and became almost extinct. However, a small spark remained that has been fanned into a flame every now and then during history, resulting in the formation of a new order of deaconesses, the most important of which are mentioned later.

As the deaconesses declined, the religious orders grew stronger. Known as monastic orders and comprised of monks and nuns (though not in the same orders), they controlled the hospitals, running them as institutions concerned more with the patients' religious problems than their physical ailments. However, monks and some nuns were better educated than most people in those times, and their liberal education may well have included some of the medical writings of Celsus and Galen.

Later, with the coming of the Renaissance in the fourteenth century, separation of hospital and church began, effecting spectacular improvement in the scientific and skillful treatment of the sick and injured. It was within the monasteries, however, that education in general progressed significantly during this earlier period.

Lay citizens banded together to form secular orders. Their work was similar to that of the monastic orders in that it was concerned with the sick and needy, but they lived in their own homes, were allowed to marry, took no vows of the church. They usually adopted a uniform, or habit. Nursing was often their main work.

The military nursing orders, known as the Knights Hospitallers, were the outcome of the Crusades, the military expeditions undertaken by Christians in the eleventh, twelfth, and thirteenth centuries to recover the Holy Land from the Moslems.

The most prominent of these three types

of orders—religious, military, and secular—during the Middle Ages are described in the following paragraphs.

The **Order of St. Benedict,** the foremost religious order, was founded by St. Benedict of Nursia (c. 480–543) on the beautiful mountain Monte Cassino, about halfway between Rome and Naples. It became a great and powerful center which sent workers throughout Europe raising standards of education and culture and providing better care for the sick and poor. St. Benedict's rule placed the care of the sick (in which bathing was stressed, a departure from the ascetic practices of some other orders) above and before every other duty of the monks. He established infirmaries within the monasteries primarily for the care of sick members of the order but also to help centralize and organize the care of pilgrims, wayfarers, and "refugees." With war, famine, and pestilence common occurrences, such service was sorely needed.

The **Knights Hospitallers,** an outgrowth of the Crusades, was the first military order of nurses. The first Crusade (there were nine in all) originated in 1095 when disorganized hordes of men and women of every age, type, and description answered Pope Urban II's call to march to Jerusalem and recover the Holy Land from the Moslems who had taken it by force from the Byzantine Empire in the seventh century A.D. Ill prepared physically and psychologically for such a journey, disorganized and inadequately equipped, the crusaders (whose symbol was an eight-pointed cross) died by the thousands along the way.

The later Crusades were essentially expeditions to assist the earlier crusaders in the Holy Land. It was during the first Crusade that the military order, the Knights Hospitallers, was established for the original purpose of bringing the wounded from the battlefield to the hospitals and caring for them there, which explains the name of the order. Later, two other branches of the Knights were formed, one to defend the wounded from the enemy while they were being brought to the hospital, and the other to defend the pilgrims when they were attacked.

There were three principal orders of the Knights Hospitallers: St. John of Jerusalem; the Teutonic Knights; and the Knights of St. Lazarus, whose principal mission was to care for victims of leprosy, one of the major health problems from the eleventh to the mid-thirteenth century. Women had their own branches of the Knights Hospitallers. They performed their services principally in hospitals to which only women patients were admitted.

The story of the Knights Hospitallers is both colorful and interesting. Wealthy and influential, these orders had their successes and failures for approximately seven centuries.

Hospital Brothers of St. Anthony was a secular order founded about 1095 by a grateful man who had been miraculously cured of St. Anthony's Fire, which was probably erysipelas. The men and women who joined the order cared only for patients with this disease in special hospitals to which no other patients were admitted. Thus they succeeded in curtailing the spread of erysipelas and no doubt became specialists of a sort in the treatment of this disease.

The Antonines later became a religious order and, when these orders were suppressed, the character of their contribution to nursing changed. They took care of patients with other illnesses, the special hospitals for St. Anthony's Fire closed, and erysipelas became a major problem for several centuries, especially among surgical and obstetric patients in general hospitals.

The **Beguines of Flanders,** believed to have been founded in about 1184 by a priest, was one of the most important secular orders. The widows and unmarried women who comprised its membersnip (at one time numbering 200,000) devoted their lives to helping others. Their nursing duties included the care of the sick in their homes and in hospitals, serving soldiers and civilians during the Battle of Waterloo, caring for victims of cholera during the dreadful epidemics of the nineteenth century, and responding to calls for assistance in times of disastrous fires, floods, and famines.

These sisterhoods spread to Germany, Switzerland, and France and became so numerous, strong, and popular that they were able to resist attempts to abolish them by monastic orders and religious leaders.

The **Third Order of St. Francis** is one of three orders founded by St. Francis of Assisi (1182–1226), probably the best known of the saints connected with nursing. A compassionate young man who loved people, birds, and animals, he was also a fanatic and ascetic with marked qualities of leadership, attracting the influential and learned as well as the humble and lowly to his orders.

The Third Order of St. Francis, also called the Franciscan Tertiaries, worked principally among the lepers. They were assisted by the women of the Order of Poor Clares, the second order formed by St. Francis, whose members were largely young women who had left their noble families for a life of service.

After the death of St. Francis at the age of forty-four, the ideals of the Franciscan friars changed considerably, improving in some respects, degenerating in others. But the friars extended their work to the sick and poor, particularly in the slum areas of Europe's large cities, and rendered remarkable service.

The Order of Poor Clares became an enclosed order, and this changed the lives of the sisters greatly. They continued their work in some ways, however. It was the Franciscan sisters who helped Dr. W. W. Mayo, a Civil War surgeon, to found the famous St. Mary's Hospital in Rochester, Minnesota, in 1889.

Order of the Holy Ghost (Santo Spirito), a secular order, was founded in Montpellier, France, in the late twelfth century. Initiated by a knight known as Guy de Montpellier, its members included both men and women. They nursed the poor in the community and assumed responsibility for all of the nursing at the Santo Spirito Hospital in Rome in 1204. They later extended their service to other large hospitals in Italy, France, and Germany. They cared for lepers in shelters outside the hospitals and for persons with other infectious diseases. The order later became monastic and eventually almost disappeared.

Guy de Montpellier established this order in connection with a medical school which had existed in Montpellier since the eighth century, and which became famous as a center of medical education, reaching its period of greatest achievement in the thirteenth and fourteenth centuries. Patients flocked to Montpellier seeking cures under the care of renowned physicians, one of the most outstanding being the surgeon Guy de Chauliac (1298–1368).

The **Grey Sisters,** an order of uncloistered nuns which originated in about 1222, ministered to the poor and the sick in home and hospital for many years. In the fourteenth and fifteenth centuries when the plague invaded Europe, they worked closely with the Alexian Orders in meeting the nursing needs.

The **Alexian Brotherhood** came into being in about 1348 in the Netherlands when the "Black Death" was sweeping Europe. The brothers took no vows, adopted no rule at the time, bending all their efforts to caring for the stricken and burying the victims of plague.

Nearly a century later, in 1431, they organized as a religious order, taking vows of obedience, poverty, and chastity and choosing as their patron saint Alexus, a man of noble birth who in the fifth century worked in a hospital in Syria. They were among the pioneers of organized nursing in Europe.

There were several outstanding personalities of the Middle Ages who were not members of orders, but who nonetheless made significant contributions to the health and welfare of the masses. Some of these were canonized, notably Elizabeth of Hungary, Catherine of Siena, and Hildegard of Bingen. The most prominent women were abbesses or members of royalty who nursed the sick, established educational programs for nurses, and sometimes wrote books and treatises. Hildegarde of Bingen (1098–1178) was educated in a Benedictine monastery and years later became its abbess. Several of her writings were related to medicine and the care of the sick, including general diseases of the body, their causes, symptoms and treatment, aspects of anatomy and physiology, and human behavior. Many of these things were unknown to physicians of the time.

Medicine

The Dark Ages on the Continent halted the promising progress of medicine, and except for Galen, who died about A.D. 200, no great physician practiced medicine in Europe during this period. The Christian church, obsessed with its belief that man's main purpose on earth was to prepare for a future life, saw little need for the science and philosophy of the Greeks or the hygienic teachings and sanitation systems of the Romans. Plagues swept Europe periodically for centuries. Medical knowledge survived and developed in only three areas.

In the eastern Roman Empire, Byzantine physicians nourished the teachings of Hippocrates and Galen, refusing to let them become obsolete; in Salerno in southern Italy, an educational ideal was fostered for medicine as well as for other areas of learning, a medical school was established, and laymen in Salerno translated many Greek manuscripts of importance in medical history; and vigorous medical activity was carried on in the Moslem empires. Although there was warfare there as in Europe, the conquerors preserved rather than destroyed the culture they found and encouraged further development. Within one hundred years they had achieved a standard of culture that took the Germanic tribes who invaded the Roman Empire ten times as long to develop.

The Arabs translated the works of Hippocrates, Galen, Aristotle, and others. Physicians adopted the Hippocratic method of careful observation of patients. One of the outstanding physicians was Rhazes (850–932) of Baghdad who was especially interested in communicable diseases and gave an accurate account of smallpox. Another and far more prominent physician was Avicenna (980–1037), a Persian whose *Canon of Medicine* was studied in the medical schools of Europe from the twelfth to seventeenth centuries. Moses ben Maimon (Maimonides), born in Moslem-controlled Spain of a Jewish family descended from King David, was an excellent clinician who became the court physician to Sultan Saladin.

Medical centers that included hospitals were founded in Cairo, Alexandria, Damascus and Baghdad. There the Arabs made advances in physiology, hygiene, chemistry, and, particularly, pharmacy. Because their religion prohibited human dissection, their knowledge of anatomy changed little during this time. Men probably gave care in these hospitals, because women were kept in seclusion.

Hospitals and Hospital Care

Hospitals in which the sick received care were established as needs increased and the wherewithal was available. At the close of the Middle Ages, there were hospitals all over Europe, particularly in larger cities such as Paris and Rome, and in England, where several hundred had been established. Most of these have long since been eliminated or abandoned, but a few have remained through the centuries. The oldest of these is the Hotel Dieu of Lyons (House of God's Charity), built in 542, in which both men and women nursed the patients.

The Hotel Dieu of Paris, founded in c. 650, has a less favorable record as far as nursing is concerned. Staffed by Augustinian nuns who did the cooking and laundry as well as the nursing, and who had neither intellectual nor professional stimulation, the hospital was not distinguished for its care of patients. In 1908 the nuns were expelled from the Hotel Dieu. The records of nursing kept by this hospital were well done, however, and have been a source of enlightenment for historians. Still in existence in Rome is the Santo

Spirito Hospital, established in 717 by order of the Pope, to care only for the sick.

Hospitals in England during the Middle Ages differed from those on the Continent in that they were never completely church-controlled, although they were founded on Christian principles and accepted responsibility for the sick and injured. The oldest and best-known English hospitals from a historical point of view are St. Bartholomew's founded in 1123; St. Thomas's founded in 1213; and, in 1247, Bethlehem Hospital, originally a general hospital that later became famous as a mental institution, referred to frequently as Bedlam.

An interesting sidelight here is the treatment of the mentally ill. In Bedlam, as in similar institutions, the inmates were treated with inhumane cruelty. Beatings and starvation were not uncommon. However, in Gheel, Belgium, reports of miraculous cures at the tomb of St. Dymphna, an Irish princess murdered by her mad father, brought the mentally ill in hope of healing. The people of Gheel took in the pilgrims as foster families and gave them care and affection. The therapy persists to this day in Gheel.

The nursing care in most early hospitals was essentially basic: bathing, feeding, giving medicines, making beds, and so on. It was rarely of high quality, however, largely because of the retarded progress of nearly all civilization and the shortsighted attitude toward women that was typical of the Dark Ages.

THE RENAISSANCE

The word *renaissance* as used in history refers to both a movement and a period of time. In years, it is generally conceded to have lasted from 1400 to 1550, the years during which there was a transitional movement toward revival of the arts and sciences in Europe, culminating in the Modern Age in which we still live. Also during this period great explorations were made, including the discovery of America.

New impetus was given to literature and art, to bookbinding, to the founding of libraries, universities, and medical schools—but not nursing schools. These came more than three centuries later. Merchants made huge fortunes in trade. Bankers likewise became wealthy through the making of loans, especially to kings and princes.

The Age of Discovery, 1450–1550, a part of this period, brought great increase in geographical knowledge. Man became excited about the world around him and about the prospect of finding gold in other lands, particularly in America. New passageways were sought to old countries, and the acquisition of new colonies and territories became extremely important to the established kingdoms and empires.

The Renaissance saw the birth and death of Leonardo da Vinci, Michelangelo, and other great artists. And to medicine it gave Paracelsus, Vesalius, and Paré.

Theophrastus Paracelsus (1493–1541), a Swiss physician and exceptional chemist, made contributions chiefly in the area of pharmaceutical chemistry.

Andreas Vesalius (1514–1564), a Belgian, made detailed anatomical studies in the universities and hospitals, disproving by his practical methods some of the classical theories of Galen and others. One of his many published works was a voluminous illustrated book, *De Corporis Humani Fabrica Libri Septem (Seven Books on the Structure of the Human Body),* in which he displayed his great fund of knowledge and also criticized and corrected Galen. For this he was berated by advocates of Galen. He gradually lost his tremendous energy and initiative and settled down to a routine physician's life.

Ambroise Paré (1510–1590), a Frenchman, served as an apprentice to a barber surgeon and later became the first of the surgeons of the Renaissance. A student of Vesalius, he became a great military surgeon who reintroduced the use of the ligature instead of the cautery to occlude blood vessels during surgery, adopted a simple technique of wound dressing to replace the oil-boiling method in wide use, improved obstetrical techniques, designed artificial limbs, and wrote books on surgery.

Barber surgeons were men in France who not only did barbering but also performed such procedures as bleeding, cupping, leeching, giving enemas, and extracting teeth—procedures that the physicians of medieval times prescribed for their patients but considered undignified to perform. The barber surgeon was required a wear a short robe, whereas the regular surgeons, of whom there were very few, were entitled to wear a long one.

There was understandable friction among the three groups—physicians, barber surgeons, and surgeons—and the problems were not completely revolved until the practice of surgery improved greatly and the Royal College of Surgeons was established in 1800.

The striped barber pole, symbol of the present-day barber, dates from the time when the patient being bled clung to a staff; the bloody bandage that covered his wound is represented by the red stripe on the barber's pole.

Nursing apparently continued in a way similar to that established in the earlier part of the Middle Ages. The charter of St. Bartholomew's Hospital called for a matron and twelve other women to make beds, wash, and attend the poor patients. They were to receive about two pounds a year and room and board, with the matron receiving more. All slept in one room at the hospital. They cared for about 100 patients. However, whether this was typical is not known.

FROM REFORMATION TO NIGHTINGALE

The Reformation was a religious movement beginning early in the sixteenth century that resulted in the formation of various Protestant churches under leaders who had revolted against the supremacy of the Pope.

Monasteries were closed; religious orders were dispersed, even in Catholic countries. Because many of these orders were involved in the care of the sick, nursing and hospital care suffered a severe setback. A startling effect was the almost total disappearance of male nurses. Almost all Catholic nursing orders after 1500 were made up of women. In Protestant countries, too, women and nursing became almost synonymous, for Protestant leaders recognized the vacuum in care of the sick and urged the hiring of nurse deaconesses and other elderly women to nurse the sick.

Also out of this era came noted Catholic orders devoted to care of the sick.

The Sisters of Charity were founded by St. Vincent de Paul (1576–1660) of France, a Catholic priest. He was ably assisted by Mlle. Louise La Gras, a woman of noble birth greatly interested in nursing and social work.

Once a prisoner himself, having been captured by pirates, St. Vincent de Paul became vitally interested in lessening the suffering of all slaves and prisoners. This interest expanded to include the sick and poor in his small country parish, and to help him in his work, he organized a society of women. This small group was so successful that similar groups were formed in other localities in France. The most famous of all, the Sisters of Charity, was organized in Paris under the direction of Mlle. La Gras. A younger group, the Daughters of Charity, was formed later. A noncloistered order, the Sisters were free to go wherever they were needed.

The Sisters of Charity were always carefully selected and from the beginning their ideals and standards were very high. Members of this order took over the nursing service in many European hospitals and came to Canada and the United States to give similar service during the early history of these countries.

In Spain, the **Brothers Hospitallers of St. John of God** was founded by a man who gave care to the sick, with special attention to the mentally ill. The order spread around the world, and they opened and staffed hospitals wherever they went, including the Americas. The care given in their hospitals in Goa as described by a sixteenth century traveller seemed to be a model of the times, perhaps even ahead of the times.

In Italy, Camillus, also to be canonized, trained and supplied nurses (men) for hospital care, and founded an order dedicated to care of the sick and dying.

In the New World, Cortez founded the first hospital (in Mexico City); within twenty years, most major Spanish towns had one. It was a hundred years later that a Hotel Dieu was founded in Sillery (Canada) and another at Montreal. In the latter, care was given by a young lay woman and three nursing sisters who came from France, but perhaps the first "nurse" in Canada was Marie Herbert Hobau in Nova Scotia, the widow of the surgeon and apothecary who accompanied Champlain.[3]

Records in Jamestown, Virginia also tell of the selection of certain men and women to care for the sick. There were numerous health problems in the early American colonies, in part, the result of the difficult living conditions. Hospitals of a type existed; one was described as accommodating fifty patients—if they slept two in a bed. (Not uncommon in Europe either.)

The seventeenth and eighteenth centuries were periods of continuing change in Europe, and scientific advances had an enduring influence on medicine and health. Of the creative scientists of those times, the following are key figures:

William Harvey (1578–1657), an English physician generally regarded as the father of modern medicine, was the first to describe completely (except for the capillary system) and accurately the circulatory system, replacing the earlier explanations which, though remarkable at the time, actually were at least partially incorrect.

Thomas Sydenham (1624–1689), an Englishman educated at Oxford and Montpellier, revived the Hippocratic methods of observa-

tion and reasoning and in other ways "restored" clinical medicine to a sound basis.

Antonj van Leeuwenhoek (1632–1723), of Holland, improved on Galileo's microscope and produced one that permitted the examination of body cells and bacteria.

William Hunter (1718–1783) and his brother **John** (1728–1793), of Scotland, obstetrician and surgeon respectively, conducted meticulous anatomical research and thus founded the science of pathology.

William Tuke (1732–1822), an English merchant and philanthropist, instituted long overdue reforms in the care of the mentally ill. Chief founder of the York Retreat (1796), he had important influence on subsequent treatment of the mentally ill.

Edward Jenner (1749–1823), an English physician, friend and pupil of John Hunter, in 1796 originated vaccination against smallpox.

Rene Laennec (1781–1826), of France, invented the stethoscope in 1891. Before this, the physician had listened to the patient's heartbeat by placing his ear against the patient's chest wall.

Even with these advances, medical education was still sketchy. Some practicing physicians had no medical education. An MD degree required apprenticeship with a physician, surgeon, or apothecary, some university classes, some dissecting at an anatomical school or hospital—or any variation of these. There were a few noted schools in Italy, Germany, and Scotland; the English colonies had none until 1765. A practical apothecary school started earlier, but most often pharmicists were also physicians.

By the end of the eighteenth century, nurses of one kind or another functioned in hospitals. Conditions were not attractive and much has been written about the drunken, thieving women who tended patients. However, some hospitals made real efforts to set standards. One set of criteria included such attributes as good health, good sight and hearing (to make pertinent observations), nimbleness, quietness, good temper, diligence, temperance and "to have no children, or other to come much after her.''[4] Already a hierarchy of nursing personnel had begun, with helpers and watchers assigned to help the sisters, as the early English nurses were called.

In other parts of Europe, nursing was becoming recognized as an important service. Diderot, whose *Encyclopedia* attempted to sum up all human knowledge, said that nursing "is as important for humanity as its functions are low and repugnant." Urging care in selection, since "all persons are not adapted to it," he described the nurse as "patient, mild, and compassionate. She should console the sick, foresee their needs, and relieve their tedium."[5]

Another progressive step was the first nursing textbook, which had been published in Vienna early in the eighteenth century.

Midwifery, too, was gaining new attention. In England in 1739, a small lying-in infirmary was started for the education of medical students and midwives, and soon other lying-in hospitals began to appear. In London, poor women also benefited in home deliveries when a famous physician began to teach medical students midwifery and also taught women to become nurse-midwives at the bedside. (His students had to contribute funds to the care and support of these women.)

Nevertheless, it should be remembered that even with the tremendous increase in hospital building at that time, most care was still given in the home by wives and mothers.

The advent of the industrial revolution in England saw the development of power-driven machinery to do the spinning, weaving, and metal work that had previously been done manually in the home. Improvement in the steam engine as a source of power improved mining procedures and also resulted in the development of factories, which the English called mills. The cotton, woolen, and iron industries grew rapidly and there was a corresponding improvement in agriculture.

The industrialization of Europe did not begin until the mid-nineteenth century when England had already assumed international leadership, her empire was growing, and British trade was the center of world marketing.

Socially, the people of means lived a most luxurious life. Graciousness and elegance prevailed, and woman's mission in life was to carry on these traditions. For this she was educated and carefully prepared by her parents.

The common women worked largely as servants in private homes or not at all. With the coming of factories, men, women, and children worked under cruel conditions. Caring for the sick in hospitals and homes were the "uncommon" women—prisoners, prostitutes—unkempt, unsavory, disinterested. Health conditions were still dreadful, with epidemics such as cholera sweeping whole countries. Children, orphaned in these epidemics were finally put in almshouses, no improvement in their lot. The situation was no different in America, but probably worst in England, and a number of social reformers began to work for change.

Culturally, great progress was made, particularly on the Continent. The demand for intellectual liberty brought marked advancement in educational facilities for men, but not for women. This was also true in the United States where, for example, Harvard University, established at Cambridge, Mass., in 1636, admitted only men, a policy it steadfastly maintained into the twentieth century. Columbia University in New York City, founded in 1754, followed a similar policy but lowered its ban on women with the founding of Barnard College in 1889. Teachers College was founded as a coeducational institution in 1888.

Out of this confused century came scientists and physicians who made dramatic breakthroughs in medical science:

Oliver Wendell Holmes (1809–1894), a Boston physician, furthered safe obstetric practice, pointing out the dangers of infection. He is author of the famous treatise "The Contagiousness of Puerperal Fever," published in 1843.

Crawford W. Long (1815–1878), an American physician, excised a tumor of the neck under ether anesthesia in 1832 but did not make his discovery public until after Dr. William T. Morton announced his in 1846. This led to one of medicine's most enduring controversies: Who should receive the credit for discovering the anesthetic properties of ether?

Ignaz P. Semmelweis (1818–1865), of Vienna, is famous for the advances he effected in the safe practice of obstetrics.

Louis Pasteur (1822–1895), of France, chemist and bacteriologist, became famous through his germ theory of disease, the development of the process known as pasteurization, and the discovery of a treatment for rabies. His work overlapped that of Robert Koch.

Lord Joseph Lister (1827–1912), English surgeon, developed and proved, in 1865, his theory of the bacterial infection of wounds on which modern aseptic surgery is based.

Robert Koch (1843–1910), of Germany, founded modern bacteriology. He originated the drying and staining method of examining bacteria. His most important discovery was the identification of the tubercle bacillus, which led eventually to tremendous reductions in loss of life from that disease.

Wilhelm Röntgen (1845–1923), a German physicist, discovered X-rays in 1895 and laid the foundation for the science of roentgenology and radiology.

Sir William Osler (1849–1919), a renowned Canadian teacher and medical historian, was associated with McGill University, the University of Pennsylvania, Johns Hopkins University, and Oxford University, England. He was knighted in 1911.

Pierre Curie (1859–1906), a French chemist, and his Polish wife, **Marie** (1867–1934), discovered radium in 1898.

NURSING IN THE NINETEENTH CENTURY

The dreary picture of secular nursing is not totally unexpected, given the times. Because proper young women did not work outside the home, nursing had no acceptance, much less prestige. Even those nurses not in the Dickens' Sairy Gamp mold or those desiring to nurse found themselves in competition with workhouse inmates, a cheaper worker for the hospital administration.

It was acceptable to nurse as a member of a religious order, when the motivation was, of course, religious and the cost to the hospital little or none.

During the nineteenth century, several nursing orders were revived or originated that had substantial influence on modern nursing. In most instances, these orders cared for patients in hospitals that already were established, in contrast to the orders of earlier times which founded the hospitals in which they worked. The most influential are described in the following paragraphs.

The **Church Order of Deaconesses,** an ancient order, was revived by Theodor Fliedner (1800–1864), pastor of a small parish in Kaiserswerth, Germany, to care for the patients in a hospital he opened in 1836. At first he had only one deaconess whom he trained in nursing. Although the training was quite superficial, the work expanded, more deaconesses joined the staff, and the deaconess institute at Kaiserwerth became famous. (Florence Nightingale obtained her only "formal" training in nursing there.) Four of the deaconesses and Pastor Fliedner journeyed to Pittsburgh, Pennsylvania, in 1849, to help establish a hospital under the leadership of Pastor William Passavant; and similar assistance was given to the founders of institutions on the Kaiserswerth plan in London, Constantinople, Beirut, Alexandria, Athens, and other localities.

Pastor Fliedner's work began with discharged prisoners (rather than the sick poor), in whom he became greatly interested through the reforms effected in England under Elizabeth Fry. Aided by both his first and second wives, he also established an orphanage and a normal school. The Kaiserswerth institute still exists and still conducts a school of nursing.

The **Protestant Sisters of Charity** was

founded by Elizabeth Fry (1780–1845) of England, whose work among prisoners and the physically and mentally ill was based on reforms that had been instituted by John Howard (1726–1790) a quarter of a century before. Mrs. Fry became interested in the deaconesses at Kaiserswerth and visited the hospital to observe how they functioned. She then organized a small group of "nurses" in London to do similar work among the sick poor. She first called the group the Protestant Sisters of Charity, later changed it to Institute of Nursing Sisters. (Unofficially they often were called the Fry Sisters or Fry Nurses.) The sisters were not affiliated with any church. Their training for nursing was extremely elementary. This group was in no way connected with the Sisters of Charity established earlier by Saint Vincent de Paul.

The **Sisters of Mercy** was a Roman Catholic society formed by Catherine McAuley (1787–1841) in Dublin, which later became an order and adopted a rule. The sisters visited in Dublin hospitals and nursed victims of a cholera epidemic in 1832; their work grew rapidly and spread throughout the world, including the establishment of several Mercy hospitals in the United States.

The **Irish Sisters of Charity,** also a Roman Catholic group, was started by Mary Aikenhead (1787–1858). The sisters visited the sick in their homes and did volunteer nursing in the community during emergencies. They had limited nurses' training and, in 1892, founded a training school for lay persons in St. Vincent's Hospital, in Dublin, in which they previously had assumed all nursing duties. They opened additional St. Vincent's hospitals in other areas of the world including the United States, to which they had come in 1855 to nurse victims of a cholera epidemic in San Francisco.

Also during this period, several nursing sisterhoods were established under the auspices of the Church of England. One of these, the **Sisters of Mercy in the Church of England,** was organized about 1850. The sisters had little, if any, formal preparation, but through practical experience acquired in district "nursing" and work in a cholera epidemic, they became quite proficient.

Another Anglican sisterhood, **St. Margaret's of East Grinstead,** was founded by a doctor in 1854. The sisters worked entirely among the sick in the community; they were not associated with hospitals in any way.

The Anglican order that did the most to improve hospital nursing during this period was **St. John's House,** founded in 1848 by the Church of England. Named for the parish in which it was located—St. John the Evangelist in St. Pancras, London—its purpose was to instruct and train members of the Church of England "to act as nurses and visitors to the sick and poor."[6] The original plan also stipulated that the order should be connected with "some hospital or hospitals, in which the women under training, or those who had already been educated, might find the opportunity of exercising their calling or of acquiring experience."[7]

The first training program was successful, as were the twenty-five subsequent ones developed by St. John's House to meet changing needs, and the graduates were always in great demand.

Progress in medicine and science during these centuries was accompanied by accelerated interest in better nursing service and nurses' training. Neither was achieved to a significant degree, however, despite the fine work of dedicated men and women who belonged to the several nursing orders of the time. Limited in numbers and inadequately prepared for their nursing functions, the members of these orders could not begin to meet the need for their services. Such care as patients received in the majority of institutions was grossly inadequate.

In the mid-nineteenth century, therefore, the time was right—perhaps overdue—for the revolution in nursing education that originated under the leadership of Florence Nightingale and which influenced so greatly and so quickly (from an historical point of view) the nursing care of patients and, indeed, the health of the world.

REFERENCES

1. Thelma Ingles, ''The Physicians' View of the Evolving Nursing Profession—1873–1913,'' *Nursing Forum,* **15**,2:141–2 (1976).
2. Committee on Medical Education, ''Nursing Education: Status or Service Oriented?'' *Bull. N.Y. Acad. Med.,* **53**:502 (June 1977).
3. Josephine A. Dolan, *Nursing in Society,* 14th ed. (Philadelphia: W. B. Saunders Company, 1978) p. 98.
4. Bonnie Bullough and Vern Bullough, *The Care of the Sick: The Emergence of Modern Nursing* (New York: Prodist, 1978), p. 57.
5. Bullough, ibid., p. 69.
6. Lucy Ridgely Seymer, *A General History of Nursing,* 4th ed. (London: Faber & Faber Ltd., 1956), p. 74.
7. Ibid., p. 75.

BIBLIOGRAPHY

Austin, Anne L. *History of Nursing Source Book.* New York: G. P. Putnam's Sons, 1957. A compilation of direct quotations from the works of many authors who have written about nursing over the centuries. Fascinating source material.

Bullough, Vern, and Bonnie Bullough. *The Care of the Sick: The Emergence of Modern Nursing.* New York: Prodist, 1978. An easily read history of nursing that contains many unusual and fascinating details not found in most other histories. Also includes some discussion of modern nursing issues and trends. Excellent bibliography.

Dolan, Josephine. *Nursing in Society: A Historical Perspective,* 14th ed. Philadelphia: W. B. Saunders Company, 1973. Describes how nurses responded over the years to the health needs of human beings, with emphasis on the activities of individuals and groups who shaped the evolution of nursing. Basic lists of sources given, as well as footnotes and references.

Ehrenreich, Barbara, and Deirdre English. *Witches, Midwives, and Nurses: A History of Women Healers.* Old Westbury, N.Y.: The Feminist Press, 1973. From a feminist viewpoint, the story of women as healers, described as the beginning of research to be done to recapture the role of women as healers in Western civilization. Points out male domination and restrictions of women healers. Interesting bibliography, about half on witchcraft.

Ellis, Harold. ''Royal Operations: A Contrast to Modern Surgery.'' *AORN J.,* 17 (May 1973), 101–108. A fascinating account of surgery done on European royalty, primarily in the eighteenth and nineteenth centuries.

Kalisch, Beatrice and Philip Kalisch. *The Advance of American Nursing.* Boston: Little, Brown and Company, 1978. An unusually detailed history with many clarifying and humanizing quotations from original sources. Fascinating reading and excellent bibliography. Primary emphasis on the United States.

Mish, Ina. ''Nursing Process—Medieval Style.'' *Nurs. Forum.* 18–2 (1979) 196–203. Interesting view of how women functioned as healers in medieval times.

The Influence of
Florence Nightingale

It has been said that Florence Nightingale, an extraordinary woman in any century, is the most written about woman in history. Through her own numerous publications, her letters, the writings of her contemporaries, including newspaper reports, and the numerous biographies and studies done of her life, there emerges the picture of a sometimes contradictory, frequently controversial, but undeniably powerful woman who probably had a greater influence on the care of the sick than any other single individual.

Called the founder of modern nursing, Nightingale was a strong-willed woman of quick intelligence who used her considerable knowledge of statistics, sanitation, logistics, administration, nutrition, and public health not only to develop a new system of nursing education and health care, but also to improve the social welfare systems of the time. The gentle caring lady of the lamp, full of compassion for the soldiers of the Crimea, is an accurate image, but no more so than that of the hard-headed administrator and planner who forced change in the intolerable social conditions of the time, including the care of the sick poor. Nightingale knew full well that tender touch alone would not bring health to the sick or prevent illness, so she set her intelligence, her administrative skills,

her political acumen, and her incredible drive to achieve her self-defined missions. In the Victorian age when women were almost totally dominated by men—fathers, husbands, brothers—and it was undesirable for them to show intelligence or profess interest in anything but household arts, this indomitable woman accomplished the following:

1. Improved and reformed laws affecting health, morals, and the poor.
2. Reformed hospitals and improved workhouses and infirmaries.
3. Improved medicine by instituting an army medical school and reorganizing the army medical department.
4. Improved the health of natives and British citizens in India and other colonies.
5. Established nursing as a profession with two missions—sick nursing and health nursing.[1]

The new nurse and the new image of the nurse that she created, in part through the nursing schools she founded, in part through her writings, and in part through her international influence, became the model that persisted for almost a hundred years. In today's light, some of her tenets for the "good" nurse seem terribly restrictive, but it should be remembered that in those times not only the image but the reality of much of secular nursing was based on the untutored, uncouth workhouse inmates for whom drunkenness and thievery were a way of life. It was small wonder that each Nightingale student had to exemplify a new image.

The Nightingale nurse had to establish her character in a profession proverbial for immorality. Neat, ladylike, vestal, above suspicion, she had to be the incarnate denial that a hospital nurse had to be drunken, ignorant, and promiscuous.[2]

These historical idiosyncrasies should not, and do not, detract from the many Nightingale precepts that are not only pertinent today, but remarkably far-sighted.

EARLY LIFE

Florence Nightingale was born on May 12, 1820, in Florence, Italy, during her English parents' travels there. She was named for the city in which she was born, as was her older sister Parthenope, who was born in 1819 in Naples (known in ancient times by the Greek name Parthenope).

The family was wealthy and well educated with a high social standing and influential friends, all of which would be useful to Nightingale later. Primarily under her father's tutelage, she learned Greek, Latin, French, German, and Italian, and studied history, philosophy, science, music, art, and classical literature. She traveled widely with family and friends. The breadth of her education, almost unheard of for women of the times, was also considerably more extensive than that of most men, including physicians. Her intelligence and education were recognized by scholars, as indicated in her correspondence with them.

Nightingale was not only bright, but, according to early portraits and descriptions, slender, attractive, and fun-loving, enjoying the social life of her class. She differed from other young women in her determination to do something "toward lifting the load of suf-

fering from the helpless and miserable."[3] Later she said that she had been called by God into His service on four separate occasions beginning when she was seventeen. This strong religious commitment remained with her, although she had increasingly little patience with organized religion or with traditional Biblical exhortations. At one point she stated, "God's scheme for us was not that He should give us what we asked for, but that mankind should obtain it for mankind."[4] Apparently, the encouragement of Dr. Samuel Gridley Howe and his wife, Julia Ward Howe (who wrote "The Battle Hymn of the Republic"), during a visit to the Nightingale family home in 1844 helped to crystallize Florence's interest in hospitals and nursing. Nevertheless, her intent to train in a hospital was strongly opposed by her family, and she limited herself to nursing family members. There is some indication that this was the genesis of her firm belief that nursing required more than kindness and cold compresses.

Later, in *Notes on Nursing* she wrote, "It has been said and written scores of times that every woman makes a good nurse. I believe, on the contrary, that the very elements of nursing are all but unknown."[5] At the same time, she added a few tart remarks about the need for education.

It seems a commonly received idea among men and even some women themselves that it requires nothing but a disappointment in love, the want of an object, a general disgust, or incapacity for other things to turn a woman into a good nurse. This reminds one of the parish where a stupid old man was set to be schoolmaster because he was 'past keeping the pigs' . . . The everyday management of a large ward, let alone of a hospital— the knowing what are the laws of life and death for men, and what the laws of health for wards (and wards are healthy or unhealthy, mainly according to the knowledge or ignorance of the nurse)—are not these matters of sufficient importance and difficulty to require learning by experience and careful inquiry, just as much as any other art? They do not come by inspiration to the lady disap-

*pointed in love, nor to the poor workhouse
drudge hard up for a livelihood.*[6]

Although remaining the obedient daughter, Nightingale found her own way to expand her knowledge of sick care. She studied hospital and sanitary reports and books on public health. Having received information on Kaiserswerth in Germany, she determined to receive training there—more acceptable because of its religious auspices. On one of her trips to the continent, she made a brief visit and was impressed enough to spend three months in training and observation there in 1851 while her mother and sister went to Carlsbad to "take the cure." (The Nightingales were considered appropriately delicate Victorian ladies, although all lived past eighty.) At the time she wrote positively about Pastor Fliedner's program, but she later described the nursing as "nil" and the hygiene as "horrible."[7] Her later effort to study with the Sisters of Charity in Paris was frustrated, although she got permission to inspect the hospitals there as she had in other cities during her tours. She examined the general layout of the hospital, as well as ward construction, sanitation, general administration, and the work of the surgeons and physicians. Apparently, these observational techniques and her analytical abilities then and later were the basis of her unrivalled knowledge of hospitals in the next decade. Few of her contemporaries ever had such knowledge.

In 1853 Nightingale assumed the position of superintendent of a charity hospital (probably more nursing home) for ill governesses, run by titled ladies. Although she had difficulties with her intolerant governing board, she did make changes considered revolutionary for the day and, even with the lack of trained nurses, improved the care. And she continued to visit hospitals. Just as Nightingale was negotiating a superintendency in the newly reorganized and rebuilt King's College Hospital in London, England and France, in support of Turkey, declared war on Russia in March 1854.

CRIMEA—THE CHANGING POINT

The Crimean War was a low point for England. Ill-prepared and disorganized in general, the army and the bureaucracy were even less prepared to care for the thousands of soldiers both wounded in battle and prostrated by the cholera epidemics brought on by less than primitive conditions. Not even the most basic equipment or drugs were available, and, as casualties mounted, Turkey turned over the enormous, but bare and filthy barracks at Scutari across from Constantinople to be used as a hospital. The conditions remained abominable. The soldiers lay on the floor in filth, untended, frequently without food or water because there was not equipment to prepare or distribute either. Rats and other vermin came from the sewers underneath the building. There were no beds, furniture, basins, soap, towels, eating utensils, and few provisions. There were only orderlies, and none of these at night. The death rate was said to be 60 percent.

In previous wars, the situation had not been much different, and there was little interest on the battle sites, for ordinary soldiers were accorded no decencies. But now, for the first time, civilian war correspondents were present and sent back the news of these horrors to an England with a newly aroused social conscience. The reformers were in an uproar; newspapers demanded to know why England did not have nurses like the French Sisters of Charity to care for its soldiers, and Parliament trembled. In October, Sidney Herbert, Secretary of War and an old friend of Florence Nightingale, wrote begging her to lead a group of nurses to the Crimea under government authority and expense. "There is but one person in England that I know of who would be capable of organizing such a scheme . . . your own personal qualities, your knowledge, and your power of administration, and, among greater things, your rank and position in society give you advantages in such work which no other person possesses."[8] Nightingale had already decided to offer her services, and the two letters crossed. In less than a week, she had assembled thirty-eight nurses, the most she could find that met her standards—Roman Catholic and Anglican sisters and lay nurses from various hospitals—and embarked for Scutari.

Even under the miserable circumstances found there, Nightingale and her contingent were not welcomed by the army doctors and surgeons. Dr. John Hall, chief of the medical staff, and his staff, although privately acknowledging the horrors of the situation, resented outside interference and refused the nurses' services. Hall and Nightingale soon developed a mutual hatred for each other. When Dr. Hall was honored with the KCB— Knight Commander of the Order of the Bath —she referred to him as "Knight of the Crimean Burial Grounds."[9]

Nightingale chose to wait to be asked to help. To the anger of her nurses, she allowed none of them to give care until one week later when scurvy, starvation, dysentery, exposure, and more fighting almost brought about the collapse of the British army. Then, the doctors, desperate for any kind of assistance, turned to the eager nurses.

Modern criticisms of Florence Nightingale frequently refer to her insistence on the physician's overall authority and her own authoritarian approach to nursing. The first criticism may have originated with her situation in the Crimean War. In mid-century England her appointment created a furor; she was the first woman ever to be given such authority. Yet, despite the high sounding title that Herbert insisted she have—General Superintendent of the Female Nursing Establishment of the Military Hospitals of the Army—her orders required that she have the approval of the Principal Medical Officer "in her exercise of the responsibilities thus vested in her. The Principal Medical Officer will communicate with Miss Nightingale upon all subjects connected with the Female Nursing Establishment, and will give his directions through that lady."[10] Although no "lady, sister, or nurse" could be transferred from one hospital to the other without her approval, she had no authority over anyone else, even orderlies and cooks. What she accomplished had to be done through sheer force of will or persuasion. Her overt deference to physicians was probably the beginning of the doctor-nurse game.

Whatever the limitations of her power, Florence Nightingale literally accomplished miracles at Scutari. Even in the "waiting" week, she moved into the kitchen area and began to cook extras from her own supplies to create a diet kitchen, which for five months was the only source of food for the sick. Later, a famous chef came to Crimea at his own expense and totally reorganized and improved military cooking. Nightingale managed to equip the kitchen and the wards by various means. One report is that when a physician refused to unlock a supply storehouse, she replied, "Well, I would like to have the door opened, or I shall send men to break it down."[11] It was opened, and he was recalled to London.

Miss Nightingale had powerful friends and control over a large amount of contributed funds—a situation that gained her some external cooperation from most physicians after a while. Through persuasion and the use of good managerial techniques, she cleaned up the hospital; the orderlies scrubbed and emptied slops regularly; soldiers' wives and camp followers washed clothes; the vermin were brought under some control. (Wrote Nightingale to Sidney Herbert, "the vermin might, if they had but unity of purpose, carry off the four miles of beds on their backs and march them into the War Office.")[12] Before the end of the war, the mortality rate at Scutari declined to 1 per cent. When the hospital care improved, Nightingale began a program of social welfare among the soldiers—among other things, seeing to it that they got sick pay. The patients adored her. She cared about them, and the doctors and officers reproached her for "spoiling the brutes." The soldiers wrote home, "What a comfort it was to see her pass even; she would speak to one and nod and smile to as many more, but she could not do it all, you know. We lay there by hundreds, but we could kiss her shadow as it fell, and lay our heads on the pillow again content." And, "Before she came, there was cussin' and swearin', but after that it was holy as a church." And, "She was all full of life and fun when she talked to us, especially if a man was a bit down-hearted."[13] News correspondents wrote reports about the "ministering angel" and "lady with the lamp" making late rounds after the medical officers had retired—which inspired Longfellow later to write his famous poem "Santa Filomena." England and America were enthralled, and she was awarded decorations by Queen Victoria and the Sultan of Turkey.

But all did not go well. The military doctors continued in their resentment and tried to undermine her. There were problems in her own ranks, dissension among the religious and secular nurses, and problems of incompetence and immorality. Later, she wrote:

Rebellion among some ladies and some nuns, and drunkenness among some nurses unhappily disgraced our body; minor faults justified pro tanto *the common opinion that the vanity, the gossip, and the insubordination (which none more despise than those who trade upon them) of women make them unfit for, and mischievous in the Service, however materially useful they may be in it.*[14]

Her problems increased with the unsolicited arrival of another group of nurses, under another woman's leadership, although the problem was eventually resolved. No doubt, Nightingale was high-handed at times, and despite praise of her leadership, she was also called "quick, violent-tempered, positive, obstinate, and stubborn."[15]

Certainly she drove herself in all she did. When the situation at Scutari was improved, she crossed the Black Sea to the battle sites and worked on the reorganization of the few hospitals there—with no better support from physicians and superior officers. There she contracted Crimean fever (probably typhoid

or typhus) and nearly died. However, she refused a leave of absence to recuperate and stayed in Scutari to work until the end of the war. She had supervised 125 nurses and forced the military to recognize the place of nurses.

From her experiences, and to support her recommendations for reform, Nightingale wrote a massive report entitled *Notes on Matters Affecting the Health, Efficiency, and Hospital Administration of the British Army,* crammed with facts, figures, and statistical comparison. On the basis of this and her later well-researched and well-documented papers, she is often credited with being the first nurse researcher. Reforms were slow in coming but extended even to the United States, when the Union consulted her about organizing hospitals. In 1859 she wrote a small book, *Notes on Nursing: What It Is and What It Is Not,* intended for the average housewife and printed cheaply so that it would be affordable. These and other Nightingale papers are still amazingly readable today—brisk, down-to-earth, and laced with many a pithy comment. For instance, in *Notes on Hospitals* written in the same year, she compares the administration of the various types of hospitals and characterized the management of secular hospitals under the sole command of the male hospital authorities as "all but crazy." And her words were prophetic: "If we were perfect, no doubt an absolute hierarchy would be the best kind of government for all institutions. But, in our imperfect state of conscience and enlightenment, publicity, and the collision resulting from publicity are the best guardians of the interests of the sick."[16]

Her knowledge was certainly respected, and she was consulted by many, including the Royal Sanitary Commission on the Health of the Army in India. When asked by the members of the Commission what hospitals she had visited, she listed those in England, Turkey, France, Germany, Belgium, Italy, and Egypt, including all hospitals in some cities, and even Russian military hospitals. Her reforms in India extended beyond the medical and nursing facilities to raising the sanitary level of India. Again, her insights were uncanny. In describing the proper method of analyzing the problem of sanitation and disease, she also suggested checking on "unwholesome trades fouling the water."

What is particularly astonishing is that all of this was done from her own quarters. On her return from the Crimea, she took to her bed or at least to her rooms and emerged only on rare occasions. There is much speculation on this illness—whether it was a result of the Crimea fever, neurasthenia, or a bit of both, or whether she simply found it useful to avoid wasting time with people she did not want to see. For she was famous now and had been given discretion over the so-called Nightingale Fund to which almost everyone in England had subscribed, including many of the troops.

THE NIGHTINGALE NURSE

In 1860, Nightingale utilized some of the 45,000 pounds of the Nightingale Fund to establish a training school for nurses. She selected St. Thomas's Hospital because of her respect for its matron, Mrs. S. E. Wardroper. The two converted the resident medical officers to their plan, although apparently most other physicians objected to the school. The students were chosen, and the first class in the desired age range of twenty-five to thirty-five years and with impeccable character references numbered only fifteen. It was to be a one-year training program, and the students were presented with what would be called terminal behavioral objectives that they had to master satisfactorily. Students could be dismissed by the matron for misconduct, inefficiency, or negligence. However, if they passed the courses of instruc-

---

Duties of Probationer under the "Nightingale Fund."
St. Thomas's Hospital, 1860.

You are required to be

Sober.	Punctual.
Honest. .	Quiet and Orderly.
Truthful.	Cleanly and Neat.
Trustworthy.	Patient—Cheerful, and Kindly.

You are expected to become skillful

1. In the dressing of blisters, burns, sores, wounds and in applying fomentations, poultices, and minor dressings.
2. In the application of leeches, externally and internally.
3. In the administration of enemas for men and women.
4. In the management of trusses, and appliances in uterine complaints.
5. In the best method of friction to the body and extremities.
6. In the management of helpless patients,, i.e., moving, changing, personal cleanliness of, feeding, keeping warm, (or cool), preventing and dressing bed sores, managing position of.
7. In bandaging, making bandages, and rollers, lining of splints, etc.
8. In making the beds of the patients, and removal of sheets whilst patient is in bed.
9. You are required to attend at operations.
10. To be competent to cook gruel, arrowroot, egg flip, puddings, drinks, for the sick.
11. To understand ventilation, or keeping the ward fresh by night as well as by day; you are to be careful that great cleanliness is observed in all the utensils; those used for secretions as well as those required for cooking.
12. To make strict observation of the sick in the following particulars: The state of secretions, expectoration, pulse, skin, appetite; intelligence, as delirium or stupor; breathing, sleep, state of wounds, eruptions, formation of matter, effect of diet, or of stimulants, and of medicines.
13. And to learn the management of convalescents.

tion and training satisfactorily, they were entered in the "Register" as certified nurses. The Committee of the Nightingale Fund then recommended them for employment; in the early years, they were obligated to work as hospital nurses for at least five years (for which they were paid).

The students' time was carefully structured, beginning at six in the morning, and ending with a nine o'clock bedtime, which included a semi-mandatory two-hour exercise period (walking abroad must be done in twos and threes, not alone). Within that time there was actually about a nine-hour work and training day (a vast difference from future American schools). This included bedside teaching by a teaching sister or the Resident Medical Officer and elementary instruction in "Chemistry, with reference to air, water, food, etc.; Physiology, with reference to a knowledge of the leading functions of the body, and general instruction on medical and surgical topics,"[17] by professors of the medical school attached to St. Thomas's, given voluntarily and without renumeration. The keys to the Nightingale school were that it was not under the control of the hospital and had education as its purpose. The Fund paid the medical officers, head nurses and matron for teaching students, beyond whatever they earned from the hospital in their other duties. Both the head nurses and matron kept records on each student, evaluating how they met the stated objectives of the program. The students were expected to keep notes from the lectures and records of patient observation and care, all of which were checked by the nurse-teachers. At King's College Hospital, run by the Society of St. John's House, an Anglican religious community, midwifery was taught in similar style and with similar regulations, again under the auspices of the Nightingale Fund Committee. And, at the Royal Liverpool Infirmary, nurses were trained for home nursing of the sick poor under a Nightingale protocol but were personally funded by a Liverpool merchant-philanthropist. As Nightingale said in 1863, "We have had to

introduce an entirely new system to which the older systems of nursing bear but slight resemblance . . . It exists neither in Scotland nor in Ireland at the present time."[18]

The demand for the Nightingale nurses was overwhelming. In the next few years, requests also came for them to improve the workhouse (poorhouse) infirmaries and to reform both civilian and military nursing in India. In her responses to these demands, Nightingale wrote many reports, detailing to the last item the system for educating these nurses and for improving patient care, including such points as general hygiene and sanitation, nutrition, equipment, supplies, and the nurses' housing conditions, holidays, salaries, and retirement benefits. (For India, she suggested that they had better pay good salaries and provide satisfactory working and living conditions, or the nurses might opt for marriage, because the opportunities there were even greater than in England.) She constantly reiterated that she could not supply enough nurses but, when possible, she would send a matron and some other nurses, who would train new Nightingale nurses. She warned that one or two could not change the old patterns. "Good nursing does not grow of itself; it is the result of study, teaching, training, practice, ending in sound tradition which can be transferred elsewhere."[19]

Although Nightingale never headed a school herself, she selected the students and observed their progress carefully; with some she carried on years of correspondence. One of her favorites, Agnes Jones, was recommended to reform nursing at the Liverpool Workhouse Infirmary which, with twelve other nurses, she did admirably, proving to the economy-minded governor that this kind of nursing also saved money. Nightingale often said that conditions there were as bad as at Scutari; and indeed her young protege died of typhus there. Nevertheless, reform of this pesthole showed England an example of what nursing care could be.

Despite her reputation and her personal acquaintance with Queen Victoria, her cabinet, and every prime minister during this time, Nightingale and her ideas ran into opposition. Although some doctors who understood what this new nurse could do were supporters, the idea of the nurse as a professional was not commonly accepted. Said one physician, "A nurse is a confidential servant, but still only a servant . . . She should be middle-aged when she begins nursing, and if somewhat tamed by marriage and the troubles of a family, so much the better."[20] Maintaining standards was a constant struggle; even St. Thomas's Hospital slipped, and Nightingale, who had been immersed in the Indian reforms, had to take time to reorganize the program. What evolved over the years, from the first program, was one of preparation for two kinds of nursing practitioners, the educated middle- and upper-class ladies who paid their own tuition, and the still carefully selected poor women who were subsidized by the Fund. The first were given an extra year or two of education to prepare them to become teachers or superintendents; a third choice was district nursing. "She must be of a yet higher class and of a yet fuller training than a hospital nurse, because she has not the doctor always at hand and because she has no hospital appliances at hand."[21] The special probationers were expected to enter the profession permanently. The second group were prepared to be the hospital ward nurses.

In Nightingale's later years, she came into conflict with the very nurses who had been trained for leadership. In 1886, some of these nurses, now superintendents of other training schools, wanted to establish an organization that would provide a central examination and registration center, the forerunner of licensure. Nightingale opposed this movement for several reasons: that nursing was still too young and disorganized; that national criteria would not be as high as those of individual schools; and that the all-important aspect of "character" could not be tested. She fought the concept with every weapon at her disposal, including her powerful contacts, and succeeded in limiting the fledgling Royal British Nurses' Association

to maintaining a "list" instead of a "register." (Nurse licensure came to South Africa before it came to England.) Nevertheless, it was a beginning and, although she was probably right about the standards, recognition of nurses was facilitated with the setting of national standards, however minimum.

Nightingale's prolific writings on nursing have survived and some of them are still surprisingly apt. Often they reflected her concern about the character of nurses and her own determination that their main focus be on nursing. For instance, in her early writings on hospitals (before the Nightingale schools), she reluctantly conceded that the nurse would have to be permitted visitors on her time off, distracting though that might be, and that spying on the nurse when she went out in her limited free time, although it had some advantages, was "no blessing in the long run and degrading to all concerned." Yet, nurses were to be held strictly to rules that limited their outside excursions to their exercise period, and it was preferred that they live adjacent to the patient wards. Her views moderated over the years, but her emphasis on morality and other personal qualities never wavered.

It was a time when salaries were low and petty thievery common, and an accepted, desirable fringe benefit of a job (also recommended by Nightingale for nurses) was a daily allowance of beer, or even wine and brandy. But a Nightingale nurse who was found to be dishonest and drunken was dismissed instantly and permanently.

One principle from which she did not swerve was that nurses were to nurse, not to do heavy cleaning ("if you want a charwoman, hire one"); not to do laundry ("it makes their hands coarse and hard and less able to attend to the delicate manipulation which they may be called on to execute"); not to fetch ("to save the time of nurses . . . all diets and ward requisites should be brought into the wards"). Then, as in many places now, status and promotion came through assumption of administrative roles,

What a Nurse Is to Be

(From a Nightingale article on "Nurses, Training of, and Nursing the Sick," in *A Dictionary of Medicine*, edited by Sir Robert Quain, Bart., M.D., 1882)

A really good nurse must needs be of the highest class of character. It need hardly be said that she must be—(1) Chaste, in the sense of the Sermon on the Mount; a good nurse should be the Sermon on the Mount in herself. It should naturally seem impossible to the most unchaste to utter even an immodest jest in her presence. Remember this great and dangerous peculiarity of nursing, and especially of hospital nursing, namely, that it is the only case, queens not excepted, where a woman is really in charge of men. And a really good trained ward "sister" can keep order in a men's ward better than a military ward-master or sergeant. (2) Sober, in spirit as well as in drink, and temperate in all things. (3) Honest, not accepting the most trifling fee or bribe from patients or friends. (4) Truthful—and to be able to tell the truth includes attention and observation, to observe truly—memory, to remember truly—power of expression, to tell truly what one has observed truly—as well as intention to speak the truth, the whole truth, and nothing but the truth. (5) Trustworthy, to carry out directions intelligently and perfectly, unseen as well as seen, "to the Lord" as well as unto men—no mere eye-service. (6) Punctual to a second and orderly to a hair—having everything ready and in order before she begins her dressings or her work about the patient; nothing forgotten. (7) Quiet, yet quick, quick without hurry; gentle without slowness; discreet without self-importance; no gossip. (8) Cheerful, hopeful; not allowing herself to be discouraged by unfavourable symptoms; not given to depress the patient by anticipations of an unfavourable result. (9) Cleanly to the point of exquisiteness, both for the patient's sake and her own; neat and ready. (10) Thinking of her patient and not of herself, "tender over his occasions" or wants, cheerful and kindly, patient, ingenious and feat.[22]

but Nightingale recognized that "many women are valuable as nurses, who are yet unfit for promotion to head nurses." Her alternative, however, would not be greeted favorably today—a raise after ten years of good service!

Nightingale also commented on other issues considered pertinent today. Continuing education was a must, for she saw nursing as a progressive art, in which to stand still was to go back. "A woman who thinks of herself, 'Now I am a full nurse, a skillful nurse. I have learnt all there is to be learned,' take my word for it, she does not know what a nurse is, and she will never know: she has gone back already."[23] Although there is no evidence that she took any action to help end discrimination against women, Nightingale believed that women should be accepted into all the professions, but she warned them, "qualify yourselves for it as a man does for his work." She believed that women should be paid as highly as men, but that equal pay meant equal responsibility. In a profession with as much responsibility as nursing, it was particularly important to have adequate compensation, or the intelligent, independent women would not be attracted to it. Until the end, she was firm on the need for nurses to obey physicians in medical matters; however, she stressed the importance of nurse observation and reporting because the physician was not constantly at the patient's bedside as the nurse was. She was adamant that a nurse (and woman) be in charge of nursing, with no other administrative figure having authority over nurses, including physicians. She knew the importance of a work setting that gave job satisfaction. In words that are a far-off echo of nurses' plaints today, she wrote:

Besides, a thing very little understood, a good nurse has her professional pride in results of her Nursing quite as much as a Medical Officer in the results of his treatment. There are defective buildings, defective administrations, defective appliances, which make all good Nursing impossible. A good Nurse does not like to waste herself, and the better the Nurse, the stronger this feeling in *her. Humanity may overrule this feeling in a great emergency like a cholera outbreak; but I don't believe that it is in human nature for a good Nurse to bear up, with an ever-recurring, ever-useless expenditure of activity, against the circumstances which make her nursing activity useless, or all but useless. Her work becomes slovenly like the rest, and it is a far greater pity to have a nurse wasting herself in this way than it would be to have a steam engine running up and down the line all day without a train, wasting coals.*

Perhaps I need scarcely add that Nurses must be paid the market price for their labor, like any other worker; and that this is yearly rising.[24]

Obviously, Nightingale is eminently quotable, in matters of health care and nursing today, in part because she was so far ahead of her time, and in part, unfortunately, because the errors of omission and commission in the field have a tendency to reappear or remain uncorrected.

Planner, administrator, educator, researcher, reformer, Florence Nightingale never lost her interest in nursing. As nearly as can be determined, her actual clinical nursing was limited to her early care of sick families, the short period at Kaiserswerth, a briefer interim of caring for victims of a cholera epidemic before the war, and then, of course, her experience in the Crimea. Yet, her perceptiveness of patient needs was uncanny for the time and frequently is still applicable today. In her *Notes on Nursing*, not only is there careful consideration of "Observation of the Sick" and crisp comments on "Minding Baby," but pertinent directions on hygiene, nutrition, environment, and the mental state of the patient. At age seventy-four, in her last major work on nursing, she differentiated between sick-nursing and health-nursing, and emphasized the primary need for prevention of illness, for which a lay "Health Missioner" (today's health educator?) would be trained.

When Nightingale died on August 13, 1910, she was to be honored by burial in Westminister Abbey. However, she had chosen instead to be buried in the family plot in Hampshire, with a simple inscription: "F.N. Born 1820, Died 1910."

REFERENCES

1. Evelyn R. Barritt, "Florence Nightingale's Values and Modern Nursing Education," *Nursing Forum,* **12,**4:10 (1973).
2. Ibid., p. 34.
3. Vern Bullough and Bonnie Bullough, *The Care of the Sick: The Emergence of Modern Nursing* (New York: Prodist, 1978), p. 86.
4. Barritt, op. cit.
5. Lucy Ridgely Seymer, *Selected Writings of Florence Nightingale* (New York: Macmillan Publishing Co., Inc., 1954) p. 124.
6. Ibid., pp. 214–15.
7. Bullough, op. cit., p. 86.
8. Josephine A. Dolan, *Nursing in Society: A Historical Perspective,* 14th ed. (Philadelphia: W. B. Saunders Company, 1978) p. 159.
9. Philip Kalisch and Beatrice Kalisch, *The Advance of American Nursing* (Boston: Little, Brown and Company) p. 37.
10. Seymer, op. cit., p. 28.
11. Dolan, op. cit., p. 161.
12. Kalisch, op. cit., p. 37.
13. Kalisch, op. cit., p. 39.
14. Seymer, op. cit., p. 28.
15. Barritt, op. cit., p. 8.
16. Seymer, op. cit., p. 222–223.
17. Seymer, op. cit., p. 244.
18. Ibid., p. 234.
19. Ibid., p. 229.
20. Dolan, op. cit., p. 169.
21. Seymer, op. cit., p. 316.
22. Seymer, op. cit., p. 351.
23. Agnes E. Pavey, *The Story of the Growth of Nursing* London: Farber & Farber Ltd., 1938, p. 296.
24. Seymer, op. cit., p. 276.

BIBLIOGRAPHY

Baritt, Evelyn. "Florence Nightingale's Values and Modern Nursing Education." *Nurs. Forum,* **12,**1 (1973), 6–47. Exploration of Nightingale values, such as nurses' need for continuing education, liberal education, economic security, and research.

Cope, Zachary. *Florence Nightingale and the Doctors*. Philadelphia: J. B. Lippincott Company, 1958. An interesting book, which points out Florence Nightingale's relationships with physicians of the period. Includes letters and data that throw additional light on Nightingale's complex character.

Levine, Myra E. "Florence Nightingale . . . the Legend That Lives." *Nurs. Forum*, **2**,4 (1963), 24–35. A fresh look at Florence Nightingale as a woman, not a myth. Her contributions to modern nursing and health care are briefly described.

Palmer, Irene. "Florence Nightingale: Reformer, Reactionary, Researcher." *Nurs. Res.*, **26** (Mar.-Apr. 1977), 84–89. Discusses significant aspects of Nightingale's beliefs and philosophy as they contributed to her character formation and the role she played in nursing history.

Seymer, Lucy. *Selected Writings of Florence Nightingale*. New York: Macmillan Publishing Co., Inc., 1954. Includes Nightingale's most important writings dealing with nursing. Extremely interesting in terms of not only learning more about this famous nurse as an individual, but also appreciating her many farsighted concepts of care.

Woodham-Smith, Cecil. *Florence Nightingale*. New York: McGraw-Hill Book Company, 1951. A well-written and discerning biography, throwing new light on the life and character of Nightingale.

See also the sections on Nightingale in the Bullough, Dolan, and Kalisch books listed in the bibliography of Chapter 1. An outstanding collection of Nightingale's writings can be found in the Adelaide Nutting Historical Nursing collection at Teachers College, Columbia University, New York. Some of her most noted works are listed below in chronological order.

The Institution of Kaiserswerth on the Rhine for the Practical Training of Deaconesses under the Direction of the Rev. Pastor Fliedner, Embracing the Support and Care of a Hospital, Infant and Industrial Schools, and a Female Penitentiary, 1851.

Notes on Matters Affecting the Health, Efficiency, and Hospital Administration of the British Army. Founded chiefly on the Experience of the Late War. Presented by Request to the Secretary of State for War, 1858.

Subsidiary Notes as to the Introduction of Female Nursing into Military Hospitals in Peace and in War. Presented by Request to the Secretary of State for War, 1858.

A Contribution to the Sanitary History of the British Army During the Late War with Russia, 1859.

Notes on Hospitals, 1859, 3rd edition, almost completely rewritten, 1863.

Notes on Nursing: What It Is, and What It Is Not, 1859.

Observations on the Evidence Contained in the Statistical Reports Submitted to the Royal Commission on the Sanitary State of the Army in India, 1863.

Suggestions on a System of Nursing for Hospitals in India, 1865.

Suggestions on the Subject of Providing, Training, and Organizing Nurses For the Sick Poor in Workhouse Infirmaries. Paper No. XVI in the 'Government Report of the Committee Appointed to Consider the Cubic Space of Metropolitan Workhouses, 1867.

Introductory Notes on Lying-In Institutions Together With a Proposal for Organising an Institution for Training Midwives and Midwifery Nurses, 1871.

On Trained Nursing for the Sick Poor, 1876.

Nurses, Training of and Nursing the Sick, from A Dictionary of Medicine, edited by Sir Robert Qwain, Bart., M.D., 1882.

Sick-Nursing and Health-Nursing (Paper read at the Chicago Exhibition 1893).

Health Teaching in Towns and Villages—Rural Hygiene (a paper read at the Conference of Women Workers, Leeds, 1893), published 1894.

NURSING IN THE
UNITED STATES

The Evolution of the Trained Nurse, 1873–1903

Nursing in the United States between the American Revolution and the Civil War was probably no better or worse than in Europe. As noted in Chapter 1, nurses from both Catholic and Protestant nursing orders came to America, and their nursing care, although semitrained, was the best offered. But there were not enough of them. Even given the occasional compassionate lady who might have ventured into hospitals to help with care in an epidemic or other emergency, the quality of lay nurses was probably about the same as in England.

Early hospitals, privately managed and funded by endowments or public subscription, were modeled after those in Europe, with no improvement in quality; the mentally ill were confined in insane asylums, or poorhouses and prisons.

Yet, by the time of the Civil War, social reforms had also reached America. One of the key figures was Dorothea Lynde Dix (1802–1887), a gentle New England schoolteacher, who became interested in the conditions under which the mentally ill existed when she went to teach a Sunday school lesson in a jail. She began to survey the needs of those forgotten people, and her descriptive reports and careful documentation even-

tually resulted in the construction of state psychiatric institutions (the first in Trenton, New Jersey), and lessening in inhumane care, if no improvement in the understanding of the illnesses.

THE CIVIL WAR

When the Civil War began in April 1861, there was no organized system to care for the sick and wounded. There never had been. In the American Revolution, for instance, such basic care as existed was given by camp followers, a few wives, women in the neighborhood, and "surgeons' mates." It is possible that some of these women were employed by the Army, for there are female names on the payroll lists as "nursing the sick."[1]

American women, considered by American men just as delicate and proper and unsuited for unpleasant service as their European counterparts, nevertheless rushed to volunteer. Within a few weeks, 100 women were given a short training course by physicians and surgeons in New York City, and Dorothea Dix, well known by then, was appointed by the Secretary of War to superintend these new "nurses." Meanwhile, members of religious orders also volunteered, and nursing in some of the larger government hospitals was eventually assigned to them because of the inexperience of the lay volunteers.[2]

Except for that group, almost none of the several thousand women who served as nurses during the war had any kind of training or hospital experience. They can be categorized as follows:

1. The nurses appointed by Miss Dix or other officials as legal employees of the Army for forty cents and one ration a day.
2. The sisters or nuns of the various orders.
3. Those employed for short periods of time for menial chores.
4. Black women employed under General Orders of the War Department at ten dollars a month.
5. Uncompensated volunteers.
6. Women camp followers.
7. Women employed by the various relief organizations.

It is estimated that some 6,000 women performed nursing duties for the Northern Armies. The South used only about 1,000, because of the attitude that prevailed for some time that caring for men was unfit for Southern ladies. (Nevertheless, a number of these ladies, such as Kate Cummings, who recorded her experiences, gave distinguished service under severe conditions in the Southern hospitals.)[4]

The American Army medical officers were no more pleased with the presence of females in their domain than were the British in Crimea. It was not that Miss Dix didn't try for the serious-minded; her recruiting specified only plain-looking women over thirty-five who wore gray, brown, or black dresses with no bows, curls, jewelry, or hoop skirts, and who were moral and had common sense. Presumably, those who did not qualify were among the many unofficial and unpaid volunteers. Some of the information on what the Civil War nurses did comes from the writings of Louisa May Alcott and Walt Whitman,

both volunteers. In her journal, Alcott described her working day which began at six. After opening the windows, because of the bad air in the makeshift base hospital, she was "giving out rations, cutting up food for helpless boys, washing faces, teaching my attendants how beds are made or floors are swept, dressing wounds, dusting tables, sewing bandages, keeping my tray tidy, rushing up and down after pillows, bed linens, sponges, and directions . . ."[5] Volunteers also read to the patients, wrote letters, and comforted them. Apparently, even the hired nurses did little more except, perhaps, give medicines. But so did the volunteers, sometimes giving the medicine and food of their choice to the patient, instead of what the doctor ordered.

By 1862, enormous military hospitals, some as large as 3,000 beds, were being built, although there were still some makeshift hospitals, former hotels, churches, factories, and almost anything else available. There was even a hospital ship, The Red Rover, a former Mississippi steamer captured from the Confederates, and staffed by nuns. Other floating hospitals were inaugurated and served as transport units, with nurses attending the wounded.[6] Discipline in hospitals was rigid for nurses and patients alike, with the latter given strict orders to be respectful to the nurses. According to one Army hospital edict, the nurses, under the supervision of the "Stewards and Chief Wardmaster," were responsible for the administration of the wards, but many of their duties appeared more related to keeping the nonmedical records of patients and reporting their misbehavior than to nursing care. If the patient needed medical or surgical attendance, the doctor was to be called.[7]

Georgeanna Woolsey wrote that the surgeons treated the nurses without even common courtesy because they did not want them and tried to make their lives so unbearable that they would leave. The surgeons were often incompetent. As a temporary expediency, contract surgeons were employed with no position, little pay, and only minimal rank. Jane, another Woolsey sister who was also a volunteer nurse, wrote that although some were highly skilled, "faithful, sagacious, tenderhearted," others were drunken, refused to attend the wounded, or injured them more because of their incompetence."[8]

It was surgeons and officers of the latter type that the formidable nurse Mary Ann (Mother) Bickerdyke attacked. She managed to have a number of them dismissed (in part because of her friendships with Generals Grant and General Sherman.) About this tough "Soldier's Friend," one physician stated, "Woe to the surgeon, the commissary, or quartermaster whose neglect of his men and selfish disregard for their interests and needs come under her cognizance."[9]

Another fighter was Clara Barton, who early in the war cared for the wounded of the Sixth Massachusetts Regiment. One story told about her is that while supervising the delivery of a wagonload of supplies for soldiers, she neatly extricated an ox from a herd intended for the Army, so that the wounded would have food.[10]

Only in recent years has attention been given to the black nurses of the Civil War. Harriet Tubman, the "Moses of her people," not only led many black slaves to freedom in her underground railroad activities before the war, but also nursed the wounded when she joined the Union Army. Similarly, Sojourner Truth, abolitionist speaker and activist in the women's movement, also cared for the sick and wounded. Susie King Taylor, born to slavery and secretly taught to read and write, met and married a Union soldier and served as a battlefront nurse for more than four years, although she received no salary or pension from the Union Army.[11]

There were other heroines, untrained women from the North and South, caring for the sick and wounded with a modicum of skills but much kindness and, as in the Crimea, the soldiers were sentimentally appreciative, if not discriminating.

Even when paid, Civil War nurses had little status and no rank. One exception was Sally Tomkins, a civic-minded Southern woman, who efficiently took charge of a makeshift hospital and was made a captain of the cavalry by Confederacy President Jefferson Davis so that she could continue her work. An investigative report by the United States Sanitary Commission noted that nurses had not been well treated or wisely used.

> They have not been placed, as they expected and were fitted to be, in the position of head nurses. On the contrary, with a very inefficient force of male nurses, they have been called on to do every form of service, have been overtaxed and worn down with menial and purely mechanical duties, additional to the more responsible offices and duties of nursing.[12]

Nevertheless, the Civil War opened hospitals to massive numbers of women, wellbred "ladies," who would otherwise probably not even have thought of nursing. Some of these, such as Abby, Jane, and Georgeanna Woolsey, later helped lead the movement to establish training schools for nurses.

THE EARLY TRAINING SCHOOLS

The nursing role of women in the Civil War, however unsophisticated, and probably the fame of Florence Nightingale brought to the attention of the American public the need for nurses and the desirability of some organized programs of training. There had been elementary efforts in this direction previously; an organized school of nursing, founded in 1839 by the Nurse Society of Philadelphia under Dr. Joseph Warrington, awarded a certificate after a stated period of lectures, demonstration, and experience at a hospital; a school of nursing for a "better type" of woman connected with Women's Hospital in Philadelphia in 1861 gave a diploma after six months of lectures.

More physicians became interested in the training of nurses and, at a meeting of the American Medical Association in 1869, a committee to study the matter stated that it was "just as necessary to have well-trained, well-instructed nurses as to have intelligent and skillful physicians." The committee recommended that nursing schools be placed under the guardianship of county medical societies, although under the immediate supervision of lady superintendents; that every lay hospital should have a school; and that nurses be trained not only for the hospital but for private duty in the home.[13]

In 1871, the editor of *Godey's Lady's Book*, the most popular woman's magazine of the time, wrote an editorial on "Lady Nurses" that was remarkably farsighted.

> *Much has been lately said of the benefits that would follow if the calling of sick nurse were elevated to a profession which an educated lady might adopt without a sense of degradation, either on her own part or in the estimation of others. . . .*
> *There can be no doubt that the duties of sick nurse, to be properly performed, require an education and training little, if at all, inferior to those possessed by members of the medical profession. . . . The manner in which a reform may be effected is easily pointed out. Every medical college should have a course of study and training especially adapted for ladies who desire to qualify themselves for the profession of nurse; and those who had gone through the course, and passed the requisite examination, should receive a degree and a diploma, which would at once establish their position in society. The graduate nurse would in general estimation be as much above the ordinary nurse of the present day as the professional surgeon of our times is above the barber-surgeon of the last century.*[14]

Unfortunately, this idea of an educated nurse with professional status was a long time in coming.

Nevertheless, in 1892, the New England Hospital for Women and Children, staffed by women physicians who were interested in the development of a school, acted upon a statement in its bylaws of 1863 "to train nurses for the care of the sick." It was a one-year program in which the students provided round-the-clock service for patients, there was no classwork (although a few lectures

were given during the winter months), and the duty extended from 5:30 A.M. to 9 P.M., with a free afternoon every second week from 2 to 5 P.M. At the end of the year, one student graduated—Melinda Ann (Linda) Richards, thereafter called America's first trained nurse, probably because of all the nurses that graduated from this primitive early program, she moved on to be a key figure in the development of nursing education. Richards, like some of the other students in the schools that evolved, had been a nurse in a hospital, although some schools would not accept them because they wanted to set a new image. This indicates that despite the frequent descriptions of criminal and thieving women who nursed, some nurses, although untrained in the later sense, must have been at least respectable, intelligent women.

Another outstanding graduate of New England Hospital for Women and Children (1879) was Mary Mahoney, the first trained black nurse. A tiny, dynamic, charming woman, she worked primarily in private duty in the Boston area but was apparently always present at national nurses' meetings. In her honor, the Mary Mahoney Medal was initiated by the National Association of Colored Graduate Nurses, and the award was later continued by the American Nurses' Association.

In 1873, three schools supposedly based on the Nightingale model, were established.[15] The Bellevue Training School in New York City was founded through the influence of several society ladies who had been involved in Civil War Nursing, including Abby Woolsey. Appalled by the conditions—900 patients, three to five occupying strapped-together beds, tended by ex-convict nurses and night watchmen who stole their food and left them in filth—these women sent a young physician to England to confer with Nightingale. Then they raised funds to set up a nurses' training class for which they were given six wards. The hospital agreed to place these students under the direction of a female superintendent, provided that they also did the scouring and cleaning that had been done by the other "nurses"; they would not hire anyone to clean. Although the school attempted to follow Nightingale principles and reported that it was attracting educated women, its overall purpose was to improve conditions in a great charity hospital, and much of the learning was on a trial-and-error basis. Nevertheless, Bellevue had a lot of interesting firsts: interdisciplinary rounds where nurses reported on the nursing plan of care; patient record keeping and writing of orders, initiated by Linda Richards who became night superintendent; the first uniform, by stylish and aristocratic Euphemia Van Rensselaer, which started a trend. And of course, two of nursing's greatest leaders were Bellevue graduates—Lavinia Dock and Isabel Hampton Robb.

The Connecticut Training School was started through the influence of another Woolsey, Georgeanna, and her husband, Dr. Francis Bacon. Through negotiation with the hospital, the superintendent of nurses was designated as separate from, and not responsible to, the steward (administrator) of the hospital, and teaching outside the wards was permitted. However, the threatened steward managed to make life so miserable for a series of superintendents that each resigned; but control remained with nursing. Meantime, all good intentions notwithstanding, the students soon were sent to give care in the homes of sick families, with the money going to the School Fund—and the school could boast that for thirty-three years it was not financed or directed by the hospital.

The Boston Training School was the last of that first famous triumvirate. Again, a group of women associated with other educational and philanthropic endeavors, spearheaded its organization, but this time for the purpose of offering a desirable occupation for self-supporting women and also to provide good private nurses for the community. After some prolonged negotiation that allowed the director of the school, instead of the hospital, to maintain control, Massachu-

setts General Hospital assigned "The Brick" building to the school because it (The Brick) "stands by itself; represents both medical and surgical departments; and offers the hard labor desirable for the training of nurses."[16] Apparently, there was rather poor leadership, and nurses continued to do dishwashing and other menial tasks with little attention to training. When Linda Richards became the third director, she reorganized the work, started classes, and set out to prove that trained nurses were better than untrained. As an example, she cared for some of the sickest patients herself. By the end of 1876, she had charge of all the nursing in the hospital.

Other major training schools that were to endure into a second century of existence were founded in the next few years, somewhat patterned after Nightingale's precepts. Their success and the popularity of their graduates resulted in a massive proliferation of training schools. In 1880, there were fifteen; by 1900, 432; by 1909, 1,105 hospital-based diploma schools. Hospitals with as few as twenty beds opened schools, and the students provided almost totally free labor. Usually, the only graduate nurses were the superintendent and perhaps the operating room supervisor and night supervisor. Students earned money for the hospital, for after a short period, they were frequently sent to do private nursing in the home, with the money reverting to the hospital, not the school. Except for the few outstanding schools, all Nightingale principles were forgotten: the students were under the control of the hospital and worked from twelve to fifteen hours a day—twenty-four if they were on a private case in a home, and lessons, if any, were scheduled for an hour late in the evening when someone was available to teach (it wasn't necessary for all students to be available). Moreover, if the "pupils" lost time because of sickness, which was almost always contracted from patients or caused by sheer overwork, the time had to be totally made up before the student could graduate. Why then did training schools draw so many applicants? Because the occupational opportunities for untrained women were limited to domestic service, factory work, retail clerking, or prostitution. Even with the strict discipline, hard work, long hours, and almost no time off, after a year or two of training (the second year unabashedly free labor to the hospitals), the trained nurse could do private duty at from $10 a week to the vague possibility of $20 (if she could collect it), a far cry from the $4 to $6 average of other women workers. Of course, on these cases, she was a twenty-four-hour servant to family and patient, lucky to have time off for a walk, and because there were necessarily months with no employment, even an excellent nurse was lucky to gross $600 a year.[17] Higher education for women was limited to typewriting or teaching, but these were seldom taught in universities. Those colleges and universities that did admit women rarely prepared them for professions. So the more famous hospital schools, particularly, had hundreds and even thousands of applicants a year. On the other hand, there were a multitude of hospitals and sanitariums of all kinds that were looking for students to meet their staffing needs, and for these, high-quality applicants were frequently lacking. Consequently, application standards were lowered rapidly. Apparently, most schools admitted a class of thirty to thirty-five[18] (in some cases determined by their staffing and financial needs). Attrition, caused in part by the tremendously high percentage of student illness and the unpleasant working and living conditions, was often 75 percent.

Student admission requirements varied, but all nurse applicants were female. Some hospitals accepted men in programs but gave them only a short course and frequently called them attendants. In 1888, at Bellevue Hospital, the Mills School was established with a two-year course, but for a long time its graduates also were called attendants. Other early schools admitting men were at Grace Hospital, Detroit; Battle Creek Sanitarium, Battle Creek, Michigan; Boston City Hospital, Carney, and St. Margaret's, Boston; Pennsylvania Hospital in Philadelphia, and the Alexian Brothers hospitals in Chicago and St. Louis.[19] At first, the minimum age for all students was about twenty-five, later lowered to twenty-one, to prevent losing young women to other fields. Eight or less years of schooling were common, but usually good health and good character were absolute prerequisites. Obedience in training was essential, and a student could be dismissed as a troublemaker if the overworked girl grumbled, talked too much, was too familiar with men, criticized head nurses or doctors, or could not get along "sweetly" wherever placed. Married women and those over thirty were frequently excluded because they could not "fall in with the life successfully." And, of course, if they were divorced, they were naturally eliminated— "too self-centered with interests elsewhere." Blacks were also generally silently excluded. Over the years, training schools for black nurses were founded, the first organized in 1891 at the Provident Hospital in Chicago.

In the 1890s, only 2 percent of nurse training was theory, containing some anatomy and physiology, *materia medica,* perhaps some chemistry, bacteriology, hygiene, and lectures on certain diseases. The leading schools developed their own institutional manuals, such as the simply written *Hand-Book of Nursing for Family and General Use,* written by a committee of nurses and physicians at the Connecticut Training School and published in 1878. The other great pioneering texts were *A Textbook of Nursing for the Use of Training Schools, Families, and Private Students,* by Clara Weeks Shaw (1885); *Nursing: Its Principles and Practice for Hospital and Private Use,* by Isabel Hampton (1893); *The Textbook on Materia Medica for Nurses,* by Lavinia Dock (1890); and the first scientific book written by a nurse, a textbook on anatomy, by Diana Kimber (1893). Almost from the beginning there were those physicians who objected to so much education for nurses and devoted considerable medical journal space to their fulminations about the "overtrained nurse."

Training, as we understand it, is drilling, and a person who is to carry out the instructions of another cannot be too thoroughly drilled. Pedagogy is another matter. We have never been able to understand what great good was expected from imparting to nurses a smattering of medicine and surgery. . . . To feed their vanity with the notion that they are competent to take any considerable part in ordering the management of the sick is certainly a most erroneous step.

The work of a nurse is an honorable 'calling' or vocation, and nothing further. It implies the exercise of acquired proficiency in certain more or less mechanical duties, and is not primarily designed to contribute to the sum of human knowledge or the advancement of science . . .[20]

One physician even suggested a correspondence course for training nurses to care for the "poor folks,"[21] and a New York newspaper editorial proclaimed, "What we want in nurses is less theory and more practice." But then, this was at a time when a leading Harvard physician held that serious mental exercise would damage a woman's brain or cause other severe trauma, such as the narrowing of the pelvic area, which would make her unable to deliver children.[22]

However, there were also farsighted physicians who supported not "teaching a trade, but preparing for a profession," as Dr. Richard Cabot noted in 1901. He listed reforms that included: (1) nurses should pay for their training and be taught by paid instructors; (2) nursing should be taught by nurses; medicine by physicians; (3) the nurse's training should not be entirely technical. He added, "Subjects like English literature and history, which tend to give us a deeper and truer sympathy with human nature, are surely as much needed in the education of the nurse, who is to deal exclusively with human beings, as in the curriculum of the chemist or engineer, who deals primarily with things and not persons."[23] But, meanwhile, students continued to live a slavelike existence, without outward complaint, poorly housed, overworked, underfed ("rations of a kind and quality only a remove better than what we might place before a beggar," said a popular journal), and unprotected from life-threatening illness (80 percent of the students in the average hospital graduated with positive tuberculins).[24] If they survived all this, no wonder they were expected to graduate as "respectful, obedient, cheerful, submissive, hard-working, loyal, pacific, and religious."[25] It was not professional education; it was not even a respectably run apprenticeship, because learning was not from skilled masters, but rather from their own peers who were but a step ahead of them. These principles of sacrifice, service, obedience to the physician, and ethical orientation are embodied in the Nightingale Pledge, written in 1893 by Lystra E. Gretter, superintendent of the school at Harper Hospital in Detroit, a pledge still frequently recited by students today.

I solemnly pledge myself before God and in the presence of this assembly;

To pass my life in purity and to practice my profession faithfully;

I will abstain from whatever is deleterious and mischievous and will not take or knowingly administer any harmful drug; I will do all in my power to maintain and elevate the standard of my profession, and will hold in confidence all personal matters committed to my keeping and all family affairs coming to my knowledge in the practice of my calling;

With loyalty will I endeavor to aid the physician in his work, and devote myself to the welfare of those committed to my care.[26]

THE NURSE IN PRACTICE

In the late eighteenth and early nineteenth centuries, the graduate trained nurse had two major career options: she could do private duty in homes, or, if she were exceptional (or particularly favored), gain one of the rare positions as head nurse, operating room supervisor, night supervisor, or even superintendent. The latter positions were, of course, much more available before the flood of nurses reached the market. Even so, in private duty, trained nurses often competed with untrained nurses who were not restrained from practicing in many states until the middle of the twentieth century. And, given the long hours and taxing physical work in home nursing, most private nurses found themselves unwanted at forty, with younger, stronger nurses being hired instead. Some of the more ambitious and perhaps braver nurses chose to go west to pioneer in new and sometimes primitive hospitals.

The practice of nursing was scarcely limited to clinical care of the patient. Job descriptions of the time appear to give major priority to scrubbing floors, dusting, keeping the stove stoked and the kerosene lamps trimmed and filled, controlling insects, washing clothes, making and rolling bandages, and other unskilled housekeeping tasks, as well as edicts for personal behavior.[27] Nursing care responsibilities included "making beds, giving baths, preventing and dressing bedsores, applying friction to the body and extremities, giving enemas, inserting catheters, bandaging, dressing blisters, burns, sores, and wounds, and observing secretions, expectorations, pulse, skin, appetite, body temperature, consciousness, respiration, sleep, condition of wounds, skin eruptions, elimination, and the effect of diet, stimulants, and medications," and carrying out any orders of the physician.[28] One of the more interesting treatments to modern nurses might be the vivid description of leeching, which included placing leeches, removing them from human orifices where they may have disappeared, and emptying them of excess blood.[29]

At the end of the nineteenth century, the growth of large cities was a phenomenon in the United States. Although the cities had their beautiful public buildings, parks, and mansions, they also had their seamy sides— the festering slums where the tremendous flow of immigrants huddled. Between 1820 and 1910, nearly thirty million immigrants entered the United States, with a shift in numbers from Northern European to Southern European by the early 1900s. Health and social problems multiplied in the slum areas. In New York, for instance, it was not unusual to house thirty-six families in a six-story walk-up on a narrow 25-× 90-foot lot. Vermin, lack of sanitation, and the fact that many immigrants converted their crowded rooms into sweatshops made it easy for epidemics to rage through the neighborhoods, and death from tuberculosis was common.[30]

Somehow, Americans did not seem to feel a great need to serve the sick poor in their homes; after all, there were public dispensaries and charity hospitals. Nevertheless, in 1877, the Women's Board of the New York City Mission sent nurses, who received their training at Bellevue, into the homes of the poor to give physical care. In 1886, the Visiting Nurse Society of Philadelphia sent nurses not only to the poor, but to those of moderate means who could pay. In the same year, the nurses of the Boston Instructive District Nursing Association formally included patient teaching in their visit—principles of hygiene, sanitation, and aspects of illness. Other such agencies followed, but, by 1900, it was estimated that only 200 nurses were engaged in public health nursing.

One of the key figures in community health nursing was Lillian Wald. After graduating from New York Hospital School of Nursing and working a short time, she decided to enter Women's Medical College. When she and another nurse, Mary Brewster, were sent to the Lower East Side to lecture immigrant mothers on the care of the sick, they were both shocked at what they saw; neither had known such abject poverty could exist. Wald left medical school, with Mary Brewster moved to a top-floor tenement on Jefferson Street, and began to offer nursing care to the poor. After a short while, the calls came by the hundreds from families, hospitals, and physicians. People were cared for, whether or not they could afford to pay. The concern of these nurses was not just nursing care, but seeing what other services could be made available to meet the many social needs of the poor. Challenging the entire community to assume responsibility for these conditions of "poverty and misery" was an attitude strongly advocated by Lavinia Dock, who wrote in 1937:

> As I recollect it, this point of view turned rather toward exploration and discovery than simply toward good works alone, when Lillian D. Wald and Mary Brewster went in 1893, free from every form of control, 'without benefit of' managers, committees, medical encouragement, or police approval, into Jefferson Street (at first, then later into Henry Street), there to do what they could do; to see what they could see; and to publicize all that was wrong and remediable by making their findings known as widely as possible . . .
>
> If I am not mistaken, it was Lillian Wald who first used the term public health nursing —adding the one word public to Florence Nightingale's phrase health nursing—in order to picture her inner vision of the possibilities of nursing services as widely and as effectively organized as were state and federal health services, and acting in harmonious cooperation with them, if not a part of them.[31]

After two years of such success, larger facilities, more nurses, and social workers were needed. In 1895, Wald, Brewster, Lavinia Dock, and other nurses moved to what was eventually called the Henry Street Settlement, a house bought by philanthropist Jacob H. Schiff. By 1909, the Henry Street staff had thirty-seven nurses, all but five providing direct nursing service. Each nurse was carefully oriented to the customs of the immigrants she served and was able to demonstrate the value of understanding the family and the environment in giving good nursing care. Each nurse kept two sets of records, one for the physician and another recording the major points of the nurse's work.[32]

The establishment of school nursing was also started by Lillian Wald, who suggested that placing nurses in schools might help solve the problem of the schools having to send home so many ill children. (Health conditions in New York Schools were so bad that in 1902, 10,567 children were sent home from school; local physicians did little in

these settings.) Wald sent a Henry Street nurse, Lina L. Rogers, to a school on a one-month demonstration, which proved so successful that by 1903 the School Board began to appoint nurses to the schools. It was not an easy job, and on occasion the schools were the sites of riots because mothers misunderstood the preventive measures that needed to be taken by the nurses. One amusing tale is found in the Children's Bureau records. On being notified that her child needed a bath, a mother wrote, "teacher, Johnny ain't no rose. Learn him, don't smell him."[33]

Industrial nursing also began to provide job opportunities for the trained nurses. Its beginnings are generally credited to the president of the Vermont Marble Company in Proctor, Vermont, who in 1895 employed a trained nurse, Ada M. Stewart, to give "district nursing" service to the employees of the company. No public health nursing service was available at that time.

Miss Stewart often traveled about the town on a bicycle, wearing her nurse's uniform and a plain coat and hat, teaching company employees and sometimes other members of the community "habits for healthy living," caring for minor injuries, calling the doctor when indicated, and, at the schoolteacher's request, talking to schoolchildren about hygiene and first aid. Miss Stewart's service was so helpful that in 1895 the marble company employed her sister, Harriet, to give similar service in other Vermont communities in which the company had mills and quarries.[34]

The century ended with another war, where again nurses proved their worth. The Spanish-American War lasted less than a year, but there was considerable loss of life. The Army was completely unprepared for it, and the hospital corpsmen were even less ready to cope with the sick and wounded. The National Society of the Daughters of the American Revolution offered to serve as an examining board for military nurses. The task of separating the fit from the unfit and the trained from the untrained among the

5,000 applicants was overwhelming. Significant of the questions asked the volunteers were, "Are you strong and healthy?" and "Have you ever had yellow fever?" Although only a small percentage of the soldiers ever left the camps in the South to fight in Cuba, at one point fully 30 percent became ill from malaria, dysentery, and typhoid. Once more, some Army surgeons, particularly the Surgeon General, objected to the presence of trained women nurses, but their efforts to recruit male nurses were unsuccessful because glory, rank, and decent salary were lacking. Consequently, nursing was done by the dregs of the infantry squads. Finally, with serious outbreaks of typhoid killing the enlistees, women nurses from many training schools took over. Wearing their own distinctive school uniforms and caps, they included superintendents of nursing on leave from their noted schools, as well as new, young graduates. Their letters and journals relate the horrible conditions under which the nurses worked. Some literally worked themselves to death in the Army Hospitals in the South.

Meanwhile, a hospital ship, the U.S.S. Relief, sailed to Cuba with supplies, medicines, and equipment—and Esther Hasson of New London, Connecticut, who would later become the first superintendent of the Navy Nurse Corps. They were just in time to receive the wounded of a naval battle, but, again, the greatest problem was disease. Among these was yellow fever, about which little useful was known. In testing out the theory that the disease was caused by a certain type of mosquito, nursing gained its first martyr. Twenty-five-year-old Clara Maas of East Orange, New Jersey volunteered to be bitten by a carrier mosquito. After being bitten several times, she died of yellow fever and is still considered a heroine in helping to prove the source of the disease.

The conditions under which soldiers and sailors were cared for continued to be horrendous, but an investigation after the war indicated that the only redeeming aspect was the quality of the services of the women nurses, even though they were insufficient in number and were forced to work inefficiently. A recommendation was made for "a corps of selected trained women nurses ready to serve when necessity shall arise, but, under ordinary circumstances, owing no duty to the War Department, except to report residence at determined intervals."[35] Still, the attitude of military authorities was hostile. One hospital commander surgeon objected to retaining women nurses, citing their "coddling" of patients, not letting the Army private (orderly) nurse, and the difficulty in preserving "good military discipline with this mixed personnel." So, although the number of women Army nurses had reached 1,158 in September 1898, by the next July, there were only 202. Despite this setback, a group of influential women, including some prominent nurses, eventually lobbied through a bill, and the Army Nurse Corps was established on February 2, 1901. Dita H. Kinney, Head Nurse of the U.S. Army Hospital at Fort Bayard, New Mexico, became the first nurse superintendent. It took longer for the Congress to act on a Navy Nurse Corps, although it had the support of the Navy's Surgeon General, but finally it too became a reality in 1908.[36]

THE IMPACT OF NURSING'S EARLY LEADERS

Perhaps it was said best by Isabel Hampton Robb as she spoke to other early nursing leaders. "We are the history makers of trained nurses. Let us see to it that we work so as to leave a fair record as the inheritance of those who come after us, one which may be to them an inspiration to even better efforts."[37]

It was an amazing period of coordinated female leadership in what was barely becoming an accepted respectable occupation in the last quarter of the century. Yet, before the new century was far along, this intrepid coterie of nurses was responsible for setting nursing standards, improving curricula, writing textbooks, starting two enduring professional organizations and a nursing journal, inaugurating a teacher training program in a university, and initiating nursing licensure. They were a mixed group, but with certain commonalities: usually unmarried, but, except for Lavinia Dock, not feminist; graduates of the better training schools, later functioning in some teaching and/or administrative capacity, most often as superintendent of a school, and involved in the early nursing organizations. Fortunately, many were also great letterwriters and letter savers as well as authors, so that there are many fascinating insights into their lives.*

Nursing's first trained nurse, Linda Richards, had a continuing impact on the training schools because she spent much of her career moving from hospital to hospital in what seems to have been an improvement campaign. In those earliest days, almost any graduate was considered a prime candidate for starting another program, and some undoubtedly lacked the intellectual and leadership qualities needed, so that the new schools, if not actual disasters, were frequently of poor quality. Linda Richards apparently had the skill and authority to upgrade both the school and nursing service which were, after all, almost inseparable. However, she seemed willing to accept school management that tied the economics of the hospital with student education, usually to the detriment of the latter.

One of the most noted nursing figures is Isabelle Hampton, who left teaching to enter Bellevue Training School in 1881. Not only was she attractive and charming, but she was "in every sense of the word a leader, by nature, by capacity, by personal attributes and qualities, by choice, and probably to some extent by inheritance and training; a follower she never was."[38] In her two major superintendencies, she made a number of then radical changes—cutting down the students' workday to ten hours and eliminating their

*See particularly the Christy series in *Nursing Outlook*, listed in the bibliography.

free private duty services. At Johns Hopkins, which she founded, she recruited fractious Lavinia Dock, who was still at Bellevue, to be her assistant. They must have made an interesting pair, for Lavinia, also a "lady," was outspoken and frequently tactless, particularly with physicians. Later, she was to say

A quite determined movement on the part of our masculine brothers to seize and guide the helm of the new teaching is . . . most undeniably in progress. Several . . . have lately openly asserted themselves in printed articles as the founders and leaders of the nursing education, which so far as it has gone, we all know to have been worked out by the brains, bodies and souls of women . . . who have often had to win their points in clinched opposition to the will of these same brothers and solely by dint of their own personal prestige as women . . .[39]

M. Adelaide Nutting graduated in that first Hopkins class, and the three became friends. Nutting followed Hampton as principal of the school when in 1894 Isabel was married to one of her admirers, Dr. Hunter Robb, and, as was the custom, retired from active nursing. (Letters of the time reveal the anger, dismay, and even sadness of her colleagues at her marriage. They were sure Dr. Robb was not nearly good enough for her, and, besides, she was betraying nursing by robbing the profession of her talents.) Nevertheless, Isabel Hampton Robb maintained her interest in nursing and continued to be active in the development of the profession. In 1893, she had been appointed chairman of a committee to arrange a congress of nurses under the auspices of the International Congress of Charities, Correction, and Philanthropy at the Chicago World's Fair. There, before an international audience of nurses, she voiced her concern about poor nursing education and that the term *trained nurse* meant "anything, everything, or next to nothing," in the absence of educational standards. At the same time, Dock pointed out that the teaching, training, and discipline of nurses should not be at the discretion of medicine. Similar themes were reiterated in other papers, as well as the notion that there ought to be an organization of nurses. Shortly after the Congress, eighteen superintendents organized the American Society of Superintendents of Training Schools for Nursing (later to become the National League of Nursing Education) to promote the fellowship of members, establish and maintain a universal standard of training, and further the best interests of the nursing profession. The first convention of the society elected Linda Richards president.

Another attendee at those early meetings was Sophia Palmer, descendant of John and Priscilla Alden and a graduate of Boston Training School, who, after a variety of experiences, organized a training school in Washington, D.C., over the concerted opposition of local physicians who wanted to control nursing education. She approved the steps that were taken but was impatient with what seemed to be blind acceptance of hospital control of schools. "She had a very intense nature and, like all those who are born crusaders, had little patience with the slower methods of persuasion . . . She was like a spirited racehorse held by the reins of tradition."[40] Within a short time, she and some of the others in the Society, including Dock and the new Mrs. Robb, recognized the need for another organization for all nurses. Although some of the training schools had alumnae associations, they were restrictive; in some cases, their own graduates could not be members, and any "outsider" could not participate. Therefore, if a nurse were to leave the immediate vicinity of her own school, there was no way in which she had any organized contact with other nurses. In a paper given in 1895, Palmer stressed that the power of the nursing profession was dependent upon its ability to organize individuals who could influence public opinion. Dock also made recommendations for a national organization. In 1896, delegates representing the oldest training school alumnae associations and members of an organizing committee of the Society selected a name for the proposed organization—Nurses' Associated Alumnae of the United States and Canada (to become the American Nurses' Association in 1911), set a time and place for the first meeting (February 1897 in Baltimore), and drafted a constitution. At the end of that February meeting, held in conjunction with the fourth annual society convention, the constitution and by-laws were adopted and Isabel Hampton Robb was elected president. Among the problems discussed at those early meetings were nursing licensure and creation of an official nursing publication.

There were a number of nursing journals: the *British Journal of Nursing,* established by one of England's nursing leaders, Ethel Gordon Fenwick; and in the United States, the short-lived *The Nightingale,* started by a Bellevue graduate; *The Nursing Record* and *The Nursing World,* also short-lived; and *The Trained Nurse and Hospital Review,* which Palmer edited for a time, and which continued for seventy years. But the leaders of the new organizations wanted a magazine that would promote nursing, owned and controlled by nursing.

For several years there was discussion but no action, until another committee on ways and means of producing a magazine was formed. In January 1900, they organized a stock company and sold $100 shares only to nurses and nurses' alumnae associations. By May, they had a promise of $2,400 in shares, and almost 500 nurses had promised to subscribe. Admittedly, they had overstepped their mandate, they reported to the third annual convention of the Nurses' Associated Alumnae, but they were given approval to establish the magazine along the lines formulated. The J. B. Lippincott Company was selected as publisher, and Sophia Palmer became editor, which she did on an unpaid basis for the first nine months. (She had become director of the Rochester City Hospital in New York). As the first issues went for mailing in October, it was discovered that the post office rules prevented its being mailed because the journal's stockholders were not incorporated. M. E. P. Davis and

Sophia Palmer assumed personal responsibilities for all liabilities of the new *American Journal of Nursing*, and it went out. The *Journal* was considered the official organ of the nursing profession, but the stock was still held by alumnae associations and individual nurses. It was Lavinia Dock who donated the first share of stock to the association, and by 1912, the renamed American Nurses' Association had gained ownership of all the stock of the American Journal of Nursing Company, which it still retains.[41]

One other major organization, the American Red Cross, was ushered into existence by a nurse, Clara Barton, the school teacher who had volunteered as a nurse and directed relief operations during the Civil War, and had served with the German Red Cross during the Franco-Prussian war in 1870. (The establishment of the International Red Cross as a permanent international relief agency that could take immediate action in time of war had occurred in Geneva in 1864 with the signing of the Geneva Convention guidelines.) After her return to the United States, Barton organized the American Red Cross and persuaded Congress in 1882 to ratify the Treaty of Geneva so that the Red Cross could carry on its humanitarian efforts in peacetime. Clara Barton, however, was not an active part of the nursing leadership that was molding the profession.

That group had another immediate goal. The Society recognized that the nurses were at a disadvantage because they had no postgraduate training in administration or teaching, so a committee consisting of Robb, Nutting, Richards, Mary Agnes Snively, and Lucy Drown was formed to investigate the possibilities. At the sixth Society convention, they reported their success. James Russell, the farsighted dean of Teachers College at Columbia University in New York, had agreed to start a course for nurses if they could guarantee the enrollment of twelve nurses, or $1,000 a year. The Society agreed. Members of the Society screened the candidates, contributed $1,000 a year, and taught the course—hospital economics. Later, the

students were also allowed to enroll in psychology, science, household economics, and biology. Anna Alline, one of the two graduates of the first class, then took over the total administration of the course.

There was one more major goal to be reached—licensure of nurses. Not only did the 432 hospital-based schools vary greatly in quality, but the market was also flooded with "nurses" who had been dismissed from schools without graduating, "nurses" from six-week private and correspondence courses, and a vast number of those who simply called themselves nurses. It was inevitable that people became confused, for when they hired nurses for private duty in their homes, the "nurse" could present one of the elaborate diplomas from a $13 correspondence course that guaranteed that anyone could become a nurse, a real or forged reference, or a genuine diploma from a topquality school. How could they judge? Consequently, because of the abysmal care given by individuals representing themselves as nurses, the public was once more disenchanted with the "nurse." Therefore, nursing's leaders were determined that there must be legal regulation, both to protect the public from unscrupulous and incompetent nurses and to protect the young profession, by establishing a minimum level of competence, limiting all or some of the professional functions to those who qualified. The idea was not new; medicine already had licensing in some states, and many aspiring professions were also moving in that direction.

In September 1901, at the first meeting of the newly formed International Council of Nurses, which was held in Buffalo, a resolution was passed, stating that "it is the duty of the nursing profession of every country to work for suitable legislative enactment regulating the education of nurses and protecting the interests of the public, by securing State examinations and public registration, with the proper penalities for enforcing the same."[42]

In the United States, such licensing was a state function, so to gain the necessary legislative lobbying power, it was recommended that state or local nurses' associations be formed. In many ways the disagreements that arose in their formation were forerunners to those that would center on the licensure process. Who should be eligible? In New York, for instance, Sylveen Nye, who became the state association's first president, thought *all* nurses should be included and the standards could be raised later. Sophia Palmer, another key figure in its formation, believed that only "qualified" nurses should be permitted to belong—those who graduated from certain types of schools. Later, the question was "Who should be eligible for licensure?"

As it was, New York had become the early leader in the licensure drive, for it had in place a Board of Regents that regulated education—and licensure. In 1897, Palmer, in a smart political move, had already presented nursing's case to another emerging group of women who were gaining power and prestige —the New York Federation of Women's Clubs. They passed a resolution supporting her licensure concept, which included two major points—need for a diploma from a school meeting certain standards, and insistence that the examining board consist only of nurses, as was true of other professions. Immediately, Palmer organized a meeting with the secretary of the Board of Regents, who then and later was helpful and supportive, suggesting guidelines for action. (For instance, this licensed nurse needed to be called something. Among the titles suggested by nurses were graduate nurse, trained nurse, certified nurse, registered nurse, and registered graduate nurse.) The Regents also suggested the formation of a state nurses' association. Once formed, the New York State Nurses' Association developed a licensure bill and embarked on a campaign to gain support for the proposed legislation. Opposition was foreordained. In a circular addressed to the women's clubs, Palmer accurately pinpointed the sources:

The New York State Nurses' Association

is preparing to apply for legislative enactments which will place training schools for nurses under the supervision of the Regents of the University of the State, with a view to securing by the authority of the law a minimum basis of education for the nurse, beyond which the safety of the sick and the protection of the public cannot be assured.

While such a law cannot prevent the public from employing untaught women as nurses, if it so desires, it will prevent such women from imposing themselves upon the public as fully trained nurses.

In this movement the Nurses' Association will meet with opposition: First, from the trained nurses of the State who are afraid to make an independent stand for their own and the public protection. Second, from all of the managers and proprietors of institutions which are not equipped for giving this minimum education, and which now conduct so-called training schools, for commercial advantages, and third, from all the vast army of so-called nurses who, without adequate nursing experience and education, undertake the grave responsibility of a nurse's work.[53]

And there was just that kind of opposition and more, for there were 15,000 untrained nurses in New York at the time, opposed to 2,500 who were trained. In addition, some physicians objected to their lack of representation on the proposed nursing board, as did some nurses, including Nye. Moreover, some physicians did not see the necessity for any fancy standards and worried about over-education of nurses. Said one, "Nursing is not, strictly speaking, a profession. Any intelligent, not necessarily educated, woman can in a short time acquire the skill to carry out with explicit obedience the physician's directions."

Nevertheless, the bill became law on April 24, 1903. It was pitifully weak by today's standards, but daring for the times. Educational standards were set. A training school for nurses had to give at least a two-year program and be registered by the Regents. The board of five nurses was to be chosen by the Regents from a list submitted by the New York State Nurses' Association. The Regents, on advice of the Board, were to make rules for the examination of nurses, and also revoke licensure for cause. The New York State Nurses' Association was given the right to institute proceedings and prosecute those violating the law, a responsibility that was not changed for some years. It should be remembered, though, that this, like all nurse licensure laws in those times, was permissive, not mandatory. That is, only the title RN was protected. Untrained nurses could continue to work as nurses as long as they did not call themselves RNs.

New York was not the first state to register nurses. On March 3, 1903, North Carolina, and on April 1, 1903, New Jersey had passed laws. It was said that both were inspired by New York's initiative. (Virginia followed New York on May 14.) However, New York's law was the strongest. For instance, New Jersey's law omitted a board of any kind; North Carolina had a mixed board of nurses and doctors and allowed a nurse to be licensed without attending a training school, if vouched for by a doctor. Partially because New York had the greatest number of trained nurses and because of the experience in regulation of the Board of Regents, the state's nurses were looked to as leaders in the further developments. The prestige, power, and authority of the Board of Regents was such that later many training schools in other states and other countries sought and received approval under New York's law—an action that also upgraded schools in those states. In fact, by 1906, more schools were registered outside the state than within.

The enactment of the first nursing licensure laws was soon followed by like actions in other states; and in a sense it was the end of one era and the beginning of another. Nursing's leaders had shown themselves to be, as a whole, dedicated, strong, and remarkably bold. They set standards for nursing at a time when standards in long-established medicine were still quite weak. Despite internal dissension and the opposition of some powerful hospital administrators and physicians, they had a licensing law

passed—at a time when women had no vote. They literally created a young profession out of a woman's occupation. But the struggle to achieve full professionalism was far from over.

REFERENCES

1. Ida C. Selavan, "Nurses in American History: The Revolution," *Am. J. Nurs.*, **74**:592–594 (Apr. 1975).
2. Josephine A. Dolan, *Nursing in Society*, 14th ed. (Philadelphia: W. B. Saunders Company, 1978), p. 175.
3. Philip Kalisch and Beatrice Kalisch, "Untrained But Undaunted: The Women Nurses of the Blue and Gray," *Nurs. Forum*, **15**,1:25–26 (1976).
4. Ibid. pp. 22–25.
5. Ibid. p. 17.
6. Anne Austin, "Nurses in American History—Wartime Volunteers—1861-1865," *Am. J. Nurs.*, **75**:817 (May 1975).
7. Kalisch, op. cit., pp. 15–16.
8. Vern Bullough and Bonnie Bullough, *The Care of the Sick: The Emergence of Modern Nursing* (New York: Prodist, 1978), p. 113.
9. Dolan, op. cit., pp. 176–177.
10. Ibid., pp. 175–176.
11. Joyce Ann Elmore, "Nurses in American History: Black Nurses: Their Service and Their Struggle," *Am. J. Nurs.*, **76**:435 (Mar. 1976).
12. Kalisch, op. cit., p. 27.
13. Dolan, op. cit., p. 194.
14. Ibid.
15. Josephine Dolan, "Nurses in American History: Three Schools—1873", *Am. J. Nurs.*, **75**:991 (June 1975).
16. Dolan, op. cit., p. 206.
17. Philip Kalisch and Beatrice Kalisch, *The Advance of American Nursing* (Boston: Little, Brown, and Company, 1978), pp. 188–189.
18. Ibid., pp. 135–136.
19. Dolan, op. cit., pp. 308–309.
20. Thelma Ingles, "The Physician's View of the Evolving Nursing Profession—1873–1913," *Nurs. Forum*, **15**,2:147 (1976).
21. Ibid., p. 148.
22. Bonnie Bullough and Vern Bullough,

"Sex Discrimination in Health Care," *Nurs. Outlook,* **23**:44 (Jan. 1975).

23. Ingles, op. cit., pp. 139–140.

24. Beatrice Kalisch and Philip Kalisch, "Slaves, Servants, or Saints (An Analysis of the System of Nurse Training in the United States, 1873–1948)," *Nurs. Forum,* **14**,3:230–231 (1975).

25. Ibid., p. 228.

26. Kalisch, *The Advance of American Nursing,* op. cit., pp. 141–142.

27. Ibid., pp. 173–174.

28. Ibid., p. 174.

29. Ibid., pp. 176–177.

30. Ibid., pp. 225–228.

31. "Our First Public Health Nurse—Lillian D. Wald," *Nurs. Outlook,* **19**:660 (Oct. 1871).

32. Kalisch, op. cit., pp. 230–236.

33. Ibid., pp. 236–240.

34. Ada Stewart Markolf, "Industrial Nursing Begins in Vermont," *Publ. Health Nurs.,* **37**:125 (Mar. 1945).

35. Kalisch, op. cit., p. 216.

36. Ibid., pp. 217–220.

37. Lyndia Flanagan, *One Strong Voice: The Story of the American Nurses' Association* (Kansas City, Mo.: American Nurses' Association, 1976), p. 292.

38. M.A. Nutting, "Isabel Hampton Robb— Her Work in Organization and Education," *Am. J. Nurs.,* **10**:19, 1910.

39. Ashley, Jo Ann, "Nurses in American History: Nursing and Early Feminism." *Am. J. Nurs.,* **75**:1466 (Sept. 1975).

40. Teresa Christy, "Portrait of a Leader: Sophia F. Palmer," *Nurs. Outlook,* **23**:746–747, (Dec. 1975).

41. Flanagan, op. cit., pp. 35–38.

42. Kalisch, p. 260.

43. Mary Lucile Shannon, "The Origin and Development of Professional Licensure Examinations in Nursing: From a State-Constituted Examination to the State Board Test Pool Examination" (unpublished Ed.D. dissertation, Teachers College, Columbia University, 1972), pp. 57–58.

BIBLIOGRAPHY

Ashley, Jo Ann. "Nurses in American History: Nursing and Early Feminism." *Am. J. Nurs.* **75** (Sept. 1975), 1465–1467. Nurse feminist writer points out how pre-World War I feminist movement failed because of lack of participation by most women, including nurses.

Ashley, Jo Ann. *Hospitals, Paternalism, and the Role of the Nurse.* New York: Teachers College Press, 1976. Traces history of nursing in hospitals and concludes that much of nursing power today has its roots in ongoing hospital and male paternalism.

Austin, Anne. "Nurses in American History: Wartime Volunteers 1861–1865." *Am. J. Nurs.,* **75** (May 1975), 816–818. Describes major individuals, groups, and incidents related to nursing in the Civil War. Interesting details.

Brand, Karen, and Laurie Glass. "Perils and Parallels of Women and Nursing." *Nurs. Forum,* **14**,2 (1975), 160–174. Presents overview of nursing history and attitudes of nurses as females in an emerging profession.

Christy, Teresa. "Liberation Movement: Impact on Nursing." *AORN J.,* **15** (Apr. 1972), 67–72. Primarily useful for the historical overview of feminism. Contains some humorous, although disturbing, statements made early in the feminist movement by the press and others.

Christy, Teresa. "Nurses in American History: The Fateful Decade, 1890–1900." *Am. J. Nurs.,* **75** (July 1975), 1163–1165. Highlights proliferation of schools, emergence of nursing leaders and of organized nursing.

Christy, Teresa. "Equal Rights for Women: Voices From the Past." *Am. J. Nurs.,* **71** (Feb. 1971), 288–293. The actions and attitudes of the astonishing Lavinia Lloyd Dock on the matter of equal rights for women.

Christy, Teresa. "Portrait of a Leader: M. Adelaide Nutting." *Nurs. Outlook,* **17** (Jan. 1969), 20–24.

Christy, Teresa. "Portrait of a Leader: Isabel Hampton Robb." *Nurs. Outlook,* **17** (Mar. 1969), 26–29.

Christy, Teresa. "Portrait of a Leader: Lavinia Lloyd Dock." *Nurs. Outlook,* **17** (June 1969), 72–75.

Christy, Teresa. "Portrait of a Leader: Isabel Maitland Stewart." *Nurs. Outlook,* **17** (Oct. 1969), 44–48.

Christy, Teresa. "Portrait of a Leader: Lillian D. Wald." *Nurs. Outlook,* **18** (Mar. 1970), 50–54.

Christy, Teresa. "Portrait of a Leader: Annie Warburton Goodrich." *Nurs. Outlook,* **18** (Aug. 1970), 46–50.

Christy, Teresa. "Portrait of a Leader: Sophia F.

Palmer.'' *Nurs. Outlook,* **23** (Dec. 1975), 746–751.

All of these Christy articles are fascinating looks at some of the great American nurses. Wonderful excerpts from letters. References include earlier biographical sources.

Dock, Lavinia. ''What We May Expect from the Law.'' *Am. J. Nurs.,* **50** (Oct. 1950), 599–600. A reprint from the first issue of A.J.N. that is remarkably timely today.

Dolan, Josephine. ''Nurses in American History: Three Schools—1873.'' *Am. J. Nurs.,* **75** (June 1975), 989–992. A brief overview of the founding of the first three American Schools for trained nurses.

Elmore, Joyce. ''Nurses in American History: Black Nurses: Their Struggle.'' *Am. J. Nurs.,* **76** (Mar. 1976), 435–437. One of the few sources of information about the background and contributions of American black nurses.

Flanagan, Lyndia. *One Strong Voice: The Story of the American Nurses' Association.* Kansas City, Mo.: American Nurses' Association, 1976. History of ANA. Includes selected speeches of all its presidents.

Kalisch, Beatrice, and Philip Kalisch. ''Slaves, Servants, or Saints? (An Analysis of the System of Nurse Training in the United States).'' *Nurs. Forum,* **14**,3 (1975), 222–263. Just what it says; extremely well-written and interesting.

Kalisch, Beatrice, and Philip Kalisch. ''Untrained

But Undaunted: The Women Nurses of the Blue and the Gray.'' *Nurs. Forum,* **15**,1 (1976), 4–33. Taken from their American history book. Detailed and vivid.

''Lavinia L. Dock: Self-Portrait.'' *Nurs. Outlook,* **25** (Jan. 1977), 22–26. Written in 1932 by Dock at the request of the American Journal of Nursing Company, but never published, this presents a rare first-person view of her life and beliefs.

''Lillian D. Wald,'' *Nurs. Outlook,* **19** (Oct. 1971), 659–660. A tribute to the first public health nurse in the United States, through a letter written by Lavinia Dock.

Marshall, Helen. *Mary Adelaide Nutting: Pioneer of Modern Nursing.* Baltimore: The Johns Hopkins Press, 1972. An excellent biography of this nursing leader, casting light on her life and career as well as on nursing of the times.

Selevan, Ida. ''Nurses in American History: The Revolution.'' *Am. J. Nurs.,* **75** (Apr. 1975), 592–594. Little-known details of who nursed the sick and wounded during the American Revolution.

Shannon, Mary Lucille. ''Nurses in American History: Our First Four Licensure Laws.'' *Am. J. Nurs.,* **75** (Aug. 1975), 1327–1329. Brief but useful review. Includes key points in first laws. Taken from author's doctoral dissertation.

See also the Bullough, Dolan, and Kalisch histories cited in the bibliography of Chapter 1, all of which have lengthy sections on this period.

The Emergence of the Modern Nurse, 1904–1965

The period between 1904 and 1965 encompasses a time of multiple changes for nursing, many again precipitated by external forces, including the Depression, two world wars, and various social movements. But the changes were created within nursing by nurses. They included major shifts in education—type, location, curriculum, student body, and alterations in practice—responsibility, economic status, and degree of autonomy. In 1903, the passage of the first nursing licensure laws set standards for nursing education and practice; in 1965, development of new nursing roles and the American Nurses' Association (ANA) position paper on nursing education opened the door for major revisions of those licensure laws and the emergence of the modern nurse.

NURSING BEFORE WORLD WAR I

After the licensure breakthrough, the leaders of nursing continued to look toward improvement of nurse training programs and, consequently, the improved practice of graduates of those programs. Most training schools remained under the control of hospitals, and the needs of the hospital superseded those of the school. For instance, it was not until 1912 that an occasional nurse received release time from hospital responsibilities in order to organize and teach basic nursing, and superintendents were warned not to "neglect" patient care in favor of the school or they would face punishment. There was little support for improvement from physicians. Before the Flexner report of 1910, the education of the physician, although different, was sometimes less organized than that for nursing. In the 1870s few of the medical schools required high school diplomas and courses were completed in two years, whereas the nurses' program was being lengthened to three years. For the next hundred years, physicians complained of "overtrained nurses." Moreover, nursing was dominated by and primarily made up of women; it was not considered a profession, in part because it was not situated in an academic, collegiate setting. But to get into that setting as women, much less nurses, was a battle in itself. In essence, then, there were no major changes in the quality of education in the years that followed licensure, once those very limited standards were met. The hours were still long, and the students continued to give free service, with "book learning" as an afterthought.

The public, beginning to be aroused by

poor conditions in factory sweatshops, showed surprisingly little interest in the exploitation of nursing students. Only in California, where an "Eight-Hour Law for Women" was passed in 1911, was there any movement to include student nurses (not even graduate nurses). Yet, when the bill was introduced in 1913, it was fought bitterly not only by hospitals, as might be expected, but also by physicians and nurses. No doubt, some were influenced by a sentiment voiced by physicians who were saying that nursing would be debased by being included in a law enforced by the State Bureau of Labor. Stated one physician to nurses, "The element of sacrifice is always present in true service. The service that costs no pains, no sacrifice, is without virtue, and usually without value." Retorted Lavinia Dock, "I think nurses should stand together solidly and resist the dictation of the medical profession in this as in all other things. Many MD's have a purely commercial spirit toward nurses . . . and would readily overwork them . . . If necessary, do not hesitate to make alliances with the labor vote, for organized labor has quite as much of an 'ideal' as the MD's have, if not more."[1] Although the bill finally passed, thanks to the persistence of Senator Anthony Caminetti, delegations of hospital representatives and physicians went to the governor to ask him to withhold his signature. When he asked where the people were who favored the law, a woman reporter told him that *they* were in the hospitals caring for the sick and unable to plead their own cause; he signed.[2] But, for years, superintendents of nursing complained about the expense of hiring nurses now necessary to do the work students had done.

While the Flexner Report was bringing about reform in medical schools, eliminating the correspondence courses and the weaker and poorer schools, Adelaide Nutting and other leaders were agitating for reform in nursing education. In 1911, the American Society of Superintendents of Training Schools for Nurses presented a proposal for a similar survey of nursing schools to the Carnegie

Foundation. Then President Pritchitt, stating that the Foundation's energies were centered elsewhere and ignoring nursing, directed a considerable amount of the Foundation funds in such studies for dental, legal, and teacher education.

Although women were having a little more success in being accepted in colleges and universities, there was only limited movement to make basic nursing programs an option in academic settings. Apparently, before 1900 there was a short-lived program at Howard University, but it was almost immediately taken over by Freedman's Hospital Nursing School. There is also some evidence that the School of Medicine at the University of Texas in 1896 "adopted" a hospital school of nursing to prevent its closing for lack of funds. However, the University of Minnesota program, founded in 1903 by Dr. Richard Olding Beard, a physician who was dedicated to the concept of higher education for nurses, became the first enduring baccalaureate program in nursing. Even this was more similar to good diploma programs than other university programs. Although eventually the students had to meet university admission standards and took some specialized courses, they also worked a fifty-six-hour week in the hospital and were awarded a diploma instead of a degree after three years. Similar programs were started by other universities which took over hospitals or started new ones, in part to obtain student services for their hospitals. Just prior to World War I, several hospitals and universities, such as Presbyterian Hospital of New York and Teachers College offered degree options. These developed into five-year programs with two years of college work and three years in a diploma school. This became a common pattern that lasted through the 1940s, but in 1916, when Annie Goodrich reported that sixteen colleges and universities maintained schools, departments, or courses in nursing education, they were an assortment of educational hybrids.

Nursing practice had also not developed to any extent, with most graduate nurses still doing private duty in homes. A nurse, unless becoming the favorite of one or more doctors who liked her work, found her "cases" through registries, established by alumnae associations, hospitals, medical societies, or commercial agencies. The first two frequently limited the better jobs to their graduates; commercial agencies not only charged the nurse a fee, but did not distinguish between trained and untrained nurses. Finally, a county nurse association gained control of a registry in Minnesota in 1904, and others followed. Nevertheless, private duty was an individual enterprise, with long hours, no benefits, and limited pay. (In 1926, some nurses were still working a twenty-four-hour day at what averaged out to forty-nine cents an hour, less than cleaning women made.)

However, in 1915, it is estimated, no more than ten percent of the sick received care in the hospitals, and the majority of people could not afford private duty nurses. From this need, a public health movement emerged that increased the demand for nurses. At first most of these nurses concentrated on bedside care, but others, like those coming from the settlement houses, took broader responsibilities. Nevertheless, there were no recognized standards or requirements for visiting nurses. Therefore, in June 1912, a small group of visiting nurses, representing unofficially some 900 agencies and almost four times that many colleagues, founded the National Organization for Public Health Nursing, with Lillian Wald as the first president.* It was an organization of nurses and lay people engaged in public health nursing and in the organization, management, and support of such work. The leaders of the group selected the term *public health nursing* as more inclusive than visiting nursing; it was also reminiscent of Nightingale's health nursing that had focused on prevention. One of its

first goals was to extend the services to working and middle-class people as well as to the poor.

The Visiting Nurse Quarterly, the first American publication dealing exclusively with public health nursing, was offered to the National Organization for Public Health Nursing (NOPHN) by its founder, the Cleveland Visiting Nurse Association. It became *Public Health Nursing,* the official journal of NOPHN until 1952–1953, when it was absorbed by *Nursing Outlook.* Also in 1912, the Red Cross established the Rural Nursing Service. Wald, at a major meeting on infant mortality, had cited the horrible health conditions of rural America, the high infant and maternal mortality rate, the prevalence of tuberculosis, and other serious health problems, and suggested that the Red Cross operate a national service, similar to that of Great Britain. Later, the name was changed to Town and Country Nursing Service in order to include small towns that had no visiting nurse service, and it was headquartered in Washington. Although the Service provided nurses to care for the sick, do health teaching, and otherwise improve health conditions, it was not wholly successful. Many communities did not choose to call in a national organization for assistance or could not afford the salaries of the nurses. (For a while, a wealthy woman contributed financial support to salaries, but withdrew funds because the rural nurses were not "ladies.") Nevertheless, the rural nurses carried on and proved to be a remarkably resourceful group, coping with an almost total lack of ordinary supplies and equipment. The service survived primarily because the Metropolitan Life Insurance Company decided to use rural nurses for services to their policyholders, for many local Red Cross chapters had no interest in or understanding of the service. (Red Cross involvement gradually decreased until, with increased government involvement in public health, it discontinued the program altogether in 1947.)

By 1916, public health nurses were being called on to be welfare workers, sanitarians,

---

*Changes had also occurred in the first two nursing organizations. In 1911, the Associated Alumnae changed its name to the American Nurses' Association (ANA) and in 1912, the Society of Superintendents adopted the name National League of Nursing Education (NLNE). Lind Richards

Isabel Hankton Robb

housing inspectors, and health teachers as well. A number of universities began offering courses to help prepare nurses to fulfill this multifaceted role, and Mary Gardner, one of the founders of NOPHN and an interim director of the Rural Nursing Service, authored the first book in the field, *Public Health Nursing*. One of the observations she made was that although broad-minded physicians recognized that public health nurses helped them produce results that would not have been possible alone, the more conservative feared nursing interference and were resentful of them. She noted that a service had a better chance of success if started with the cooperation of the medical profession and pointed out ways nurses could avoid friction with physicians and still be protected from the incompetents.

Another outstanding public health nurse of that period was Margaret Higgins Sanger. She became interested in the plight of the poorly paid industrial workers, particularly the women. Herself married with three children when she decided to return to work in public health, she was assigned to maternity cases on the Lower East Side of New York, where she found that pregnancy, often unwanted, was a chronic condition among the women. One of her patients died from a repeated self-abortion, after begging doctors and nurses for information on how to avoid pregnancy. That was apparently a turning point for Sanger. After learning everything she could about contraception, she and her sister, also a nurse, opened the first birth control clinic in America in Brooklyn. She was arrested and spent thirty days in the workhouse, but continued her crusade. She fought the battle for free dissemination of birth control information for decades, against all types of opposition, until today, it is generally accepted as the right of women and one of the roles of nursing.

A new specialty for nurses that endured was anesthesia. In 1889, Edith Graham began to give anesthesia at Mayo Clinic. After she married Charles Mayo, another nurse was trained to take over, for the Mayos had found a nurse more useful than an intern who was also trying to learn surgery. In 1909, a course for nurse anesthetists was established in Oregon, as were others, and these nurses were promptly as exploited by the hospitals as their sisters. It was not until 1917 that the question was officially raised as to whether nurse anesthetists were practicing medicine, and it was ruled then that they were not, if paid and supervised by a physician. However, the answer to legality was murky for more than sixty years, and the education of nurse anesthetists remained under the control of hospitals and doctors.[4]

NURSES AT WAR

The first World War was different from other wars fought by the United States, both because of its international proportions and the kinds of weapons that were used. Immediately, the demand for nurses was increased. The Army Nurse Corps expanded greatly, as did the Navy Nurse Corps (although to a lesser extent). As the war continued, recruitment standards dropped, and applicants were accepted from nursing schools attached to hospitals with less than 100 beds. All nurses needed was certification of moral character and professional qualifications by their superintendent of nurses—and, of course, they had to be unmarried. Once more untrained society girls were clamoring to be Red Cross volunteer nurses, without knowing what training was required or being willing to train for it. Afraid that Army nursing would fall into untrained hands as it had in Europe, Nutting, Goodrich, Wald, and others formed a Committee on Nursing to devise "the wisest methods of meeting the present problems connected with the care of the sick and injured in hospitals and homes; the educational problems of nursing; and the extraordinary emergencies as they arise."[5] Some weeks later, the committee was given governmental status and limited financial backing; most funds were contributions from nursing. The committee was able to estimate the number of available nurses and those in training, but, obviously, these were insufficient for both military and civilian needs.

The American Red Cross served as the unofficial reserve corps of the Army Nurse Corps. When these nurses, as well as those that were part of total multidisciplinary base units originating in hospitals, went to Europe, the home situation became desperate. Recruiting efforts were stepped up, first to attract educated women into nursing and then to encourage schools of nursing to somehow increase their capacity, even if it meant the unheard of—having local students live at home for part of their training. Interestingly enough, even though there were male nurses, and they did volunteer, they were usually put in regular fighting units and their skills went unused. Neither, apparently, did the Army choose to use black nurses. Only in mid-1917 would the Red Cross accept them, and then only if the Army Surgeon General agreed. Their eventual acceptance is credited to the efforts of Adar Thom, a black nurse.

Even with the patriotic fervor generated by the war, it was not easy to entice young women into nursing. High school students, queried about their interest in nursing, objected to the life of drudgery, strenuous physical work, poor education, severe discipline, lack of freedom and recreation as a student, and what they saw as limited satisfactory options of employment. However, schools did increase their capacity some 25 percent, and the pressures of the war brought about some educational changes. One of the more daring experiments of the time was the Vassar Training Camp. The idea came from a Vassar alumna and member of the board of trustees to establish at Vassar in the summer of 1918 a preparatory course in nursing, from which the students would move to selected schools of nursing to complete the program in little more than two additional years. As attested by graduates of the program, it was the spirit of patriotism that attracted more than 400 young women

aged fourteen to forty, schooled in many professional fields, and representing more than 100 colleges. They were to be known as Vassar's Rainbow Division because the students wore the various colored student uniforms of the schools they had selected. A large percentage of the women completed the program and entered the nursing schools they had selected, and many of nursing's leaders arose from this group. Soon, five other universities opened similar prenursing courses and also admitted high school students. Because these programs were generally of considerably higher quality than those of the training schools, the move of nursing education toward an academic setting received another nudge.

Meanwhile, nursing conditions in American military camps were reported as atrocious, and the Committee on Nursing convinced the Surgeon General to appoint Annie Goodrich to evaluate the quality of nursing service. Miss Goodrich, then an assistant professor at Teachers College, had had experience inspecting training schools for New York State. She minced no words in her report—conditions were much worse than in civilian hospitals, because there were not enough nurses to care for the patients, and they found it impossible to deal with a constantly changing group of disinterested corpsmen. Goodrich recommended that nurse training schools be set up in each military hospital, where the students, under careful supervision, would give better care than aides or corpsmen. The suggested Army School of Nursing was to be centralized in the Surgeon General's Office under the supervision of a dean. After some dispute, but with the support of the nursing organizations and influential Frances Payne Bolton of Cleveland, the Army School was approved in May 1918, with Annie Goodrich appointed Dean. The three-year course was based on the new *Standard Curriculum for Schools of Nursing*, published by the National League of Nursing Education. Unlike civilian hospitals, duty hours did not exceed six to eight hours. The military hospitals provided all medical and surgical experience, and gynecology, obstetrics, diseases of children, and public health were provided through affiliations in the second and third year. The response to the school was overwhelming, and it attracted many more students than it could accommodate.

The service of the nurses in the nightmarish battle conditions of World War I, coping with the mass casualties, dealing with injuries caused by the previously unknown shrapnel and gas, and then battling influenza at home and abroad, is a fascinating and proud piece of nursing history.[6]

BETWEEN THE WARS

In the twenty-three years between wars, nursing was affected by two major events, the Great Depression and adoption of the Nineteenth Constitutional Amendment in August 1920, granting women the right to vote. Of the two, the latter had the least immediate impact. Nurses showed relatively little interest in fighting for women's rights, and only one, Lavinia Dock, can be called an active feminist. "Dockie" was a maverick of the times. A tiny woman who loved music and was an accomplished pianist and organist, she also seemed to take on the whole world in her battle for the underdog. Early she decided that nurses could have no power unless they had the vote. Her speeches and writings were brilliant, but she did not move her colleagues. Nevertheless, she devoted a good part of her life to working for women's rights. In England, she joined the Pankhursts and landed in jail. Back in the United States, she picketed the White House, seizing the nearest, if not most appropriate, banner, "Youth to the Colors" (she was almost sixty then). Wrote her colleague, Isabel Stewart, "They all went into the cooler for the night. I think it just pleased her no end."[7]

For all her devotion to women's rights, Dock remained committed to nursing. She was editor of the *Journal's* Foreign Department from 1900 to 1923, during which she quarreled regularly with Editor Sophia Palmer and managed to ignore World War I because she was a pacifist. She was also involved with the International Council of Nursing and was the author of a number of books, including *Health and Morality* in 1910, in which she discussed venereal disease. She was equally outspoken on the forbidden subject in open meetings. A number of nurses had become infected because physicians frequently refused to tell nurses when patients had the disease. Dock also regularly castigated her profession for withholding its interest, sympathy, and moral support from "the great, urgent throbbing, pressing social claims of our day and generation."[8]

But nursing had problems of its own. Immediately after the war, there was a shortage of nurses, because many who had switched careers "for the duration" returned to their own field, and others appeared not to be attracted. In part, it was an image problem, one that was to continue to haunt nursing,* but another quite real aspect was that nursing education was in trouble. As Isabel Stewart said, "The plain facts are that nursing schools are being starved and always have been starved for lack of funds to build up any kind of substantial educational structure."[9] Later, this problem was clearly pinpointed by a prestigious committee. In 1918, Nutting had approached the Rockefeller Foundation to seek endowment for the Johns Hopkins School of Nursing, stressing the need for improvement in the education of public health nurses. The meeting resulted in a committee to investigate the "proper training" of public health nurses, an investigation that quickly concluded that the problem was nursing education in general. The findings of the Goldmark Report (presented in more detail in Chapter 5) concluded that schools of nursing needed to be recognized and supported as separate educational components with not just training in nursing, but also a liberal education. Although the report had

_____

*See Chapter 11.

little immediate impact, it did result in Rockefeller Foundation support for the founding of the Yale School of Nursing (1924), the first in the world to be established as a separate university department with its own dean, Annie Goodrich. Although a few other such programs followed, progress lagged, for many powerful physicians reached the public media with their notions that nurses needed only technical skills, manual dexterity, and quick obedience to the physician. Charles Mayo, for instance, deciding that city-trained nurses were too difficult to handle, too expensive, and spent too much time getting educated, wanted to recruit 100,000 country girls.[10] But even popular journals recognized that student nurses were being exploited by hospitals and that the kind of student being encouraged into nursing by school principals was one seen as not too bright, not attractive enough to marry, and too poor to be supported at home.[11]

A study following close on the heels of the Goldmark Report soon reaffirmed the inadequacy of nursing schools and practicing nurses. *Nurses, Patients, and Pocketbooks* (see Chapter 5) pointed out that the hasty postwar nurse recruiting efforts had not improved the lot of the patient or nurse; in 1928, problems included an oversupply of nurses, geographic maldistribution, low educational standards, poor working conditions, and some critically unsatisfactory levels of care.

How could education be so poor with licensure in effect? Ten years after the passage of the first acts, thirty-eight states had also passed such laws, but all were permissive, and although the title RN was protected, others could designate themselves nurses and work.* At one point, Annie Goodrich cited a correspondence school that turned out 12,000 "graduates" in ten years. In addition, hospital schools of all sizes felt no need to meet standards that might deprive them of free student labor. Even those

schools that chose to follow state board standards found them not too difficult, and follow-up was almost totally absent; most were approved on the basis of paper credentials. The states that did employ nurse "inspectors" ran into problems in withholding approval; members of the boards of nurse examiners were frequently as poorly qualified as the heads of schools, and the political pressures to avoid embarrassing hospitals were overwhelming.

Even in New York State where the state board was considered a model, the pressures and responsibilities of board members who also held jobs was unbelievable. They not only wrote all the licensing examination questions, but corrected all the papers and traveled all over the state to give the practical exams. Writing about grading the lengthy open-end questions, one board member complained, "The monotony is horrible; it stultifies the brain and one finds it impossible to work long at a sitting. So tiresome is it that one welcomes the diversion of a stupid answer."[12] By 1940, New York Board members were each forced to grade 1,994 tests as well as the practicals. Not until 1943 were exams scored by machine. Aside from grading fatigue, neither the test-writing skills of the authors or the state of the art of testing gave any assurance that state boards guaranteed minimum safe and effective practice for the newly licensed practitioner. Many nursing leaders were calling for grading of training schools as a starting point, but the Depression aborted any such action, although there were continued efforts to strengthen the licensing laws.

Unemployment after the stock market crash of 1929 also affected nursing. People who had no jobs could not afford private-duty nurses. It was estimated that 8,000 to 10,000 graduate nurses were out of work, and notices warning nurses not to come to find work in specific areas became frequent in the *Journal*. A 1932 campaign by ANA to promote an eight-hour day for nurses, hiring of nurses by hospitals, and discontinuance of some nursing schools met a cold reception.

---

*The first mandatory law was passed in New York in 1938, and implemented in 1944.

Even though complaining of the cost of training students, hospital administrators clung to the schools, perhaps because, despite financial figures to the contrary, students were obviously an economic asset. If one compared what the American Hospital Association said the students gave to hospitals in service—$1,000—with an average of 7,000 hours that the students gave—the hospital seemed to be crediting their contribution at about fourteen cents an hour. This was of questionable accuracy at best.[13] However, even directors of nursing showed a reluctance to hire graduate nurses, and 73 percent of hospitals employed no graduates at all on floor duty. By 1933, the desperate straits of unemployed nurses finally led to many working in hospitals for room and board. Even then, although some administrators believed this was taking advantage of unfortunate nurses, others thought that they were not worth food and lodging.

Some help finally came with the Roosevelt Administration, when relief funds were allocated for bedside care of the indigent and nurses were employed as visiting nurses under the Federal Emergency Relief Administration (FERA). Ten thousand unemployed nurses were put to work in numerous settings under the Civil Work Administration (CWA) in public hospitals, clinics, public health agencies, and other health services. The follow-up Works Progress Administration (WPA) then continued to provide funds for nurses in community health activities. A few nurses also entered a new field that opened—airline stewardess.

By 1936, the number of diploma nursing schools had decreased from more than 2,200 in 1929 to a little less than 1,500 state-accredited programs. There were about seventy "collegiate" programs, most merely of the liberal arts plus hospital school pattern. Many were still floundering. At this point, the NLNE presented its third revision of the *Curriculum Guide for Schools of Nursing*, with input from thousands of nurses around the country. A guide that was to endure (probably beyond optimum usefulness), its

major assumptions were that the primary function of the school was to educate the nurse, and that the community to be served extended beyond the hospital. Numbers of academic and clinical hours as well as content were suggested.

An obvious problem was the lack of qualified teachers; even in so-called university programs, nurses did not meet the usual requirements for teaching rank. One outcome was that baccalaureate programs for diploma nurses began to offer specialized degrees in education, administration, or public health nursing. The other was a very slow move to graduate education. For years, most of the graduate degrees held by nurses were in education, in part because Teachers College and other universities began to accept baccalaureate graduates for graduate preparation in education. In fact, some of the greatest leaders in nursing education either graduated from Teachers College or held teaching positions. One such was Isabel Stewart who arrived in 1908 for one semester and stayed for 39 years.[14] She succeeded M. Adelaide Nutting, who was the first nurse ever to receive a professorship in a university (1910) and who remained until 1925.[15] As early as 1932, Catholic University offered graduate courses in nursing, but that was uncommon. Apparently, the first, or nearly first, nurse to earn a doctoral degree was Edith S. Bryan; it was in psychology and counseling from Johns Hopkins.

Another slow starter in American nursing was nurse-midwifery. In the 1920s, legislation such as the Sheppard-Tanner Act paid for nurses to give maternity and infant care, but nurse-midwives were not included. Still, a considerable amount of maternity care, particularly deliveries, was done by lay midwives, some competent, some dangerously incompetent. When, in 1925, Mary Breckenridge founded the Frontier Nursing Service in rural Kentucky, the FNS staff was a mix of British nurse-midwives and American nurses trained in midwifery in Britain. (The rule was that if the husband could reach the nurse, the nurse could make it back to the patient by some means.) The outstanding services of the nurses on horseback (later in jeeps), who gradually increased their services to other aspects of primary care, is an ongoing success story.[16] The FNS also founded one of the early nurse-midwifery schools (1936); the first was at the maternity center of New York City in 1932. Also formed was a professional association (see Chapter 27).

Of all the entrants into nursing, two groups particularly got short shrift—men and blacks. The prejudice against men was specifically related to nursing and has persisted to some extent (see Chapter 11). As the distorted image of the female nurse evolved, men did not seem to fit into the concepts held by the power figures in and out of nursing. Therefore, although men graduated from acceptable nursing schools, usually totally male, and attempted to become active members of ANA, even forming a men's section, their numbers and influence remained small until the post-World War II era.

Black nurses, on the other hand, were caught in the overall, common prejudice against their race. Individual black nurses, as noted earlier, broke down barriers in various nursing fields. As early as 1908, they organized the National Association of Colored Graduate Nurses (NACGN), both to fight against discriminatory practices and to foster leadership among black nurses. Although ANA had a nondiscriminatory policy, some state organizations did not, and a rule that the nurse must have graduated from a state-approved school to be an ANA member eliminated even more black nurses.* In 1924, it was reported that only fifty-eight state-accredited schools admitted blacks, and most of these were located in black hospitals or in departments caring for black patients in municipal hospitals. Of these schools, 77 percent were located in the South; twenty-eight states offered no opportunities in nursing ed-

ucation for black women. Most of the southern "schools" that trained black nurses were totally unacceptable, and many of those approved barely met standards. Moreover, there were some 23,000 untrained black midwives in the South, but no one made the effort to combine training in nursing and midwifery, which would have been a distinct service. In 1930, there were fewer than 6,000 graduate black nurses, most of whom worked in black hospitals or public health agencies that served black patients. Opportunities in other fields either were not open to them or they did not, understandably, have the advanced preparation necessary. Middle-class black women were usually not attracted to nursing, because teaching and other available fields offered more prestige and better opportunities. It was not until a 1941 Executive Order and the corresponding follow-through that any part of the federal government made any effort to investigate grievances and redress complaints of blacks. The subsidized Cadet Nurse Corps of World War II also proved to be a boon for black nurses. Of the schools participating, twenty were all-black and enrolled 600 black students; the remaining 400 were distributed among twenty-two integrated schools. However, it was clear that approved black schools were being held to lower standards for an assortment of reasons, some political. There were also overt and covert methods in the North and South to prevent the more able black nurses from assuming leadership positions—some as simple as advancing the least aggressive. And for all the desperate need for nurses, the armed forces balked at accepting and integrating black nurses. Not until the end of the war and after some aggressive action by NACGN and the National Nursing Council for War Service did this change.[17]

THE EFFECTS OF WORLD WAR II

Not just black nurses, but nurses in general found that exigencies of war created

---

*Finally, in 1951, NACGN was absorbed into ANA, and ANA required nondiscrimination for all state associations as a prerequisite for ANA affiliation.

new opportunities, freedom, and also problems for nurses that proved to be long-lasting. As usual in wartime, nurses were in demand in the armed services. There were not enough nurses for both the home front and the battlefield, even with stepped-up efforts to encourage women to enter nursing programs. Finally, legislation was passed in 1943 establishing the Cadet Nurse Corps. The Bolton Act, the first federal program to subsidize nursing education for school and student, was a forerunner of future federal aid to nursing. For payment of their tuition and a stipend, students committed themselves to engage in essential military or civilian nursing for the duration of the war. The students had to be between seventeen and thirty-five years old, in good health, and have a good academic record in an accredited high school. This new law brought about several changes in nursing. For instance, it forbade discrimination on the basis of race and marital status and set minimum educational standards. The first, theoretically accepted, was not always implemented in good faith. The latter, combined with the requirement that nursing programs be accelerated from the traditional thirty-six months to thirty, forced nursing schools to reassess and revise their curricula.

Two other major efforts to relieve the nursing shortage had long-range effects in the practice setting. One was the recruitment of inactive nurses back into the field. For the first time, married women and others who could work only on a part-time basis became acceptable to employers and later became part of the labor pool. The other was the training of volunteer nurse's aides. Although such training was initiated by the Red Cross in 1919, it was discouraged later by nurses, particularly during the Depression. During World War II, both the Red Cross and the Office of Civilian Defense trained more than 20,000 aides. First, they were used only for nonnursing tasks, but the increasing nurse shortage forced them to take on basic nursing functions. After the war, with a continued shortage, trained aides were hired as a

necessary part of the nursing service department. Their perceived cost-effectiveness stimulated the growth of both aide and practical nurse training programs and eventually increased federal funding for both.

Finally, major changes occurred within the Armed Forces. Nurses had held only relative rank, meaning that they carried officers' titles but had less power and pay than their male counterparts. In 1947, full commissioned status was granted, giving them the right to manage nursing care. At the same time, as noted previously, discrimination against black nurses ended but, oddly enough, in the male-controlled Armed Services, it was not until 1954 that male nurses were admitted to full rank as officers.

As in all previous wars, nurses proved themselves able and brave in military situations. Many were in battle zones and some became Japanese prisoners of war. Their stories have been told in films, books, plays, and historical nursing research, and are well worth reading. (See bibliography.)

TOWARD A NEW ERA

The usual postwar nurse shortage occurred after World War II, but this time for different reasons. Only one of six Army nurses planned to return to her civilian job, finding more satisfaction in the service. Poor pay and unpleasant working conditions discouraged civilian nurses as well. In 1946, the salary for a staff nurse was about $36 a week, for a forty-eight-hour work week, less than that for typists or seamstresses (much less men). Salaries were supposed to be kept secret, and hospitals, particularly, held them at a minimum, with such peculiarities as a staff nurse earning more than a head nurse. Split shifts were common, with nurses scheduled to work from 7 to 11 and from 3 to 7 with time off between the two shifts. The work was especially difficult because staffing was short and nurses worked under rigid discipline. It was small wonder that in one survey only about 12 percent of the nurses queried planned to make nursing a career; more than 75 percent saw it as a pin-money job after marriage, or planned to retire altogether as soon as possible. Unions were beginning to organize nurses, so in 1949 the ANA approved state associations as collective bargaining agents for nurses. However, because the Taft-Hartley Act excluded nonprofit institutions from collective bargaining, hospitals and agencies did not need to deal with nurses. In addition, the ANA no-strike pledge took away another powerful weapon.

As noted previously, one answer that administrators saw was hiring of nurse's aides. Use of volunteers and auxiliary help—that is, anyone other than licensed or trained nurses, practical nurses, aides, or orderlies —increased tremendously.

One group of workers that proliferated in the postwar era was practical nurses, defined by ANA, NLNE, and NOPHN as those trained to care for subacute, convalescent, and chronic patients under the direction of a physician or nurse. Thousands who designated themselves as practical nurses had no such skills and their training was simply in caring for their own families, or, at most, aide work. Whereas the first school for training practical nurses appeared in 1897, by 1930 there were only eleven, and in 1947, still only thirty-six. With the new demand for nurse substitutes, 260 more practical nurse schools opened by 1954, mostly in hospitals or long-term care institutions, and a few in vocational schools. Aiding the movement was funding from federal vocational education acts. There were, unfortunately, also a number of correspondence courses and other commercialized programs that did little more than expose the student to some books and manuals and present her a diploma. By 1950, there were 144,000 practical nurses, 95 percent of them women, and, although their educational programs varied, their on-the-job activities expanded greatly—to doing whatever nurses had no time to do. By 1952, some 56 percent of the nursing personnel were nonprofessionals, and some nurses be-

gan to fear that they were being replaced by the less expensive, minimally trained workers.

Nevertheless, with working and financial conditions not improving, the nursing shortage persisted. Soon, a team plan was developed with a nurse as a team leader, primarily responsible for planning patient care, and less-prepared workers carrying it out. Although the plan persisted for years, it did little to improve patient care; rather, it kept the nurse mired in paper work, away from the patient, or required to make constant medication rounds. Often, practical nurses carried the primary responsibilities for patient units on the evening and night shift, with the few nurses available stretched thin, "supervising" these workers.

There were more nurses than ever at mid-century, but there were also tremendously expanded health services, a greater population to be served, growth of various insurance plans that paid for hospital care, a post-war baby boom with in-hospital deliveries, new medical discoveries that kept patients alive longer, and a spread of the nurses into other areas of health care. Hospitals still weren't the most desirable places to work, and economic benefits were slow in coming. Moreover, there were now more married nurses who chose to stay home to raise families. Studies done in 1944, 1947, and 1948,* all of which pointed out some of the economic and status problems of nurses, particularly in hospitals, went largely ignored.

When the Korean War broke out in 1950, the Army again drew nurses from civilian hospitals, this time from their reserve corps. War nursing on the battlefront was centered to an extent on the Mobile Army Surgical Hospitals (MASH), located as close to the front lines as possible. Flight nurses, who helped to evacuate the wounded from battlefront to military hospitals, also achieved recognition. When that war was over and nurse reservists returned to their civilian jobs, it is

*See Chapter 5.

possible that their experiences increased the discontent with working situations at home.

This was also a period of great medical and scientific discoveries, and physicians became increasingly dependent on hospitals for supportive services. As physicians cured or prolonged the lives of patients, the corollary care required of nurses became more complex. It was not just a matter of patient comfort, but crucial life-and-death judgment. In the 1950s, Frances Reiter began to write of the nurse clinician, a nurse who gave skilled nursing care on an advanced level. This concept emerged into the clinical specialist,* a nurse with a graduate degree and specialized knowledge of nursing care, who worked as a colleague of physicians. At the same time, the development of coronary and other intensive care units called for nurses with equally specialized technical knowledge, formerly the sole province of medical practice.* In Colorado, in 1965, a physician, in collaboration with a school of nursing, was pioneering another new role for nurses in ambulatory care. As the nurses easily assumed responsibility for well-child care and minor illnesses, they called upon their nursing knowledge and skills as well as a medical component. What emerged was the "nurse practitioner."†

Nursing education was also going through a transition period in those decades. In the years immediately after World War II, the quality of nursing education was under severe criticism. There was no question that in the diploma schools, where most nurses were educated, there were frequently poor levels of teaching, inadequately prepared teachers, and a major dependence on students for services; often, two thirds of the hours of care were given by students.

The Brown Report* in 1948 and a follow-up study in 1950* that attempted to implement that report made clear that nursing education was anything but professional. It was on the basis of findings of the latter report

---

*See Chapter 15.
† See Chapter 5.

that national accreditation for nursing by nursing was strengthened.

With the reorganization of the nursing organizations, the National League for Nursing (NLN) assumed the responsibility for all accrediting functions in nursing. Dr. Helen Nahm, director of the accrediting service for the first seven years, saw it as the culmination of all previous efforts to raise nursing education standards—and as a last chance. Those schools who chose to go through the voluntary process and met the standards were placed on a published list, which, for the first time, gave the public, guidance counselors, and potential students some notion of the quality of one school as compared with another. Eventually, accreditation proved a significant force in improving good schools and closing poor ones (although it has also been accused of rigidity throughout the years).

An impetus for collegiate nursing education was an advisory service funded by the Russell Sage Foundation for institutions of higher learning that were interested in enriching and improving their programs. The 1953 report by Dr. Margaret Bridgman, "Collegiate Education for Nursing," helped to stimulate baccalaureate nursing programs to improve academically. In many cases, they were still quite similar to diploma programs, whose quality had improved considerably in the 1950s. The slow rate of growth of collegiate programs resulted in part from the uncertainty of nursing about what these programs should be and how they should differ from diploma education and in part from the anticollegiate faction in nursing that saw no point in higher education—a faction that was cheered and nurtured by a large number of physicians and administrators. At times, it seemed to be a moot question whether any nurses were necessary. A postwar survey of the American College of Surgeons indicated that the vast majority believed, with few exceptions, that the needs of the sick could be met by nurse's aides, or, at most, by practical nurses, and administrators were not averse to the "cheap is best" concept.

Introduction of a different kind of nurse was a startling breakthrough. The development of the nurse technician in community colleges was the most dramatic change in nursing education since its beginning. Based on a study by Dr. Mildred Montag at Teachers College, and funded by the W. K. Kellogg Foundation, pilot programs were established in a number of sites around the country in 1952. It was an idea whose time had come, for not only were community colleges the most rapidly expanding educational entities of the time, but the late bloomer, the mature man and woman, and the less affluent student found this opportunity for a career in nursing and a college degree highly desirable. Follow-up studies showed that these nurses performed well in what they were prepared to do—provide care at the intermediate level in the continuum of nursing functions as defined by Montag. It was probably partially the influence of the associate degree (AD) programs, which were nondiscriminatory and generally nonpaternalistic in their relations with students, that helped loosen the tight restrictions on nursing students' personal lives in both diploma and some baccalaureate programs. Still, even into the late 1960s some diploma schools excluded married students and men. The growth of AD programs ultimately outran all others in nursing except practical nurse programs.

Graduate education for nurses progressed slowly. Most degrees continued to be in education, in part because of the great shortage of teachers of nursing with graduate degrees and in part because graduate schools of education had part-time programs. In 1953, only 36 percent of nursing faculties had earned master's degrees, and some had no degree at all. In 1954, it was estimated that 20 percent of the positions held by nurses should require master's degrees and at least 30 percent, baccalaureate. Yet, only 1 percent of all nurses held master's and about 7 percent baccalaureate degrees, many not in nursing.

Part of the problem, of course, was financial and, although private foundations, such as the Commonwealth Fund, provided some support for graduate education, federal funding made the crucial difference. It also controlled the direction of nursing education. Its funding for the study of public health nursing from 1936 on created more baccalaureate-prepared nurses in public health than in any other field; its support of psychiatric nursing increased the volume of nurses educated in that field.[18] In 1956, the passage of the Federal Nurse Traineeship Act, which authorized funds for financial aid to registered nurses for full-time study to prepare for teaching, supervision, and administration in all fields, opened the door for advanced education for nurses at both the baccalaureate and graduate level. Short-term traineeships also provided for continuing education programs. Another boost was the 1963 Surgeon General's Report* that specifically pointed out differences in the quality and quantity of nurses and their education and recommended both recruitment and advanced education. Following this, there was a new surge of federal aid to nursing. Nurse Traineeship programs continued to be enacted until the present, although the struggle for funds, depending on the administration, was sometimes most difficult (see Chapters 12 and 19).

Master's programs for nurses still tended to focus on administration or education even in schools of nursing, and not until the 1960s did clinical programs develop. Clinical doctoral programs in nursing were nonexistent until the 1960s.

Nursing research also tended to take a slow path. Although there were studies of nursing service, nursing education, and nursing personality, most were done with or by social scientists. When nurses assisted physicians and others in medical research, it was just that—assisting. Nursing leaders realized that nursing could not develop as a profession unless clinical research focusing on nursing evolved. One of the first major steps in that direction was the 1952 publication of *Nursing Research*, a scholarly journal that

---

*See Chapter 5.

reported and encouraged nursing research. The other was ANA's establishment of the American Nurses' Foundation* in 1955, for charitable, educational, and scientific purposes. The Foundation conducts studies, surveys, and research, funds nurse researchers and others, and publishes scientific reports.

In 1956, the federal government also began to fund nursing research. Federal support in the 1960s provided research training through doctoral programs, including the nurse scientist program, and funding for individual and collaborative research efforts.

In all of these changes, it can be seen that the professional organizations of nursing had varied influence. At the same time, as organizations, they too were examining their roles and relationships. A study to consider restructuring, reorganizing, and unifying the various organizations was initiated shortly after World War II. In 1952, the six major nursing organizations, ANA, NLNE, NOPHN, NACGN, the Association of Collegiate Schools of Nursing (ACSN), and the American Association of Industrial Nurses (AAIN) finally came to a decision about organizational structure. Two major organizations emerged, the ANA, with only nurse members, and the renamed National League for Nursing, with nurse, non-nurse, and agency membership. The AAIN decided to continue, and the National Student Nurses' Association was formed (practical nurses had their own organization). (See Chapters 24, 25, 26, and 27 for details of the organizations.) Although there was an apparent realignment of responsibilities, the relationships between ANA and NLN ebbed and flowed; sometimes they were in agreement and sometimes they were not; sometimes they worked together, at other times each appeared to make isolated unilateral pronouncements. Some nurses longed for one organization, but there seemed to be mutual organizational reluctance to go in that direction. Yet, it must be said that in those chang-

ing times each had some remarkable achievements—NLN in educational accreditation; ANA in its lobbying activities, its development of a model licensure law in the mid-1950s, and its increased action in nurses' economic security.

Then, in 1965, ANA precipitated (or inflamed) an ongoing controversy. After years of increasingly firm statements on the place of nursing education in the mainstream of American education, ANA issued its first Position Paper on Education for Nursing. It stated, basically, that education for those who work in nursing should be in institutions of higher learning, that minimum education for professional nursing should be at least at the baccalaureate level; for technical nursing, at the associate degree level; and for assistants, in vocational education settings.

Although there had been increased complaints by third party payors about diploma education, and diploma schools had declined as associate and baccalaureate degree programs increased, there was an outpouring of anger by diploma and practical nurses and those involved in their education. It was a battle that persisted and became another divisive force in nursing. But, then, so was the beginning of the nurse practitioner movement. There were nurses who feared it or saw it as pseudomedicine, detracting from pure nursing professionalism. The issues remain unresolved.

Therefore, whether or not 1965 can be considered the gateway to a new era of nursing, it was the beginning of dramatic and inevitable changes in the education and practice of nursing and in the struggle for nursing autonomy.

REFERENCES

1. Philip Kalisch and Beatrice Kalisch, *The Advance of American Nursing* (Boston: Little, Brown and Company, 1978), pp. 285–286.
2. Ibid., pp. 281–284.
3. Ibid., pp. 398–406.
4. Vern Bullough and Bonnie Bullough, *The Care of the Sick: The Emergence of Mod-*

---

*See Chapter 25.

ern Nursing (New York: Prodist, 1978), pp. 201–202.

5. Kalisch, op. cit., p. 297.
6. Ibid., pp. 295–325.
7. Teresa E. Christy, "Portrait of a Leader: Lavinia Lloyd Dock," *Nurs. Outlook*, **17**:74 (June 1969).
8. Ibid.
9. Kalisch, op. cit., p. 332.
10. Bullough, op. cit., p. 156.
11. Dorothy D. Bromley, "The Crisis in Nursing," *Harper's Magazine*, **161**:159–160, (July 1930).
12. Mary Lucille Shannon, "The Origin and Development of Professional Licensure Examinations in Nursing: From a State-Constituted Examination to the State Board Test Pool Examination," Unpublished Ed.D. dissertation, Teachers College, Columbia University, 1972, p. 127.
13. Beatrice Kalisch and Philip Kalisch, "Slaves, Servants, or Saints? An Analysis of the System of Nurse Training in the United States, 1873–1948," *Nurs. Forum*, **14**,3:248 (1975).
14. Teresa Christy, "Portrait of a Leader: Isabel Maitland Stewart," *Nurs. Outlook*, **17**:44–48 (Oct. 1969).
15. Teresa Christy, "Portrait of a Leader: M. Adelaide Nutting," *Nurs. Outlook*, **17**:20–24 (Jan. 1969).
16. Helen Tirpak, "The Frontier Nursing Service: Fifty Years in the Mountains," *Nurs. Outlook*, **23**:308–310 (May 1975).
17. Kalisch, *The Advance of American Nursing*, op. cit., pp. 553–569.
18. Ibid. p. 591.

BIBLIOGRAPHY

Breckinridge, Mary. *Wide Neighborhoods: The Story of the Frontier Nursing Service.* New York: Harper and Rowe, Publishers, 1952. The history of the service, by its founder. Now out of print, but found in many libraries.

Bullough, Bonnie. "Nurses in American History: The Lasting Impact of World War II on Nursing." *Am. J. Nurs.*, **76** (Jan. 1976), 118–120. An overview of the long-lasting changes that World War II brought in nursing. Good bibliography.

Dreves, Katharine Densford. "Nurses in American History: Vassar Training Camp for Nurses." *Am. J. Nurs.*, **75** (Nov. 1975), 2000–2002. One of nursing's leaders, a recruit to the Vassar Camp, reminisces about her experience. An interesting insight.

Fitzpatrick, M. Louise. "Nurses in American History: Nursing and the Great Depression." *Am. J. Nurs.*, **75** (Dec. 1975), 2188–2190. The major effects of the Depression on nursing are presented succinctly. Useful bibliography.

Kalisch, Beatrice and Philip Kalisch. "Nurses in American History: The Cadet Nurse Corps—in World War II." *Am. J. Nurs.*, **76** (Feb. 1976), 240–242. A detailed review of the Bolton Act that provided federal aid to nursing education in World War II and consequently also initiated improvements in nursing education.

Kalisch, Beatrice and Philip Kalisch. "Nurses Under Fire: The World War II Experience of Nurses in Bataan and Corregidor." *Nurs. Research*, **6** (Nov.–Dec. 1976), 409–429. Experiences of Army, Navy, and civilian nurses in the Philippines during World War II are described in extraordinary detail, citing personal letters and memoirs. Engrossing. Extensive bibliography.

Monteiro, Lois. "Lavinia L. Dock (1947) on Nurses and the Cold War." *Nurs. Forum*, **17**,1 (1978), 46–54. Astonishing and brave letters written to General Marshal and the USSR ambassador.

Watson, Joellen. "The Evolution of Nursing Education in the United States: 100 Years of a Profession for Women." *J. Nurs. Ed.* **16** (Sept. 1977), 31–38. Relates women's movement to nursing education.

See also the Ashley, Brand, and Kalisch articles cited in Chapter 3 bibliography, as well as the Bullough, Dolan, and Kalisch histories.

Major Studies of the Nursing Profession

Although a great many of the studies in nursing that have been done in this country have helped to advance the profession as well as to solve local or immediate problems, comparatively few have marked a definite trend or greatly influenced the progress of nursing. Described here are the reports of research and studies that have guided nursing in the past and will always be considered milestones in the development of nursing.

The Educational Status of Nursing (1912). Conducted under the leadership of M. Adelaide Nutting, chairman of the education committee of the American Society of Superintendents of Training Schools for Nurses, and published by the U.S. Bureau of Education, the 1912 report on the Educational Status of Nursing resulted from a questionnaire study of what schools of nursing throughout the country were actually teaching their students at that time and the techniques employed. It also covered the students' working and living conditions. Although this study revealed many appalling practices, it did not create the stir in nursing or in the public that it should have. However, it did begin to establish nursing as a profession and to set a precedent for later studies. It also highlighted the need for con-

tinued investigation of educational practices in nursing, and—even as early as 1912—the need for schools of nursing to be independent from hospitals.

Nursing and Nursing Education in the United States. The Goldmark Report (1923). Also stimulated by Nutting, the Rockefeller Foundation funded a Committee for the Study of Nursing Education to investigate "the proper training of the public health nurse." It was chaired by Dr. C.E.A. Winslow, professor of public health, Yale University, and included ten physicians (2 of whom were hospital superintendents), six nurses (Nutting, Goodrich, Wald, Clayton, Beard, and Ward), and two lay representatives. Secretary and chief investigator was Josephine Goldmark, who had already done recognized field study. It soon became apparent that the scope of the study needed to be expanded to encompass nursing education in general. Goldmark gathered and synthesized the opinions of leading nurse educators and also surveyed and studied twenty-three schools of nursing and forty-nine public health agencies, seeking answers to questions about the preparation of teachers, administrators, and public health nurses, clinical and laboratory experience for students, financing of schools of nursing, licensure for nurses, and the development of university schools.

As the study pointed out, education of nurses was still on an apprenticeship basis, a method abandoned by other professionals. Moreover, the quality of the teachers was poor; formal instruction was erratic, uncoordinated, and frequently sacrificed to the needs of the hospital, and students were often poorly selected. In essence, there was little training and almost no education. The conclusions of this landmark study did not result solely from the survey but also from the firm opinions of its prestigious committee members and the opinions of nursing leaders interviewed. Because some have still not been implemented, they have a remarkably contemporary ring:[1]

Conclusion 1. That, since constructive health work and health teaching in families is best done by persons:

(a) capable of giving general health instruction, as distinguished from instruction in any one specialty; and

(b) capable of rendering bedside care at need; the agent responsible for such constructive health work and health teaching in families should have completed the nurses' training. There will, of course, be need for the employment, in addition to the public health nurse, of other types of experts such as nutrition workers, social workers, occupational therapists, and the like.

That as soon as may be practicable all agencies, public or private, employing public health nurses, should require as a prerequisite for employment the basic hospital training, followed by a post-graduate course, including both class work and field work, in public health nursing.

Conclusion 2. That the career open to young women of high capacity, in public health nursing or in hospital supervision and nursing education, is one of the most attractive fields now open in its promise of professional success and of rewarding public service; and that every effort should be made to attract such women into this field.

Conclusion 3. That for the care of persons suffering from serious and acute disease, the safety of the patient and the responsibility of the medical and nursing professions demand the maintenance of the standards of educational attainment now generally accepted by the best sentiment of both professions and embodied in the legislation of the more progressive states; and that any attempt to lower these standards would be fraught with real danger to the public.

Conclusion 4. That steps should be taken through state legislation for the definition and licensure of a subsidiary grade of nursing service, the subsidiary type of worker to serve under practising physicians in the care of mild and chronic illness, and convalescence, and possibly to assist under the direction of the trained nurse in certain phases of hospital and visiting nursing.

Conclusion 5. That, while training schools for nurses have made remarkable progress, and while the best schools of today in many respects reach a high level of educational attainment, the average hospital training school is not organized on such a basis as to conform to the standards accepted in other educational fields; that the instruction in such schools is frequently casual and uncorrelated; that the educational needs and the health and strength of students are frequently sacrificed to practical hospital exigencies; that such shortcomings are primarily due to the lack of independent endowments for nursing education; that existing educational facilities are on the whole, in the majority of schools, inadequate for the preparation of the high grade of nurses required for the care of serious illness and for service in the fields of public health nursing and nursing education; and that one of the chief reasons for the lack of sufficient recruits of a high type to meet such needs lies precisely in the fact that the average hospital training school does not offer a sufficiently attractive avenue of entrance to this field.

Conclusion 6. That, with the necessary financial support and under a separate board or training school committee, organized primarily for educational purposes, it is possible, with completion of a high school course or its equivalents as prerequisite, to reduce the fundamental period of hospital training to 28 months, and at the same time, by eliminating unessential, noneducational routine, and adopting the principles laid down in Miss

Goldmark's report, to organize the course along intensive and coordinated lines with such modifications as may be necessary for practical application; and that courses of this standard would be reasonably certain to attract students of high quality in increasing numbers.

Conclusion 7. Superintendents, supervisors, instructors, and public health nurses should in all cases receive special additional training beyond the basic nursing course.

Conclusion 8. That the development and strengthening of university schools of nursing of a high grade for the training of leaders is of fundamental importance in the furtherance of nursing education.

Conclusion 9. That when the licensure of a subsidiary grade of nursing service is provided for, the establishment of training courses in preparation for such service is highly desirable; that such courses should be conducted in special hospitals, in small unaffiliated general hospitals, or in separate sections of hospitals where nurses are also trained; and that the course should be of 8 or 9 months' duration; provided the standard of such schools be approved by the same educational board which governs nursing training schools.

Conclusion 10. That the development of nursing service adequate for the care of the sick and for the conduct of the modern public health campaign demands as an absolute prerequisite the securing of funds for the endowment of nursing education of all types; and that it is of primary importance, in this connection, to provide reasonably generous endowment for university schools of nursing.

Although the recommendations related to education are usually given the most attention, the Goldmark Report did not neglect its original focus on public health nursing. Among other things, it was concluded that both bedside nursing care and health teaching for preventive care could be combined in one generalized service, as opposed to the separated services and agencies that were more common at the time.

Although the 500-page report was published, it did not have the wide dissemination, interest, or impact of the Flexner Report.

Only a few of the recommendations were given serious consideration on a wide scale at the time. One important result of the study, however, was the establishment of the Yale University School of Nursing in 1923, financed by the Rockefeller Foundation. This represented a significant forward step in education for nursing.

Nurses, Patients, and Pocketbooks (1928). This study was conducted by the Committee on the Grading of Nursing Schools composed of twenty-one members representing the American Nurses' Association, National League of Nursing Education, National Organization for Public Health Nursing, the American Medical Association (which later withdrew), American College of Surgeons, American Hospital Association, American Public Health Association, and representatives of general education. Nurses contributed about one-half of the $300,000 needed to finance the study; the remainder came from foundations and friends of nursing, such as Frances Payne Bolton, who also served on the committee. May Ayres Burgess, a statistician, directed the study.

The committee focused on three separate studies: supply and demand of graduate nurses; job analysis of nurses; and grading of nursing schools. The first report, *Nurses, Patients, and Pocketbooks,* showed that there was an oversupply of nurses, with serious unemployment problems, that there was a geographic maldistribution, with most nurses remaining in large cities; that salaries and working conditions were poor, and that although in general both patients and physicians were satisfied with nurses' services (which were, of course, primarily in the private duty sector), there was evidence of some serious incompetence.

An Activity Analysis of Nursing (1934). This is a report of the second study sponsored by the Committee on the Grading of Nursing Schools. The principal purpose of this study, conducted by Ethel Johns and Blanche Pfefferkorn at the committee's request, was to gather facts about nurses' activities that could be used as a basis for improving the curricula in schools of nursing. It represents the first large-scale attempt to find out what nurses were actually doing on the job—in hospitals, in public health agencies, and on private duty—and this focused attention on nursing service as well as on nursing education and encouraged a closer correlation of theory and practice.

Nursing Schools Today and Tomorrow (1934). This was the final report of the eight years of study conducted under the auspices of the Committee on the Grading of Nursing Schools. It gave statistics on the numbers of "trained and untrained" nurses and answered such questions as: What should a professional nurse know and be able to do? How can hospitals provide nursing service? It described the nursing schools of the period and recommended essentials for a basic professional school of nursing.

A number of startling facts were brought to light. For instance, 42 percent of teachers in schools of nursing had not even graduated from high school; only 16 percent had a year or more of college. Again, it was pointed out that nursing was the only profession in which the student essentially provided all the service for her "learning" institution. Moreover, a large number of the existing schools were so small that student education was totally inadequate. Most certainly, the need for consistent evaluation of programs was urgent.

A Study on the Use of the Graduate Nurse for Bedside Nursing in the Hospital (1933). This was the first study done by the NLNE Department of Studies, which was established in 1932, with Blanche Pfefferkorn as its director. Prompted by previous findings of the Grading Committee, Miss Pfefferkorn and her co-workers made a comparative study of the bedside activities of the graduate and student nurse in the hospital to lend support to the gradually emerging belief (somewhat reluctantly accepted by hospital administrators) that nursing care should be given principally by graduate staff nurses, not by nursing students. The study helped clarify the issues and laid a foundation for further progress toward reduction in the number of noneducational assignments given to students of nursing.

A Curriculum Guide for Schools of Nursing (1937). Although in style and format this publication does not appear to be a report of a study, the content was so much influenced by a study that it is sometimes referred to as such. The purpose of the study, directed by Isabel Stewart, chairman of the NLNE Committee on Curriculum, was to

> . . . gather, evaluate, and present in usable form the most progressive ideas and practices in relation to the basic nursing curriculums that have been successfully tried out or are considered by competent judges to be suitable for use and practicable in nursing schools.

The need for this study was recognized following the issuance of two NLNE publications recommending curriculum content and method: *Standard Curriculum for Schools of Nursing,* 1917; and *A Curriculum for Schools of Nursing,* 1929. Although it was extremely helpful to directors and others responsible for schools of nursing, the curricula advocated in these first two publications proved to be too rigid to meet the changing emphasis on broader education for nurses. The word *guide* in the 1937 publication was, therefore, highly significant. The new guide, intended, according to Stewart, for students of professional caliber, preparing themselves for a profession, placed much greater emphasis on application of the sciences. The role of the clinical instructor was stressed, and all faculty were encouraged to use newer and more creative methods of teaching. The Guide was never revised again but was used in many schools for another quarter-century.

Study of Incomes, Salaries and Employment Conditions Affecting Nurses (Exclusive of Those Engaged in Public Health Nursing)

(1938). The American Nurses' Association initiated this questionnaire survey, which was launched in 1936 and conducted through state studies sponsored by the twenty-three state nurses' associations that agreed to participate. The data obtained from more than 11,000 private duty, institutional, and office nurses were presented in the published report as state summaries, national findings, and recommendations. This study undoubtedly had considerable bearing on the development of the ANA's economic security program.

Administrative Cost Analysis for Nursing Service and Nursing Education (1940). Blanche Pfefferkorn directed this study, which was sponsored jointly by NLNE and AHA in cooperation with ANA. The major obectives of the study, as stated in the report (p. 4), were

1. To find out the cost to an individual hospital of
    a. Operating the nursing service without a school;
    b. Operating the nursing service with a school.
2. To develop methods and criteria which will make possible a valid comparison of costs in one institution with the costs in another.

This study, which focused on the purely business side of nursing service and education, produced some interesting and potentially usable data on the cost to the hospital of conducting a school of nursing and the economic value of the service rendered by nursing students, estimated in terms of graduate service. Hospital administrators and nurse educators were greatly enlightened by this study, although it appears doubtful that many institutions actually adopted cost accounting for nursing education and service at that time.

The General Staff Nurse (1941). As it became more and more common for hospitals to employ graduate professional nurses to provide bedside nursing care, formerly given almost entirely by students, the organizations most concerned—ANA, NLNE, AHA, and CHA—felt the need to determine the status of general staff nurses as seen by directors of nursing, the nurses themselves, and others. A joint committee of these organizations was formed to make such a study. The report indicates that general staff nurses had little status at the time. This was reflected in their hours of duty, their salaries, and personnel policies. This study gave impetus to a movement to try to upgrade the status of the general staff nurse.

Hospital Care in the United States (1947). Although this study conducted by the Commission on Hospital Care, a national group appointed by the AHA representing a wide variety of occupations and professions, was primarily concerned with hospitals in this country, it necessarily touched upon nurses and nursing because they are such an integral part of hospitals and the services they render.

An introductory statement noted:

We have boasted of our fine institutions, of the number of hospital beds per unit of population, and of the high standards of hospital care that exist in the United States. Yet, both physical facilities and the arrangements under which they operate leave much to be desired. Many of our hospitals are old and outmoded. Some are housed in makeshift adaptations of buildings designed for other purposes. In many urban communities, there is wasteful duplication of facilities created and continued by special interests, individual ambitions, and prejudices. There are many regions in the United States in which hospital care is quite inadequate. It is wholly lacking in some rural areas.

The survey was far-reaching in scope and recommendations, many of which applied to nursing service and education. The findings were of great interest to legislators, and it is generally agreed that the Hill-Burton Hospital Construction Act was influenced by this study. The report, published by the Harvard University Press for the Commonwealth

Fund, is still considered a valuable source book.

Nursing for the Future (1948). Esther Lucile Brown, PhD, a social anthropologist with the Russell Sage Foundation, conducted this study for the National Nursing Council, a large group of representatives of many health organizations and services, which had functioned under other titles before and during World War II to recruit nursing students and coordinate military and civilian nursing needs.

The study, funded by the Carnegie Foundation for the Advancement of Teaching and the Sage Foundation (which published it), was to analyze the changing needs of the profession. Brown, who had already studied nursing as an emerging profession, gathered data by visiting nursing schools, attending workshops, and consulting with individual physicians and hospital administrators, as well as using both a nursing and a lay advisory committee.

The report of her findings was ironically not much different from those of earlier studies, indicating the slow progress of nursing education. At one point, Dr. Brown pondered "why young women in any large numbers would want to enter nursing as practiced, or schools of nursing as operated today."[2] Once more, the same inadequacies were pointed out and, once more, the closing of the several thousand small, weak schools was urged. In particular, Brown emphasized the necessity for official examination of all schools, publication and distribution of lists of accredited schools, and public pressure to eliminate the nonaccredited schools.[3]

In addition, she strongly recommended "that effort be directed to building basic schools of nursing in universities and colleges, comparable in number to existing medical schools, that are sound in organizational and financial structure, adequate in facilities and faculty, and well-distributed to serve the needs of the entire country."[4] Noting that many diploma schools still operated

for the staffing benefit of the hospital, she found nursing education not professional.

Although Brown was undoubtedly also influenced by her nursing advisors, many of whom had already made similar statements, the report was the first to make the point that nursing education, as a whole, not just an elite part, should be part of the mainstream of education, and that nurses could be divided into professional and practical levels.

The report received mixed reviews. Many nurses felt threatened, and some physicians and hospital administrators considered it a subversive document, fearing that it had economic security implications for nurses. (Nor did they appreciate the fact that the authoritarianism of hospitals was pinpointed, as was the dilemma of the nurse caught between the demands of physicians and administrators.)

Therefore, although the Brown report prompted a re-examination of beliefs and attitudes about professional education and practice, relationships with practical nurses, and discrimination in selection of students based on race, religion, sex, marital status, and economic background, in 1970, Lysaught found that many of the recommendations were still unfulfilled—and still valid.

A Program for the Nursing Profession (1948). Actually an account of the extended deliberations and thinking of a Committee on the Functions of Nursing rather than a report of study or research, this report was accorded the attention and had the immediate influence of a scientific presentation. Under the direction of Eli Ginzberg, a professor of economics at Columbia University, the committee, which originated in the Division of Nursing Education of Teachers College, Columbia University, with representatives from nursing, medicine, and the social sciences, undertook to identify the problems confronting nursing and to suggest their solutions. The group found the shortage of personnel to be the outstanding problem in nursing at that time and attributed that shortage to minimal economic incentives in nursing, the public's increasing need for health care and more nurses, the "apparent financial weakness" of voluntary hospitals, and inefficient use of available nursing personnel. The committee recommended a number of broad and specific solutions related to both nursing education and service, encompassing both practical and professional nurses.

Nursing Schools at the Mid-Century (1950). Current national accreditation procedures for schools of professional nursing were influenced by the findings of this study of practices (in 1949) in more than 1,000 schools of nursing. The study represented one attempt to implement the Brown Report, previously described. Conducted under the auspices of the National Committee for the Improvement of Nursing Services (a committee of the joint board of the six national nursing associations in existence at that time), the study covered such areas as organization of the schools, the cost of nursing education, curriculum content, clinical resources, student health, and others. The report contained statistics, tables, and graphs that schools used to evaluate their own performance as compared with that of others.

Patterns of Patient Care (1955). This study was conducted under the direction of Frances L. George and Dean Ruth Perkins Kuehn of the University of Pittsburgh. Its main purposes were to determine how much nursing service was needed by a group of nonsegregated medical and surgical patients in a large general hospital and how much of this service could safely be delegated to nursing aides and other nonprofessional personnel. The report, published by Macmillan Publishing Co., Inc., New York, contained much practical information about staffing patterns and the allocation of duties which was helpful to other nursing service administrators and of interest to all nurses. Variations of these suggested staffing patterns were used in a number of hospitals for years.

Twenty Thousand Nurses Tell Their Story (1958). This is a report of a five-year program

of studies of nursing functions, initiated by the American Nurses' Association and the American Nurses' Foundation, made possible by the financial support of individual nurses throughout the country, and made meaningful by the 20,000 nurses who were "guinea pigs" in one way or another for the study. The report of results, prepared under the direction of Everett C. Hughes, professor of sociology at the University of Chicago, who also helped with some of the thirty-four studies, was published by J. B. Lippincott Company, Philadelphia.

These studies, intended to effect better care for patients, revealed what nurses actually were doing on the job, their attitude toward their role as they saw it, and their satisfaction in their work.

The results formed the basis for the development of stated functions, standards, and qualifications of nurses prepared by each ANA section for its members. The studies also indicated that further research was needed in many rapidly developing areas of nursing practice, both clinical and nonclinical.

Community College Education for Nursing (1959). Mildred Montag wrote Part I of this report of a five-year Cooperative Research Project in Junior-Community College Education for Nursing. Part II was written by Lasser G. Gotkin. The project was sponsored by the Institute of Research and Service in Nursing Education at Teachers College, Columbia University, New York, and the report was published by McGraw-Hill Book Company, New York.

This was an "action research" project in that a program was developed with methods of evaluating its effectiveness built into the planning. Seven junior/community colleges cooperated in the study by establishing two-year programs leading to an associate degree in nursing. Dr. Montag participated in the planning of all programs.

Part II of the report gives data obtained from 811 graduates of the junior/community colleges, presenting persuasive arguments for the establishment of more associate degree programs to prepare nurses for first-level positions in nursing.*

Toward Quality in Nursing: Needs and Goals (1963). The Consultant Group on Nursing, a twenty-five-member panel of representatives from nursing, medicine, hospital administration, other areas of the health field, and the public, was appointed in 1961 by the Surgeon General of the U.S. Public Health Service to advise him on nursing needs and to identify what role the federal government should take in assuring adequate nursing services for the nation. The report of this group discussed major problem areas and recommended a number of measures for their solution.

Quantitative and qualitative shortages of various levels of nursing personnel were emphasized; deficiencies in the system of educational preparation for nursing were summarized; recruitment needs to assure adequate personnel by 1970 were projected; problems in attracting, retaining, utilizing, and upgrading personnel through improved nursing administration were identified; and the need for augmentation and support of nursing research was stressed.

One recommendation urged the nursing profession, with the aid of federal and private funds, to begin a study of the present system of nursing education; the remaining recommendations were directed specifically toward areas requiring federal financial assistance.

An Abstract for Action (1970). The study titled *An Abstract for Action* was a direct result of a recommendation by the Surgeon General's Consultant Group on Nursing in its 1963 report, *Toward Quality in Nursing.* These experts recommended a national investigation of nursing education with special emphasis on the responsibilities and skills required for high-quality patient care. Although provision of funds for such a study

---

*See Chapter 13 for more detail on the original Montag dissertation and its effect on nursing education.

was also recommended, no government funds were forthcoming.

Shortly thereafter, the American Nurses' Association and National League for Nursing established a joint committee to determine ways to conduct and finance such a study. The scope of the proposed study was enlarged to examine not only the changing practices and educational patterns of current nursing, but also probable future requirements. Confident that the problems of nursing ranged beyond the manpower problem, which the President's National Advisory Committee on Health Manpower was about to investigate, the American Nurses' Foundation in the fall of 1966 voted to grant up to $50,000 to help launch a study. Impressed by this willingness of nursing to back its conviction that the study was needed, both the Avalon Foundation and Kellogg Foundation granted $100,000 each to support the investigation. At the same time, an anonymous benefactor contributed $300,000.

In a meeting with the proposed head of the study, W. Allen Wallis, president of the University of Rochester and of the joint committee, it was decided that the study group to be set up would be an independent agency, functioning as a self-directing group with the power to plan and conduct its investigations as it saw fit. No participants would be selected to represent an interest group or a particular position, but would be chosen for their broad knowledge of nursing, their skills in related disciplines, such as medicine and health administration, or their competency in relevant fields, such as economics, education, management, and social research. By January 1968, the new National Commission for the Study of Nursing and Nursing Education (NCSNNE) was fully established with twelve commissioners (three of whom were nurses); a project director, Jerome P. Lysaught; an associate director, Charles H. Russell; and a small staff. A timetable for the three-year study was set, including the provision for a contingency operation (until January 1971) to initiate implementation of the recommendations.

Basically, the study focused on supply and demand for nurses, nursing roles and functions, nursing education, and nursing careers. After reviewing the emerging trends affecting the health care system, the commission set as its major objective to "improve the delivery of health care to the American people, particularly through the analysis and improvement of nursing, and nursing education." To meet the objective, two general approaches were used—the analysis of current practices and patterns and the assessment of future needs.

The methods of study included observational and descriptive tasks, combined with collection and analysis of findings from other studies. The findings and recommendations, plus projections for the future, were then subjected to the scrutiny of groups and individuals involved in the delivery of health care. The project staff likened this approach to the work of Flexner in his study of American medicine, refined by the experience of professional studies conducted in the last quarter century. A nursing advisory panel of ten was appointed to advise on plans for the study, suggest locations for site visits, and generally review and criticize each stage of the study. In addition, a health professions advisory panel, consisting of individuals with broad experience and understanding, was selected to ensure a rounded analysis of each content area. The two panels also provided a means for determining consensus and reasonable compromise in terms of the needs of the health field when rival solutions to problems were presented.

Overall, there was an extensive search of the literature, questionnaires and surveys, 100 site visits, and a number of invitational conferences and meetings involving leaders in nursing service, nursing education, medicine, health administration, consumer groups, and third-party payors, to react to preliminary recommendations.[5] The final report, entitled *An Abstract for Action*, was published in mid-1970, followed by a second volume of *Appendices* in 1971. A total of some fifty-eight specific recommendations

and some subsumed recommendations emerged from the report, with four priorities cited:

Increased research into the practice of nursing and education of nurses; improved educational systems and curricula based on the results of that research; clarification of roles and practice conjointly with other health professions to insure the delivery of optimum care; and increased financial support for nurses and for nursing to ensure adequate career opportunities that will attract and retain the number of individuals required for quality health care in the coming years.[6]

The report concluded with four central recommendations:

1. *The federal Division of Nursing, the National Center for Health Services Research and Development, other government agencies, and private foundations appropriate grant funds or research contracts to investigate the impact of nursing practice on the quality, effectiveness, and economy of health care.*
2. *Each state have or create, a master planning commmttee that will take nursing education under its purview, such committees to include representatives of nursing education, other health professions, and the public, to recommend specific guidelines, means for implementation, and deadlines to ensure that nursing education is positioned in the mainstream of American educational patterns.*
3. *A National Joint Practice Commission, with state counterpart committees, be established between medicine and nursing to discuss and make recommendations concerning the congruent roles of the physician and the nurse in providing quality health care, with particular attention to the use of the nurse clinician; the introduction of the physician's assistant; the increased activity of other professions and skills in areas long assumed to be the concern solely of the physician and /or the nurse.*
4. *Federal, regional, state and local governments adopt measures for the increased support of nursing research and education. Priority should be given to construction grants, institutional grants, advanced*

traineeships, and research grants and contracts. Further, we recommend that private funds and foundations support nursing research and educational innovations where such activities are not publicly aided. We believe that a useful guide for the beginnings of such a financial aid program would be in the amounts and distribution of funds authorized by Congress for fiscal 1970, with proportional increases from other public and private agencies. [7]

The report was received with mixed reactions, and continued to be controversial. Some stated that the research was poorly done; others that many of the recommendations were not valid; still others that there was little that was new.

Eventually, however, all the major nursing organizations, the AMA, AHA, and other health groups either published a statement of support for the report or endorsed it "in principle." An NLN Task Force studied the National Commission report in depth and in early 1973 its report was published. Each recommendation had been evaluated and either endorsed or revised and restated, with a rationale for the suggested revision. The greatest concerns were with the concept of "episodic" and "distributive" care and specific recommendations for nursing education. [8]

The determination of the commission and the project staff to begin implementation of the recommendations resulted in a commitment of funds for one year of implementation by ANA and NLN. Thereupon the Kellogg Foundation agreed to underwrite the project for two years and share with nursing the support for a third year, a total of $361,000 of Kellogg support and $25,000 each from ANA and NLN. In 1973 the status of the implementation effort was reported in *From Abstract into Action.*

At the beginning of this new phase, there was a reconstitution of the commission, which had fulfilled its task, with some members moving to a National Advisory Board. Leroy C. Burney, MD, president of the Mil-

bank Memorial Fund, became president of the commission. In addition, five advisory committees of varied makeup, including other disciplines, were also established. Nine target states were designated to begin involvement and demonstration of the practical tasks of implementation, and regional associates were appointed to aid in these efforts. The priority items of implementation were set as nursing roles and functions, nursing education, and nursing careers.

The timetable of the staff included emphasis on educational and informational activities for various "publics" the first year, development of a National Joint Practice Commission between nursing and medicine and state counterparts the second year, and concentration on generation of statewide master planning committees and changes in patterns of education and practice the third year.

During the first year, numerous articles, reviews, and commentaries were written about the report, the recommendations, and implementation by staff and interested individuals. Sixteen pamphlets were developed and printed by NCSNNE on particular concerns that grew out of the implementation phase. There were also frequent general speaking engagements and meetings with target state groups. By the summer of 1971, a newly organized National Joint Practice Commission (NJPC) had been established with ten nurses and ten physicians, each a practitioner engaged in direct patient care approximately 50 per cent of the time. The group developed a number of specific objectives, focused on the basic charge of the commission's recommendation. Subsequently, NCSNNE attention was given to models of "episodic" and "distributive" care in education and practice, study of new utilization patterns, and progress in nursing research. In terms of educational changes, much interest was focused on open curriculum, preparation of nurses in the expanded role, and some aspects of graduate education. In terms of careers, the commission looked at economic and social satisfactions, new approaches to extend the horizons of nursing, the impact of organizations, and the licensure dilemma.[9]

In summarizing the effect of the National Commission report on nursing and health care, it is necessary to recognize that it is difficult to differentiate between changes that may have occurred through a normal process of evolving trends and those that could have been a direct result of NCSNNE recommendations. For instance, there has been an upsurge of action in continuing education, open curriculum programs, and increase in AD and baccalaureate programs. It is entirely possible that the report at least accelerated, if it did not initiate, action.

One specific action that occurred was the formation of the National Joint Practice Commission and its counterparts on the state, local, and institutional levels. Most states began, or continued, formalized nurse-physician dialogue, although some eventually dissolved, frequently because of lack of physician interest or inadequate organization. The national organization, funded in part by the Kellogg Foundation, early on made important statements.[10] It remained active until 1981. (See Chapter 27.)

Other NCSNNE interests did not have as long-lasting an impact. Many statewide master planning committees were formed, but actual results of their planning are not as evident. A few diploma programs made progress toward becoming independent educational programs; a limited number of educational programs revised their curriculums to incorporate the concepts of episodic and distributive care. Particularly disappointing was that, after the major increase in federal support to nursing in 1972, there was a totally negative attitude on the part of the administration and a consequent cutback of funds.

Lysaught concluded that there was still much to be accomplished but indicated "faith and hope" that continued progress would ensue.

In 1977, he conducted a national survey of nursing service directors to determine how much progress had been made on four selected projections of the final report: joint practice committees, a reward system for increased nursing competence, enhancement of career perspectives through recognition of advanced clinical competence, and increase of ties and joint responsibilities between nursing education and nursing service. The results showed minimum progress toward these goals on the grass-roots level. Perhaps remembering that the Commission repeated some of the recommendations of Brown's report, Lysaught suggested that the next years "should be characterized not by further search but by accomplished fulfillment."[11]

Extending the Scope of Nursing Practice: A Report of the Secretary's Committee to Study Extended Roles for Nurses (1971). At the request of the Secretary of Health, Education, and Welfare, a multi-disciplinary committee was formed to study potential and actual new roles for nursing. The committee, which was chaired by Dr. Roger O. Egeberg, then Special Assistant for Health Policy at HEW, consisted of thirteen physicians and thirteen nurses, as well as administrators and trustees of hospitals, administrators of schools of allied health, and knowledgeable HEW staff. The purpose was to "examine the field of nursing practice, to offer some suggestions on how its scope might be extended, and to clarify the many ambiguous relationships between physicians and nurses."[12] The committee elected to view the subject from the perspective of the consumers of health services. The preface of the report ended with the statement:

> We believe that the future of nursing must encompass a substantially larger place within the community of the health professions. Moreover, we believe that extending the scope of nursing practice is essential if this nation is to achieve the goal of equal access to health services for all its citizens. . ."[13]

The report reviewed many current responsibilities of nurses, from simple tasks to expert, professional techniques necessary in acute life-threatening situations, and noted the nurse's role on the health team, as leader of the nursing team, and in counseling, teaching, planning, and assessing. The committee delineated major elements of nursing practice in primary, acute, and long-term care, indicating those elements for which nurses already had primary responsibility, those for which responsibility was exercised by either physicians or nurses or a member of the allied health professions, and those responsibilities for which some nurses were already prepared and others could be prepared. Although recognizing that most nurses were not currently educationally prepared to assume extended roles and that some were reluctant to accept these roles, the committee arrived at certain conclusions and recommendations it believed significant in achieving extended roles for nursing. Legal considerations of the role were also reviewed (see Chapter 20).

Because of the impact of the report and the specific recommendations on both nursing practice and education, and subsequent HEW financial support to programs and individuals willing to carry out these recommendations, they are cited here:

> Health education centers should undertake curricular innovations that demonstrate the physician-nurse team concept in the delivery of care in a variety of settings under conditions that provide optimum opportunity for both professions to seek the highest levels of competence. Financial support should be made available for programs of continuing nurse education that could prepare the present pool of over one million active and inactive nurses to function in extended roles. The continuing education of nurses should be structured to encourage professional advancement among and through all nursing education programs and to encourage the use of equivalency examinations to evaluate competence, knowledge, and experience.
>
> Increased attention should be paid to the commonality of nursing licensure and certification and to the development and acceptance of a model law of nursing practice suita-

ble for national application through the States. The nursing profession should undertake a thorough study of recertification as a possible means of documenting new or changed skills among practicing nurses.

> Collaborative efforts involving schools of medicine and nursing should be encouraged to undertake programs to demonstrate effective functional interaction of physicians and nurses in the provision of health services and the extension of those services to the widest possible range of the population. The transfer of functions and responsibilities between physicians and nurses should be sought through an orderly process recognizing the capacity and desire of both professions to participate in additional training activities intended to augment the potential scope of nursing practice. A determined and continuing effort should be made to attain a high degree of flexibility in the interprofessional relationships of physicians and nurses. Jurisdictional concerns per se should not be permitted to interfere with efforts to meet patient needs.
>
> Cost-benefit analyses and similar economic studies should be undertaken in a variety of geographic and institutional settings to assess the impact on the health care delivery system of extended nursing practice.* Toward the same objective, attitudinal surveys of health care providers and consumers should be conducted to assess the significance of factors that might affect the acceptance of nurses in extended care roles which they do not now normally occupy.

The Study of Credentialing in Nursing: A New Approach (1979). There were two major considerations that precipitated a study of credentialing in nursing: an ongoing disagreement and/or confusion between ANA and NLN on their respective roles in credentialing nurses, which was becoming somewhat acidulous by the mid-1970s, and increased activity by state and federal governments, presumably indicating public disaffection on the whole matter of health manpower credentialing. (See Chapter 20.) It was the action of the 1974 ANA House of

---

*An appendix to this paper listed more than thirty locations in which nurses were being prepared for or were practicing in extended roles at that time.

Delegates "to examine the feasibility of accreditation of basic and graduate education" that stimulated two conferences on credentialing, under the sponsorship of the ANA Commission on Education. The outcome of these conferences, in which NLN and the American Association of Colleges of Nursing (AACN) were also involved, was a recommendation that the scope of a feasibility study should encompass more than accreditation to include assessment of credentialing mechanisms for organized nursing services, certification, and licensure, and "to formulate a proposal for studying the adequacy of these mechanisms, and to recommend future directions."[14]

In August 1975, ANA contracted with the Center for Health Research, College of Nursing, Wayne State University to complete a proposal that had been developed in draft form at the second credentialing conference. The proposal that was developed had as its stated purposes: (1) to assess the adequacy of current credentialing mechanisms in nursing, including accreditation, certification, and licensure, for providing quality assurance to the public served, and (2) to recommend future directions for credentialing in nursing. The study was to include nursing service and nursing education, but was not to attempt to demonstrate the relationship between credentials and the quality of care. The proposal was accepted by the ANA Board of Directors in December 1975. When the NLN declined to co-sponsor the study, the ANA proceeded to do so alone in August 1976. At that time, the Committee for the Study of Credentialing in Nursing (CSCN) was appointed—ten nurses and five others, with the later addition of Dr. Margretta Styles, former dean of the Wayne State College of Nursing as chairperson. A project director, Inez G. Hinsvark, professor in the School of Nursing, University of Wisconsin, Milwaukee, was selected as project director. The twenty-four-month contract negotiated by ANA provided that the study committee have responsibility for the program, and the university, the administrative responsibility.

The purposes of the study remained essentially the same, with the addition of "to suggest ways for increasing the effectiveness of credentialing." It was a complex task of some magnitude. The study began with a comprehensive review of the literature and information, position papers, documents, and laws that were offered by various state agencies, nursing associations, and credentialing agencies. Groups of nursing and related health organizations and agencies concerned about nursing credentialing were invited to participate as cooperating groups and became a useful source of information. A model was constructed, composed of three areas identified for analysis: governance, policy, and control of credentialing within nursing; credentialing in the job market, and credentialing in nursing education. In addition, a set of principles appropriate to guide all credentialing endeavors was created, and current issues in credentialing and barriers to change were identified with position statements formulated. The methodologies used in the study included interviews, meetings, a modified Delphi technique, content analysis of written materials, and surveys.

The committee's final recommendations encompassed principles to be applied to credentialing in nursing; positions concerning definitions of nursing, entry into practice, control and cost of credentialing, accountability and competence; credentialing definitions and their application to nursing (licensure, registration, certification, educational degrees, accreditation, charter, recognition, approval), the establishment of a national nursing credentialing center, and a statement that "the professional society in nursing, currently called the American Nurses' Association, make provision for categories of memberships for credentialed nursing personnel and students of nursing."[15] Plans for follow-up were also suggested.

The impact of these recommendations is

still being determined. However, in 1979, an independent task force for implementation of the report was established by the ANA Board of Directors. Despite stated concerns by some members of the 1980 House of Delegates that the independence of the task force threatened the possibility of ANA "control" of nursing credentialing, a resolution was passed supporting implementation "based on continuing review, development, and necessary modification" as well as cooperation of appropriate nursing groups. The task force of fifteen distinguished individuals (eleven nurses) began its work with funding from ANA, one SNA and some specialty nursing organizations.

Other Studies. In the last decade, the number of studies about and important to the nursing profession have increased. A number of them are national studies that are federally funded and include such topics as the career patterns of nurses, trends in RN supply, job availability for new graduates, and the distribution, salaries, and job responsibilities of nurse practitioners. For instance, one major study of this kind, *Analysis and Planning for Improved Distribution of Nursing Personnel and Services,* which was contracted to the Western Interstate Commission for Higher Education by HEW in 1975, was geared to strengthen nurses' abilities to analyze and plan for improved distribution of nursing personnel and services, explore ways to reduce uneven distribution, and involve nurses in health planning.[16] One of the most complex activities was to develop a state model for planners to project nursing manpower resources and requirements—a major breakthrough in the field. Other studies and surveys that are regional or statewide still have implications for the total profession. Because of this, data, recommendations, and other pertinent aspects of specific studies are included throughout this book, as they relate to particular topics.

REFERENCES

1. Josephine Goldmark, *Nursing and Nursing Education in the United States* (New York: Macmillan Publishing Co., Inc., 1923).
2. Esther Lucile Brown, *Nursing for the Future* (New York: Russell Sage Foundation, 1948), p. 45.
3. Ibid., pp. 132–170.
4. Ibid., pp. 48, 178.
5. Jerome Lysaught, *An Abstract for Action* (New York: McGraw-Hill Book Company, 1970), pp. 1–23.
6. Ibid., p. 155.
7. Ibid., pp. 156–161.
8. "Report of the Task Force," *Nurs. Outlook,* **21**:111–118 (Feb. 1973).
9. Jerome Lysaught, *From Abstract into Action* (New York: McGraw-Hill Book Company, 1973), pp. 1–21.
10. "Nurse and Medical Practice Acts Must Permit Flexibility, NJPC Says," *Am. J. Nurs.,* **74**:602 (Apr. 1974).
11. Jerome Lysaught, and others, "Progress in Professional Service: Nurse Leaders Queried," *Hospitals,* **52**:120 (Aug. 16, 1978).
12. U.S. Department of Health, Education, and Welfare, *Extending the Scope of Nursing Practice* (Washington, D.C.: The Department, 1971), p. 2.
13. Ibid., p. 4.
14. "The Study of Credentialing in Nursing: A New Approach," a report of the Committee, (Jan. 1979), p. 3.
15. Ibid., pp. 82–92.
16. Jean Lum, "WICHE Panel of Expert Consultants Report: Implications for Nursing Leaders," *J. Nurs. Admin.* **9**: 11–19 (July 1979).

BIBLIOGRAPHY

In the text of Chapter 5, the publisher and date of publication are cited for the older studies that were widely available. Many of these reports are now out of print. However, some libraries have photocopies, and microfilmed editions of most of them are also available. For information on the latter, address inquiries to University Microfilms, 313 North First Street, Ann Arbor, Mich.

Christy, Teresa, et al. "An Appraisal of 'An Abstract for Action,'" *Am. J. Nurs.,* **71** (Aug. 1971), 1574–1581. Authors criticize quality of research in "Abstract," particularly on historical facets.

"Credentialing in Nursing: A New Approach," *AJN:*79, 674–683 (April, 1979). (Also in *Nursing Outlook:* 27, 263–271 (April, 1979). A brief report of the study's findings.

Krekeler, Sister Kathleen. "The Detrimental Side of Tradition," *Sup. Nurs.* **9** (Mar. 1978), 47–51. Reviews the self serving reactions to famous nursing studies.

Lysaught, Jerome. *An Abstract for Action.* New York: McGraw-Hill Book Company, 1970. The report of the NCSNNE with recommendations for action.

Lysaught, Jerome. *An Abstract for Action: Appendices.* New York: McGraw-Hill Book Company, 1970. A helpful supplement to the report, containing a variety of materials providing background for the study.

Lysaught, Jerome. *From Abstract into Action.* New York: McGraw-Hill Book Company, 1973. The follow-up report of the NCSNNE, detailing implementation and making recommendations for further action. Appendix A of *From Abstract into Action* provides an extensive list of publications related to the NCSNNE study.

Lysaught, Jerome. "From Abstract into Action," *Nurs. Outlook,* **20** (Mar. 1972), 173–179. A progress report from the NCSNNE concerning the implementation of recommendations of the original report.

Lysaught, Jerome, et al. "Progress in Professional Service: Nurse Leaders Queried," *Hospitals,* **52** (Aug. 16, 1978), 93–98ff. A follow-up survey to determine the status of some of the NCSNNE recommendations shows a disappointing lack of progress.

"National Commission for the Study of Nursing and Nursing Education: Summary Report and Recommendations," *Am. J. Nurs.* **70** (Feb. 1970), 279–294.

"Report of the Task Force," *Nurs. Outlook,* **21** (Feb. 1973), 111–118. An NLN task force reviews the recommendations of the NCSNNE, stating agreement or opposition, with rationale.

Rawnsky, Marilyn. "The Goldmark Report: Midpoint in Nursing History," *Nurs. Outlook,* **21** (June 1973), 380–383. The background of the report, early problems and educational issues of the times. Similarities to today's problems are noted. Excellent reference list of journals of the time.

The Study of Credentialing in Nursing: A New Approach, Vol. I and Vol. II (Kansas City, Mo: American Nurses' Association, 1979). Volume I presents background of credentialing study and recommendations. Volume II is a compilation of outstanding papers on credentialing that provide excellent references on the topic.

CONTEMPORARY
PROFESSIONAL
NURSING

THE
HEALTH CARE
SETTING

The Impact of Social and Scientific Changes

As a part of society, and as one of the health professions, nursing is affected by the changes, problems, and issues of society in general as well as those that specifically influence the health care scene. Some of the changes, such as the civil rights of minority groups and women, have been developing for almost 100 years but seem to have reached the point of real action. Others, such as the new life-styles and technological and scientific advances, have appeared to emerge on the scene with a suddenness that has created what Toffler calls "future shock," the shattering stress and disorientation induced in individuals when they are subjected to too much change in too short a time.[1]

Surrounded by constant change, nurses (and others, for that matter) are tempted to ignore the potential effects on the profession, or at best to cope with the problems only when they become inescapable. Professions that ignore the pervasiveness of social trends find themselves scrambling to catch up, rather than planning to advance; reacting, rather than acting. When the public justifiably accuses the professions of unresponsiveness to their needs, it is, in part, because those professions have not been acute enough to observe patterns of future development or have been too insular to see the

necessity to become a part of them. It is a luxury that no profession, least of all nursing with its intimate person-to-person contact, can afford. The purpose of this chapter, therefore, is to review some of the major changes in the last decade or two to determine their impact on nursing.

POPULATION: GROWTH AND CONTROL

For a number of years, the increase in world population growth has been of some concern. By mid-1971, the world's population had reached a total of 3.71 billion, an increase of 74 million over 1970. If the present rate of population growth remains at 2 per cent, as reported at that time, world population will have doubled by the year 2006.[2] The greatest rate of growth has been in Africa, Asia, and Latin America, where poverty, disease, and starvation are also common.

According to the estimates of Ehrlich, a key figure in the study of population, there are between three and seven times more people than Earth can possibly maintain over a long period of time. The only reason they are sustained now (mostly living in misery) is because we are burning our capital—nonrenewable resources being exhausted at a fantastic rate, with an accompanying destruction of the capability of the planetary ecosystem to replenish the supply of renewable substances.[3] He noted that between 1 and 2 billion people are undernourished or malnourished today—that is, receiving too few calories or inadequate nutrients in their diet—which, when it occurs in pregnancy, infancy, and early childhood, may result in permanent stunting of growth and damage to the brain. Moreover, it is estimated that in 1970, 10 to 20 million people starved to death, some in the United States.

In the hunger belt of the world's southern hemisphere live 2.5 billion citizens in undeveloped countries. It is estimated that almost all are ill-fed, at least 60 per cent are malnourished, and 20 per cent more are starving.

In part for these reasons, population control, on a worldwide basis, has received increased attention. Whereas once most such activities were funded by private groups, the designation by the United Nations of 1974 as World Population year signified a change in population control activities to international organizations (the UN, the Organization for Economic Cooperation and Development, and the World Bank). One expert made the following observation:

> This organization expansion has been facilitated by the weakening of traditional sources of resistance to population control policies. Marxist, Nationalist, and Catholic opposition has been countered by arguments about the importance of population control for economic development, and the increase of freedom of choice. Furthermore, the proliferation of family planning activity in rural Chinese communes and American ghettos suggests that family planning is becoming "internationalized" and "depoliticized"[4]

The development of pills, injections, intrauterine devices (IUD's), and societal acceptance of (and sometimes governmental pressure for) sterilization and abortion have also had an impact. Research in these areas continues, but there is also social service research devoted to understanding the sources of resistance to family planning and methods of overcoming it, particularly in the seriously overpopulated and poverty-stricken cultures. Although world population has decreased slightly, overpopulation is still a serious health and social problem.

In the United States, the census clock at the Commerce building in Washington recorded more than 220 million Americans the year before the official 1980 census. The clock adds a person every nineteen seconds, taking into account the birth rates, death rates, and patterns of movement of people in and out of the country.

After the spectacular two-decade population explosion of post-World War II, the birth rate in the United States has also gradually declined, and the rate of growth slowed. But the fact that those who are already poor, undernourished, undereducated, and underemployed tend to have the most children brings international emphasis down to national and local practical concerns, particularly those related to health. For instance, the most economically depressed of the population have converged in the urban areas. As the middle class made a hasty exodus from the deteriorating inner cities, blacks, Spanish-speaking persons, and the poor from Appalachia moved into the urban areas. For some, it was merely an exchange of rural poverty with fresh air to urban poverty with polluted air. These groups not only lack adequate housing, nutrition, and jobs, but have a multitude of health problems for which they may not seek help until there is a serious need. A whole series of specific needs related to health emerged because of their particular social-ethnic-economic problems. The need is for readily available health services, such as neighborhood family health centers, health workers who understand the problems of the people and are able to communicate with them, understandable health teaching, and coordination of the multiple services required. Some of the more urgent health needs that have been cited are preventive, diagnostic, referral, and counseling services for pregnant women, infants, and preschool children, and community mental health services to alleviate problems or redirect deviant behavior of individuals, families, or groups.

Population control and family planning are also issues in the United States. Although the concept is acceptable to most in the abstract, the specific methods are controversial for various reasons. Use of contraceptive measures may be against the moral, religious, or cultural mores of a group, and there is particular opposition by some to any form of sterilization. Abortion, made legal for the first triad of pregnancy by a Supreme Court decision, has been bitterly opposed by the Catholic Church and various Right-to-Life groups. Their single-mindedness has had definite political impact where governmental funding is concerned. In each Congressional session and in many state legislatures since the 1973 decision, there have been pressures and subsequent actions to restrict severely the cases in which abortions are paid for by tax dollars. In 1977, the Supreme Court ruled that states were under no obligation to pay for elective abortions with Medicaid funds and that municipal hospitals were not required to provide elective abortions. When more states then chose not to fund abortions with Medicaid, a series of additional ethical-legal problems arose—why should the poor woman be discriminated against when abortion was legal and available to those who could pay? The issue is far from settled, for, according to various 1976 polls, 67 percent of the general public agreed that the right of a woman to have an abortion should be left up to the woman and her doctor; yet, they do not seem to press the majority view aggressively. The struggle goes on, but there has already been a decrease in the number of Medicaid abortions sought.

One serious concern is the rate of teen-age pregnancies. In 1978, teen-age pregnancy was rated as the No. 1 population problem in the United States by the president of the Planned Parenthood Federation. One million young women were becoming pregnant each year, and two thirds of the pregnancies were unwanted. Of the total number, 370,000 ended in abortion (one third of the total number of abortions), some 235,000, in illegitimate births, and 100,000 in hastily legitimized marriages likely to end in divorce. Others have pointed to the increased morbidity and mortality rates of the young mother and child, besides the economic and social disadvantages that accrue to both. In addition, the rights of the young woman, her parents, the father, the unborn child, and society itself have become both ethical and legal issues. (See Chapter 22.)

Nevertheless, birth control measures of all kinds are being used increasingly by those who for personal or sociological reasons (such as opposition to further population increase) choose to limit the number of children they have. One report states that one in six American couples of child-bearing age has had a sterilization operation, and the trend is expected to continue. Sterilization has become the first choice of couples over thirty years old; contraceptive pills are second. Although most of these measures are used by middle-class families, a major social issue in the early 1970s was the use of sterilization and abortion for low-income groups, under federal auspices. The question arose as to whether the very young and/or mentally defective and their families understood fully when an informed consent was signed. Some blacks also see these measures as deliberate black genocide by the white population.

The acceptance of contraceptive measures and abortion is considered responsible for the new low of birth and fertility rates in the United States. For health care it has meant the appearance of community abortion centers and abortion units in hospitals as well as more surgery for sterilization and a tremendous growth of federal and private family planning centers. (Some nurses are becoming specialists in the field.) For the nurse opposed to these measures, it is a disturbing time. There are arguments for legal abortion:

the right of a woman to choose whether she wishes to bear a child; the number of neglected, mistreated, unwanted, and undernourished children; the real overpopulation problem; and finally, the fact that illegal abortions will be performed unsafely and sometimes fatally on the poor women who cannot afford expensive safe abortions, if legal abortion does not exist. On the other side is the moral-religious belief that the act is murder, even early after conception, and that all fetuses have the right to life. The decision of the nurse is obviously a personal one, but those who decide that they want no part of any of these measures, must take into consideration the philosophy of their place of employment.

There are still other problems of overpopulation that affect health care. Besides depletion of all resources, because of overuse and poor use, environmental pollution is unbelievably high. Aside from industrial pollution, litter, garbage dumps, automobiles, furnaces, and incinerators pollute air, land, and water. There is evidence that all of these contribute to the morbidity and mortality of people. Moreover, the tensions of modern life and availability of potent drugs of all kinds, particularly psychotropic drugs, result in drug abuse to the point where accidents and suicides are reaching new highs. In fact, whereas there were declines in deaths from the nine leading diseases (for unknown reasons), suicides, homicides, and accidents were on the increase in the 1970s, if nothing else a signal that better mental health services are necessary.

TECHNOLOGICAL, SCIENTIFIC, AND MEDICAL ADVANCES

There is little question that the technological advances of the last quarter century have been extraordinary and, combined with scientific—medical advances, the beginnings of a new health care system have been emerging. Some of the most significant technologi-

cal changes affecting patient care facilities can be categorized as

1. Developments in diagnosis and patient care, such as automated clinical laboratory equipment, artificial human organs, improved surgical techniques and equipment, and the use of the electronic computer in diagnosis.
2. Hospital information handling—mainly coming from application of the electronic computer for patient billing, accounting, medical research, and diagnostic applications. These are being developed to control the flow of information so that health practitioners can have ready access to necessary data and have information transmitted quickly and accurately to all affected departments. (In the area of community health, a complete physical with all necessary laboratory and other diagnostic tests is possible in less time and usually for less cost than by traditional methods—all with the help of computers.)
3. Developments affecting hospital supply and services, such as widespread adoption of plastic and other inexpensive materials, adoption of improved materials and such equipment as specialized carts, conveyers, and pneumatic tubes.
4. Improvement in the management and structural design of health facilities—all aimed toward more efficient utilization of personnel, equipment, and space. This involves improved concepts of management and construction of health facilities, putting into effect concepts of progressive patient care and other advances in organizing health services.
5. Mass communication, making possible speed of health information and new knowledge, and exerting a powerful influence in molding public opinion. It can bring about positive results, such as providing information on communicable diseases and ways in which to get help; it can provide knowledge about other social and health problems, and even provide

formal educational programs. Unfortunately, entertainment for the masses appears to take overwhelming precedence over any kind of positive teaching-learning process.

Although there is undeniable progress in health care directly attributable to technology, there is also great fear that the more machines do, the less human interaction there will be. In addition, the fear of loss of privacy becomes particularly acute with revelations of how the government and others could gain access to information about an individual's private life. Some sociologists predicted a few years ago that man would soon carry one card, a record of his name, age, address, date and place of birth, blood type, IQ, religion, marital status, salary, credit rating, political affiliation, and personality traits, all carefully coded and stored by a computer (accurately, one hopes). Actually this exists today in Sweden, with almost all of these data correlated with the citizen's personal number, which is given at birth. However, it was recently shown that almost any number of people had access to this information, and some changes were demanded. (See Chapter 22.) With the sophistication of computers (some of which are capable of 400 trillion computations per hour) and the American tendency to use computerized information, their increased use in health care institutions is inevitable. Only the initial cost is a deterrent for some hospitals now. For nurses this means learning to use the new technology for the benefit of the patient, but continually maintaining the emphasis on individuality and human contact, which no machine can provide, as well as protecting the patient's privacy.

Scientific and medical advances have gone beyond the imagination of science fiction. Theoretically, with the isolation of DNA and the process of cloning (production of genetically identical copies of an individual organism), a human being could be created by artificial means. Even the possibility is rather frightening to man and raises many ethical issues. In 1978, the birth of the first test-tube babies with the ovum fertilized outside the mother's body created a worldwide furor. The replacement of nonfunctioning human parts with artificial substitutes or human transplants is also a reality. Already there are implanted or attached titanium and polyethylene thigh bones; cords of woven Dacron for tendons; plastic, steel, and metal-alloy joints; orlon and Dacron blood vessels; plastic and titanium heart valves; and artificial voice devices. Moreover, progress has been made in electronic stimulation of the brain for hearing and seeing, artificial hearts, and miniaturized versions of the artificial kidney. More controversial is the use of human parts from a dead or dying individual to maintain life in another person with nonfunctioning vital organs. Corneal transplants have been readily accepted, because the donor is already dead. The transplant of hearts, kidneys, and livers taken from an individual whose heart is still beating because of artificial life-maintenance techniques has produced not only ethical but legal problems (see Chapter 22). There are two major problems. First, the tremendous cost of using all of these transplant techniques means that, in almost all cases, someone must make a selection of those who will have surgery and a chance to live. Sometimes the poor risk or simply the poor have no access to these new techniques. Second is the question of whether it is morally right to precipitate the death of the person kept alive artificially by disconnection of machinery in order to use his vital parts for someone else. Only a few states and a few judges have chosen to make a definitive statement of when death occurs —at the cessation of brain functioning or heart functioning. This ability to prolong life artificially has been extremely disturbing to many in the health field and certainly to the families concerned. And the more sophisticated the techniques of survival, the more complex the decision. Legal aspects aside (Chapter 22), the decisions of when, or if, life-sustaining measures should be discontinued for a terminal patient and who should decide this (patient, family and/or physician, or court) are not easily made. All who see a patient suffer intolerably or simply exist, without hope of regaining any brain function, find that they must struggle with this issue. Nurses are not immune and must seek a solution with which they can live.

Other aspects of progress in the health field, although not as dramatic, are just as meaningful. Interest in acupuncture is rising in the United States, and a number of doctors and others are learning the techniques. New knowledge of cancer and other killer diseases, communicable diseases, and the destructive mental illnesses not only prolongs life but requires new techniques of treatment. One of the challenges for nurses inherent in such progress is development of *nursing* techniques to add to the knowledge and skills related to new drugs and other therapies. Moreover, the survival of the young and the very old, both of whom require extensive and different nursing care, suggests needs for research and major activity in these fields. Health teaching also comes to the forefront, because many of the diseases, particularly communicable diseases, can be controlled only through use of preventive measures, which must be communicated adequately to the public. (The apparently successful eradication of smallpox in the world in 1978 was a great milestone.) That "simple" health teaching has not been altogether successful is indicated, in part, by the fact that venereal disease reached what was called epidemic proportions in 1979. Moreover, it has been said that most of the major health problems requiring current and future attention are man-made: Americans' growing cigarette smoking habits, alcohol-centered socializations, high-fat, high-calorie diets, fast and powerful automobiles, air and water pollution, pesticide-dependent agriculture, and exposure to radiation and as yet unknown pollutants. The government, recognizing the great need for all aspects of health teaching of the public, has stated its intention to give increased priority to funding for health teaching and prevention. In ad-

dition, patient teaching is being given impetus because some insurance plans are now reimbursing the cost of such teaching. But there is much that is not known about effective health teaching—or behavior modification.

EDUCATION

Trends in education affect nursing in a number of ways: (1) the kind, number, and quality of students entering the nursing programs and the background they bring with them; (2) the development of educational technology, which frequently becomes a part of nursing education; and (3) the social impact of demands on education, which are eventually also extended to educational specialties, such as nursing.

In the 1970s, schools and colleges found that they had overexpanded in the baby boom era, and their overproduction created a pool of unemployed college graduates. Many, both men and women, usually over twenty and with one or more degrees in hand, turned to nursing—in all types of programs; so did other college students. Although there have always been college students who entered nursing, this large influx raised new questions for nursing education. Should some universities limit their admissions to college graduates? If so, for what degree? Should such students be given priority? Would the trend continue? (In 1979, there seemed to be the beginning of a decline.) Other service fields attracting the same group were also asking these questions. And the public asked why such misjudgment of needs and resources had occurred.

The diversity of students that both high schools and colleges were graduating has also become a public issue. Many high school graduates seem to fit into two extreme groups: those who, for whatever reason, cannot adequately read, spell, write, or do arithmetic and somehow still manage to graduate, and those who have sophisticated knowledge in mathematics and science, are articulate in writing and speech, and have learned to be questioning and independent. The fact that some students and parents have sued schools because the student has not learned basic skills has added fuel to public reaction. Some states tried to institute competency tests before the diploma could be given, with some resistance from educators and nonachieving students. The issue is not closed, for, with the increasing cost of education at all levels, there is a corollary call for educational accountability. In higher education, particularly, the government has questioned the quality of teaching, the precedence of research over teaching, the usefulness of tenure, and teacher productivity. Although some students are content to simply "get through" college, others are demanding participation in curriculum decision making and improved quality in both the content and teaching of their courses. Meantime, with the open-door policies of many colleges, a heterogeneous group of individuals continues to enroll. For educators this poses an immediate problem (or challenge) to sort out, assist, support, encourage, or accelerate such a diversity of students.

This same diversity of age, background, education, and life experience in those seeking advanced education has been an important factor in both social and political pressures for more flexibility in higher education. One focus is on liberalizing ways by which individuals can receive academic credit for what they know, regardless of when, where, or how they acquired that knowledge. Credentials are viable currency in the struggle for upward mobility, and those in the health field are as eager as others in society to be a part of this movement. In general education, the concepts of independent study and credit by examination have been explored by an increasing number of colleges, and a variety of testing mechanisms are being used to grant credit, including teacher-made tests and standardized tests, which have wide acceptance. One example of the latter is the College Level Examination Program

(CLEP), which was developed by the Educational Testing Service and funded by the Carnegie Corporation. It includes tests of general education and numerous examinations in individual courses for which about 500 colleges and universities award credit.

Pressure toward a more open curriculum has also been exerted on general and nursing education through recommendations in reports made by prestigious groups and foundations. For example, the Carnegie Commission on Higher Education conducted a series of studies that seemed to voice the complaints of the public about limitations imposed by higher education. In its special report, *Less Time, More Options: Education Beyond the High School* (1971), several recommendations were of particular importance to nursing education. In recommending that "professions, wherever possible, create alternate routes of entry other than full-time college attendance, and reduce the number of narrow, one-level professions which do not afford opportunities for advancement," the commission stated a particular concern with the "growth of horizontal professions in the health services that impede vertical mobility." It further recommended that "a degree (or other form of credit) be made available to students at least every two years in their careers (and in some cases every year.)"[5] An earlier report on medicine and dentistry had already recommended a health science core that could lead to training in a variety of health-related professions—a move toward horizontal mobility.[6] At the same time, two other national reports made recommendations in the same vein.[7,8]

It was predicted that an aid to these new educational or flexible patterns was the use of all types of audio-visual media, programmed learning, and other new techniques that can enhance the teaching-learning process. Although these methods appear to be generally successful, they are expensive, and there is some argument as to whether the learning acquired is superior to that gained by more traditional methods. One great asset appears to be that learning can be individualized more easily through use of these techniques and also that satisfactory learning can occur in places other than in the classroom and in the teacher's presence—even to the point of checking out these learning tools as books are checked out from the library. The latter is particularly pertinent with a rising demand for continuing education in all professional fields, an aspect of the demand for current competence.

The kinds of actions taken by nursing education as a result of, or perhaps as a corollary to, these pressures are discussed in Chapter 12. It is important, however, to recognize that influences on general education have affected, and will continue to affect, nursing education as well.

THE WOMEN'S RIGHTS MOVEMENT

Nursing, from its American beginning, was primarily made up of women, and some nurses have always been involved in the women's rights movement to some degree, but not nearly as much as one would expect. The suffragette route was not easy for women in the late nineteenth and early twentieth centuries, and often women did not support the movement. That may have been caused, in part, by the negative, even vindictive, portrait newspapers painted of those in the movement, as illustrated by a few typical quotes:[9] "organized by divorced wives, childless women, and sour old maids," "unsexed women," "entirely devoid of personal attractions . . . these maiden ladies who perhaps have been disappointed, having found it utterly impossible to induce any young or old man into the matrimonial noose," "personally repulsive," "laboring on the heels of strong hatred towards men." Whether the opposition resulted from the fear of overthrowing "the most sacred of our institutions (marriage)" or "Are we to put the stamp of truth upon the feeling that men and women in the matrimonial relationship are to be equal?" is a moot point. Legal discrimination against women has not ended,

even with the passage of women's suffrage in 1921. (See Chapter 17.) There are also other manifestations of discrimination that are psychological rather than legal.

That many women in other occupations and professions as well as housewives have felt just as strongly is indicated by the resurgence of the "women's lib" movement, called by some one of the major phenomena of the last decade. As in any other movement there have been extremists who have become famous (or infamous) but in general, the movement is becoming increasingly organized and powerful. Among the most active groups is the National Organization for Women (NOW), founded in 1966 and made up of women and men who support "full equality for women in truly equal partnership with men" and ask an end to discrimination and prejudice against women in government, industry, the professions, churches, the political parties, the judiciary, labor unions, education, science, medicine, law, religion, and every other field of importance in American society. NOW activities are directed toward legislative action to end discrimination, and it attempts to promote its views through demonstrations, research, litigation, and political pressure. Among actions taken are development of a model rape law, endorsement of health education for women in self-help clinics, and support of women in training of health care personnel. Both NOW and other groups often organize consciousness-raising sessions for women to make them aware of their potential and aid them in achieving a better understanding of themselves and their role in society. The impact of the movement can be observed in newspaper reports, which show that both legal and social changes are occurring, slowly but surely, in relation to women's roles. A sudden overwhelming about-face by men (and women) in terms of what women are, and can be, is not expected; attitudes are too deeply embedded. Forty years ago, psychoanalyst Karen Horney, who defied Freud's negative and degrading views on women, wrote, "The view that women are infantile and emotional creatures, incapable of responsibility and independence, is the work of the masculine tendency to lower women's self respect." The literature of psychiatry and, it is charged, the attitudes of many psychiatrists, are still influenced by Freud's notions. There is also insurmountable evidence that children are socialized into stereotyped male and female roles by books, use of toys and influence of parents, teachers, and others—a problem being given special attention by feminists.*

Certainly these attitudes are not merely American. A 1974 UN report indicated that sexist attitudes were found around the world (and frequently held by UN delegates).

In 1975, the International Women's year culminated in a UN-sponsored conference in Mexico City, intended to develop a ten-year plan to improve the status of women, particularly stressing education and health care. More than 1,000 UN delegates and 5,000 other feminists and interested spectators attended, but at the end of the week, despite a document of official recommendations, the highly politicized meeting was not as successful as had been hoped. The UN allotted considerably less money to this conference than to others, and the preordained president of the conference was the male attorney general of Mexico. More serious was the division of interests of the women. The caucus of Third World Women, for instance, showed little interest in the concerns of Western women. Equal pay and day care centers were not issues in countries where most women have no voting or property rights. When 500 million of the 800 million illiterates in the world are women, they are

not upset at the use of sexual stereotypes in books. The recommendations that emerged were a mixture and focused on encouraging governments to ensure equality in terms of educational opportunities, training and employment, to ameliorate the "hard work loads" falling on women in certain economic groups and in certain countries, to improve access to health services, better nutrition and other social services, to ensure that women have equal rights with men in voting and participating in political life, and that both men and women have the right to determine the number and spacing of their children.

There was even greater anticipation by American women for the three-day National Women's Conference in Houston in 1977. Again, there was dissension on specific issues, particularly ratification of the Equal Rights Amendment, abortion rights, and sexual preference (lesbian) rights. It was said that the major breakthrough was the end of the psychological isolation constraining feminist activities.

The 1,442 delegates, elected at 56 state and territorial meetings that were open to the public included just about all races and cultures in the United States (including four Eskimos) and a variety of the political and apolitical, rich and poor, housewives and career women. Their point of agreement was that they were tired of second-class citizenship and craved greater social and economic equality. It was an ebullient but tightly run proceeding. Said one news report,

*According to NOW, "A feminist is a person who believes women (even as men) are primarily people; that human rights are indivisible by any category of sex, race, class or other designation irrelevant to our common humanity; a feminist is committed to creating the equality (not sameness) of the sexes legally, socially, educationally, psychologically, politically, religiously, economically in all the rights and responsibilities of life." Wilma Scott Heide, "Nursing and Women's Liberation: A Parallel," *Am. J. Nurs.,* **73**:824 (May 1973).

The conference was run with more efficiency and dispatch, more zest and panache than most conventions dominated by men . . . No one could accuse the participants of being any less adroit, canny or Machiavellian than men . . . What had not been clear was whether women who were eager to improve their lot, but had never been involved in the political process before, could be kept in order long enough even to discuss, let alone vote, on all these issues. Order was achieved by the kind of discipline any male politician would give his eyeteeth to attain.[10]

Although there were some protests that the majority ruled so firmly that the minority did not have full say, the final twenty-five-point National Plan for Action was passed by convincing majorities. Included in the final document were substantive resolutions calling for passage of the ERA, encouragement and recruitment of women for political office and appointments, full and equal employment rights, support of human rights, peace and disarmament (the women's rights logo is a stylized dove), extension of Social Security benefits for housewives, federal rural plans to overcome problems of isolation, poverty, and underemployment, a strong focus on minority women, welfare and poverty as women's issues, and equal rights for lesbians (considered the most sensitive issue in terms of public acceptance). Included in the health-related area were protection of and support for battered women, children, and rape victims, a national health insurance plan with special provisions for women, expansion of research on contraceptive drugs, alcohol, and drug abuse, emphasis on safety of all drugs, participation of women in governmental health planning and policy groups, and funding to encourage women to enter the health professions.*

For all the high hopes of the women, however, President Carter's follow-up the next year was slow and inadequate, and when the women protested, he strongly indicated his displeasure with their criticisms of his policies, particularly in what he saw as not specifically women's issues. In the period that followed, it was a win some, lose some situation. On the winning side was the extension of ERA ratification until June 30, 1982. A new organization, ERAmerica, was formed to spearhead the first nationwide effort to ratify the proposed equal rights amendment. In addition, various legal suits to fight discrimination in promotion, pay, retirement benefits, among other things have culminated in new case law.

---

*Details on these resolutions are in the March 1978 issue of *Ms.*, pp. 19–21; 81–84.

The matter of women's rights is closely related to the problems, activities, and goals of women working in the health service industry. From 75 percent to 85 percent of all health service workers are women, and the largest health occupation, nursing, is almost totally female. These women-dominated occupations are also expanding most rapidly, but, as one writer indicated, "Health service is women's work but not women's power . . . The health service industry is run by a small minority. It is run primarily by physicians, who have traditionally held the power, but also by the increasingly powerful hospital administrators, insurance company directors, government regulators, medical school educators, and corporation managers. Most of these people are men."[11] According to Brown, the reasons for so many women in health care is that, first, they are an inexpensive source of labor; second, they are available; and third, they are safe, that is, no threat to physicians who, in order to expand their power and income, "must be assured of subordinates who will stay subordinate."[12] Whether or not these points are valid, it is certainly accurate to say that for many of the women in the field today, these were the best jobs available and the salaries were incredibly low for a long time.

Navarro attributes the traditionally low status of women in the work force to the social role of the woman in the family, in which the wife has the job of taking care of home and family at no salary. The employer of the husband, in essence, gets the work of two for the price of one. The wife has "emotional rewards," a concept carried over to other kinds of caring work. One of the ascribed virtues of womanhood is seen as being a good homemaker, and even now, to do something else may be criticized as neglecting home and family, woman's real work.[13]

That labor force is now changing. More women continue to work despite childbearing; they have become more militant about pay and conditions of work; and they are beginning to fight for position. More women are looking to the health field for a career, not just a stop-gap job. Yet, a HEW study points out that male-female stereotypes in the health field are still as much reality as assumption. "The majority of women select and continue to pursue traditionally female occupations and roles. Most employed women, whatever their occupations, must struggle with conflicts between family obligations, personal desires and ambitions, and the demands and limitations of their work."[14] It has also been noted elsewhere that a woman who has a career (or simply a job) as well as a family still tends to do two jobs, with most of the responsibility of home still hers.

This HEW study supported the conclusion of others about the role and the problems of women in health. Among the major issues cited were sex stereotyping and friction with male professionals. These are familiar problems to nurses, especially in doctor-nurse relationships. Dr. Leonard Stein has characterized this as the *doctor-nurse game,* in which the nurse must communicate recommendations to the physician without appearing to do so and the physician must request recommendations from nurses without appearing to be asking for them. Dr. Stein concludes that, "The game is basically a transactional neurosis, and both professions would enhance themselves by taking steps to change the attitudes which breed the game."[15] Virginia Cleland, an activist nurse, agrees. "Today, there is no doubt in my mind that our most fundamental problem in nursing is that we are members of a woman's occupation in a male-dominated culture."[16]

More than any other factor, the absence of professional autonomy for nurses (see Chapter 16) is considered a direct result of sex discrimination in nursing, with the end result that the patient/client ultimately suffers. The movement of nurses toward seeking autonomy is seen partially as the result of the women's movement, and the struggles in achieving autonomy have certainly enhanced interest in the movement. The fight against sexual discrimination has a new impetus in

nursing, as well as in other segments of society and has spilled over to include in the consumer movement the entire issue of women's health.

THE CONSUMER REVOLUTION

The consumer revolution said to have begun when Theodore Roosevelt signed the first Pure Food and Drug Act in 1906, has been an accelerating phenomenon since the 1950s. Although various interpretations are put on the term, it might be broadly defined as the concerted action of the public in response to a lack of satisfaction with the products and/or services of various groups. The publics are, of course, different, but often overlapping: a woman unhappy about the cost and quality of auto repairs might be just as displeased by the services of her gynecologist, the cost of hospital care, or the use of dangerous food additives. One well-known health consumer advocate calls the increasing confrontations between consumer and provider just the "tip of the iceberg" of some major changes in American society. She says:

> The growth of "consumerism" has something to do with the transition from an economy of scarcity to one of abundance, with increasing education and income. It has a lot to do with television, faster communications, and rising levels of expectation . . . Very importantly, consumerism involves, in one way or another, all income levels and all social groups, not just the poor, the blue collar workers, or the rich.[17]

There have probably always been dissatisfied consumers, but the major difference now is that many are organized in ad hoc or permanent organizations and have the power, through money, numbers, and influence, to force providers to be responsive to at least some of their demands. The methods vary but include lobbying for legislation, legal suits, boycotts, and media campaigns. One of the most noted, albeit highly criticized, consumer activists is Ralph Nader, whose Center for Study of Responsive Law produced a blitz of study group reports in the early 1970s that exposed abuses in a wide range of fields. Currently, his Health Research Group is one of the most influential in health consumerism. And there is an increasingly strong force moving in that direction. Consumers, who first concentrated their efforts against the shoddy workmanship and indifferent services offered in material goods, have now turned to the quality, quantity, and cost of other services, particularly in health care. Fewer patients/clients are accepting without protest the "I know best" attitudes of health care providers, whether physician, nurse, or any of the many others involved in health care. The self-help phenomenon, in which people learn about health care and help each other ("stroke clubs" and Alcoholics Anonymous, for instance), has extended to self-examination and self-help preventive medicine— sometimes through classes sponsored by doctors, nurses, and health agencies. A less positive development, the increase in malpractice suits, has been attributed in part to poor rapport and inadequate communication between provider and consumer, with the result of mutual misunderstanding—the human dimension, rather than any aspect of medical treatment.[18]

The dehumanization of patient care, which is contrary to all the stated beliefs of the professions involved, is repeatedly castigated in studies of health care. Although complaints often are directed to the care of the poor, too often it is a universal health care deficiency. The concerted action of organized minority groups led to the development of the American Hospital Association's Patient Bill of Rights,* which received widespread attention in 1973, followed by a rash of similar rights statements specifically directed to children, the mentally ill, the elderly, pregnant women, the dying, the handicapped, patients of various religions, and others. In some cases, presidential conferences and legisla-

*See Chapter 22.

tion have followed. The whole area of the rights of people in health care, which focuses to a great extent on patients' rights to full and accurate information so they can make informed decisions as appropriate in their care, has major implications for nurses (see Chapter 22).

An excellent example of the rise of a health consumer group is the Women's Health Movement that emerged from women's disenchantment with their personal and institutional health relationships. Their complaints centered on physicians' attitudes toward women, which seem to be the result of both medical education and professional socialization. Not only are there the Freudian concepts but such recent gems as, "The traits which compose the core of the female personality are feminine narcissism, masochism, and passivity."[19] The fact that women's complaints of the health care system are neither isolated nor trivial is attested to by the attention given by lay and professional media to such problems as unnecessary hysterectomies. However, the impetus toward organization is credited to the women's consciousness-raising groups of the 1960s in which women shared their medical experiences and found support for taking action. The Women's Health Movement, identified as a grass-roots organization, came into existence around 1970 and by 1975 had increased to 1,200 identified groups providing direct services, and tens of thousands of women who considered themselves activists or participants. Groups are also active in Canada, Europe, South America, Australia, and New Zealand.[20] Their activities are centered on changing consciousness, providing health-related services, and working to change established health institutions. Specific and well-known (as well as controversial) entities are the various feminist health centers and their know-your-body and self-help courses and books. The organizations' scope of functions is increasing to include not only primary care, but nutritional, psychological, gerontologic, and pediatric services. Without doubt, those involved see the need for women to control their own essential femaleness as simultaneously related to the wider issues of female equality and liberation. "The health care system has been an agent of social control as equally restrictive as any political or economic system. Women seek to dissolve the power it exercises over them."[21]

Other consumers are also concerned with the power issue and are insisting on such rights as participation in governing boards of hospitals and other community health institutions, accrediting boards, health planning groups, and licensing boards. A revision of national legislation (PL93-641, National Health Planning and Resources Act of 1974, discussed in Chapter 19) and changes in licensure laws (discussed in Chapter 20) point out their increased success, in both the consumer revolution and the "rights" movement. What lies ahead in terms of more regulation, such as an overall federal consumer protection law, is not yet clear.

GOVERNMENTAL INTERVENTION AND REGULATION

Although governmental action is presumably a manifestation of the voice of the people, there is almost always some group that is alienated by the laws or regulations. "Governmental interference" is criticized by the average citizen, as well as by industry, unions, and other large and influential groups. Some of the objections may be attributed to a natural American tendency not to want to be regulated any more than necessary, but also a factor is potential abuse, that is, governmental control for the benefit of the elected or appointed.

A frightening example was revealed in 1979 when newly disclosed White House documents showed that President Nixon and some of his appointees had attempted to control public broadcasting in order to purge it of commentators considered hostile to the president and reorganize it so it might serve the Administration's aims. Among the methods used were tampering with the board of directors of the Corporation for Public Broadcasting (CPB), using federal appropriations as a device to reorganize the system along desired lines, and using the trade press by leaking misinformation. New legislation to revise tax laws to make them punitive to the industry was temporarily dismissed as not enough of a sure thing. There is evidence that the board was indeed made a Nixon advocate, and the plan might have succeeded altogether had Nixon not been forced to resign.[22]

Another point that can be made by this example is that this information might never have come to light had the *New York Times* and the Carnegie Commission, which was studying the PBS, not received the documents through a Freedom of Information Law request. The 1966 Freedom of Information Act (FOIA) was an attempt at more open government and laid down the general rule that documents are to be made public unless they are covered by any of nine specific exemptions, such as defense secrets, medical files, trade secrets, investigatory records, or internal policy memos. The federal bureaucracy did not want the law and undermined its enforcement by excessive processing fees, response delays, and pleas of ignorance for documents in terms other than an exact title. This and some court cases led to a Congressional revision that tightened up the law so that agencies were given deadlines by which time to respond, excessive copying fees were banned, and the exemptions were narrowed. The bill was vetoed by President Ford at the behest of an alarmed executive branch but was passed over his veto in 1974. The Privacy Act, also signed into law in 1974, had similar requirements for action, but allows an individual to see his/her own records, in whatever governmental agency they may be, if identifiable to him/her in some way: name, social security number, fingerprints, or picture. It also puts strict limits on access by third parties (a point alluded to earlier in relation to computerized records), providing both civil and criminal sanctions against agency employees for un-authorized release of records. These laws are discussed in more detail in Chapter 19, and their effect on health care is discussed in Chapter 22.

Since the 1974 amendment went into effect, a variety of previously secret governmental documents have been demanded and released, and the contents made public. Often, this only confirmed the public's feeling that considerable bureaucratic action regulating their lives was not necessarily in their best interest. That many had been previously convinced is evident in the number of FOI laws passed in states relating to state records, as well as the "sunshine" or open meeting laws that require meetings of all bodies at all levels of government to be conducted before citizen or media spectators (with certain exemptions). However, even where these laws are in effect, they are frequently violated. For instance, an "unofficial" meeting is held and decisions are made preceding the formal open meetings. Whether this type of action can be controlled by legislation is debatable, but, no doubt, consumer pressure will lead to further tightening of the open government laws at all levels.*

Governmental regulation of some kind may well be inevitable in the complex American industrial system. The argument given for increasing the regulation of so many businesses, industries, and professions is their apparent inability to regulate and/or discipline themselves. Obvious examples are unsafe and shoddy workmanship of materials and goods sold to the public, dangerous additives to food, false or misleading advertising, unsafe or dangerous working conditions, pollution of the environment, unnecessarily high costs of goods or services, incompetent practitioners, and general unresponsiveness to public needs or complaints. In some cases, governmental agencies that have been in existence for some time have widened their scope of authority. For example, the Federal Drug Administration that already keeps a firm hand on the manufacture and distribution of drugs plans to expand into the area of nutrition to prevent exploitation of the public by sale of ineffective health foods and vitamins, a move that was prompted by the discovery that a cancer-producing dye was commonly found in food. Opponents claim such expansion represents empire building. FDA control has already been expanded by law to include medical devices. As another example, enforcement of the Occupational Safety and Health Act (OSHA), a law that obtained new rights for workers, is being stepped up because of a flood of complaints of endangerment of worker safety and health, particularly in cases of radiation and industrial pollutants. Yet, there are also complaints that inspectors' concentration on minute violations is causing serious problems for small companies. In relation to medicine, the Federal Trade Commission has filed restraint of trade suits and made rulings on a variety of AMA activities: controlling health-provider supply, inhibiting HMO development, fee setting, and its stand on physician advertising.[23] There is considerable effort by lobbyists in industry, business and medicine to limit the powers of the FTC.

The cynical say that regulation is ineffective because those with power and influence can circumvent any law's intent. In part, that is true, because strong representation of a regulated group on a regulatory board is not uncommon. Those who also do effective lobbying (and that is frequently an industry's priority), can either prevent or weaken regulatory laws.

The health care system is a prime example of the regulation game. The education of health service workers of all kinds is subsidized to a large extent by state or federal government, and an increasing amount of the Gross National Product (GNP) goes to pay for health care services. Yet, there are complaints that health care costs are rising with-

---

*A good source of information about this issue is the Freedom of Information Center, Box 858, Columbia, Mo. 65201. Copies of reports and special papers are available at nominal cost.

out satisfactory manifestation of improved care or professional accountability; in fact, there is continued evidence of self-indulgent administration and spending and even outright corruption. But government's control of the purse strings has the ability to force reform when it is not forthcoming. New governmental largesse is often coupled with controls, with negative as well as positive results and some neat evasions of the intent. There are numerous examples. Medicare and Medicaid regulations have been proliferating in an attempt to ensure that this vast amount of money is properly spent. Yet, the massive amount of required documentation, some say, takes more time then the appropriate care, and may well substitute for the care in some instances, if some nursing homes are an example. In nursing, regulations of the 1975 Nurse Training Act specified how and for what nurse practitioners should be trained, a good attempt at setting standards, but preventing a certain amount of innovation. The Professional Standards Review Organizations (PSROs) are intended to monitor the quality of care of Medicare patients through peer review; yet, there is already evidence of cover-up by these physician-controlled groups that is being ignored. In all cases, there was resistance on the part of the recipient of funds, but seldom did they not want or need governmental funding enough to accept the money and, presumably, the control. How health manpower credentialing will be influenced through the power of the purse strings is discussed in Chapter 20.

Is there any alternative to regulation? Some have suggested that harnessing the forces in the competitive market would increase productivity, lower cost, and improve quality in health care. But are other industries such good examples? Others say that self-regulation is not a realistic expectation, but that external regulation could be made more workable and more palatable, with more consumer control over the bureaucracies. Still others say it simply requires finding the middle ground between under- and over-regulation. No immediate plan appears on the horizon, and it seems that governmental involvement is increasing. When national health insurance becomes a reality, the governmental regulatory process will surely escalate even more.

For several years, some form of national health insurance has been in the making, but the wide variation of benefits and subsequent cost, the debate over whether such care should come from the private or governmental sector, what the responsibility of the citizen should be, and simple political maneuvering delayed final action. The plan eventually adopted cannot help but be complex, but its effect on all health care, including nursing, will be overwhelming. It can be a major determinant of utilization, education, and compensation for nursing, affecting the numbers and kinds of nurses who will be providing services. Nursing has had some input into proposed laws, and both ANA and NLN have made statements on what they consider necessary components of any form of national health insurance. These components include a guarantee of comprehensive health services for all people, meaning the total range of health care services: preventive, health maintenance, diagnostic, treatment, protective, emergency, primary care, and community health; high-level utilization of nurses and other health personnel; provisions for quality or peer review; and joint participation of consumers and providers. However, often the interpretation and implementation of the law through governmental agencies is an even more important factor, and nurses must continue to participate at this level.

OTHER FACTORS

The history of nursing makes clear the influence of socioeconomic factors on the profession. It is no different today. Double-digit inflation has already had an impact on the cost and support of nursing education, nurse supply and demand, and, perhaps, quality of care. Cost containment will probably be one of the leading health issues in the next decade. Nurses who do not choose to make the effort to understand the hows and whys of cost benefit may find themselves at a loss to justify their utilization in a particular setting.

Also related to economics is the power of unions. Labor was said to be at a crossroads in 1978, with membership down to a 41-year low, with loss of bargaining elections at nearly 52 percent in 1977, its legislation repeatedly blocked by newly potent business lobbies and inflation-wary legislators; its aging leaders inspiring less public confidence than in any other American institution. In part, this was the result of an inability to adjust to postwar work patterns—a growth switch from industry to white collar, wholesale and retail trade, and service industries. Women, now making up almost half of the work force, do not identify with the union hard hat image. In order to recoup their losses and regain their momentum of the 1940s and 1950s, unions are now turning to or beefing up other potential sources of union activity, such as the health care industries. This includes professionals and nonprofessionals, as demonstrated by the 1978 announcement of the American Federation of Teachers to concentrate efforts on organizing nurses and other health workers.

Still another social change is in the lifestyles of people, especially the young. The tendency for many of the young, regardless of social class, to seek escape from the ideas of their elders has resulted in acceptance of exotic religions, new food idiosyncrasies, commune living and other approaches to family living, with or without benefit of legal marriage. The number of illegitimate children appears to be rising, and the single parent, whether through marriage or adoption, is becoming more common—and more or less acceptable. To some extent, there is also more acceptance of homosexuality as a right of personal choice. Less acceptable and often tragic is the dependence on psychotropic drugs, whose long-term effects on current and future generations is still not known. All of these become factors that nurses must

consider when these individuals or families seek health care. Approving or not, nurses cannot isolate themselves from the needs of these groups. Nurses may, in fact, be one of their few resources, through the increasingly popular neighborhood free clinics. The health teaching alone is a tremendous responsibility, for neither the "establishment" nor its advice is readily acceptable to these groups. Still, the health of at least a part of future generations may depend on how well the health care system can interact with those whose culture and life-style have little meaning to the traditionalist providers—to some, a moral as well as cultural discrepancy.

Today, just as in the middle of the nineteenth century, there seems to be an upswing of social concern for society's outcasts. Like other health professionals, nurses are also identifying their roles in meeting the health needs of the derelicts, the discharged mental patients in unsupervised boarding houses, the neglected and lonely in rundown SROs (single-room occupancy hotels), the juveniles in trouble, and prisoner inmates. These people have not been able to cope with society's pressures, morals, and laws, and they present health problems as well, a virtually untouched area of need in which nursing can make a real contribution.

Seldom do these changes start with health care as a focus; they are a part of the fabric of society. Nurses must be alert to the many changes occurring in society and their potential impact on the profession. It is not as if nurses can afford to simply stand aside, observe, and react after the fact. As part of society, nurses should also be change agents in their profession to meet society's needs and, in the long run, perhaps their own as well.

REFERENCES

1. Alvin Toffler, *Future Shock* (New York: Random House, Inc., 1970), p. 2.
2. *The Official Associated Press Almanac* (Maplewood, N.J.: Hammond Incorporated, 1974), p. 2.

3. Paul Ehrlich, "The Population Crisis: Where We Stand," in *Population, Environment, and People,* edited by Noel Hinrichs (New York: McGraw-Hill Book Company, 1971).

4. Reid Reynolds, "Some Political and Ethical Problems in the Development of Family Planning," *International Journal of Health Services,* 3:592 (1973).

5. Carnegie Commission on Higher Education, *Less Time, More Options: Education Beyond the High School* (New York: McGraw-Hill Book Company, 1971).

6. Carnegie Commission on Higher Education, *Higher Education and the Nation's Health* (New York: McGraw-Hill Book Company, 1970), p. 53.

7. Department of Health, Education, and Welfare, "Report on Licensing and Related Health Credentialing" (Washington, D.C., The Department, 1971).

8. Jerome Lysaught, *An Abstract for Action* (New York: McGraw-Hill Book Company, 1970).

9. Teresa Christy, "Liberation Movement: Impact on Nursing," *AORN J.,* 15:67–68 (Apr. 1972).

10. "What Next for U.S. Women," *Time,* 111:21 (Dec. 5, 1977).

11. Carol A. Brown, "Women Workers in the Health Service Industry," *Internatl. J. of Health Services,* 5:173 (1975).

12. Ibid., p. 174.

13. Vicente Navarro, "Women in Health Care," *New Eng. J. Med.,* 292:400 (Feb. 20, 1975).

14. Department of Health, Education and Welfare, *Executive Summary: A Story of the Participation of Women in the Health Care Industry Labor Force.* DHEW Publication No. (HRA)77–644, p. i.

15. Leonard Stein, "The Doctor-Nurse Game," *Arch. Gen. Psychiat.,* 16:699–703 (June 1967).

16. Virginia Cleland, "Sex Discrimination: Nursing's Most Pervasive Problem," *Am. J. Nurs.,* 71:1542 (Aug. 1971).

17. Nancy Quinn and Anne R. Somers, "The Patient's Bill of Rights: A Significant Aspect of the Consumer Revolution," *Nurs. Outlook,* 22:243 (Apr. 1974).

18. Department of Health, Education, and Welfare, *Medical Malpractice: Report of the Secretary's Commission on Medical Malpractice* (Washington, D.C.: The Department, 1973), pp. 67–81.

19. J.R. Wilson, et al., *Obstetrics and Gynecology* (St. Louis: C. V. Mosby Company 1971), as quoted in Marieskind, "The Women's Health Movement," p. 219.

20. Helen Marieskind, "The Women's Health Movement," *Intl. J. of Health Services,* 5(2): 218 (1975).

21. Ibid., p. 219.

22. "Files Show the Nixon White House Tried to Mold Public TV Politically," *New York Times,* 128:1, 9 (Feb. 24, 1979).

23. Joseph Avellone and Francis Moore, "The Federal Trade Commission Enters a New Arena: Health Services," *N. Eng. J. Med.,* 293:478–483 (Aug. 31, 1978).

BIBLIOGRAPHY

Abernathy, Virginia. "Illegitimate Conception Among Teenagers," *Am. J. Pub. Health,* **64** (July 1974) 662–665. Includes high risk characteristics and strategic considerations for averting illegitimate teen-age pregnancies.

Atwater, John. "Adapting the Venereal Disease Clinic to Today's Problem," *Am. J. Pub. Health,* **64** (May 1974), 433–435. The problems of venereal disease clinics in responding to the current epidemic are discussed, stressing particularly the need for personalized care, the need to reduce the number returning with avoidable infections, and the need to improve patient acceptability of services.

Becker, Marshall, Robert Drachman, and John Kirscht. "A New Approach to Explaining Sick-Role Behavior in Low-Income Populations," *Am. J. Pub. Health,* **64** (Mar. 1974), 205–216. This study examines a behavioral model related to reasons for noncompliance of low-income populations with medical instructions, as related to mothers and children. Included are attitudes toward medical authority, general health concern, family experience, and demographic variables.

Brink, Pamela, Ed. *Transcultural Nursing: A Book of Readings.* Englewood Cliffs, N.J.: Prentice-Hall, Inc., 1976. Intended for nurses and other health care workers interested in patients from other cultures. Includes childrearing, language, value systems, personality.

Brown, Carol. "Women Workers in the Health Service Industry," *Intl. J. of Health Services,* **5**(2) (1975), 173–183. A thought-provoking look at the conflicts of women in the health field and the pressures under which they work.

Brownmiller, Susan. *Against Our Will: Men, Women, and Rape.* New York: Simon & Schuster, Inc., 1975. Traces the use and meaning of rape in war, rape laws, analyzes false myths about rape, and examines the "female victim psychology."

Bullough, Bonnie, and Vern Bullough. *Poverty, Ethnic Identity, and Health Care.* New York: Appleton-Century-Crofts, 1972. Comprehensive description of the multiple forces and factors underlying health problems among poor and certain ethnic groups. Examples of health problems given and solutions suggested.

Bumbalo, Judith, and Delores Young. "The Self-Help Phenomenon," *Am. J. Nurs.,* **73** (Sept. 1973), 1588–1591. How self-help groups function and what nurses can learn from them are described. List of names and addresses of some self-help groups is given.

Butler, Robert. *Why Survive? Being Old in America.* New York: Harper & Row, Publishers, 1973. Dr. Butler thoroughly documents the grim reality of being old and poor, the patchwork systems of bureaucratic services, and the negative attitude of the public.

Cook, Rebbeca, and Bernard Dickens. "A Decade of International Change in Abortion Law: 1967–1977." *Am. J. Pub. Health,* **68** (July 1978), 637–644. New laws are focusing on health and social welfare of women and their families as indications for termination of pregnancies, but regulations for delivery of services are still often restrictive.

Cropp, G. J. "Effects of Air Pollution on Health," condensed and reprinted from *J. Environmental Health* (May–June 1973), in *Nurs. Digest,* **1** (Oct. 1973), 32–35. A brief review of the air pollutants affecting health and some suggestions for amelioration.

Culclasure, David. "Medical Benefits from Space Research." *Am. J. Nurs.,* **74** (Feb. 1974), 275–278. The manager of the NASA Biomedical Applications Team discusses some of the devices and techniques adapted from space technology to improve patient care.

Dean, Patricia. *"Toward Androgeny."* *Image,* **10** (Feb. 1978), 10–14. Notes characteristics and stereotypes of women and suggests women maintain the important skills in which they have been socialized and also add positive skills, usually considered part of male role.

de Beauvoir, Simone. *The Second Sex.* New York: Vantage Books, 1974. Retraces the historical evolution of the role and position of women. Quotable comments on current status.

Donabedian, Avedis. "Issues in National Health Insurance." *Am. J. Pub. Health,* **66** (Apr. 1976), 345–350. Author notes that health insurance affects volume, content, and distribution of services and their prices. Any system should have objectives that include efficacy, quantitative and qualitative adequacy and efficiency.

Echeveste, Dolores, and John Schlacter. "Marketing: A Strategic Framework for Health Care," *Nurs. Outlook,* **22** (June 1974), 377–381. The need for health care providers to monitor consumer-client needs and desires and adjust their services is pointed out. Included are the kinds of health care publics, their perceptions of health, and how providers can communicate effectively with them.

Ethnicity and Health Care. New York: NLN, 1976. Deals with specific health needs of Chinese-Americans, Mexican-Americans, American Indians, Jews, and Afro-Americans.

Fee, Elizabeth. "Women and Health Care: A Comparison of Theories," *Intl. J. of Health Services,* **5**(3) (1975), 397–415. Also reprinted in *Nurs. Dig.,* **4,** (Winter 1976), 74–78. Feminists and the health care system.

Foster, Marie B., and Phyllis P. Paxton. *Providing Safe Nursing Care for Ethnic People of Color.* New York: Appleton-Century-Crofts, 1976. Book was planned and developed by ethnic nurses of color to provide specific information and guidance in care of these groups.

Frankle, Reva, and F. K. Heussenstamm. "Food Zealotry and Youth: New Dilemmas for Professionals," *Am. J. Pub. Health,* **64** (Jan. 1974), 11–18. Description of some of the eating patterns and diets adopted by young people that may lead to poor nutrition and/or adult conflict.

Frantz, Rita. "Computers in Nursing Education: Implications for the Future," *Image,* **8** (June 1976), 23–26. Although applied to nursing education, has pertinent points related to state of the art of computer use, problems, and ethical considerations.

Friedan, Betty. *The Feminine Mystique.* New York: W. W. Norton & Company, Inc., 1963. The feminist book that first attracted modern attention to attitudes and beliefs about women.

Fuchs, Victor. *Who Shall Live?* New York: Basic

Books, 1974. A noted economist surveys every aspect of the health care system and finds that health in the United States has less to do with what is spent on health care than on heredity, environment, and life-style.

Gager, Nancy, ed. *Women's Rights Almanac, 1974*. Bethesda: Elizabeth Cady Stanton Publishing Company, 1974. The world's first reference guide about and for women, includes considerable general data about women as well as an overview of the international women's movement.

Gordon, Edmund, and Derek Green. "An Affluent Society's Excuses for Inequality: Developmental, Economic, and Educational," *Am. J. Orthopsychiatry*, **44** (Jan. 1974), 4–18. A review of some of the contrasting theories in relation to the factors affecting educational achievement of the disadvantaged.

Gornick, Vivian, and Barbara Moran, Eds. *Women in Sexist Society: Studies in Power and Powerlessness*. New York: Basic Books, 1971. Interesting to note universality of sexism in various cultures.

Greenleaf, Nancy, Ed. "The Politics of Self-Esteem," *Nurs. Digest*, **6**(3) (Fall, 1978). Entire issue. Series of articles directed toward women's consciousness-raising. Good annotated bibliography.

"Health Care Regulation," (a series of articles). *Hospitals*, **52** (Sept. 1978), 5–8, 71. Various viewpoints on pertinent aspects of increasing governmental regulation.

Heide, Wilma. "Nursing and Women's Liberation—A Parallel," *Am. J. Nurs.*, **73** (May 1973), 824–826. A former NOW president and nurse points out some of the symptoms of oppression of women that have a parallel in nursing and believes that nurses, with heightened consciousness of the feminist role, can make the health care system more humanistic.

Hennig, Margaret, and Anne Jardin. *The Managerial Woman*. Garden City, N.Y.: Anchor Press, 1977. Excellent research on successful women in management. Begins with socialization of boys and girls into male-female roles. Includes strategies for action.

Higginson, John. "A Hazardous Society? Individual versus Community Responsibility in Cancer Prevention," *Am. J. Pub. Health*, **66** (Apr. 1976), 359–371. Discusses environmental factors in cancer and the responsibility of both community and individual to reduce risks.

Huber, Joan, ed. *Changing Women in a Changing Society*. Chicago: University of Chicago Press, 1973. Twenty-one research reports ranging from such topics as the historical investigation of the women's movement to the success of black women and married career women. Written mostly by women.

Janeway, Elizabeth. *Man's World, Woman's Place: A Study in Social Mythology*. New York: Dell, 1971. Attitudes and ideas about male-female roles; suggestions for changing.

Klerman, Gerald, "The Therapeutic Future of Mind-Altering Drugs," condensed and reprinted from *J. School Health* (Feb. 1973) in *Nurs. Digest*, **1** (Oct. 1973), 73–79. Background of discovery of these drugs and their effect, and implications for the future.

Knowles, John. "The Health System and the Supreme Court Decision—An Affirmative Response," *Family Planning Perspectives*, **5** (1973), 113 reprinted in *Nurs. Digest*, **1** (Oct. 1973), 36–46. A well-known physician and health leader presents the many ramifications of the Supreme Court decision on abortion. Clearly and thoughtfully expressed.

Kosnik, Rev. Anthony. "Theological Reflections on Criteria for Defining the Moment of Death," *Hosp. Prog.*, **54** (Dec. 1973), 64–69. Some of the clinical and legal definitions of death are reviewed, and recommendations are made for their improvement.

Kowalski, Karren. Ed. *Women's Health Care*, entire issue of *Nurs. Dim.* **7** (Sept. 1979). Reprints of major articles on issues in women's health care. Includes annotated bibliography.

Lamb, Karen. "Freedom for Our Sister, Freedom for Ourselves: Nursing Confronts Social Change," *Nurs. Forum*, **4** (Fall 1973), 328–352. The thesis of this article is that nursing and the Women's Rights movement are inextricably bound together, that nurses cannot achieve real professionalism, become innovators, and develop career orientation unless the position of women and nurses is raised.

Levine, Carol. "Sharing Secrets: Health Records and Health Hazards," *Hastings Center Report*, **7** (Dec. 1977), 13–15. Discusses abuses of confidentiality, research, and consent.

Levinson, Richard. "Sexism in Medicine," *Am. J. Nurs.*, **76** (Mar. 1976), 426–439. Sociologist accuses medicine of perpetuating "illness" role of women by perpetuating idiological myths. Good bibliography.

"Liberation Movement: Impact on Nursing," *AORN J.*, **15**:67–84 (April, 1972). Panel presentation by various individuals including history, aspects of the doctor-nurse game, and psychosocial implications of discrimination.

Marieskind, Helen. "The Women's Health Movement," *Intl. J. of Health Services.* **5**(2) (1975) 217–223. Good overview of the origin, purposes, and activities of the movement.

Mauksch, Ingeborg. *National Health Insurance.* Entire issue *Nurs. Dim.* **7** (Fall, 1979). Good overview of issues influencing policies related to NHI. Compilation of articles.

Milio, Nancy. "A Framework for Prevention: Changing Health–Damaging To Health Generating Life Patterns". *Am. J. Pub. Health,* **66**: 435–439 (May, 1976). A set of propositions is offered for proposed strategies to improve healthful behavior.

Milio, Nancy. *The Care of Health in Communities: Access for Outcasts.* New York: Macmillan Publishing Co. 1975. Portrays the care of health in U.S. and compares U.S. health care with other countries. Analyzes U.S. care in context of concern for environmental problems and planning and implementing personal health care services.

Murphy, Raymond, and Kenneth Bird. "Telediagnosis: A New Community Health Resource," *Am. J. Pub. Health,* **64**:113–119 (February, 1974). A report on the use of a two-way audiovisual microwave circuit to increase availability of medical services, including illnesses treated, validity of diagnosis, patient acceptance, and use of nurse clinician.

Nathanson, Constance. "Illness and the Feminine Role: A Theoretical Review". *Nurs. Digest.* **4** (3) (Summer, 1976). 73–77. Describes explanatory model of female illness, which always make the assumption that women's illness behavior is related to their being women.

Models for Health Care Delivery: Now and for the Future. Kansas City, Mo.: Am. Nurses Association, 1975. Interesting paper given at an American Academy of Nursing meeting.

Navarro, Vicente. "The Underdevelopment of Health of Working America: Causes, Consequences and Possible Solutions." *Am. J. Pub. Health,* **66**: (June 1976), 538–547. Presents the health conditions of workers and possible solutions. Extensive references.

Navarro, Vicente. "Women in Health Care." *N. Eng. J. Med.* **400** (Feb. 20, 1975), 398–402. Presents evidence showing discrimination against women in the health care work force.

Olesen, Virginia, ed. *Women and Their Health: Research Implication for a New Era.* DHEW Pub. No (HRA) 77–3138. 1975. Proceedings of conference include interesting paper on the various facets of the subject.

Proceedings of the International Conference on Women in Health. DHEW Publication No. (HRA) 76–51. June, 1975. Papers given at conference describe roles and status of women in health care in various countries.

Prussin, Jeffrey. "National Health Insurance: a Political Issue at the Crossroads." *Nurse Educator,* **3** (Nov.- Dec. 1978), 23–27. Reviews key issues and problems.

Quinn, Nancy, and Anne Somers. "The Patient's Bill of Rights: A Significant Aspect of the Consumer Revolution," *Nurs. Outlook,* **22** (Apr. 1974), 240–244. A discussion of this significant AHA statement and similar statements with a prediction that consumers will expect and receive greater participating rights in their health care.

Redman, Barbara, Ed. "Patient Teaching." *Nurs. Digest,* **6**(1) (Spring 1978), entire issue. Series of articles devoted to various aspects of patient teaching, beginning with recommendations of President's Committee on Health Education. Good annotated bibliography.

Reeder, Leo. "The Patient-Client as a Consumer." *J. of Health and Social Behavior,* **13** (Dec. 1972), 406–412. Also condensed in *Nurs. Dig.* (Sept. 1973), 56. Interesting perspective for health providers.

Reynolds, Reid. "Some Political and Ethical Problems in the Development of Family Planning." *Int'l. J. of Health Services* **3**(4) (1973), 591–595. Explores, in part, concern that family planning can be accompanied by exploitations of underprivileged.

Roberts, Joan, and Thetis Group. "The Women's Movement and Nursing." *Nurs. Forum,* **12** (Summer 1973), 303–322. Attitudes of nurses concerning sex discrimination in nursing are explored, with some history of discrimination of women health workers reviewed.

Schneir, Miriam, Ed. *Feminism: The Essential Historical Writings.* New York: Vintage Books, 1972. Interesting excerpts from the literature, beginning in the eighteenth century, includes several nurses.

Women's Role in Contemporary Society. The Report of the New York City Commission on Human Rights. New York: Discus Books, 1970. Includes well-prepared papers by noted feminists on topics such as women in the labor force; various kinds of discrimination; women and blackness; women and social services.

Slavinsky, Ann, and Vivian Romoff. "Consumer Participation," *J. Nurs. Admin.,* 2 (May–June 1972), 14–18. Participation of patients in their care, in this case, the chronically ill, is described as both an administrative and therapeutic measure.

Strolie, Frances et al. *Nursing and the Social Conscience.* New York: Appleton-Century-Crofts, 1970. A provocative book that pleads with nurses to do more for the social sick. Describes specific problem areas.

Szasz, Thomas. "Illness and Indignity," *JAMA,* 227 (Feb. 4, 1974), 543–545. Physician notes the ways in which a patient is forced to lose dignity and self-determination and urges changes in the situation.

Tanis, Julia. "Recognizing the Reasons for Contraceptive Non-Use and Abuse." *Mat. Child. Nurs.,* 2 (Nov.-Dec. 1977), 364–369. Reviews major reasons why contraceptives are not used appropriately, with useful guidelines to help.

"The Modern Men of Parts," (Medicine) *Time,* 108 (Mar. 18, 1974), 73–74. Interesting illustrated update on artificial body parts.

Toffler, Alvin. *Future Shock.* New York: Bantam Books, 1970. Describes what is happening to people overwhelmed with change and projects some of the changes for tomorrow. Includes physical and psychological dimensions.

Turner, Castellano, and William Darity. "Fears of Genocide Among Black Americans as Related to Age, Sex, and Religion," *Am. J. Pub.* *Health,* 63 (Dec. 1973), 1029–1034. The results of this study indicate that black Americans, particularly young black males, are suspicious that genocide is the aim of family planning programs controlled by whites, although black women are more positively inclined. The ambivalence created by fear of genocide and desire to use family planning methods is discussed.

Uhley, Herman. "Automatic Monitoring for All Patients," *Hospitals,* 47 (Nov. 1, 1973), 101–102. An automatic system making routine monitoring of all hospital patients a practical reality is discussed.

Vladeck, Bruce. "Interest Group Representation and the HSAs: Health Planning and Political Theory." *Am. J. Pub. Health,* 67 (Jan. 1977), 23–29. Examination of PL 93–641 concerning the composition of HSA's suggests that expectations of substantial change may be unrealistic.

Weisbruch, Jonathan. "Public Health Professionals and Prison Health Care Needs," *Am. J. Pub. Health,* 67 (Aug. 1977), 720–722. Overview of prison health, history, necessary elements, constraints. Article in same journal describes use of excorpsman in prison health.

Minority Groups in Nursing 1976—A Bibliography. Kansas City, Mo.: ANA, 1976. Reference resource to literature on minorities in nursing and other health care professions.

See also a special report by the National Health Council (New York, June 1978), *Antitrust and Health Service: A Second Look,* and *Awareness Papers,* volume one of White House Conference on Handicapped Individuals, held May 23-27, 1977 in Washington, D.C.

Health Care Delivery: Where?

Health care today is given in a variety of settings: in more than 7,000 hospitals, about 4,000 extended-care facilities, some 23,000 nursing homes, an increasing number of health maintenance organizations (HMOs), community health centers, state or city clinics, and the homes of patients/clients. Involved in this care are more than 4 million workers, of which approximately 3 million are employed in hospitals. The size and complexity of the health care system alone creates problems in the quality of services provided.

It is generally agreed that some of the essential elements of optimum health services in the community include a unified, cooperative team approach to care; a spectrum of services, including diagnosis, treatment, rehabilitation, education, and prevention; a coordinated community and/or regional system incorporating these services; continuity of care given by the hospital, community, physician, and other health agencies; a continuum of health services; and a program of evaluation and research concerning adequacy of services in meeting patient and community needs. This chapter and the next are intended to present an overview of current health care delivery, its organization, and its workers. Specific details on how the nurse

may function in these various settings are presented in Chapter 15.

DEFINITIONS

In recent years it has become popular to refer to health care delivery as being comprised of several levels: self-care, primary care, secondary care, tertiary care. Another differentiation is primary, acute, and long-term care. Definitions vary and are somewhat hotly debated, but the following will provide a frame of reference.

Primary care: *"(a) a person's first contact in any given episode of illness with the health care system that leads to a decision of what must be done to help resolve his problems; and (b) the responsibility for the continuum of care, i.e., maintenance of health, evaluation and management of symptoms, and appropriate referrals."*[1] *It is at this level that basic medical and other health care services are provided.*

Millis, a layman who has had long-standing relationships with the health professions, puts it this way: "To me, primary care includes all the health services needed by a given population that are not provided by secondary and tertiary care. It includes health services as well as sickness services. It includes response to self-limiting disease, minor disability, and chronic and incurable disease. It includes prevention of disease, health maintenance, and public health. Most important, it includes self-care and thus addresses itself to those health problems that currently account for so much morbidity—automobile accidents, obesity, alcoholism, drug abuse, iatrogenic disease, and environmental hazards.[2]

Acute care: *". . . those services that treat the acute phase of illness or disability and has as its purpose the restoration of normal life processes and functions."*[3]

Long-term care: *"those services designed to provide symptomatic treatment, maintenance, and rehabilitative services for patients of all age groups in a variety of health care settings."*[4]

Secondary care: *the point where consulting specialty and subspecialty services are provided in either an office (group practice) or community hospital inpatient setting.*

Tertiary care: *the point where highly sophisticated diagnostic, treatment, or rehabilitation services are provided, frequently in university medical centers or equivalent institutions.*

The definition of self-care, the first level of care, is self-explanatory. Its interpretation varies, chiefly in relation to whether it excludes all physician or other health professional involvement completely, even as a volunteer consultant to a self-help group.

SELF-CARE

Obviously, most people spend most of their lives in a relative state of health or at a level of self-care. The constitution of the World Health Organization (WHO) defines health as a "state of complete physical, mental, and social well-being, and not merely the absence of disease or infirmity," which, although it serves as a broad philosophical declaration, is more an optimum goal than a reality. Nevertheless, it does point out that an individual has some degree of "illness" even in the best of times. Self-care is not new and ranges from a simple matter of resting when tired, to a more careful judgment of

selecting or omitting certain foods or activities, or a semiprimary care activity of taking one or more medications self-prescribed or prescribed by a physician at some other point of care. Health care advice comes gratuitously from family, friends, neighbors, and the media (often with a product to sell). People also seek actively, although informally, information or advice from the same groups or a health professional acquaintance, but their self-care often becomes a matter of trial and error. Increasingly, a new consumer mentality has included in the public's self-care armamentarium the help of others with similar conditions or concerns (see Chapter 6), so that the individual has support and reinforcement as needed but also can detect at what point he/she needs professional help. In some cases, a person may have had some level of professional care previously and may again, but a certain amount of informed self-diagnosis is not only less expensive for the public, but may also serve a useful purpose for the individual. For instance, a mother who has been taught to take her child's temperature can give much more accurate information to a doctor or nurse practitioner (or avoid a call altogether if she also knows how temperature relates to a child's well-being). A blood pressure reading taken properly at home is more likely to identify a hypertension problem quickly than is a yearly physical. Dr. Kenneth Sehnert of Georgetown University developed an entire program for what he called the activated patient, teaching in an organized course format specific knowledge and skills that a lay person could learn and use. Included were such aspects as taking vital signs, use and abuse of medications, and when to call a doctor.[5] The program has aroused interest and is being used by others as well.

Norris has described seven areas of activity in self-care:

1. *Monitoring, assessing, diagnosing— breast self-examination, and other monitoring for cancer, and diagnosing minor illnesses and communicable diseases.*

2. *Supporting life processes—teeth brushing, bathing, and other ritualistic habits.*
3. *Therapeutic and corrective self-care—care of minor illness and chronic illnesses, even such serious conditions as kidney disease that require dialysis.*
4. *Prevention of disease and maladjustment states—taking into consideration risk factors for certain illnesses such as cardiac conditions; and methods of maintaining psychological well-being.*
5. *Specifying health needs and care requirements—youths demanding that their particular health needs be met as they perceive them.*
6. *Auditing and controlling the treatment program—women and minorities demanding better care.*
7. *Grass roots or self-initiated health care—using peers as therapists (Weight-watchers; smoking programs).*[6]

Because it has been determined in the last few years that life-style has a major influence on most of the serious illnesses of people, those who know what the risk factors are at least have the choice of deciding toward better health. Thus, prevention and health teaching have a large part in maintenance of health. Although more information is reaching the population through the various forms of communication media, health professionals as sources of knowledge have the potential for being influential in educating the public as patients or nonpatients. Their frequent neglect to do so has something to do with attitude and the reimbursement and reward system. Teaching is not telling; it takes time, patience, and follow-up. At best, only partial results are visible, because long-term outcome may be many years away. Therefore, although given much lip service, patient teaching, let alone health teaching, by health professionals, is not as ubiquitous in health care as might be expected. It should also not be equated with self-care.[7]

On the other hand, there are constant political promises of mass effort toward prevention and teaching. In Canada, which has a national health system, a plan to help peo-

ple to keep healthy includes strategies for health promotion and regulation in its 74 points, as well as educational campaigns, support of physical recreation activities, and regulation of advertising, food content, and pollution.[8] This is not an inexpensive undertaking and could not be implemented fully, but the philosophy and comprehensive efforts have been commended in the United States and elsewhere. In fact, in 1979, among the top federal priorities for better health care in the United States were prevention and health teaching.

A philosophical point that is raised frequently is whether a government has the right to legislate individual choice. Attempts to mandate the use of seat belts and motorcycle helmets have not been successful. The more complex problems of smoking, drug use, and pollution control have not only personal but economic ramifications. The bottom line is most often self-care or self-caring by the individual.

Primary health care is delivered through a variety of modes. It is not practical to discuss the institutions involved in the various types of health care delivery under those particular headings because there is considerable overlap of functions. For instance, hospitals and health maintenance organizations (HMOs) may deliver all levels and types of care, even encouraging or sponsoring self-care activities on the part of individuals and community groups. Therefore, institutions and agencies are presented as units.

PHYSICIAN PRIVATE PRACTICE

The first step in primary care is ambulatory care, that is, health service given to a person who is not a bed patient in a health care institution. Currently, most of this care involves physician-patient contact. Various sources indicate that the vast majority of care given by physicians is on an ambulatory basis; only about 10 percent of the people seen are admitted to a hospital. There are two major categories of ambulatory care, private and institutional (that in organized settings). The latter include hospital-based ambulatory services, neighborhood health centers, HMOs, organized home care, prison health services, emergency medical services, prepaid health groups, and health department clinics. The vast bulk of visits is in solo, partnership, or private group practice, on a fee-for-service basis, which is the major mode of organization for physicians and other health care providers generally acknowledged to be licensed to practice independently, such as dentists, chiropractors, podiatrists, and optometrists. Although there is a growing acceptance of nurses practicing independently, most people must be educated to that concept.

Physicians in private practice provide a range of health services and operate on a contractual basis (usually unwritten) with the patient—certain services for a certain fee. When a patient requires hospitalization, he/she pays the hospital for services provided there, except for the physician, who maintains an independent status and is paid directly on a separate fee basis. If a referral is made to specialists (secondary care), those specialists receive their fees, and the primary care physician picks up the patient again when specialist services are no longer warranted.

About 60 percent of all active physicians are in office practice, and most patient visits to physicians are made in the office. If an emergency arises, the patient may be seen in a hospital emergency room where the physician has staff privileges. Few make house calls. A small percentage of physicians (usually in the urban areas) do not have hospital staff privileges, in which case the patient may be seen in the hospital by a referred colleague. From a business and tax viewpoint, private practice may be a corporation or partnership, or hold some other designation.

There is little known about how physicians distribute their time in office practice among history taking and examinations, diagnosing, therapy, teaching or counseling, supervising or teaching staff, and paper work; most appear reluctant to have outsiders looking into their work. Nor is there much information on how doctors interact, what the doctor-patient relationship consists of, how decisions are made, how quality is monitored; how much traveling and meeting time is devoted to continuing education.[9] What is known is that approximately 75 percent of doctors in office practice classify themselves as being in some kind of specialty (not family practice), with the highest number in general internal medicine, general surgery, obstetrics and gynecology, and pediatrics. Patients who can choose their own point of admission into the health care system usually start with a physician office visit, and there is increasing concern that, for all the importance of that choice, people do so on an unsophisticated and relatively uninformed basis—someone's recommendation, proximity to home, or at best a blind choice from a list provided, at request, by the local medical society. Frequently, people do a preliminary diagnosis of their own symptoms and choose a specialist on the basis of the organ that seems to be involved. Because that physician may have no contact with the other specialists the individual has chosen at random, continuity and comprehensiveness of care is generally lacking.

A physician's private practice setting may consist of only himself/herself (solo practice) and some full-time or part-time clerical help and/or medical assistant, office nurse, physician's assistant (PA), any of whom may also be a family member, to a group practice with one other physician in the same specialty or a multiple physician specialty conglomerate with all of the workers previously cited plus X-ray and laboratory facilities with the appropriate personnel, and other supportive health professionals and services such as health education and physical therapy. More and more of these practice modes also include nurse practitioners as employees or as full partners (see Chapter 15). Most private practitioners are paid by the patient or some form of third-party insurance. In recent years, those serving primarily Medicaid patients in ghetto areas have been labeled "Medicaid mills", in part because of the poor quality of care and physician-encouraged overuse of services.

Prepaid group practices (PPGP) are still relatively few but have received considerable attention. They are broadly defined as a medical care delivery system that accepts responsibility for the organizing, financing, and delivery of health care of a defined population.[10] At least 50 percent of the patients are covered by prepayment for as broad a range of services as possible. Two prominent PPGPs are Kaiser-Permanente on the West Coast, and the Health Insurance Plan (HIP) of Greater New York, both of which also operate in other areas of the country.

NURSE PRIVATE PRACTICE

Nurses have been in private practice since formal nursing programs were started. (See Chapters 3 and 4.) In a manner of speaking, private duty nursing was and is a professional practice for which the individual has professional and financial responsibility. However, at one time, fees and hours were set by hospitals, registries, or the professional associations, even though the nurse and patient or family essentially had a private contract with each other. Because of the Federal Trade Commission's tendency to consider fee-setting as restraint of trade, the practitioner has more control over the fee now; however, to a great extent the nursing care is given to a bed patient in the hospital or home for at least eight hours a day with certain physician orders to be considered.

In an emerging concept of nurse private practice, (see Chapter 15) the nurse has an office where patients are seen, although he or she may also make house calls. In this form of independent practice, nurses have the same economic and managerial requirements as physicians, with the added concern that reimbursement by third-party payors is still greatly limited. Some insurance companies reimburse, and some laws have been passed to allow for reimbursement of certain practitioners, particularly nurse-midwives and psychiatric clinical specialists. However, because much nurse reimbursement requires a physician's order or supervison, nurses are often dependent on patients' paying their own bills. Although some groups of nurses and a few individuals working in independent practice are surviving financially, frequently, they also hold other positions, such as teaching posts. There are, of course, nursing faculty who carry a private practice as an enhancement of their faculty role and are not dependent on that income. It should be noted that these nurses do not necessarily have medical diagnosis and treatment skills.

In a somewhat hybrid situation are the nurse practitioners who practice in an isolated area and are the sole source of health care to that population. These nurses are usually trained as family nurse practitioners (see Chapter 15). They may work under specified protocols, be in telephone contact with backup physicians, have arrangements with local pharmacists about prescriptions, have admitting privileges in some hospitals, or any combination of these. The nurses may be paid by the community, state, or by some other special arrangement. The primary care given is whatever is within the scope of that nurse's practice.[11]

HEALTH MAINTENANCE ORGANIZATIONS (HMOs)

Health Maintenance Organizations are sometimes equated with Prepaid Group Practices, but others believe that there is a distinct difference. An early HEW statement describes the HMO organizational base.

An HMO can be organized and sponsored by either a medical foundation (usually organized by physicians), by community groups who bring together various interested leaders or organizations, by labor unions, by a governmental unit, by a profit or nonprofit group allied with an insurance company or some other financing institution, or by some other arrangement. The HMO may be hospital-based, medical school-based, or be a free-standing outpatient facility or group of such facilities. [12]

According to the 1972 Social Security amendments, health maintenance organizations (HMOs) provide to enrollees, on the basis of a predetermined fixed cost or rate, comprehensive health services without regard to the extent or frequency of services. These services may be given directly or through arrangements with others, and include the services of primary care and specialty physicians and institutional services. When in 1972-1973, some organizations received federal funding for HMO development, the AMA voiced strong opposition to what it called unwarranted federal competition in the practice of medicine. Nevertheless, the 1973 HMO Act was passed and authorized federal grants and loans over a five-year period. To be included were physician care, inpatient and outpatient care, medically necessary emergency health services, short-term evaluations and crisis intervention, mental health services, medical treatment and referral services for the abuse of or addiction to alcohol and drugs, diagnostic laboratory and diagnostic and therapeutic radiological services, and preventive services; and dental care and prescription drugs could be contracted for. Services had to be available on a twenty-four hour, seven-day-a-week basis, with subscribers paying nothing or only a minimum copayment at the time of service. [13]

Care may be given at the HMO or at an institution with which it has an arrangement to cover what the HMO does not have. For instance, an HMO may have medical services and/or multiphasic diagnostic services in one building, but not inpatient services, or it may actually function in a large hospital. However, a major emphasis is on prevention and health teaching, and nurse practitioners are involved in these as well as other aspects of primary care at HMOs.

For all their apparent benefits, HMO growth has been slow. One reason is that there is still physician reluctance to change practice modes or their outright opposition, another that start-up and other costs of the comprehensive services are high, sometimes making HMOs noncompetitive with Blue Cross/Blue Shield, and the third that HEW regulations were originally so restrictive and complex as to create problems in implementation. Other problems are also cited: a scandal in California, where prepaid health plans contracting to provide comprehensive medical services for Medicaid patients were found to enroll subscribers without informed consent, to provide inadequate and depersonalized care, and to misuse funds; complaints about skimping on health services to cut costs; and some inaccessibility. The HMOs must overcome these problems and develop marketing techniques to woo subscribers. There is little research showing that HMOs actually deliver superior care, and, in most, quality assurance mechanisms are not yet in place.

Nevertheless, there is clear evidence that total medical costs for HMO enrollees are 10 to 40 percent lower than for those of comparable individuals with health insurance. [14] To a great extent that is due to a 30 percent lower hospitalization rate. Because hospitalization is a major health care cost, HMOs also lowers the national cost of health care. Perhaps because of Congressional resistance to soaring health costs, the 95th Congress passed a reauthorization for federal grants and loans for HMOs, although the fraud scandals had scaled down the original enthusiastic administrative proposals and spurred financial disclosure mechanisms. Also added were provisions for new financial support for outpatient services, and certain service requirements were relaxed for the early and financially difficult years.

There is no expectation that HMOs will replace private practice unless national health insurance makes these plans more attractive to physicians; however, the competitiveness of the HMO presence in a community has already been shown to lower the cost of health care for those who prefer other forms of primary care.

NEIGHBORHOOD HEALTH CENTERS
(NHCs)

Out of the social unrest of the 1960s and early 1970s emerged the neighborhood health center, an ambulatory facility "based on the concepts of full-time, salaried physician staffing, multidisciplinary team health practice, and community involvement in both policy making and facility operations."[15] The NHC movement was stimulated by funding from the Office of Economic Opportunity (OEO) during the Johnson administration. In many ways, they were similar to the early charitable dispensaries, which were established because of the hospitals' lack of interest in ambulatory care and disappeared in the 1920s because of poor financing, poor staffing, and physician disapproval.

NHCs are primarily found in medically underserved urban areas, where the minority poor and various ethnic groups have relied on hospital ambulatory services for primary care. In many cases, the hospital clinic service and emergency service, often expensive, overcrowded, fragmented, and disease-oriented, are inappropriately used. The emergency room, particularly, is found to be more used for nonemergency primary care than for emergencies because of its twenty-four-hour availability. Complaints of activist representatives of the poor are that care is also disinterested and depersonalized. Although attending physicians are usually present at one point or another, much care is given by a rotating house staff, with no continuity of care. Even when nurse practitioners participate, care is usually episodic, and most do not carry a stable case load (although they could and want to). The reasons that hospital ambulatory care has not improved much, despite much visibility, are complex[16] and there does seem to be some slow progress. However, their effectiveness

is a major reason for the rise of the NHCs, called by some one-stop health shopping at acceptable, affordable prices, with interest in providing wholistic health care. Often, they are at least partially staffed by the ethnic group served, so communication is improved, and a real effort is made to provide services when and where patients/clients need them, in an atmosphere of care and understanding.

Although much of the health care given by NHCs is excellent, their problems have caused a drop in number from the peak development of the 1970s. The problems include tensions between community advisory boards and administrators of the center and/ or the back-up hospitals and funding. Starting and maintaining NHCs are extremely expensive, and most patients can pay only through Medicare/Medicaid, if at all. With the demise of OEO in the 1970s and other governmental cutbacks, NHCs were forced to scramble for private foundation funds and to rely on Medicare/Medicaid funding. When external funds were not available, severe program and personnel cuts were often necessary. The future of NHCs remains uncertain, in part because of a sociological question: are they perpetuating a separate kind of care for the poor? However, it is possible that a national health insurance program may revitalize NHCs; their patient- and family-centered approach is a model for private health care.

GOVERNMENTAL FACILITIES

In the federal government, at least twenty-five agencies have some involvement in delivering health services. Those with the largest expenditures in direct federal hospital and medical services are the Veteran's Administration, which operates the largest centrally directed hospital and clinic system in the United States, the Department of Defense (members of the military and dependents), and the Health Services Administration of DHHS.* Two major agencies that provide direct services from HHS are the Health Services Administration (HSA), which operates the Public Health Service hospitals, and the Indian Health Service hospitals, health centers, and field stations. A variety of other HHS agencies provide indirect funding or contracts for clinics, drug and alcohol rehabilitation centers, maternal-child and family planning, neighborhood health centers, and the National Health Service Corps. In direct federal hospital and medical services, HHS spends the largest amount of money, primarily because of Social Security's Medicare/Medicaid and the Social and Rehabilitation Service.

State and local governments also have multiple functions and multiple services in health care delivery, directly through grants and funding to finance their own programs, and indirectly as third party payors. Although most states have some version of a state health agency (SHA) or department, health services are often provided through other state agencies, a situation that creates territorial battles, duplication, and gaps. In most states, operation of mental hospitals and the Medicaid program, two of the most important state health functions, is by departments other than the SHA. In direct services, some states operate mental, tuberculosis, or other hospitals, alcohol and drug abuse programs, provide noninstitutional mental health services, fund public health nursing programs and laboratories, provide services for maternal and child health, family planning, crippled children, immunization, tuberculosis, chronic respiratory disease control, and venereal disease control. All are considered traditional public health services, in addition to environmental health activities.

On a local level, services offered by a health department depend a great deal on the size, needs, and demands of the constituency. There appears to be little information about local health departments or health officers. Those with considerable visibility are in large urban centers where health problems are complex and generally unresolved.

Some large municipalities operate hospitals that provide for the indigent or working poor who are not covered by Medicaid or private insurance. Some health departments run school health services and screening programs. Some duplicate services offered by the state. There is little data to identify how much state and local agencies coordinate their services to avoid duplication or omission, but lack of coordination or cooperation is not uncommon. Although there is a great deal of criticism of most local health services in relation to high cost, waste, corruption, and poor quality, attempts to terminate any of them, particularly hospitals in medically underserved areas, become political conflicts, with representatives of the poor complaining that no other services are available and that the loss of local jobs will create other hardships. With all the politically sensitive issues involved, most health care experts are pessimistic about reorganization or major improvement of the health systems at any governmental level.

HOME HEALTH CARE

Home health care is probably more of a nurse-oriented health service than any other, originating with Florence Nightingale's "health nurses" and the pioneer efforts of such American nurses as Lillian Wald. Nevertheless, what Wald worked for in the late nineteenth century, comprehensive services for the patient and family that extend beyond simple care of the sick, is even more pertinent today. The National League for Nursing, which in cooperation with other groups accredits home health agencies, defines home health services as:

an array of health care services provided to individuals and families in their places of residence or in ambulatory care settings for pur-

---

*The Department of Health, Education and Welfare (DHEW) became the Department of Health and Human Services (DHHS) in 1980.

poses of preventing disease and promoting, maintaining or restoring health, or minimizing the effects of illness and disability. Services appropriate to the needs of the individual and his family are planned, coordinated and made available by an organized health agency—through the use of agency-employed staff, contractual arrangements, or a combination of administrative patterns. Medical services are primarily provided by the individual's private or clinic physician although in some instances agencies will employ or contract for physician's services.

These services must be available to the total population and must include all service components necessary to ensure the health and safety of those for whom such services are appropriate.[17]

The League gives particular attention to the types of services that make up home health care. Listed as basic, essential services are home health aide–homemaker, medical supplies and equipment (expendable and durable), nursing, nutrition, occupational therapy, physical therapy, speech pathology services, and social work. Other essential services, which may be provided through combined coordinated efforts of agency and community, include audiological services,* dental services, home-delivered meals, housekeeping services, information and referral services, laboratory services,* ophthalmological services,* patient transportation and escort services, physician's services,* podiatry services,* prescription drugs, prosthetic/orthotic services,* respiratory therapy services, and X-Ray services.* In addition, environmental/social support services such as barber/cosmetology services, handyman services, heavy cleaning services, legal and protective services, pastoral services, personal contact services, recreation services, and translation services are highly desirable, and some might be developed as volunteer efforts.[18]

Agencies that provide home care have various organizational bases. As noted earlier, some cities, counties, and states provide

---

*Can be arranged for by the agency.

home health care, but the general trend emphasizes services related to case-finding, health teaching, and well-baby care, much of which is clinic-based now. Visiting Nurse Associations (of various names), which are voluntary agencies, have been the classic providers of home care. Depending on location and resources, the spectrum of services varies greatly, but includes personal health services and patient/family teaching. New entrants into the field are hospital-based home health services, the "hospital without walls" concept. A prototype program at Montefiore Hospital in New York City in the late 1940s provided nursing, medical, social, housekeeping, transportation, medication, occupational therapy, physical therapy, and diagnostic services. Since then, a large number of hospitals have initiated such programs, but the number of services may be limited. In some cases, most services are contracted for, including nursing, by using established voluntary or proprietary agencies already in operation. At times, the program is little more than a coordination of services for continuity of care, which is nevertheless a vast improvement over what is still most common—discharge with no follow-up except for a clinic or physician appointment.

Most aggressive in providing services are the large number of proprietary agencies that are springing up throughout the country. Some offer comprehensive services; others concentrate efforts on training and deploying of home workers and home health aides. In these agencies, operated for profit, marketing is brisk and sophisticated. Although there have been numerous complaints of poor-quality care, the readily available services on a twenty-four-hour day, seven-day week basis have proved to be highly competitive.

One reason for the increase in interest is the financial support of Medicare/Medicaid. On the other hand, as in the HMOs, the complex restrictiveness of the regulations, particularly in relation to reimbursable services, leads to quality problems and severe financial burdens for the homebound patient. Determining the need for home care is not a simple matter and varies both in terms of the patient and the environment. Cheating is not difficult, and cases of fraud have naturally appeared. It is ironic that the voluntary agency that provides monitored, comprehensive care is less likely to be reimbursed adequately than are proprietary agencies that provide strictly limited services to only those who can pay. Yet, comprehensive home health care is being hailed as both less expensive than institutional care and as a more effective, humane approach, especially for the elderly and chronically ill. Whether it is indeed cheaper may depend on what supportive services are needed. Is only health care needed or a variety of social services? And what of the difficulty of coordinating physician, agency, and patient, much less other entities? Consideration must also be given to the need for close planning and participation of family; if family or significant others are absent in a patient's life or they are unwilling to take on the necessary responsibility, home care may not be the most desirable approach for dependent individuals. On the other hand, with the participation of those health professionals who have a commitment to this aspect of health care, reasonable assurance of quality, and adequate financing, home health care has tremendous potential for filling a health care gap.

HOSPITALS

Hospitals are generally classified according to size (number of beds, exclusive of bassinets for newborn); type (general, mental, tuberculosis, or other special, such as maternity, orthopedic, eye and ear, rehabilitation, chronic disease, alcoholism, or narcotic addiction); ownership (public or private, including the for profit investor-owned proprietary hospital or not for profit voluntary hospital, which may be owned by religious, fraternity, or community groups), and length of stay (short-term, average stay less than thirty days or long-term, thirty days or

more). Hospitals vary from less than twenty-five to more than 2,000 beds. The most common type of hospital is the voluntary, general short-term hospital, followed by the local government, general short-term hospital, although this might be changing as a result of the financial pressures on cities and towns. The two major groups in terms of size are short-term general hospitals, averaging 160 beds, and long-term hospitals averaging 900 beds. The term *teaching hospital* is applied to those in which medical students and/or residents and specialty fellows (house staff) are taught and does not include those that provide educational programs or experiences for other health professionals or allied health workers. These 9 percent of hospitals usually have more than 400 beds and are in medical centers proximate to the medical school (in which case, they are often tertiary care centers).

Because of all these variations, it is difficult to draw one picture of the hospital as an entity. However, the diagram on p. 119 shows a common organizational pattern of a large general hospital, which will illustrate both the line of authority and the kinds of services available. Obviously, smaller hospitals may not have as many diverse clinical services and few, if any, education programs, but almost always there are business and finance departments, physical plant (maintenance of all kinds), laundry, supplies and storeroom, dietary and food services, clinical nursing units (inpatient and outpatient), and the other professional service units, such as laboratories, radiology, other diagnostic and treatment units, pharmacy, and perhaps social service. Some hospitals are now purchasing or sharing laundry and food services in the belief that this is less expensive in the long run. The physical layout of a hospital varies from one-story to high-rise, and may include large or small general or specialized patient units, special intensive-care units, operating rooms, recovery rooms, offices (sometimes including doctors' private offices), space for diagnostic and treatment facilities, storage rooms, kitchen

HOSPITAL ORGANIZATION

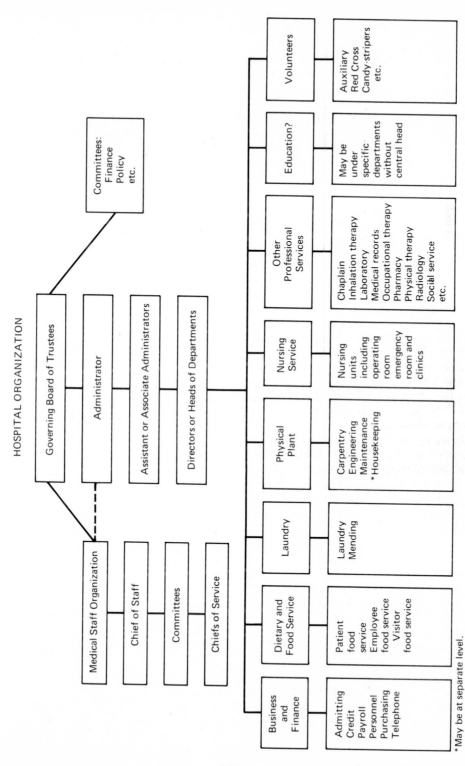

* May be at separate level.

and dining rooms, maintenance equipment, storage and work rooms, meeting rooms, classrooms, chapel, waiting rooms, and gift and snack shops. Most hospitals have some form of emergency services, such as an emergency room, but many no longer maintain their own ambulance services. A great many have outpatient or ambulatory services and perhaps an extended-care unit for patients not needing major nursing service; some provide home care.

Nursing service has the largest number of personnel in the hospital, in part because of round-the-clock, seven-day-a-week staffing. Other departments, such as radiology and clinical laboratories, may maintain some services on evenings and weekends and be on call at nights. There is some trend toward having other clinical services available on weekends, at least. For instance, a patient who needs rehabilitation exercises or other treatments in the physical therapy department lacks this necessary care in the evening and weekends when that department follows the usual 8-to-5, Monday-through-Friday staffing pattern.

The primary purpose of hospitals is to provide patient services. However, many also assume a major responsibility for education of health personnel in basic educational programs or in in-service programs, and participate in health research. Frequently they are associated with schools of health professions and occupations and provide the setting for health education and research, even though they do not finance such programs.

Hospitals are licensed by the state and presumably are not permitted to function unless they maintain the minimum standards prescribed by the licensing authority. ("Presumably" because the process of closing a hospital because of inadequate facilities and/or staff is a long, difficult, and not always successful process.) However, to be eligible for many federal grants, such as Medicare, and to be affiliated with educational programs, including medical residency programs, accreditation is necessary. Accreditation by the Joint Commission on Accreditation of Hospitals (JCAH) is voluntary and is intended to indicate excellence in patient care. Specific standards, usually more rigorous than those of the state, are set to measure hospital efficiency, professional performance, and facilities and must be met in all facets of health care services (including nursing). Visits are made by an inspection team that may or may not have a multidisciplinary makeup, review various records and minutes of meetings, interview key people, and generally scrutinize the hospital. Reports are made that include criticisms and recommendations for action. Accreditation may be postponed, withheld, revoked, granted, or renewed on the basis of the inspection and review of the hospital's report and self-evaluation. Nurses are now usually included on the inspection team, and there is nursing input into the standards for nursing service. To be eligible for an accreditation survey by JCAH, the hospital must be registered or listed by the American Hospital Association (AHA), have a current unconditional license to operate as required by the state, and have a governing body, organized medical staff, nursing service, and other supporting services. JCAH is made up of key medical and hospital organizations, but not ANA or other health professional groups. Neither does it include consumers, a fact that has caused some anger from consumer groups. To placate these groups, some JCAH visitors have had open hearings to receive consumer input about the institution being inspected. Just how much weight is given to this evidence is not known. Again, change may be forthcoming, particularly because there has been public criticism that accreditation cannot be equated to excellence or even safety in patient care.

Voluntary hospitals are usually organized under a constitution and by-laws that invest in the board of trustees the responsibility for all aspects of hospital operation, including ultimate responsibility for medical care. This governing board is generally made up of individuals representing various professional and business groups interested in the community. Although unsalaried and volunteer (except for proprietary hospitals, where members are often stockholders), board members are usually extremely influential citizens and are often self-perpetuating on the board. This type of membership originated because at one time administrators of hospitals did not have a business background, and because of the still-present need to raise money to support the hospital. (Most trustees still see recovery of operating costs as their most crucial hospital problem.) Some consumer groups have complained that most members are businessmen, bankers, brokers, lawyers, and accountants, with almost nonexistent representation of women, consumers in general, and labor. Physicians also complain of lack of medical representation, although they work closely with the board and are only subordinate to it in certain matters. Because of these pressures, boards are gradually acquiring broader representation.

It is also possible that there will be some lessening of trustee power as hospitals adopt the corporate model, integrating the board of trustees and the administration of the hospital, with the board having full-time and salaried presidents and vice-presidents. The growth of mergers, consortia, and holding companies that are creating new business-oriented hospital systems may also change the role of trustees.

Public hospitals usually do not have boards of trustees. Hospital administrators are directly responsible to their administrative supervisors in the governmental hierarchy, which may be a state board of health, a commissioner, a department (as the Veteran's Administration) or some public corporation with appointed officials. Presumably, all are ultimately responsible to the public.

The hospital administrator, the direct agent of a governing board, implements its policies, advises on new policies, and is responsible for the day-to-day operations of the hospital. Some years ago physicians and nurses frequently became hospital administrators, but increasingly, this position is filled by a lay person with management background and possibly a master's degree in hospital administration or business administration. Hospital or health administration, like any other, encompasses planning, organizing, directing, controlling, and evaluating the resources of an organization. In large institutions the administrator (the vast majority of whom are men) has a staff of assistants or associates, each responsible for a division or group of departments. Forward-looking hospitals have recognized that the nurse administrator should hold one of these positions in order to participate in the policy-making decisions that inevitably affect the largest hospital department. Department heads or supervisors are next in the line of authority; these individuals also are gradually becoming specialists by education and experience in their area of responsibility.

The medical staff is an organized entity made up of selected physicians and dentists who are granted the privilege of using the hospital's facilities for their patients. They, in turn, evaluate the credentials of other physicians who wish to join the staff and recommend appointment to the hospital's governing board, which legally makes the appointments. A typical classification of medical staff includes honorary (not active), consulting (specialist), active (attending physicians), courtesy (those not wishing full status but wanting to attend private patients), resident (house staff of residents and fellows). Through their committees, including the Credentials Committee, the medical staff is an impressive power in the hospital, for it is often in a position literally to control not only medical practice, but all patient care in the hospital. (The medical staff organization is parallel to and not subordinate to that of hospital administration.) However, where the medical staff is more progressive, there are nurses and other representatives on medical committees concerned with patient care, and decisions are made jointly. Moreover, legal pressures, such as the *Darling v. Charleston Com. Mem. Hospital* decision (see Chapter 21), increased malpractice suits, community pressures, and governmental pressures, through the Medicare amendments (see Chapter 19), are focusing on the responsibility of medical staffs to monitor carefully the medical care given and to institute immediately necessary improvements. The utilization review committee, required for Medicare reimbursement, reviews records to determine that the patient's admission is valid, treatment is appropriate, and discharge is in a reasonable time. The Professional Services Review Organization (PSRO) looks at these and other factors even more carefully. Nurses have been participating in these committees and are even employed full-time in some instances.

One problem for nurses in the organization of hospitals as it now stands is in dual responsibility. It has generally been understood that nurses are responsible to the administration by whom they are employed, but also to the physicians who have been considered responsible overall for patient care. When the two authorities differ, which is not uncommon, the nurse is caught in the middle (and so is the patient). Now the nurse's legal responsibility to the patient is receiving new attention and nurses are becoming more aggressive in seeking autonomy (see Chapter 16). Neither administrators nor physicians seem to show much enthusiasm for this trend.

EMERGENCY MEDICAL SERVICES

Ambulance services, originally a profit venture of funeral directors, are a vital link in transporting accident victims or those suffering acute overwhelming illnesses (such as myocardial infractions) to a medical facility. In most cases, providing for such services, either directly or through contracts, is now the responsibility of a community, a responsibility that is not consistently assumed. The unnecessary deaths because of delayed and/ or inept care have received considerable attention, which was probably responsible for some important federal legislation. The Fed-

eral Highway Safety Act of 1966 contained performance criteria for Emergency Medical Services (EMS) and required states to submit EMS plans. The Emergency Medical Service Act of 1973 authorized three years of funding to states, counties, and other nonprofit agencies to plan, expand, and modernize EMS's with special consideration to be given to rural areas. Under these laws, Emergency Medical Technicians (EMTs) have been trained and staff many ambulance services. Between 1973 and 1978, the Robert Wood Johnson Foundation funded fortyfour health departments and other entities to improve emergency medical services. An evaluation done at the end of that time concluded that both the quality and efficiency of the services had been upgraded. Considered responsible for some of the improvement was the training of paramedics, giving medical directions to ambulance teams by radio or protocol, centralizing emergency dispatch throughout a region, and setting up telephone numbers for all emergencies. The study also called for more support for such programs from all governmental levels.

EXTENDED CARE FACILITIES

With the enactment of Medicare/Medicaid in 1965, one of the benefits received was coverage of care rendered by a certified nursing home. Certification was obtained by compliance with federal regulations. Since that time interest in care of the elderly and disabled in nursing homes has increased considerably and regulations have changed to meet new needs and problems. This legislation was probably a key factor in the development of extended care facilities (ECFs), usually nursing homes, to which hospitals send recuperating patients no longer needing intensive nursing and medical attention but still requiring skilled nursing care. Medicare will not pay for a patient kept in a hospital beyond a certain point of need for hospital services, and other third-party payors, as well as individuals, found that it was less expensive to move a patient to an ECF. Four out of five patients are admitted from another health care facility, usually a hospital; the rest come directly from the community.

Because it was necessary to fulfill specific Medicare requirements in order to receive ECF status (and Medicare payment), many nursing homes upgraded their facilities and care to qualify. Some of these requirements included a utilization review plan, rules drawn up by at least one physician and one nurse, nursing service directed by an RN, in-service education, and licensure of the nursing home administrators. Theoretically, some ECFs are short-term facilities with an expected patient stay of less than 100 days, but in reality most shelter long-term patients. Most of the patients are white, female, widowed, with a chronic health problem. The median age of all patients tends to be 82 or slightly older, although the age spectrum includes 20 and under.

In 1974, a HEW survey revealed that about 45 percent of the 16,000 plus nursing homes participating in the Medicare/Medicaid programs were certified as skilled nursing facilities (SNFs) for patients requiring skilled nursing and rehabilitation services on a daily basis to help them achieve an optimum level of functioning, and about 4 percent were considered intermediate care facilities (ICFs), providing health related services to individuals not requiring the degree of care and treatment that an SNF makes available, but more than just room and board. Optimum nursing home care was described as preventive, protective, restorative, and supportive, meeting the medical, nursing, psychosocial, and rehabilitation needs of the individual. Unannounced visits that provided data for that report indicated that the degree of compliance varied a great deal, with particular laxity in adhering to safety standards, in meaningful participation of the physician, and in meeting the health care needs of patients and residents in the areas of rehabilitation and nutrition. Drug abuse and misuse and violation of patients' rights were also found. More regulations were promulgated to deal with these problems, and remedial projects were developed, among them—training nursing home surveyors, and upgrading the knowledge and skills of personnel, including doctors and nurses.

The organizational structure of a nursing home is often much like that of a hospital, but the number of diagnostic and therapeutic departments are usually fewer, depending on the major purpose of the institution. It may or may not be associated with a particular hospital. Some extended care facilities have expansive services providing a continuum of care from skilled nursing to home care. One popular approach is day care, which gives an individual supervision, companionship, meals, and even health care while the family members are at work (or even if they are not). Providing a break from constant care of an elderly or handicapped person often helps to keep the individual at home.

With an expanding older population often outliving their good health, nursing homes are proliferating. Much is still being reported in the media about lack of care and the tendency to allow patients to vegetate at the least, and to neglect or abuse them at the worst. Although this kind of treatment has been documented, there are many nursing homes where programs of physical, mental, and social activity and reality orientation are an innate part of the care. A new interest in geriatrics and gerontology, as well as government requirements and JCAH accreditation promise a continued upgrading of care in nursing homes.

OTHER HEALTH CARE FACILITIES

As new needs in health care arise, innovative ways of meeting those needs are developed. Some last; some do not. Others seem to be a reincarnation from earlier times, or at least a variation. For instance, some women again want to have their babies at home, with a nurse midwife in attendance, and are doing so. But an intermediate approach is the

Childbearing Center or Birth Center, where a woman can have a natural birth in warm, homelike surroundings, with the baby's father and siblings present if desired—and at less expense than at a hospital. How easily such a center is licensed seems to depend largely on the attitude of physicians in the area, and standards vary greatly.

Another return in time is the hospice movement, pioneered in Great Britain by Dr. Cicely Saunders at St. Christopher's in London. The first widely recognized hospice in the United States was Hospice, Inc., established in 1971 in New Haven, Connecticut. Modeled after St. Christopher's, its concentration was on improving the quality of patients' last days or months of life so that they could "live until they die." Two thirds of the patients die at home, surrounded by their families and free of technological, life-prolonging devices. Functioning on a twenty-four-hour, seven-day-a-week basis, backup medical, nursing, and counseling services are always available. Symptom control is a vital first step, and pain-relieving medications are not withheld.

Because third-party payors do not always cover such comprehensive care, increased public interest spurred experimental programs. HEW regulations that funded demonstration projects in 1978 described the hospice concept:

> The goal of hospice care is to help terminally ill patients continue life with minimal disruption in routine activity, including working and remaining in the family environment. Hospice uses a multidisciplinary approach to delivering social, psychological, medical, and spiritual services through the use of a broad spectrum of professional and voluntary care givers with a goal of making the patient as physically and emotionally comfortable as possible. Integral to the hospice concept is the philosophy that pain is preventable and can be controlled through the use of drugs.
>
> The hospice experience in the United States has placed emphasis on home care. It offers physician services, specialized nursing services, and other forms of care in the home in order to enable the terminally ill patient to remain at home in the company of family and friends as long as possible. Inpatient hospice settings have been utilized primarily where there is no one in the patient's home to assist in the care of the patient, the patient's pain and symptoms must be closely monitored in order to be controlled, or the family needs a rest from the tedium and stress in caring for the patient (respite care).

A hospice may be physically in a separate building, or a unit within a hospital, but, in reality, it is a concept, an attitude, a belief that involves support of the family as well as the dying patient. It can be carried out in an ordinary hospital setting, with extraordinary perceptions.

Other variations of health care are really programs carried out to meet the needs of specific populations, but utilizing health care delivery modes that are already in effect. Some examples are: a hospital satellite clinic to serve a particular cultural group; an experimental high school clinic focusing on specific needs of adolescents; "free" clinics; multipurpose clinics geared to the counterculture groups, including youth; rural health centers that meet the needs of isolated areas; and the whole gamut of posthospital (or preventive) mental health services that include mental health clinics, halfway houses, day centers, and semisupervised living services.

As these new approaches become acceptable and the services become reimbursable, the entire health care delivery system is affected.

ISSUES IN HEALTH CARE DELIVERY

Today's health care system is frequently condemned as a nonsystem focused on sick care.

Two critics described the medical care system as:

> That great impersonal, Hydra-headed technological monster clonking across the landscape, gobbling up the Gross National Product and excreting computerized bills, neither

curing nor caring, growing two new hospital wings and a cobalt radiation unit for every general practitioner that is lopped off, engineered by greedy villians.[19]

Today's health care crisis is a miasma of vested interests, obsolescence, malpractice, incompetence and questionable social concern. While some groups may be more guilty than others, few can properly throw the first stone.[20]

Citizens of the United States now spend more than 8 percent of the Gross National Product on health care—more than any other nation in the world, and costs are rising by more than 10 percent a year. There are more physicians and nurses per capita (twice as many surgeons) than in most Western nations plus millions of other health workers. The technology available was inconceivable three decades ago, and still we are not as healthy as we could be. Ironically, part of the problem is the result of the praiseworthy technology. "People just didn't used to be sick as much as they are today," an old Negro sharecropper is quoted as saying. "They died when they got sick and didn't live sick." Many other reasons are given. There is no question that much of the lack of health is caused by the socioeconomic environment, which is crucial to health for both the affluent and the poor. The poor have limited access to basic needs, including health care and/or knowledge of how to use it. For the affluent, despite abundant access to medical care, poor health often results from their very ability to fulfill their needs and wants, or from their selected life-style.

The major health care delivery problems identified by consumers relate to high costs, fragmentation of services, maldistribution of health personnel, overspecialization of practitioners, unavailable, inaccessible, or limited access to care, inadequate quality, depersonalization, and loss of personal control within the system. Blame is distributed freely: among various levels of government for the lack of consistent standards and the proliferation (or deficiency) of facilities and manpower, and among the practitioners for

their self-serving attitudes and inability or unwillingness to discipline incompetents and to provide high-quality care. Everyone is blamed for high cost. The complaints are justified, but the resolution of complaints is not an easy matter. As noted in Chapters 6, 20, and 22, the consumer revolution is bringing about changes in some aspects of care, particularly in patients' rights, but this gradual process is also part of a new general "rights" philosophy. Other concerns have multiple facets. The public demand for improved health services, translated into legislation, paid for added health care facilities and showed an early willingness to pay for each facility in order to have the newest, best, and most complete collection of technological equipment. The cost became astronomical. When it was clear that the "experts" had misjudged the number and kind of health care facilities that would actually be needed and that new equipment would always be supplanted by the newer with higher price tags, enthusiasm became condemnation.

Today there is recognition that hospitals are overbedded, and because of their cost, the financial necessity to fill these beds contrasts strangely with the lip-service commitment to health teaching, prevention, and home care. There is some indication that there are administrators who are less than enthusiastic when good patient teaching in the clinics or home lowers patient admission or patient days. There is some progress in hospitals sharing equipment, facilities, or services, partially because they are no longer affordable on a small scale. There are also mandated curtailments. In 1979, Blue Cross stated that it would no longer pay for routine admission laboratory tests, unless specifically ordered by a physician. In most states, governments are also keeping the reimbursement formula low enough to bring angry protests from administrators—along with more budgetary slashes.

The public is somewhat ambivalent about all this—people want cuts in costs, including taxes, which pay for many of these services, but they also want full, high-quality health care. Are both possible? Alternative health delivery services, discussed earlier, are still controversial, and there is no indication of public willingness to abandon traditional services or to change life-styles.

Meanwhile, government regulation increases, even while legislators aver the need for decreases. The practitioners resent this governmental control, but because neither education nor practice is free from the need for government funds, there is little expectation that control will lessen.

Health care experts and policy makers have suggested remedies, but like the economic pundits, their "guesstimates" of future trends are not totally reliable. Some place great faith in some sort of national health insurance, but the difficulty of assessing the cost and outcome of the assorted proposals has made the Congress slow to act.

Both in current practice and future predictions, health manpower is a major consideration and a serious issue.

REFERENCES

1. U.S. Department of Health, Education, and Welfare, *Extending the Scope of Nursing Practice* (Washington, D.C.: The Department, 1971), p. 8.
2. John Millis, "Primary Care: Definitions of and Access to . . ." *Nurs. Outlook,* **25**:443 (July 1977).
3. US DHEW, op. cit., p. 10.
4. US DHEW, op. cit., p. 11.
5. K.W. Sehnert, and J.T. Nocerino, *Activated Patient: A Course Guide,* (Washington, D.C.: Center for Continuing Health Education, Georgetown University), 1974.
6. Catherine Norris, "Self-Care," *Am. J. Nurs.,* **79**:486–489 (Mar. 1979).
7. Lowell Levin, "Patient Education and Self-Care: How Do They Differ?" *Nurs. Outlook,* **26**:170–175 (Mar. 1978).
8. Marc Lalonde, *A New Perspective on the Health of Canadians,* (Ottawa: Government of Canada), 1974.
9. Steven Jonas, et al., *Health Care Delivery in the United States* (New York:

Springer Publishing Co., Inc.), 1977, pp. 122–123.
10. Ibid., p. 141.
11. Anne Warner, ed., *Innovations in Community Health Nursing* (St. Louis: C.V. Mosby Company), 1978.
12. USDHEW, *Health Maintenance Organizations: The Concept and Structure,* (Washington, D.C.), 1971.
13. Jonas, op. cit., pp. 143–144.
14. Harold S. Luft, "How Do Health Maintenance Organizations Achieve Their 'Savings'?" *New Eng. J. Med.,* **293**: 1336–1343, (June 15, 1978).
15. Jonas, op. cit., p. 146.
16. Ibid., pp. 125–135.
17. *Proposed Model for the Delivery of Home Health Services* (New York: National League for Nursing, 1974).
18. Ibid.
19. H. Jack Geiger, "Who Shall Live?" (Book Review), *New York Times* Book Review Section, Mar. 2, 1972, p. 1.
20. Martha Rogers, "Nursing Is Coming of Age-Con," *Am. J. of Nurs.,* **75**:1842 (Oct. 1975).

BIBLIOGRAPHY

Aiken, Linda. "Primary Care: The Challenge for Nursing". *Am. J. Nurs.,* 77 (Nov. 1977), 1828–1832. Author urges nurses to participate in primary care, pointing out some important dimensions for nurses.

Anthony Amado et al. "Cost of Terminal Care: Home Hospice vs. Hospital," *Nurs. Outlook,* 27 (Aug. 1979), 522–526. A Blue Cross-funded demonstration program confirms the cost-effectiveness of home care services for the dying.

Andreoli, Kathleen. "The Ambulatory Health Care System," *Nurs. Digest.,* 5 (Spring 1977), 16–21. Looks at current ambulatory care system with consideration of those requiring, those controlling, and those providing care. Role of nurse practitioner in the system is reviewed.

Ballistella, Roger and Thomas Rundall, eds. *Health Care Policy in a Changing Environment.* Berkeley, Calif.: McCutchan Pub. Corp., 1978. Describes and analyzes current status of health care. Identifies major issues that must be confronted in making new policy decisions.

Belsky, Marvin, and Leonard Gross. *How to Choose and Use Your Doctor.* New York: Arbor House, 1975. Physician-author maintains that only informed patient is smart patient. Gives guidelines on how to be true partner in one's own health enterprise.

Colt, Avery et al. "Home Health Care Is Good Economics." *Nurs. Outlook*, **25** (Oct. 1977), 632–636. Many elderly patients can be maintained at home at roughly one third the cost of institutional care, with supportive services.

Corey, Lawrence, Steven Saltman, and Michael Epstein. *Medicine in a Changing Society*. 2nd ed. St. Louis: The C. V. Mosby Company, 1977. Today's health care system as viewed by various contributors. Includes history, discussion of health insurance, primary care, Medicare and Medicaid, community health centers, and health planning.

Craven, Joan and Florence Wald. "Hospice Care for Dying Patients." *Am. J. Nurs.*, **15** (Oct. 1975), 1816–1822. Founder of hospice movement in the United States describes concept. Excellent bibliography.

Duff, Raymond, and August Hollingshead. *Sickness and Society*. New York: Harper & Row, Publishers, 1968. The authors describe the relationship between the care of hospitalized patients and the social environment of a university medical center. One of the classic studies showing that patients' care is not what it should be. Fascinating reading, with excellent examples. Although some things have changed since it was written, many of the attitudes and situations still prevail.

Elwood, Paul. "Concept, Organization and Strategies of HMO's." *J. Nurs. Admin.*, **3** (Sept.-Oct. 1973), 29–34. The HMO system as a competitive alternative to conventional health care arrangements is explored, including an evaluation of the performance of existing HMOs.

Friedman, Kenneth and Stuart Rakoff, Eds. *Toward a National Health Policy*. Lexington, MA: D.C. Heath and Co., 1977. Series of readings related to health policy and costs. Includes discussion of major legislation.

Hillman, Bruce, and Evan Charney. "A Neighborhood Health Center: What Patients Know and Think of Its Operation." *Med. Care*, **10** (July-Aug. 1972), 336–344. Data indicates that the central issues determining satisfaction are availability and quality of care, as well as attitudes of personnel.

"HMO's: Are They the Answer to Your Medical Needs?" *Am. Lung Assn.*, **61** (Mar. 1975), 3–9. A reprint from the Oct. 1974 *Consumer Reports* explores the HMO phenomenon, arguments for and against, and offers consumer guidelines for choosing a good one.

Jonas, Steven. *Health Care Delivery in the United States*. New York: Springer Publishing Co., Inc., 1977. An excellent book of readings that includes an overview of health manpower, ambulatory and hospital care, government, health planning, and other major topics.

Joselow, Morris. "Occupational Health in the U.S.—The Next Decades." *Am. J. Pub. Health*, **63** (Nov. 1973), 929–930. A prediction of future developments in the care of workers, involving labor, federal legislation. Anticipated is a greater merging with general health services.

Krause, Elliott. *Power and Illness*. New York: Elsenier North-Holland, Inc. 1977. A controversial analysis of medical care, indicting the present system.

Kress, John and James Singer. *HMO Handbook*, Rockville, Md.: Aspen Systems Corp. 1975. Describes HMOs and provides guidelines on how to start one. Useful in understanding organization of HMOs.

Law, Sylvia, et al. *Blue Cross: What Went Wrong?* New Haven: Yale University Press, 1974. A scathing condemnation of the activities of Blue Cross as the fiscal intermediary for Medicare. One hundred pages of appended notes and documentation show that the formula for determining hospital charges is reasonable by neither marketing or accounting standards. Proposals for improvement are made by the University of Pennsylvania Health Law Project (co-authors) and implications for national health insurance are pointed out.

Lebow, Joy. "Consumer Assessments of the Quality of Medical Care." *Med. Care*, **12** (Apr. 1974), 328–337. Studies using consumer evaluations are reviewed.

Leininger, Madeline. "An Open Health Care System Model." *Nurs. Outlook*, **21** (Mar. 1973), 171–173. Author proposes a model that will allow the clients various routes of entry and exit, and allow them to receive the services of the professionals who can best meet their particular needs.

Levin, Lowell. "Patient Education and Self-Care: How Do They Differ?" *Nurs. Outlook*, **26** (Mar. 1978), 170–175. Author believes the biggest difference is that in self-care education, the learner determines own needs and goals.

Lewis, Charles, et al. *A Right To Health*. New York: John Wiley & Sons, Inc., 1976. An examination of the paradoxes and dilemmas of primary health care in the United States; identification of problems and policy options of the future.

"Life and Death and Medicine." *Sci. Am.* (Sept. 1973). Entire issue on topics such as varied interventions for illness, the hospital, the medical school, organization of medical care, and so on.

Libow, Leslie, et al. "Symposium—Delivery of Geriatric Community Care." *The Gerontologist,* **14** (Aug. 1974), 286–288. Explores issues of leadership and models of delivery.

Lippit, Gordon. "Hospital Organization in the Post-Industrial Society," *Hosp. Prog.,* **54** (June 1973), 75–78. Lists some characteristics of hospital organization in the future, as well as social, philosophical, and psychosocial forces that will influence such change.

Luft, Harold. "How Do Health Maintenance Organizations Achieve Their 'Savings'?" *New Eng. J. Med.,* **91** (June 15, 1978), 1336–1343. Reviews data on HMO costs to enrollees and explores why hospitalizations are fewer.

Lubic, Ruth, and Eunice Ernst. "The Childbearing Center: An Alternative to Conventional Care." *Nurs. Outlook* **26** (Dec. 1978), 754–760. Meeting needs of childbearing families through an out-of-hospital facility, staffed by a health care team who view childbirth as a normal process.

Miller, C. Arden, et al. "A Survey of Local Public Health Departments and Their Directors." *Am. J. Pub. Health,* **67** (Oct. 1977), 931–939. Describes health services rendered by health departments, problems, and constraints.

Mulligan, Joan. "There's an HMO in Your Future: Is Your Future in the HMO?" *J. Nurs. Admin.,* **3** (Sept.-Oct. 1973), 35–38. The type of nurse suitable for an HMO and issues faced by nurse administrators are described.

Navarro, Vicente. "A Critique of the Present and Proposed Strategies for Redistributing Resources in the Health Sector and a Discussion of Alternatives." *Med. Care.,* **12** (Sept. 1974), 721–742. A thought-provoking article that describes physician distribution, current strategies for change implicit in health legislation, and alternative strategies.

Norris, Catherine. "Self Care." *Am. J. Nurs.,* **79** (Mar. 1979), 486–489. Excellent article tracing growth of self-care movement and giving components of self-care.

Nursing and Long-Term Care: Toward Quality Care For The Aging. Kansas City, Mo.: Am. Nurses' Assn., 1975. Document prepared in response to Senate Committee includes recommendations on manpower and options for health care.

Ornstein, Sheldon. "A Nursing Home Is Not a Hospital," *Nurs. Outlook,* **21** (Jan. 1973), 28–31. Differences between hospitals and nursing homes are described, with emphasis on the differing purposes.

Osterweis, Marion and Daphne Champagne. "The U.S. Hospice Movement: Issues in Development," *Am. J. Pub. Health* **69** (May, 1979), 492–496. Overview of issues such as utilization of existing resources, regional planning, standards, licensure and reimbursement.

Pierotte, Doris. "Day Care for the Elderly." *Nurs. Outlook,* **25** (Aug. 1977), 59–523. Describes varied responsibilities of nurses in providing care to the elderly to reverse effects of isolation, dependence, and depression.

Roman, Stanford. "Health Maintenance Organizations: Are They for Inner Cities?" *J. Comm. Health,* **1** (Winter 1975), 127–31. Identifies areas of HMO legislation that may adversely affect inner-city care.

Sloane, Robert, and Beverly Sloane. *A Guide To Health Facilities,* 2nd ed. St. Louis: C.V. Mosby Company, 1977. Concentrates on hospitals, but describes various departments thoroughly. Inaccuracies in nursing section.

Snyder, Lilja. "We Care Enough to Come to You," *Nurs. Outlook,* **22** (Mar. 1974), 168–171. A nurse director of a county nursing service describes how she developed a program of extended health care to small towns and villages via a mobile health van.

Somers, Anne, and Herman Somers. *Health and Health Care: Policies in Perspective.* Germantown, Md.: Aspen Systems Corp., 1977. Divided into four parts of new and earlier writings of authors in historical, critical, and projective views of most facets of health care system. Authors are noted for thoughtful observations of the health care scene.

Somers, Herman. "Health and Public Policy." *Inquiry,* **12** (June 1975), 87–96. A review of federal legislation passed to deal with manpower and organizational health care problems and some political observations on possible new directions.

Smith, David and Arnold Kaluzny. *The White Labyrinth.* Berkeley, Calif.: McCutchan Pub.

Corp. 1975. Provides a systematic understanding of how the U.S. health system and its organizations work.

Shepard, Katherine, and Louise Borsotti. "Family Focus—Transitional Health Care." *Nurs. Outlook,* 23 (Sept. 1975), 574–577. Families and patients learn to cope with problems they will face at home by practicing in simulated home.

Stull, R. J. "Many Concepts Mold Multiinstitutional System." *Hospitals,* **51** (Mar. 1, 1977), 43–45. New organizational patterns of merger and consortia have major implications for hospitals.

Toynbee, Polly. *Patients.* New York: Harcourt Brace Jovanovich, Inc., 1977. A popular bestseller book, originally published in England as *Hospital,* presents a study of an "institution with an absolute grip on the lives of those who pass through it."

Ward, Barbara. "Hospice Home Care Program." *Nurs. Outlook,* **26** (Oct. 1978), 646–649. How the special needs of a dying patient and his family can be met at home.

Warner, Anne. *Innovations in Community Health Nursing.* St. Louis: C.V. Mosby Company, 1978. Exciting first-person accounts by nurse practitioners in a variety of settings from Alaska to Maine.

Widmer, Geraldine, et al. "Home Health Care: Services and Cost," *Nurs. Outlook,* **26** (Aug. 1978), 488–493. Findings of this study document type of services needed to maintain chronically ill patients at home, and cost.

Wilson, Florence and Duncan Neuhauser. *Health Services in the United States.* Cambridge, Mass.: Ballinger Company, 1976. Useful reference on United States health system, including information on health legislation.

See also related books and articles in Chapter 6, as those by Fuchs and Milio. Other good reference sources for current issues, problems, and trends in institutions are *Hospitals,* the *AHA Journal, Hospital Progress,* the CHA journal and other journals in the field, which always include nontechnical articles.

Best sources of current comprehensive data on health resources, although usually several years behind, is the U.S. Department of Health and Human Services (formerly DHEW). Many publications come from the National Center for Health Statistics and are available from the U.S. Government Printing Offices. Good examples: *Health Resources Statistics* and *Health—United States—1976-1977.* The journal *Family and Community Health* puts great emphasis on innovative health care delivery. Almost every issue has several pertinent articles.

Health Care Delivery: Who?

A hundred years ago, trained health manpower consisted of physicians, dentists, some pharmacists, and nurses. Now there are more than 250 acknowledged health occupations, with more being developed every day. Of the five million plus active personnel, the vast majority are in "allied health," defined broadly by HEW to include

> all those professional, technical, and supportive workers in the fields of patient care, public health, and health research who engage in activities that support, complement, or supplement the professional functions of physicians, dentists, and registered nurses, as well as personnel engaged in organized environmental health activities who are expected to have some expertise in environmental health.[1]

Not included in any category are faith healers, root doctors, or certain untrained healers who rely on herbs, meditation, or other semi-self-care techniques of healing. Nor does it include certain supportive services. Health care facilities, as other places of business, employ secretaries, clerks, accountants, receptionists, messengers, and others to carry on business operations. In addition, they need laundry workers, dietary workers, cooks, plumbers, electricians, carpenters, maids, porters, and similar kinds of

employees to function in the hotelkeeping aspect of their services. However, the overwhelming growth of personnel is in direct health services. Many of the health occupations and suboccupations have emerged because of increased specialization in health care, others on the peculiar assumption that several lesser-prepared workers can substitute for the scarcer professional. Some of these workers can be employed in almost any health setting—hospitals, nursing homes, clinics, doctors' offices, occupational health, and school health. Some work primarily in one setting. Most of these workers are not licensed; many are trained in on-the-job programs and even more are trained in a variety of programs with no consistent standards. Others have standardized programs approved by the American Medical Association and/or health organizations.

When health care is equated with medical care, a functional structure emerges, consisting of independent practitioners, dependent practitioners, and supporting staff. Jonas, although acknowledging that the lines separating the groups are unclear at times, describes the independent practitioners as those permitted by law to provide a delimited range of services to anyone who wants them (identified as physicians, dentists, chiropractors, optometrists, and podiatrists); dependent practitioners as those permitted by law to provide a delimited range of services under the supervision and/or authorization of independent practitioners (nurses, social workers, pharmacists, dental hygienists, physicians' assistants, and various therapists); and supporting staff as those carrying out specific tasks authorized by and under the supervision of independent and dependent practitioners, frequently without specific legal delineation of tasks or authority.[2] As Jonas readily agrees, the scope of practice and autonomy of the dependent practitioners are a great source of conflict, particularly because many have an area of expertise not within the knowledge and skills of the independent practitioner. Moreover, the gray areas of overlapping practice are becoming greater; what a particular practitioner does may be legitimately within his/her scope of practice in certain circumstances and just as legitimately that of another in other circumstances. The legal lines drawn also waver when it comes to supportive workers; there are tasks done by nurses' aides or practical nurses that are first of all part of a nurse's responsibility; in times and places of nurse shortages, they are even done with almost no supervision. With a rising acceptance of medical care as a component of health care but not its totality, the independent-dependent status concept of health practitioners will undoubtedly undergo considerable revision.

Credentialing of the health care providers and their educational programs is under a variety of auspices: the state, a single professional organization, or a coalition of professional organizations. As of 1979, the educational programs of twenty-three allied health occupations are accredited by the Committee on Allied Health Education and Accreditation (CAHEA), a collaborative effort of national health organizations and medical specialty organizations with the American Medical Association (AMA). This accreditation process begins with acceptance of minimal requirements for entry into the occupation, labeled the "Essentials," which must be adopted both by the AMA Council on Medical Education and the particular collaborating organizations concerned. Other occupations follow other procedures with their accrediting group. Allied health education programs are most frequently found in or under the auspices of medical schools, universities, colleges, junior colleges, hospitals, and the military.

Practitioners who are not licensed may become certified or registered on a voluntary basis by the occupation's national organization or a parent medical group. The inconsistency of these various processes is the focus of some of the complaints about health care credentialing. In 1977, DHEW listed the following as health personnel licensed in every state: nursing home administrators, chiropractors, dentists, dental hygienists, embalmers, environmental health engineers, practical nurses, professional nurses, optometrists, pharmacists, physical therapists, physicians (MD and DO), podiatrists, psychologists and veterinarians. This does not necessarily mean that licensure is required, only that it is available (see Chapter 20).

Compared to other nations, the United States has a more than ample supply of health workers, even in physician-population ratio. (In some countries, it is the nurses who are in shortest supply). Types of American health workers are also considerably more diverse; other nations have experimented more with such physician substitutes as the Russian feldsher or Chinese barefoot doctor. The largest categories of health workers, in order, are nursing (all types, including aides), physicians, dentists and their allied services, clinical laboratory workers, pharmacists, and radiological technicians. As feminists are the first to point out, manpower is a misnomer; from 75 to 85 per cent are women. However, they are, or have been, in the lower-paid and less powerful positions. Physicians, dentists, administrators, and others in policy making positions are overwhelmingly male.

Except for the independent practitioners who are primarily self-employed, the mass of health workers are employed in institutions and agencies, with the greatest number concentrated in hospitals.

It would be unrealistic to attempt to describe all the professional and technical workers with whom nurses work or interact. However, an introduction to the most prevalent health occupations should provide a better understanding of the complex relationships in health care.

The organization of this chapter is primarily alphabetical, although on occasion two closely related groups may be described in logical succession. The education of RNs and practical nurses is described in Chapters 12 and 13, and the practice of nursing in Chapters 15 and 16.

Administration

Health service administrators manage organizations, agencies, institutions, programs, and services within the health care delivery system. They may work in any setting but are probably more visible in hospitals, nursing homes, neighborhood health centers, and community health agencies. The principles of management can be applied to any setting, and the role of the hospital administrator, described in Chapter 7, is a reasonable example of role and functions. Nurses are usually the administrators of nursing services, but a number also hold positions as top administrators, particularly in community health agencies. Although they may retain their nursing identity, they should be functioning as administrators and have the necessary educational background. Usually, the appropriate credential is a master's degree in health services administration, hospital administration, or, recently, business administration. There are a few baccalaureate programs that prepare for beginning middle management positions.

Other positions in the operation of health facilities and plants are the usual business positions, finance, data processing, personnel, public relations, and admissions, with all types of jobs and educational levels.

Chiropractic

Chiropractic is described by the American Chiropractic Association as "a branch of the healing arts which is concerned with human health and disease processes. Doctors of chiropractic are physicians who consider man as an integrated being, but give special attention to spinal mechanics and neurological, muscular, and vascular relationships." Chiropractors use standard diagnostic measures, but treatment methods, determined by law, do not include prescription drugs and major surgery. Essentially, treatment includes "the chiropractic adjustment, necessary dietary advice and nutritional supplementation, necessary physiotherapeutic measures, and necessary professional counsel."

By 1978, nine chiropractic colleges were either accredited or eligible for accreditation by the Council in Chiropractic Education (CCE), and enrollment was increasing. Successful completion of a minimum of four years of study in the sciences, public health, clinical disciplines, and chiropractic principles and practice, including clinical practice, preceded by two professional years of college, results in a Doctor of Chiropractic diploma. The practitioner may be designated *Doctor of Chiropractic, Chiropractic Physician,* or *Chiropractor.* Most are in private practice. They are licensed in all states, the majority of which require continuing education for relicensure. All fifty states and the District of Columbia and Puerto Rico recognize chiropractic as a health profession and authorize chiropractic services as part of their worker's compensation program, as do many federal health benefits; services are also reimbursable under Medicare and Medicaid. However, in the past, both the AMA and the American Public Health Association (APHA) have passed resolutions in opposition to chiropractic, the AMA defining it as an unscientific cult. Referring patients to chiropractors or accepting referrals was considered unethical. On the other hand, one of the complaints about chiropractic has been that some practitioners continue to treat for diseases such as cancer that are seen as beyond their scope of practice. Nevertheless, there are other physicians who, noting the continual educational upgrading, see the eventual integration of chiropractic into the field of medicine, just as were homeopathy and osteopathy, also once considered unacceptable. Meanwhile, chiropractic is a portal to the health care system for thousands of people who prefer treatment that stresses personal counseling and attention and no use of drugs.

Clinical Laboratory Sciences

There are a number of technicians or technologists working in the clinical laboratories in such specialties as immunohematology, hematology, clinical chemistry, serology, microbiology, and histology. The physician in charge is a pathologist, although technologists may have specific responsibilities for technicians. *Medical technologists'* preparation includes three years of college science plus a year of professional course work in a CAHEA-accredited school covering all phases of clinical laboratory work. Certification is granted by the Board of Registry of Medical Technologists of the American Society of Clinical Pathologists, after successful completion of a board examination. The initials *MT (ASCP)* may then be used. Most states do not require licensure. Additional appropriate education and experience qualify a medical technologist for specialist certification in blood banking, chemistry, microbiology, cytotechnology, or nuclear technology.

Certified laboratory assistants, who perform routine laboratory tests, and *histologic technicians,* who prepare body tissues for microscopic examination by pathologists, are usually prepared in one-year hospital programs, also CAHEA-accredited. Certification is granted after passing an ASCP examination.

Dietary Services

Dietary services may include *dietitians* with general dietary background, those with preparation in medical dietetics, and a host of dietary assistants and other workers. Medical or therapeutic dietitians are responsible for selection of appropriate foods for special diets, patient counseling, and sometimes management of the dietary service.

Clinical dietitions work with patients not in the hospital, but perhaps in clinics, neighborhood health centers, or in their own home. These include pregnant women, diabetics, and those with other nutritional problems.

A baccalaureate program with majors in food, nutrition, and food management is usually basic, with the possible addition of a dietetic internship program approved by the American Dietetic Association. Certification is granted by ADA.

Food service supervisors may be prepared in junior college programs. Two thirds of the approximately 45,000 are employed by hospitals and related institutions. Most are women, although more men are entering the field, which is considered a shortage area.

Dentistry

Dentists treat oral diseases and disorders. They may fill cavities, extract teeth, and provide dentures for patients. Ten per cent of dentists specialize. Specialists are oral surgeons, pedodontists (work with children), orthodontists (correct irregularities of teeth and jaws), periodontists (gum disease specialists), endodontists (root canal therapy). These specialties require two or more additional years of training, and a specialty board examination. Dental school is preceded by two to four years of college with specific science courses; most entering students, however, are college graduates. The dental school curriculum is a three- to four-year course leading to a DDS (Doctor of Dental Surgery) or a DMD (Doctor of Dental Medicine) degree. All dental schools must be approved by the American Dental Association.

Dentists are licensed in all states by taking a state board examination or a National Board of Dental Examiners exam. In some states, specialists must pass a special state examination. Nine out of ten dentists are in private practice; the others practice in institutions, the armed forces, and health agencies, teach, or do research. Most are located in large cities.

Dental Hygienists, almost all women, provide dental services under a dentist's supervision. They examine and clean teeth, give fluoride treatments, take X-rays, and educate patients about proper care of teeth and gums. In many states, hygienists' responsibilities have been expanded to include duties traditionally performed by dentists, such as giving local anesthetics. They are licensed in all states through the National Board of Dental Examiners examinations and are the only ancillary personnel permitted by law to clean teeth. An RDH is awarded after passing a written and practical certification examination.

Education is comprised of a four-year program leading to a BS or a two-year certificate program. Those dental hygienists with master's degrees may be teachers or administrators. The vast majority of dental hygienists practice with dentists in offices. However, in recent years, a few have set up separate private practices, a move strongly opposed by dentists but approved in some states by court decision or attorney general rulings. A degree of resistance to dentist domination over their practice is emerging.

Dental Assistants maintain supplies, keep dental records, schedule appointments, prepare patients for examinations, process X-rays, and assist the dentist at chairside, but the function of dental assistants is also expanding. Most assistants complete a one- or two-year program at a community college or vocational-technical school. These programs award a certificate, diploma, or associate degree.

Health Educators

Community health educators help identify the health learning needs of the community, particularly in terms of prevention of disease and injury. They may then plan, organize, and implement appropriate programs, for example, screening devices, health fairs, classes, and self-help groups. Some health educators are employed by the state as consultants, others by insurance companies, voluntary health organizations such as the Heart Association, the school system (school health educators), and, occasionally, industry. Unfortunately, as governmental funding fluctuates, programs may expand or contract, and health educators may be eliminated or spread thin, as has happened in school health. A number of hospitals are employing *patient educators* or health educators to develop and direct programs of both patient education and community health education. Frequently, these people are nurses with or without training in health education and administration. Health educators usually have baccalaureate or master's degrees in health education, public health, or community health education. Master's degrees may include an administration component.

Medical Records

Medical record administrators are responsible for preparation, collation, and organization of patient records, maintaining an efficient filing system, and making records available to those concerned with the patient's subsequent care. They may also classify and compile data for review committees and researchers. CAHEA accredits both four-year baccalaureate programs and one-year hospital-based programs preceded by a baccalaureate degree. After completion of these programs the candidate qualifies for certification administered by the American Association of Medical Record Librarians. *Medical record technicians* assist the physician and the administrator in preparing reports and transcribing histories and physicals, and work closely with others using patient records. CAHEA-accredited programs are nine months in length and include theoretical instruction and practical hospital experience. *Medical record transcriptionists* have specialized courses in terminology in addition to typing and filing.

Medicine

Doctors of medicine and osteopathy practice prevention, diagnosis, and treatment of disease and injury. *Doctor of medicine degrees (MDs)* are awarded in some 120 medical schools in the United States and are considered the first professional degree. Some physicians may later decide to acquire advanced degrees (master's or doctorates) in an advanced science or public health. Admission into medical schools, after four, occasionally three, years of preprofessional college work is considered highly selective. Programs are usually four years in length with required basic sciences and clinical studies. In the last two years students have clinical clerkships, usually in hospitals, but also in clinics or doctor's offices. In this first contact with patients, they are usually supervised and taught by attending physicians or residents as they apply their clinical and scientific knowledge. Generally, physicians and professors of science are the teachers in medical school, although others include ethicists, sociologists, and, occasionally, a nurse (not usually on a full-time basis). In one medical school, nurse instructors have responsibility for teaching medical students in the clinical clerkship.[3] In most cases, medical education has little interdisciplinary focus, and contacts with other health profession students are seldom formalized, although sometimes students in a multidisciplinary setting develop interactional opportunities of their own.[4]

The formalized program of education after the doctoral (M.D.) degree is titled graduate medical education and consists primarily of the residency, which is preparation for specialties, a period of two to five years. At one time, a one-year internship, usually rotating through the various clinical services, was the norm, but after years of debate and two major reports,[5] in the mid-1960s several changes occurred. Family practice was recognized as a specialty, both the rotating and the free-standing internship (almost a general

working apprenticeship) were abolished, and residencies in hospitals with at least minimal university affiliations were developed. Almost all residency programs now are in such hospitals, but there is still a dichotomy—education on one hand and a functional hospital apprenticeship on the other. Residencies seem to have three distinct components: acquisition of knowledge, skills, and professional behavior. At completion of the specified years of residency, the physician may take certification exams in the specialty and is board-certified; if exams are not taken (or failed), he/she is board-eligible.

For a number of years, there were more first-year residency positions than American medical school graduates, and graduates from foreign medical schools, including Americans, filled positions. In some states, the vast majority were foreign medical graduates (FMGs). Because of differences in the quality of education and language and cultural differences, problems often occurred. Now, however, it is anticipated that there will be so many American medical school graduates that they may have difficulty finding suitable residencies for the specialties desired, and the Congress has cut drastically the number of FMG's. An attempt by the Congress to force medical schools to save places for a certain number of Americans from foreign medical schools was not successful, even with the threat of withholding funds. Although most American physicians choose specialties as their field of practice,* the need for more general practitioners is being met by designation of the field (thus the residency) as a specialty and heavy federal funding for those selecting that field. There is now some concern that by 1985 there may be too many family practitioners as well.

In medical centers, a "fellow" is a postresidency physician who enters even more advanced, highly specialized, or research-or-

---

*The AMA recognizes thirty-four different specialties; the most common are internal medicine, surgery, obstetrics and gynecology, psychiatry, pediatrics, radiology, opthalmology, and pathology.

iented programs, although presumably still involved in teaching and patient care. Graduate medical education is under the direction of medical school faculty recognized as specialists or subspecialists. An irony in medical education is typified by pediatrics. A pediatrician's practice will consist primarily of normal children, some with minor illnesses; yet, his/her education in a medical center is focused on tertiary care patients, whom he/she would not encounter or at least not be in position to care for in the average community hospital that does not have the resources for such complex care. It is partly because of this that nurse practitioners evolved. In some cases, nurse practitioners are also part of the teaching faculty for medical students and residents.[6]

Physician licensure is mandatory in every state, some of which require continuing education for relicensure. Students may choose two routes to licensure, the National Board Examinations given by the National Board of Medical Examiners, for which they must be students or graduates of an American or Canadian medical school, or the Federal Licensing Examination (FLEX) given by the Federation of State Medical Boards. Parts I and II of the Boards are given during the medical school years, with Part III given after the first year of graduate medical education; FLEX may be taken only after the first year of graduate medical education. The individual is not usually fully licensed until after one or the other of these exams is passed; before that, practice is covered by a temporary license or is on a student basis, just as it is with nurses until they have passed state boards. All but two states endorse the National Board certificate for licensure, and all now accept FLEX. Among the physicians not holding a license in any state, besides first-year residents, are the inactive and those engaged in medical teaching, research, or administration.

The major modes of medical practice are described in the preceding chapter, but there are, of course, physicians in every setting where medical care is provided, as well as in medical or public health education, public health practice, and research. Some positions such as that of a medical director are primarily administrative and are beginning to be recognized as such.[7]

Doctors of Osteopathy (DO)

Doctors of Osteopathy (DO) are qualified to be licensed as physicians and to practice all branches of medicine and surgery. DOs graduate from colleges of osteopathic medicine, accredited by the Bureau of Professional Education of the American Osteopathic Association (AOA). Admission to the colleges requires at least three years of preprofessional education at an accredited college or university. The DO degree usually requires four academic years of education; three of the nine accredited colleges have adopted an interdisciplinary approach, allowing for three years. Required basic sciences, anatomy, physiology, biochemistry, pathology, microbiology and pharmacology, are much the same as those in medical schools, as are the clinical courses of medicine, surgery, pediatrics, obstetrics, gynecology, radiology, and preventive medicine. The major difference is the integration of osteopathic principles dealing with the interrelationship of all body systems in health and disease and special training in osteopathic palpatory diagnosis and manipulative therapy. After graduation, almost all DOs serve a twelve-month rotating internship, with primary emphasis on medicine, obstetrics/gynecology, and surgery, conducted in an approved osteopathic hospital. Those wishing to specialize must serve an additional three to five years of residency. Continuing education is required by the AOA for all DOs in practice.

Osteopathic physicians are considered separate but equal in American medicine; they are licensed in all states and have the same rights and obligations as allopathic (MD) physicians. The "something extra" they claim is emphasis on biological mechanisms by which the musculoskeletal system interacts with all body organs and systems in both health and disease. They prescribe drugs, use routine diagnostic measures, perform surgery, and selectively utilize accepted scientific modalities of care. DOs comprise about 5 percent of all physicians; some are general practitioners who provide primary care, usually in towns and cities of less than 50,000 population. The 230 osteopathic hospitals (134 accredited), located in thirty states, usually offer a full range of services. Nursing in osteopathic hospitals is comparable to that in any other hospital.

Physician's Assistants (PAs)

In 1965, Dr. Eugene A. Stead, Jr. inaugurated a program for *physician's assistants,* later called physician's associates, designed to assist physicians in their practice, either to enable them to expand that practice, or to give them time to pursue continuing education, or to have more time for themselves and their families. The students in the Duke University program came from a variety of backgrounds and included nurses and former military corpsmen. Shortly afterward, a series of programs, called MEDEX, developed specifically for ex-corpsmen, were funded by the federal government.

In the early years of these programs, there was a great deal of confusion about the education role, legality, and scope of practice of the PA. Educational programs ran the gamut from a few months of on-the-job training to five years. Formalized programs prepared assistants to the primary care physician as well as in a range of specialties, particularly urology and orthopedics.

In 1970, the National Academy of Sciences categorized the PA in three broad functional areas.

> The Type A assistant is capable of approaching the patient, collecting historical and physical data, organizing these data, and presenting them in such a way that the physician can visualize the medical problem and determine appropriate diagnostic or therapeutic steps. He is also capable of assisting the physician by performing diagnostic and therapeutic procedures and coordinating the roles of other, more technical, assistants. While he functions under the general supervision and responsibility of the physician, he might, under special circumstances and under defined rules, perform without the immediate surveillance of the physician. He is, thus, distinguished by his ability to integrate and interpret findings on the basis of general medical knowledge and to exercise a degree of independent judgment.
>
> The Type B assistant, while not equipped with general knowledge and skills relative to the whole range of medical care, possesses exceptional skill in one clinical specialty or, more commonly, in certain procedures within such a specialty. In his area of specialty, he has a degree of skill beyond that normally possessed by a Type A assistant and perhaps beyond that normally possessed by physicians who are not engaged in the specialty. Because his knowledge and skill are limited to a particular specialty, he is less qualified for independent action. An example of this type of assistant might be one who is highly skilled in the physician's functions associated with a renal dialysis unit and who is capable of performing these functions as required.
>
> The Type C assistant is capable of performing a variety of tasks over the whole range of medical care under the supervision of a physician, although he does not possess the level of medical knowledge necessary to integrate and interpret findings. He is similar to a Type A assistant in the number of areas in which he can perform, but he cannot exercise the degree of independent synthesis and judgment of which Type A is capable. This type of assistant would be to medicine what the practical nurse is to nursing.[8]

Differing levels of education were also recommended for the three groups, from short-term certificate programs to baccalaureate education.

The type A assistant gradually became today's PA; types B and C are in relatively limited or nonjudgmental categories and are considered assistants by various names, but not PAs. Although the AMA generally defines PAs as persons qualified by academic and clinical training to provide patient services under the supervision of a licensed doctor of medicine, a more comprehensive and legally oriented definition, once suggested by Nathan Hershey, is:

> *An individual, not a physician, providing health services as an employee of a physician, or a health care institution such as a hospital or health center, who, under medical supervision and direction, engages in a range of activities and decision making that does not fall completely within the scope of activities of any of the traditional, currently licensed health professions or occupations, and whose range of health care activity includes some tasks and functions now reserved to physicians, and not recognized by laws as within the area of practice of any other health profession or occupation.*

Continued federal funding after 1972 not only encouraged the growth of programs, but pointed in certain directions: training for delivery of primary care in ambulatory settings, placement of graduates in medically underserved areas, and recruitment of residents from these areas as well as minority groups and women. Several changes in programs occurred after that, primarily a concentration on assistants for primary care physicians (fifty-three AMA-accredited programs by 1977), and a disappearance of specialty programs. Only two prepare surgical assistants; there are no other formal accredited programs.[9] Some seventy programs had been listed in 1974, up from twelve in 1972, but most probably did not meet standards for approval that the AMA had set in the early 1970s.

Currently, PA programs range from twelve to forty-two months with the majority being twenty-four months in length. The noted MEDEX program requires twelve to fifteen months of study—three months didactic, followed by a nine- to twelve-month preceptorship with a practicing physician. Upon completion, a student receives a certificate. The university medical center-based program usually consists of nine to twelve months of didactic work in basic and clinical sciences, followed by twelve to fifteen months of various clinical rotations in a tertiary care center and preceptorships with

physicians in private practice. On completion, a student receives a certificate and/or baccalaureate degree. In the college or university program (nonmedical school), nine to twelve months of basic and clinical didactic work is followed by ten to fifteen months of clinical rotations in an affiliated teaching hospital and community-based preceptorship. Upon completion, a student receives a certificate, or an associate or baccalaureate degree.[10] PA programs have been accredited by AMA's Council on Medical Education since 1974.

Although the quality of educational programs was coming under approval mechanisms as early as 1972, there was no evaluation of the products. A certification mechanism was developed under the aegis of the National Board of Medical Examiners (NMBE), and the first exam was given in 1973. NMBE then cooperated with twelve other professional groups to form the free-standing independent National Commission on Certification of Physician's Assistant (NCCPA) in 1975, which has the responsibility for PA certification, including publishing yearly lists by states, of certified PAs, and periodically recertifying PAs through continued demonstration of competency.[11] Since 1976, when approximately 3,000 PAs were certified, about 1,000 a year have taken, or are expected to take, the certifying exam. Only about 10 percent of employed PAs are not certified, particularly because more states are requiring certification for practice.

A joint statement issued in 1972 by the National Board of Medical Examiners and the Association of Physician Assistant Programs identified more than 500 health care functions as those physician's assistants should definitely be skilled in performing. However, generally, PAs are presumed to perform only medical services that are a part of the clinical specialty of the physician supervising them, and these differ according to each specialty. The health services performed by the assistant to the primary care physician include, but are not limited to (1) receiving patients, obtaining case histories, performing appropriate physical examinations, and presenting meaningful resulting data to the physician; (2) performing or assisting in laboratory procedures in the practice setting; (3) giving injections and immunizations; (4) suturing and caring for wounds; (5) providing patient counseling services and referring patients to other health services; (6) responding to emergency situations within their range of skills and experience; (7) assisting the employing physician in all settings—the physician's office, hospitals, extended-care facilities, nursing homes, and so on.

The legality of PA practice was a particularly hot issue in the early 1970s, but by 1979, most states permitted PAs to practice. Most have specific statutes that authorize varied groups of nonphysicians to qualify as PAs and authorize qualified physicians to delegate medical tasks; a smaller number use the medical practice act's exemption clause, which allows physicians to delegate certain activities to selected others under their supervision. PAs are *not* licensed, but the state usually keeps a registration list. The major difference between a PA and a nurse practitioner is that the PA, in all cases, *must* function under the supervision of a physician and cannot function independently. Physicians are legally responsible for their PAs and frequently must include the PAs in their own malpractice insurance.

A 1976 survey reveals some pertinent information about PAs. Most are white males (except MEDEX graduates, who include more minorities), but more women and minorities are being admitted to programs. Thirty percent had been corpsmen, although the next largest, 11.5 and 5.4 percent were RNs, and LPNs respectively. PAs are employed in all fifty states (in some states where their practice has not been legalized, they may be in federal service); one third were in the South. Their major practice settings, according to frequency, were in physician's offices, and the next largest number were in hospitals, although figures overlap and some go to hospitals for or with their employing physician and are not employed by the hospital. Most are in some form of primary care. Apparently, about half work more than forty hours a week, and take call, a fact that is used to explain why their salaries are frequently higher than those of nurse practitioners, even those with master's degrees. The employment rate of PAs is about 95 percent.[12]

There are still many unresolved issues related to PA practice, particularly in relation to role and functions. The American Hospital Association has published a statement on PAs in hospitals, which, overall, indicates that the medical staff and administration should formulate guidelines under which the PA can operate, with the request for the PA to be permitted to practice in the hospital being handled by the medical staff credentials committee. Emphasis is on medical supervision; however, current reality has shown that PAs go unsupervised in busy urban hospitals where they handle many emergency and other ambulatory patients. This has created a problem for nurses, for the authority of PA vis-a-vis nurse is frequently not clear. Although the nurses' associations, some state boards, some courts, and attorneys general have indicated that nurses do not take PA orders, in other states the rulings are the reverse. Because the PA usually functions according to a protocol specified by the employer-physician, there may be an operational agreement reached similar to the basis on which a nurse carries out standing orders or some verbal orders from the physician. Nevertheless, there is frequently interdisciplinary conflict when roles are not clarified.

The future of PAs is uncertain. There is no upward mobility in the field, except for teaching; medical schools are not giving them any special advantages toward admission. Tighter federal funding may put pressure on these programs. Costs are higher than for preparing master's degree nurse practitioners, and PAs have a much more limited scope of practice. To many people, however, including health professionals, the differences between PA and NP are minimal.

Although the expanded role of the nurse has been evolving for some time, it was not until about 1970 that it was clearly defined and that any reasonable number of nurse practitioners were functioning. This was particularly unfortunate in that the PA had, as a new health worker with considerable governmental support, received a great deal of public attention. The fact that both nurse practitioners and PAs performed some of the same medically oriented functions added to the confusion. At the end of 1971, the ANA issued a statement declaring that the term *physician's assistant* should not be applied to any of the nurse practitioners being prepared to function in expanded nursing roles. Other key points that are still valid were:

Several types of assistants are being prepared and utilized to function under the medical direction to extend physicians' services. None of these assistants are prepared to be substitutes for nurses, because nursing practice is more than performance of delegated medical nursing activities. Neither are these assistants acceptable substitutes for physicians. This development is of concern to the nursing profession. Physician's assistants working in a setting where nursing practice is an essential element of health care present problems that flow from the legal and ethical relationships between physicians and nurses. Therefore, nurses and physicians together must clarify the situation. . . .

As other groups have done in the past, physician's assistants are becoming organized in an effort to secure licensure, certification, and other forms of recognition as a distinct health occupation. Until the functions of the physician's assistant are more clearly identified, and generally acceptable standards for training and practice are evident, licensure for their practice by the states should not be attempted. . . .

Because the economic status of each group involved in health care is part of the economic environment of every other group, the American Nurses' Association has a stake in the economic status of the emerging physician's assistant. The ANA reemphasizes that in establishing salary systems, recognition must be given to the character of responsibilities carried, and to requirements for educa-

tion, experience and clinical expertise. In establishing the relationships between salaries of nurses and those of physician's assistants, the differences in their responsibilities, preparation and experience should be taken into account.

Concern about the economic status of nurses and PAs was, and is, realistic. Although nurse practitioners can offer services to the public beyond any that the PA can offer, frequently nurse and PA may be competing for the same job. For a number of reasons the PA not only may be the one employed, but, as noted before, will also receive a higher salary than would be offered to the nurse practitioner. Despite the fact that most physicians tend to say that they prefer nurses to PAs, the truth is that too often doctors have inadequate or no knowledge about the nurse practitioner's capabilities. What they are talking about is a nurse as a physician's assistant. A number of nurses have made this choice, which is certainly theirs to make, although it has caused some negative reaction from other nurses and nursing associations. It is possible that the situation will clarify as more nurse practitioners are prepared in standardized educational programs.

What impact the PA will have on nursing practice remains to be seen. It might be well to consider this warning:

If the physician's assistant becomes, in fact, a foreclosure on the development of increased, enhanced role functioning in nursing, then we think we are making a very serious mistake in terms of the long-run needs of the country. And we would hazard to suggest it will be a serious mistake for the profession of medicine as well as nursing and the health system generally.[13]

However, the crucial question lies in supply and demand. If MDs, NPs, and PAs all continue to be produced at the current rate and the predicted oversupply becomes reality in the next five years, who will survive?

Medical assistants (MAs) are usually employed in physicians' offices where they perform a variety of administrative and clinical tasks to facilitate the work of the doctor; however, some do work in hospitals and clinics. They perform tasks required by the doctor, in accordance with specific state laws, and are supervised by the doctor. The medical assistant, among other things, answers the telephone; greets patients and other callers, makes appointments; handles correspondence and filing; arranges for diagnostic tests, hospital admissions, and surgery; handles patients' accounts and other billings; processes insurance claims, including Medicare; maintains patient records; prepares patients for examinations or treatment; takes temperatures, height, and weight; sterilizes instruments; assists the physician in examining or treating patients; and if trained, performs laboratory procedures.

Requirements for CAHEA-accredited programs include high school graduation or its equivalent and one- (Grade I MA) or two-year (Grade II MA) programs, usually in community colleges, with some practical experience in a physician's office. For a medical assistant in pediatrics, a two-year program is required, and the MA adds to the activities cited previously, special knowledge and skills related to care of children. There are also accredited programs for *ophthalmic medical assistants* who perform routine procedures, such as simple vision testing, obtaining patient histories, changing eye dressings, and administering eye drops or oral medications. Technicians perform more complex duties and may also assist the ophthalmologist in surgery. Assistants complete a one-year program; technicians a two-year associate degree or its equivalent.

Emergency Medical Care

Emergency Medical Technicians (EMTs) respond to medical emergencies and provide immediate care to the critically ill or injured. They may administer cardiac resuscitation, treat shock, provide initial care to poison or burn victims, and transport patients to a health facility. EMTs do not determine the extent of illness, but set priorities in emergency care at the scene of the emergency, and monitor victims on the way to a hospital,

often functioning under doctor or nurse voice directions or protocols. They are also responsible for the ambulance and supplies. EMTs are trained in a U.S. Department of Transportation (DOT) course, offered under various auspices (police, hospitals, health departments). There is a National Registry of EMTs. Many serve as volunteers on ambulances, but, as noted in Chapter 7, paid EMT services are increasing. Some EMTs also have training as dispatchers.

Paramedics, a popular term that seems to encompass other allied health workers, is also applied to EMTs with advanced training, working at a more sophisticated level in emergency situations. They may defibrillate, administer intravenous fluids, do gastric lavage, and give medications by injection, also acting under physician/nurse voice direction when necessary. Completion of an EMT course and an additional 500 hours or more in paramedic program classes and clinical training is generally expected.

Nursing Support Personnel

Nursing assistants, nurses' aides, orderlies, and attendants functioning under the direction of nurses are all part of the group of ancillary workers prepared to assist in nursing care, performing many of the simple nursing tasks, as well as other helping activities besides nursing. As a rule, training has been on the job and geared to the needs of the particular employing institution, but there is some increase in public school programs within vocational high school tracks or as outside public education services. The program may vary in length from six to eight weeks or more and costs little or nothing. Commercial programs usually cost the student an unreasonable amount, make unrealistic promises of jobs, and frequently give no clinical experience; therefore these "graduates" are seldom employed. Sometimes students dropping out of certain practical nurse programs after six weeks receive a certificate as aides. In-service education during employment is relatively common. It should be remembered that the difference in training, patient care assisgnment, and ability may be enormous on both an individual and institutional basis. These workers are not licensed or certified.

Community Health Aides of various kinds are found in ambulatory care settings. "Indigenous" health aides evolved because not enough physicians or public health nurses were available to help families described as disadvantaged to identify and correct their multiple, related medical and social problems. In addition, professionals do not always communicate effectively with disadvantaged minority clientele. Therefore, in those areas of service, community people are sometimes recruited and trained as health aides. Many are women, not previously trained as vocational nurses or hospital aides. There is usually a limited didactic period with ongoing supervision and on-the-job instruction. Certain technical skills are learned, such as auditory and visual screening, but, primarily, the purpose is to identify health problems or deficiencies, such as lack of immunization, poor oral hygiene, dermatological problems, child development problems, and to assist and encourage families to seek and continue necessary medical, nursing, and other services. Although specific changes in the health status of the community are difficult to measure, on an anecdotal basis, evaluation seems to be positive. These workers may be based in a clinic, neighborhood health center, or other ambulatory care facility, and may also go into the community to do case-finding rather than wait for the client to appear in the formal health facility.

As more attention is focused on keeping people at home rather than in institutions, the services of *homemaker/home health aides* have become reimbursable by Medicaid and Medicare under certain circumstances. The National Council for Homemaker/Home Health Aide Services, which has developed a program of basic standards, defines this worker as a trained, supervised person who works as a full-fledged member of a team of professional and allied workers providing health and/or social services. The aide is assigned to the home of a family or individual when home life is disrupted by illness, disability, or social disadvantage, or if the family unit is in danger of breakdown because of stress. Specific tasks include parenting, performing or helping in household tasks, providing personal care such as bed baths, or helping with prescribed exercises, and providing emotional support. Educational programs are usually developed by the employing agency, and an NCHHHAS-approved program requires a minimum of forty hours of classroom and laboratory instruction to prepare the individual for on-the-job functioning. Most are women who already have housekeeping skills; even so, there is some question as to how effectively they can really be prepared in the limited time suggested. There is an increasing tendency for proprietary agencies to have homemaker/home health care services, and to contract these workers out to voluntary agencies. Although there is evidence that a well-trained, conscientious home/health aide can be extremely helpful to a sick person or disrupted family, there are also some serious problems in the selection of workers, the quality of training, and supervision. There are also some reimbursement problems when the homemaking part of the aide's function is reimbursable and the health part is not, or vice versa. However, the homemaker/home health aide is usually one person doing whichever aspect of the job is needed and is reimbursed in a particular situation. The term *home health aide*, introduced in the Medicare Act in 1965, was added to the older term *homemaker*. The first homemaker services were made available in 1923 to substitute for a hospitalized mother. In the Depression, "housekeeping aides" were subsidized by the government to provide work for needy women. They were assigned to assist families with children, the aged, or the chronically ill. Most often, a combination of the services is needed by the client. Ongoing assessment by health professionals is intended to evaluate the need of the family/client for specific services.

The lack of reimbursement often prevents the use of homemaker/home health aides, for full service from a proprietary agency can cost hundreds of dollars a month. Still, it is less costly health service than institutional care, and the National Council places the need at 300,000 as opposed to some 50,000 now available.

Operating room technicians (ORTs), or *surgical technicians,* or *surgical technologists* have increased considerably in the last fifteen years. They function particularly in the operating room and, sometimes, the delivery room. ORTs, under the direction of the operating room supervisor, an RN, perform required tasks, such as setting up for surgery, preparing instruments and other equipment before surgery, "scrubbing in" for surgery (assisting the surgeons by handing instruments, sutures, and so on), and otherwise assisting in the operating room.

Educational programs are most frequently offered by hospitals and some community colleges. It is recommended that they be at least a year in length, although some hospitals prepare ORTs in a short-term, intensive program plus on-the-job training. Teachers are usually operating room nurses, preferably with teaching background. Programs had been approved by the Association of Operating Room Nurses, but in 1972, AMA assumed some accrediting functions; many programs are now CAHEA-accredited. Courses include orientation to the operating room, some basic sciences, safe patient care, surgical procedures, and clinical practice. The Association of Operating Room Technicians has started a program for certifying ORTs, and the number of employers expected to require this certification will increase in the next few years.

The *psychiatric technician* works in psychiatric and general hospitals, community mental health centers, and the home, working with the mentally disturbed, disabled, or retarded under the direction of a physician and/or nurse. In hospitals, he or she is concerned with the patient's daily life affecting his physical, mental, and emotional well-being, including eating, sleeping, recreation, development of work skills, adjustment, and individual and social relations. In the community, focus is on social relationships and

adjustments. In the hospital, psychiatric technicians are expected to give some routine and emergency physical nursing care, but their close contact with patients makes observation and reporting of the patient's behavior particularly important. In some institutions they function almost independently in group therapy and counseling, seeking consultation as necessary. They may be skilled in nursing, communication techniques, counseling, training techniques, and group therapy. The educational program has generally been one year long but an emerging standard seems to be a two-year associate degree program, which includes social and physical sciences, health education, laboratory work in group and interpersonal processes, and clinical experience. In some states psychiatric technicians have the opportunity to become licensed, sometimes under the Nursing Board.

Ward (unit) clerks or *ward (unit) secretaries* are usually trained on the job in an in-service program to assist in the clerical duties involved in the administration of a nursing unit. Ward clerks order supplies, keep certain records, answer telephones, take messages, attend to the massive amount of routine paper work and, in some cases, copy doctors' orders. This relieves the charge nurse to concentrate on administration of patient care instead of paper work. In the more advanced hospitals, unit clerks are on duty at least on the day and evening shifts and sometimes at night.

Unit managers take even broader responsibilities in the management of a patient unit (usually in a larger institution) and may report directly to hospital administration instead of nursing service administration. Unit clerks often function under the direction of unit managers. In some institutions, unit management is an early step in an administrative career, and managers have full administrative responsibilities.

Podiatry

Podiatrists, doctors of podiatric medicine (DPM) (once called chiropodists), are professionally trained foot care specialists who diagnose, treat, and try to prevent diseases, injuries, and deformities of the feet. Treatment may include surgery, medication, physical therapy, setting fractures, and preparing orthoses (supporting devices which mechanically rearrange the weight-bearing structures of the foot). Podiatrists may note symptoms of diseases manifested in the feet and legs and refer the patient to a physician.

Podiatrists complete a four-year program of classroom and clinical work in a college of podiatry after a minimum of two years of college. The National Board of Podiatry Examiners gives examinations that satisfy the requirements for licensure in more than forty states. Other states use their own examinations; some require an internship, and an increasing number are requiring continuing education.

Most podiatrists are in private practice; others practice in institutions, agencies, the military, education, and research.

Public Health—Environment

Industrial hygienists deal with how noise, dust, vapor radiation, and other hazards common to industry affect workers' health. They are usually employed by industry, laboratories, insurance companies, or government to detect and correct these hazards. Their education may include a baccalaureate in environmental health, engineering, or a physical or biological science.

Sanitarians, sometimes called environmentalists, apply technical knowledge to solve problems of sanitation in a community. They develop and implement methods to control those factors in the environment that affect health and safety, such as rodent control, sanitary conditions in schools, hotels, restaurants, areas of food production and sales. Most work in government, under the direction of a health officer or administrator. Education is generally a BS in public health or the physical or biological sciences.

Pharmacy

Pharmacists are specialists in the science of drugs and require a thorough knowledge of chemistry and physiology. They may dispense prescription and nonprescription drugs, compound special preparations or dosage forms, serve as consultants, and advise physicians on selection and effects of drugs.

With the increase of prepackaged drugs, pharmacists in hospitals and clinics are particularly interested in a more patient-oriented approach to their practice. They may be involved in patient rounds, patient teaching, and consultation with nurses and physicians. In many hospitals, pharmacists are assisted by aides. The educational program of pharmacists is usually a five-year baccalaureate program including two or more years of professional course work. Five-year programs give the bachelor's degree; six-year programs, the Pharm D (Doctor of Pharmacy). Pharmacists are licensed in every state.

Radiology

Radiologists are physicians dealing with all forms of radiant energy, from X-rays to radioactive isotopes; they interpret radiographic studies and prescribe therapy for diseases, particularly malignancies. A number of technicians work under the direction of a radiologist in radiology departments.

The *radiologic technologist,* sometimes called *X-ray technician* or *radiology technician,* is concerned with the proper operation of X-ray equipment, preparation of patients for X-rays and therapy, developing of film, and some clerical work. Programs are usually two-year CAHEA-accredited hospital certificate programs, sometimes affiliated with a college or university. The graduate may become registered (AT) after passing an examination given by the American Registry of Radiologic Technicians. Two states licensed radiology technicians in 1977.

The *radiation therapy technicians* or *technologists* assist the radiologist in treatment of disease by exposing affected areas of the patient's body to prescribed doses of radiation, operating and controlling complex equipment and devices, and maintaining records. A twelve-month CAHEA-accredited program requires that the student be an RN with a college-level course in radiation physics or a radiologic technologist.

A *nuclear medicine technologist* works with radioactive isotopes administered to patients for diagnosis and treatment. He or she positions and attends to patients, abstracts data from records, assists in the operation of scanning devices using isotopes, and has responsibility for safe storage of radioactive materials and disposal of wastes. CAHEA accredits both AD programs for technicians and baccalaureate programs for technologists. The latter must first be medical or radiological technologists or nurses.

Psychology, Psychotherapy and Mental Health

Psychology is the scientific study of mental processes and behavior and psychotherapy refers generally to techniques for treating mental illness by psychological means, primarily through establishing communication between the therapist and the patients as a means of understanding and modifying behavior. In the field of mental health there is a great overlapping of therapists treating the patient with various kinds of mental problems. Besides the physician (the psychiatrist), clinical psychologists, psychotherapists, nurses, social workers, and a variety of semiprofessionals trained in mental health participate in individual and group therapy. *Psychologists* may also give and interpret various personality and behavioral tests, as might a *psychometrician*, who is skilled in the testing and measuring of mental and psychological ability, efficiency, potentials, and functions. Education for psychologists and psychotherapists is often at the master's or doctoral level. Clinical psychologists have training in a clinical setting.

Rehabilitation Services

Occupational therapy is concerned with the use of purposeful activity in the promotion and maintenance of health, prevention of disability, evaluation of behavior, and as treatment of persons with physical or psychosocial dysfunction, using a wide spectrum of treatment procedures based on activities of a creative, social, self-care, educational, and vocational nature. One important responsibility is helping patients with activities of daily living. *Occupational therapists*, the professional workers, and *occupational therapy assistants and aides* are usually employed in hospitals. However, OTs may also be in private practice or work for nursing homes or community agencies. Professional education for the occupational therapists is a baccalaureate program or a postbaccalaureate program and six to nine months of field experience leading to a certificate or master's degree. There are about sixty professional programs accredited by the CAHEA.

The American Occupational Therapy Association certifies for the professional entry level occupational therapist registered (OTR) or certified occupational therapy assistant (COTA). In some institutions, professional occupational therapists are assisted by OT assistants or aides, who may be trained in community colleges or on the job. They participate directly in the patient's activities.

Physical therapy is concerned with the restoration of function and the prevention of disability following disease, injury, or loss of body part, and sometimes physical therapy is concerned with diagnosis. The goal is to improve circulation; strengthen muscles; encourage return of motion; train or retrain the patient, with the use of prosthetics, crutches, walkers, and so on, exercise, heat, cold, electricity, ultrasound, and massage. Most *physical therapists and PT aides* work in hospitals, but PTs may also work in private practice or for other agencies. The physical therapist designs the patient's program of treatment, based on the physician's stated prescription of objectives. He or she may participate in giving the therapy and/or evaluate the patient's needs and capacities and provide psychological support. The aides work directly under the physical therapist's supervision, with limited participation in the therapeutic program. As in occupational therapy, education for the PT is on the baccalaureate or postbaccalaureate level, leading to a certificate or master's degree, which may be CAHEA-accredited. Registration is possible through the American Registry of Physical Therapists, and all states now license PTs. There has been some limited effort to require licensure of physical therapist assistants, whose education is usually at the assciate degree level.

Prosthetists make artificial limb substitutes. *Orthotists* make and fit braces. Both work with physicians and other therapists and have direct patient contact to promote total rehabilitation services. A bachelor's degree in prosthetics or orthotics plus one year of clinical experience is usual; for those with a bachelor's degree, special four- to eight-month programs in hospitals or special university courses and clinical experience are available. Orthotic/prosthetic technicians make and repair devices but usually have no patient contact. Education is primarily in vocational/technical schools.

Rehabilitation counselors help people with physical, mental, or social disabilities begin or return to a satisfying life, including an appropriate job. They may counsel about job opportunities and training, assist in job placement, and help the person to adjust to a new work situation. The usual requirement is a two-year master's degree. Others assisting in patient rehabilitation include *art therapists, dance therapists,* and *music therapists* who work primarily with the emotionally disturbed, mentally retarded, or physically handicapped. *Recreational therapists* or *therapeutic recreationists* may plan and supervise recreation programs that include athletics, arts and crafts, parties, gardening, or camping. Professional status usually requires a master's degree, although some therapists have only a bachelor's degree; assistants are generally prepared at the associate degree level.

Respiratory Therapy

Respiratory (formerly inhalation) therapy personnel perform procedures essential in maintaining life in seriously ill patients with respiratory problems and assist in treatment of heart and lung ailments. Under medical supervision the *respiratory therapy technician* administers various types of gas, aerosol, and breathing treatments, assists with long-term continuous artificial ventilation, cleans, sterilizes, and maintains equipment, and keeps patient records. The *respiratory therapist* may be engaged in similar tasks, but his/her more extensive knowledge of sciences and clinical medicine allows for the exercise of more judgment and acceptance of greater responsibility in performing therapeutic procedures. Respiratory therapy personnel usually work in hospitals and clinics.

A CAHEA-accredited program for technicians is one year long; certification is available. A therapist program, also CAHEA-accredited, may culminate in an associate or baccalaureate degree, with a minimum of two years required. The baccalaureate programs sometimes build on the AD program and prepare for supervision and teaching. Respiratory therapists may be registered, but were licensed in only one state as of 1977.

Social Work

The *social worker* attempts to help individuals and their families resolve their social problems, utilizing community and governmental resources as necessary. Social workers are employed by community and governmental agencies as well as hospitals, clinics, and nursing homes. If the social worker's focus is on patients and families, he or she may be called a *medical* or *psychiatric social worker.* A master's degree is required for full professional status of social workers, and membership in the National Association of Social Workers is open only to social workers graduated from, or students of, accredited schools of social work. Certification is granted by the Academy of Certified Social Workers after other criteria are met.

Social workers also have assistants and aides, who sometimes carry a client load in certain agencies. There may be only on-the-job training available for these workers, but in order to move upward they must acquire additional education. Some employers prefer a two-year associate degree in human or social services, even for this assisting level.

Speech Pathology and Audiology

Speech therapists and *audiologists* are specialists in communication disorders. Speech pathologists or therapists diagnose and treat speech and language disorders that may stem from a variety of causes. Speech therapists are particularly valuable in assisting patients whose speech has been affected by a cerebrovascular accident or patients with laryngectomies. Audiologists often work with children and may detect and assist with the hearing disorder of a child who has been mistakenly labeled retarded. Education for both specialties is at a master's level. There is some activity toward requiring state licensure. The American Speech and Hearing Association offers a Certificate of Clinical Competence after specific criteria are fulfilled.

Vision Care

Ophthalmologists are physicians who treat diseases of the eye and perform surgery, but they may also examine eyes and prescribe corrective glasses and exercises. *Optometrists*, doctors of optometry (OD), are educated and clinically trained to examine, diagnose, and treat conditions of the vision system, but they refer clients with eye diseases and other health problems to physicians. After a variety of diagnostic tests, they may prescribe corrective lenses, contact lenses, and special optical aids as well as corrective eye exercises to provide maximum vision. Some may specialize in such areas as prescribing and fitting contact lenses.

A minimum of six years' education is required, with two years of college before optometry school. About twelve schools and colleges are accredited by the American Optometric Association Council. All states require licensure by state board examinations; some states accept the National Board of Optometry examinations.

The majority of optometrists are in private office practice; others are in group practice, hospitals, public health agencies, research institutions, manufacturing organizations, the military, other government agencies, or are teaching and doing research in colleges and universities. There is an increasing role for optometrists in large hospitals. It is predicted by the profession that future emphasis will be in preventive optometry.

Optometric assistants assist optometrists by performing simple office and patient care duties. *Technicians* may also assist in office tasks, but usually assist in vision training and testing. Assistants complete a one-year certificate or diploma program; technicians, a two-year associate degree in paraoptometrics, given by vocational-technical institutes, two- and four-year colleges, colleges of optometry, and the military.

Opticians grind lenses, make eyeglasses, and fit and adjust them. Both AD programs or on-the-job apprenticeship qualify individuals for this job. *Optical laboratory technicians and mechanics* may be involved in polishing and grinding lenses.

Other Health Workers

There are a number of other health workers not described in this chapter, such as those in science and engineering—anatomists, biologists, biostaticians, biomedical engineers (who design patient care equipment such as dialysis machines, pacemakers, heart-lung machines), and biomedical technicians (who maintain and repair the equipment); technicians dealing with instrumentation—diagnostic medical sonographers, electrocardiograph (EKG/ECG) technicians, electroencephalographic (EEG) technologists and technicians; specialists in dealing with the visually handicapped; biological photographers; medical illustrators, patient advocates (see Chapter 22), acupuncturists, and health science librarians, to name just a few. In addition, volunteers provide many useful services. That this list is not complete and is expanding may help to explain, no matter how valuable individual services may be, why the public often becomes angered by the fragmentation of services. Even health professionals may be unsure as to who does

TABLE 8–1
Estimated Number of Persons Employed in Selected Occupations Within the Health Care Field, 1976

Health Field	Number	Health Field	Number
Total*	5,051,050 to 5,088,950		
Administration of Health Services	48,200	Midwifery	4,350
Anthropology & Sociology	1,900	Nursing & Related Services	2,484,000
Automatic Data Processing	4,300 to 5,400	Occupational Therapy	17,000 to 18,000
Basic Sciences	65,000	Opticianry	12,000
Biomedical Engineering	13,000	Optometry	25,100 to 25,300
Chiropractic	18,200	Pharmacy	121,500
Clinical Laboratory Services	193,000	Physician Extender Services	5,000
Dentistry & Allied Services	321,300	Physical Therapy	32,100
Dietetic & Nutritional Services	77,000	Podiatric Medicine	7,100
Economic Research	500	Psychology	71,000
Environmental Sanitation	23,000 to 25,000	Radiologic Technology	100,000
Food & Drug Services	51,100	Respiratory Therapy	25,000
Funeral Directors & Embalmers	50,000	Secretarial/Office Services	275,000 to 300,000
Health & Vital Statistics	1,350	Social Work	47,300
Health Education	23,000	Special Rehab. Services	13,700
Health Info. & Communication	8,400 to 10,000	Speech Pathology/Audiology	30,000
Library Services	10,300	Veterinary Medicine	36,000
Medical Records	65,000	Vocational Rehabilitation	18,000
Medicine & Osteopathy	393,700	Miscellaneous Health Services	355,450 to 360,950

*Each occupation is counted only once. For example, all physicians are in the medicine and osteopathy category.
 Statistics are not available on what percentage of the estimated 215,000 physical scientists are employed in the health field.
Source: Adapted from U.S. Dept. HEW: *Health Resources Statistics,* 1976-77 edition.

what or when for the client's well-being. Yet, this list is not exaggerated; all are part of what the federal government calls health manpower and allied health manpower, for which federal funds are often distributed for educational programs.

It is clear that if the public is to receive the services it requires, expects, and deserves, there must be direction given through the health care delivery maze.

ISSUES IN HEALTH MANPOWER

Many of the most serious issues in health manpower—numbers, distribution, proliferation, and especially quality of care have become issues focused on credentialing. This multifaceted process, which has become a major concern of the state and federal governments, is given full attention in Chapter 20.

However, the problem of health man-

power planning transcends or, perhaps, precedes credentialing. The blame for proliferation of manpower is difficult to pinpoint. Is it the practitioners or administrators who see the immediate need for quickly prepared assistants? Or is it the federal government that encourages proliferation through education and reimbursement support? The health care industry (and it *is* one of the largest industries in the United States) is labor-intensive. Health manpower frequently creates its own demands: if a certain type of practitioner is available, the availability of that service to the consumer expands—and, as the critics say, adds to the total cost of care.

Predicting demand and supply is no easy matter: development of health manpower resources may take as little as a few months or as long as ten years; in that time both demand and supply may shift rapidly; decisions on whether to expand or contract either education programs or health services frequently depend on uncontrollable external factors, such as the economy; current manpower data are inexact and usually out of date. Thus, it is not surprising that even the most educated guesses of demand and supply often err. What *is* left behind all too frequently is a mass of undereducated, poorly paid, non-cost-effective workers with little job mobility, poor motivation, and built-in anger. The result is increased union activity, and labor unions are accused of causing escalating costs. It is true that in the 1960s improved salaries were a major budget item, and the need to move from what were often below-poverty wages to living wages was largely responsible for the jump. Since that catch-up period, the masses of workers have a new aggressiveness that affects not only monetary considerations, but power issues. Some are not necessarily in the best interests of the consumer. Nevertheless, one of the trends widely predicted is aggressive action by unions to organize every type of health worker—professional, technical, aide, clerical, maintenance, and housekeeping.

The issue of maldistribution is also not easily resolved. Maldistribution of professionals, toward attractive urban and suburban areas and away from isolated, poor, or ghetto areas, is a major problem. In some cases, nurses, physician's assistants, physician-nurse, or physician-PA and/or nurse teams are giving as good or better care than solo practitioners, but the service gap still exists. Even federal intervention, such as requiring service in medically underserved areas (about 30 percent of the United States) in return for supporting the practitioners' education has had only short-term results—practitioners leave after their required service.

Health manpower education is a major issue. How many? What kind? Prepared where? Financed by whom? The education for all levels of health service practitioners is under scrutiny. Why is this education so costly? Could institutions develop more economical teaching-learning methods? Are minority groups being actively recruited? Are the types of workers in proper proportion?

Should the government continue to subsidize the education of high-earning professionals? How much should any health profession be subsidized, and for whom—the programs or students? Are the practitioners appropriately prepared to give safe and effective care?

Another concern is the workability of the health care team. It is naive to expect that by bringing together a highly diverse group of people and calling them a team that they will behave as a team. One obvious gap is their lack of communication and "practice" together, either as students or full practitioners. Sports teams practice together intensively for long periods of time, both to develop a team spirit and to enhance and coordinate their individual skills to produce a functioning unit. Not only do health care teams not have (or take) time to practice together, but often there are serious territorial disputes as areas of practice overlap more and more. As for patients, who should be members of the team, unless they are assertive, their only participation is as recipients of care. Theoretically, legally clear distinctions of each profession would be helpful; practically, it is impossible. Successful coordination depends on collegial behavior and trust and full, frequent, open communication; otherwise, valuable participants in health care will continue to be underutilized. It has also been said that "society can no longer afford to use the physician as gatekeeper to control the flow of patients in and out of the health system."[14] Physician services should be saved to assist patients who need that level and domain of services. In other words, there must be other fully acknowledged practitioners in primary health care.

One overriding issue is, who has power or should have power to make these decisions? The consumer? But, who advises the consumer? All too often, the power figures in health care make policy, even if indirectly, by their input into legislation or major influential groups. For instance, a 1978 study report on manpower policy for primary health care by the prestigious Institute of Medicine of the National Academy of Sciences showed noticeable incongruities between the body of the report, based on numerous informational and analytical papers, and the recommendations. Whereas the data indicated a need for preventive care and health teaching, and the body of the report emphasized the importance of teamwork, equal reimbursement, and accountability of all professionals, there was no mention of prevention in the recommendations. Most related to physician education and reimbursement, and one specifically stated that nurse practitioners should be supervised by physicians if providing any medical services. Physicians on the committee outnumbered by three to one any other represented group. However, one nurse on the committee, pointed out the discrepancies in what was titled "Comment" at the end of the report.

If there are any clear answers to these questions and issues, they have not been found or accepted. Consumers' restlessness with professional indecision and evasion of their concerns and complaints is reaching a critical stage. Even so, the action or nonaction of health planning groups, with major consumer input, shows that the politics of health care influences the behavior of both the practitioners and the consumers.

REFERENCES

1. Maryland Pennell and David Hoover, *Health Manpower Source Book 21: Allied Health Manpower Supply and Requirements 1950–1980* (Bethesda, Md.: US-DHEW, 1970), p. 3.
2. Steven Jonas, *Health Care Delivery in the United States* (New York: Springer Publishing Co., Inc., 1977), p. 69.
3. Cathy Luginbill, "Nurse Instructors for Medical Students," *Am. J. Nurs.*, **78**: 868–870. (May 1978).
4. Lynda Boyer, et al., "A Student–Run Course in Interprofessional Relations," *J. Med. Ed.*, **52**: 183–189 (Mar. 1977).
5. Rosemary Stevens, "Graduate Medical Education: A Continuing History," *J. Med. Ed.*, **53**: 1–18 (Jan. 1978).
6. Len Hughes Andrus, et al., "A New Teacher in Medical Education: The Family Nurse Practitioner," *J. Med. Ed.*, **52**: 896–900 (Nov. 1977).
7. K. J. Williams, "The Role of the Medical Director," *Hosp. Prog.* **59**: 50–57 (June 1978).
8. Report of the Ad Hoc Panel on New Members of the Physician's Health Team of the Board of Medicine of the National Academy of Sciences, *New Members of the Physician's Health Team: Physician's Assistants* (Washington, D.C.: National Academy of Sciences, 1970).
9. Judy Light, et al., "Physician Assistant: A Profile of the Profession, 1976," *P.A.J.* **7**: 109–123 (Fall 1977).
10. D. W. Fisher and S. Horowitz, "The Physician's Assistant: Profile of a New Health Profession," in *The New Health Professionals*, ed. by Ann Bliss and Eva Cohen. (Germantown, Md.: Aspen Systems Corp. 1977), pp. 42–43.
11. D. Glazer, "National Commission on Certification of Physician's Assistants: A Precedent in Collaboration," in *The New Health Professionals*, ed. by Ann Bliss and Eva Cohen (Germantown, Md.: Aspen Systems Corp., 1977), pp. 86–92.
12. Light, op cit., 109–123.
13. *Nurse Clinician and Physician's Assistant: The Relationship Between Two Emerging Practitioner Concepts* (Rochester, N.Y.: The National Commission for the Study of Nursing and Nursing Education, 1971).
14. Virginia Cleland and Dawn Zagornik, "Appropriate Use of Health Professionals," *J. of Nurs. Admin.*, **1**:39 (Nov.-Dec. 1971).

BIBLIOGRAPHY

Barkin, Roger. "Need for Statutory Legitimation of the Roles of Physician's Assistants." *Health Service Reports* **89** (Jan.-Feb. 1974), 31–36. Reviews three types of PAs and reviews some legislation and court decisions relating to MD and PA functions.

Beckhard, R. "Organizational Issues in the Team Delivery of Comprehensive Health Care," *Milbank Memorial Fund Quarterly*, **50** (July 1972), 287–316. Analyzes some of the issues in making health teams an effective means of primary family health care. Problems of role definition, decision making, communication, and goal setting must be resolved if health teams are going to work.

Bellin, Lowell. "Should a Paper on the Administration of Chiropractic Have Been Published in *Medical Care?* With Comments on Derivative Questions," *Medical Care,* **11** (Sept.-Oct. 1973), 441–448. An MD professor of public health comments on negative reaction of physicians to Dintenfass article cited later here.

Bistrov, V. "The Education of Medical Personnel in the USSR," *Am. J. of Pub. Health,* **64** (Feb. 1976), 149–154. An interesting discussion of how the Russians train their health personnel at various levels. Of particular comparative interest is their use of "core" curricula.

Bliss, Ann, and Eva Cohen, ed. *The New Health Professionals.* Germantown, Md.: Aspen Systems, Inc., 1977. Excellent series of papers on role, functions, determinants of practice, and evaluative research on PAs and NPs.

Challenor, Bernard, et al. "An Educational Program for Allied Health Personnel," *Am. J. of Pub. Health,* **62** (1972), 223–228. Detailed discussion of training of family health workers in Boston in joint model cities-university program.

Cleland, Virginia, and D. Zagornik. "Appropriate Utilization of Health Professionals," *J. of Nurs. Admin.* **1** (Nov-Dec. 1971), 37–40. Thoughtful consideration of utilization of health professionals and need for collegial relationships.

Dintenfass, Julius. "The Administration of Chiropractic in the New York City Medicaid Program." *Medical Care,* **11** (Jan-Feb 1973), 40–51. Describes historical evaluation, administration, level of participation and legal problems.

Edwards, Charles C. "A Candid Look at Health Manpower Problems." *J. of Med. Ed.,* **49** (Jan. 1974), 19–26. Raises somewhat unconventional questions such as, "Aren't there too many physicians?" and "Shouldn't we allow the Health Professions Education Act to lapse?"

Fenninger, L. D. "Health Manpower and the Education of Health Personnel." *Inquiry,* **10** (Mar. 1973), Suppl: 56–60. With health personnel being input, not output, how should education be paid for? How can the federal government coordinate its many manpower programs and assure quality education, not just numbers of graduates?

Fink, Paul Jay. "A Question of Identity: Physician Versus Physician's Assistant." *J. of Med. Ed.,* **50** (Feb. 1975), 190–191. Interesting short article on physician and PA identity. Makes a statement about nurses and why physicians want PA to be different from nurse.

Friedson, Eliot. *Profession of Medicine.* New York: Dodd, Mead & Company, 1970. Classic book looking at medicine from sociological point of view.

Gale, Charlotte. "Walking in the Aide's Shoes," *Am. J. of Nurs.,* **73** (Apr. 1973), 628–631. A nurse masquerading as an aide learns why aides become angry and frustrated by their work, often because of lack of recognition by nurses.

George, Madelon, Ide Kazuyaski, and Clara Vambery. "The Comprehensive Health Team: A Conceptual Model," *J. Nurs. Admin.,* **1** (Mar.-Apr. 1971), 9–13. Description of a model to assist health professionals to identify the specific functions and shared responsibilities of team members as they relate to patient-family needs.

Giacalone, Joseph, and James Hudson. "Primary Care Education Trends in U.S. Medical Schools and Teaching Hospitals." *J. Med. Ed.,* **52** (Dec. 1977), 971–981. Survey data indicate continued emphasis on education in ambulatory care, less interest in HMOs, more schools with affiliated generalist residency programs, and about the same number of PA and NP programs.

Gortner, Alan, and Frank Riessman. "New Training for New Services," from *Social Work* (Nov. 1972), in *Nurs. Digest,* **1** (July 1973), 69–78. Notes the need for consumer-centered human services and how individuals may be trained for such services more rapidly and efficiently through similation.

Greenfield, Sheldon et al. "Efficiency and Cost of Primary Care by Nurses and Physician Assistants." *N. Eng. J. Med.,* **298** (Feb. 9, 1978), 305–309. A prospective study in an HMO indicates that PAs and NPs save physicians time and reduce costs.

Grenvik, Ake. "Role of Allied Health Professionals in Critical Care Medicine." *Crit. Care Med.,* **2** (Jan.-Feb. 1974), 1–10. Discusses role of respiratory therapists, PTs, radiology technologists, and a variety of other technicians and technologists.

Handschu, S.S. "Profile of the Nurse's Aide: Expanding Her Role as Psychosocial Companion to the Nursing Home Resident." *Gerontologist,* **13** (Oct. 1973), 315–317. A study of more than 200 nurse's aides working in nursing homes reveals that most have minimal salaries, little training, no built-in rewards to the job. Recommended are better utilization and opportunity for upward mobility.

Heath, Sister Mary Clare. "The Medical Technologist's Changing Environment." *Hosp. Prog.*, **54** (Oct. 1973), 82–85. The new role of the medical technologist is described as one performing preventive as well as confirmatory and diagnostic procedures and correlating findings with other health professionals.

Holmes, Jean. "The Physical Therapist and Team Care." *Nurs. Outlook*, **20** (Mar. 1972), 182–184. Stresses the importance of effective communication between physical therapists and nurses in a community health setting.

Isler, Charlotte. "Day Hospitals for the Chronically Ill?" *RN*, **37** (Apr. 1974), 36–39. Report of a three-year project in which chronically ill, disabled elderly people attended a rehabilitation day care center. Nurses act as coordinators and help provide support and teaching for patients and family.

Kinsinger, Robert. "What This Country Doesn't Need Is a Left Carotid Artery Technician or a Career-Based Response to the 'New Careers' Scramble." *J. Allied Health* **2** (Feb. 1973), 10–15. A look at the problems created by the tremendous fragmentation of tasks in the tendency to create more specialized health technicians and some suggestions for change.

Lewy, Robert. "The Emergence of the Family Practitioner: An Historical Analysis of a New Specialty." *J. Med. Ed.*, **52** (Nov. 1977), 873–881. Describes how this new specialty area arose to replace the general practitioner and the difference between GPs and FPs.

Light, Judy, et al. "Physician Assistant: A Profile of the Profession, 1976." *PAJ* **7** (Fall 1977), 109–123. Summary of findings of national survey. Includes demographic data, types and numbers of programs, certification, hours worked, and salary.

Lippard, Vernon, and E. Purcell, eds. *Intermediate-Level Health Practitioners*. New York: Josiah Macy Jr. Foundation, 1973. Report of a conference focused on development and utilization of PAs and NPs.

Love, Judith et al. "Medical Manpower Models: Need, Demand and Supply." *Inquiry* **12** 97–125. Describes six methods of determining whether physician shortage exists, with emphasis on surveying health status of population. Extensive bibliography.

Moeller, Dade, et al. "Trends in University Environmental Health Research and Training." *Am. J. of Pub. Health*, **68** (Feb. 1979), 125–129. Survey of 150 college and university programs shows major increase in environmental health programs. Types of training and job selection are discussed.

Mosey, Anne. "Meeting Health Needs," from *Am. J. Occup. Ther.*, (Jan. 1973), in *Nurs. Dig.*, **2** (May 1974), 93–96. Stresses the importance of meeting the individual's general health needs, not only those of illness.

Musser, A.W. "Equivalency Testing: A Partial Solution to the Health Manpower Problem." *J. of Med. Ed.*, **48** (June 1973), 579–580. Like college "life experience" credits, health providers need equivalency testing. Tentative beginnings in the laboratory area.

Navarro, Vicente. "Women in Health Care." *New Engl. J. of Med.*, **292** (Feb. 20, 1975), 398–407. Statistics on women in health show few women at well-paid "top" but many at underpaid "bottom" of ladder. Calls for change.

Nelson, Eugene, Arthur Jacobs, and Kenneth Johnson. "Patients' Acceptance of Physician's Assistants." *JAMA*, **228** (Apr. 1, 1974), 63–67. Survey of 900 patients indicated good acceptance of PA. Certain attitudes are found to be related to patients' age, social class, and access to medical services.

Parlapiano, Martha. "Role Differentiation: OR Nurse-OR Technician." *AORN J.*, **15** (Mar. 1972), 30–44. Three views of the OR technician are given in relation to the past, the present, and predictions for the future. The OR nurse is seen in a leadership role, functioning with technicians on the team on a one-to-one basis. Still useful.

Pluckhan, Margaret. "Professional Territoriality —A Problem Affecting the Delivery of Health Care." *Nurs. Forum*, **11** (Summer 1972), 300–310. An interesting comparison of the concept of territoriality, common in animals, including man, and the tendency of health professionals and subgroups within the profession to protect their own territory to the detriment of health care.

Pomrinse, S. David. "The Crisis in the Health Care System." *Hosp. Admin.*, **19** (Winter 1974), 10–29. The author considers what is good and bad about our complex health care system and how it can be improved.

Rosinski, Edwin. "Education and Role of the Physician." *JAMA*, **222** (Oct. 23, 1972), 473–475. A redefinition of the role of the physician is described, with categories of medical practitioner, medical clinician, and medical scientist.

Routh, Thomas. *The Volunteer and Community Agencies*. Springfield, Ill.: Charles C. Thomas,

Publisher, 1972. An overview of, and basic orientation to, use of volunteers in service programs of community agencies.

Richter, R., et al. "The Community Health Worker: A Resource for Improved Health Care Delivery." *Am. J. of Pub. Health,* **64** (Nov. 1974), 1056–1061. Detailed discussion of recruitment, training, and utilization of community workers for screening, treatment, and follow-up of persons with hypertension and related diseases.

Roemer, Ruth. "Manpower: How Five Nations Respond to the Issues." *Hospitals,* **48**(22) (Nov. 16, 1974), 41–46. Australia, Canada, Belgium, and Norway are compared to the United States on issues of new types of personnel, effective utilization, education, regulation, and licensure. Licensure is much more important in the United States than elsewhere where all graduates are registered.

Rothberg, June. S. "Nurse and PA: Issues and Relationships." *Nurs. Outlook,* **21** (Mar. 1973), 154–158. Gender and professional jealousy have caused strained relations between these two groups.

Sadler, Alfred, Blair Sadler, and Ann Bliss. *The Physician's Assistant—Today and Tomorrow.* New Haven, Conn.: Yale University School of Medicine, 1972. Written by a physician, lawyer, and nurse, all involved with a PA program, this book presents an overview of issues, problems, and promises related to the preparation and utilization of the PA as seen at that time.

Scheffler, Richard, et al. "A Manpower Policy for Primary Health Care." *New Engl. J. of Med.,* **298** (May 11, 1978), 1058–1062. This article abstracts the major findings and recommendations of the National Academy of Sciences report, *A Manpower Policy for Primary Care,* but does not acknowledge Ford's objections cited in this chapter. Original report should be read to get total picture.

Smith, Richard A. "MEDEX." *J. AMA,* **211** (Mar. 16, 1970), 1843–1845. Discussion of conception and development of MEDEX program in Washington. Fifteen ex-corpsmen began the first class in June 1969.

Somers, Anne, and Florence Moore. "Homemaker Services—Essential Option for the Elderly." *Pub. Health Reports,* **91** (Aug. 1976), 354–359. Describes tasks and qualifications of homemakers, standards, accreditation, costs, financing, and needs.

Soroka, Mort. "Optometry in the Hospital: An Evolving Profession." *Am. J. of Pub. Health,* **68** (Apr. 1978), 404–406. Discusses increase of optometry in institutional settings and appropriate utilization.

Stevens, Rosemary. "Graduate Medical Education: A Continuing History." *J. Med. Ed.,* **53** (Jan. 1978), 1–18. Describes issues of definition of graduate medical education, control, responsibility, role in hospitals, distribution.

Torrey, F. et al. "The Family Health Worker Revisited: A Five-Year Follow-up." *Am. J. of Pub. Health,* **63** (Jan. 1973); 71–74. Problems of role expectation, lack of self-esteem, lack of mobility, and pressures for licensure are discussed.

Vanable, Eleanor. "The Professional Role of the General Hygienist as Viewed by Accreditation Commissioners and Consultants." *J. Dent. Ed.,* **41** (Dec. 1977), 730–734. As an interesting corollary to medicine and nursing, dentists see the ideal dental hygienist as skilled technician, willing to serve patients and dentists, leaving decisions regarding the practice of dental hygiene to dentists.

Way, Peter, et al. "Foreign Medical Graduates and the Issue of Substantial Description of Medical Services." *New Engl. J. of Med.,* **299** (Oct. 5, 1978), 745–751. Estimates effect of federal legislation that limits number of FMG's and makes suggestions for transition.

Wingert, Willis, et al. "Effectiveness and Efficiency of Indigenous Health Aides in a Pediatric Outpatient Department." *Am. J. Pub. Health,* **65** (Aug. 1975), 849–857. The effectiveness of indigenous health aides in providing health care supervision and coordination for indigent families is asserted and compared with that of PHNs.

Young, Lucie. "Physician's Assistants and the Law." *Nurs. Outlook,* **20** (Jan. 1972), 36–41. Review of existing legislation for the physician's assistant, including various approaches to legalizing the role. Basic information still useful.

See also Jonas, and Sloane & Sloane, and DHEW publications listed in Chapter 7, and footnoted citations in Chapter 8. For more information on specific occupations, the journals of that occupation are useful resources. For additional background on PAs, see the medical, hospital, and nursing journals of the late 1960s and early 1970s, which have a variety of articles that particularly address the emerging roles and the controversies.

NURSING IN THE HEALTH CARE SCENE

Nursing as a Profession

DEFINITIONS OF NURSING

Because the word *nurse* has certain connotations and because there are long-lived public images of nursing, concepts of the profession of nursing not only differ, but are contradictory and frequently inaccurate. Nursing implies a mother-child relationship, tending, watching over. Schulman notes that nursing's long historical orientation has been based upon a concept of "mother-surrogate," a role "characterized by affection, intimacy, and physical proximity, with an orientation for meeting the needs of a dependent ward," providing for protection and identification. The other nursing role he sees as contradictory, even antagonistic— the "healer, change-oriented, dynamic, discontinuous, and fragmentary."[1]

There seems to be a public concept of equating nursing with illness. Current dictionaries define *nurse* as someone trained to care for sick people. Moreover, since the proliferation of nurses' aides and practical nurses after World War II, the public is even more confused as to who is the nurse. It is not unusual for patients to call anyone in a uniform, who gives them personal care, nurse. Perhaps life was simpler when it was protocol for only the registered nurse to wear a white, long-sleeved uniform, white shoes and stockings, and, most important, the starched white cap and special pin of the nursing school, or, at least, the easily identified navy blue of the public health nurse. It was a symbol, a tradition, an image that came packaged with preconceived notions of what that uniformed figure could do. (Never mind that years ago, one key nursing figure described the uniform as a housedress and the cap as a dust cap).

Nurses tend to cherish a traditional image, even as they move into new roles and live uncomfortably with a blurred self-image. Kramer points out that nursing students enter schools with the concept that "real" nursing is bedside care, and that nursing programs can seldom remove that image, even if they try.[2] But, says one outspoken nurse, "real" nurses also engage in research, deliver babies, teach health, do psychotherapy, administer anesthesia, hang out a shingle, diagnose patients and clients; "real" nurses work not only in hospitals, but in jails, homes, clinics, colleges, schools, industry, and in the most rural as well as urban areas. And most of all, "real" nurses use their brains as well as their hands and feet.[3]

There are many interpretations of nursing. Why not? There are many facets to nursing,

156

and perhaps it isn't logical or accurate to settle on one point of view. All nurses must eventually determine their own philosophies of nursing, whether or not these are formalized. The public and others outside nursing will probably continue to adopt a concept or image that is nurtured by contact, hearsay, or education about the profession, and the first may be the most powerful determinant. This chapter seeks to present an overview of the components of nursing, examined in the light of professionalism, legal, and other definitions, nursing process, nursing theory, nursing diagnosis, and nursing standards.

PROFESSIONS AND PROFESSIONALISM

Almost everyone talks about the nursing profession in the sense of an organized group of persons, all of whom are engaged in nursing (the phrase is used often throughout these pages). But another question discussed both within and without the ranks of nursing is whether or not nursing as a whole is an occupation, rather than a profession in the same sense that medicine, theology, and law have been called professions since the Middle Ages. (Crossword puzzles in a distinguished newspaper consistently use *hospital aide* for the crossword that spells out *nurse.*)

Professions have been historically linked with universities or other specialized institutions of learning, implying a certain high level of scholarly learning and study, including research. The specific criteria for a profession vary and are spelled out more fully in some of the bibliography for this chapter. There is fairly general agreement, however, that professionalism centers on specialized expertise, autonomy, and service. A profession:

1. Provides services vital to human and social welfare.
2. Has it own special body of knowledge (theory) on which its skills and services are based, and continually expands this body of knowledge through continuing investigation, analysis, and research.
3. Involves essentially intellectual operations, accompanied by considerable individual responsibility.
4. Educates its practitioners in institutions of higher education.
5. Establishes and controls its own policies and activities, that is, its practitioners have relative independence in performance of their functions and activities.
6. Attracts individuals whose primary motivation is service, rather than personal gain, and who conceive of their occupation as a lifework.
7. Has a code of ethics that guides the conduct of its practitioners.
8. Has an association that fosters and ensures quality of practice.

It should be pointed out, however, that the term *profession* is essentially a social concept and has no meaning apart from society. Society decides that for its needs to be met in a certain respect a body undertaking to meet these particular needs will be given special consideration. The contract is, however, that the individuals of that favored group continually use their best endeavor to meet those obligations, constantly re-examining and scrutinizing their functions for appropriateness, and maintaining competence. When they fail to honor these obligations and/or slip into demanding status, authority, and privilege that have no connection with carrying out their professional work satisfactorily, society may reconsider. A profession is seen as a body of individuals voluntarily subordinating themselves to a standard of social morality more exacting than that of the community in general. "Only so far as this implicit contract is observed will a profession *as a profession* survive."[4] That violation of this code eventually brings retribution from society is evidenced today in the tightening of laws regulating professional practice and reimbursement. Certain behaviors, such as unprofessional conduct, may be specifically punished by removal of the practitioner's legal right to practice—licensure. What comprises unprofessional conduct may, again, vary from state to state, and also in time, particularly on such points as immorality. This is discussed more fully in Chapter 20.

Because professionalism obviously brings with it certain real advantages, practitioners of all kinds of occupations seek professional status. Many seek it through licensure which confers some of the privileges (and responsibilities) of professionalism. An interesting model of professionalism has been described as a "spectre" in which occupations are classified by degrees of professionalism, from unskilled employees upward to independent practitioners. In the "crown" of professionalism are the independent practitioners. Surrounding them are the employed professionals, and, holding a part of the pool or core of professional attributes, the semi-professional employees. Further down are skilled and unskilled employees. The lines between all of these are broken to show the possibility of mobility over time, both as individuals move upward and as occupations may move toward professional status. The further away from the crown the worker is, the less independent of the organization or bureaucracy.[5] On the other hand, despite the prestige of professionalism, many concepts that were traditionally held are fading. For instance, collective bargaining, unionism, and strikes, once seen as the antithesis of professionalism, have been gradually accepted as legitimate activities by professionals who are employed. Physicians, nurses, teachers, social workers, and others have chosen that route as the only means left to gain certain concessions from employers. Obviously, the very fact that more professionals are employed, and thus lack a degree of autonomy, has precipitated this change.

In addition, there is an increasing tendency to use the term *professional* in another context to describe one who has an assured competence in a particular field or occupation, such as a hairdresser, or someone who participates in an activity for pay as opposed to an amateur—a musician, artist, baseball player. It is particularly interesting to note the changes in dictionary definitions over the

years to include the last two concepts. Looking at it in the "pure" sense, however, the idea of professionalism has been called the most important and powerful in the belief system of nursing. But this ideology does not seem to provide all nurses with common beliefs and ideals about the profession.[6]

The Nature of Nursing: Some Definitions

In *Notes on Nursing: What It Is and What It is Not,* Florence Nightingale states in the most basic terms that nursing is to "put the patient in the best condition for nature to act upon him." Since that time, a number of other definitions have evolved, but the emphasis on care has not diminished, even in the scientific era. Definitions of nursing vary according to the philosophy of an individual or group, and interpretations of roles and functions vary accordingly.

One contemporary nurse says, "Nursing is the art of helping people feel better—as simple and as complex as this."[7] Another includes a spiritual component:

> *Nursing in its broadest sense may be defined as an art and science which involves the whole patient—body, mind, and spirit; promotes his spiritual, mental, and physical health by teaching and by example; stresses health education and health preservation as well as ministration to the sick; involves the care of the patient's environment—social and spiritual as well as physical; and gives health service to the family and the community as well as to the individual.*[8]

A new graduate said that nursing means technical skill, but also caring, understanding, supporting, teaching, and, most of all, being there.[9]

A classic definition used by nurses internationally is that of Virginia Henderson, a distinguished American nursing educator and writer.

> *The unique function of the nurse is to assist the individual, sick or well, in the performance of those activities contributing to health or its recovery (or to peaceful death) that he would perform unaided if he had the necessary strength, will or knowledge. And to do*

this in such a way as to help him gain inde-
pendence as rapidly as possible. This aspect
of her work, this part of her function, she
initiates and controls; of this she is master.
In addition she helps the patient to carry out
the therapeutic plan as initiated by the physi-
cian. She also, as a member of a medical
team, helps other members, as they in turn
help her, to plan and carry out the total pro-
gram whether it be for the improvement of
health, or the recovery from illness or support
in death. . . .[10]

Many other of today's nursing leaders hold
similar concepts, worded somewhat differently or expanded into other configurations.
Schlotfeldt states:

Nursing is an essential service to all of
mankind. That service can be succinctly de-
scribed in terms of its focus, goal, jurisdic-
tion, and outcomes as that of assessing and
enhancing the general health status, health
assets, and health potentials of all human
beings. It is a service provided for persons
who are essentially well, those who are in-
firm, ill, or disabled, those who are develop-
ing, and those who are declining. Nurses
serve all people—sometimes individuals and
sometimes collectives. They appropriately
provide primary, episodic, and long-term
care and, as professionals, are independently
accountable for the execution and conse-
quences of all nursing services.[11]

Rogers noted that "nursing's first line of
defense is promotion of health and prevention of illness. Care of the sick is resorted to
when our first line of defense fails."[12] In the
ANA position paper of 1965, the terms *care,*
cure, and *coordination* were used as part of a
definition of *professional practice* (see Chapter 12), and this phrase has been used numerous times, with individual interpretation of
the components.

As nurses expand their functions into the
new nurse practitioner role, *cure* has acquired a different meaning for some nurses,
as management of the patient's care, which
includes aspects of what has been medical
diagnosis and treatment. Some nurses, like
Rogers, feel that such medical (not nursing)
diagnosis and treatment diminishes the role

of the nurse as a nurse. (The same opponents
also usually reject the term *nurse practi-*
tioner.) However, Ford, a pioneer of the
nurse practitioner movement, calls this
"semantic roulette" and adds, "I'm not so
concerned about the words. I'm convinced
that nursing can take on that level of accountability of professional practice that involves the consumer in decision making in
his care and also demands sophisticated clinical judgment to determine levels of illness
and wellness and design a plan of management."[13] Ingeborg Mauksch voices similar
sentiments,[14] as did the multidisciplinary
group reporting to the Secretary of HEW.[15]
This group addressed itself to the need for
extending the scope of nursing practice in
primary, acute, and long-term care. However, the role of nursing in primary care,
with or without medically oriented skills, is
receiving major attention. Fagin maintains
that primary care has been the academic discipline of nursing, since its public health evolution in the early days of nursing.

Nursing is defined as including the promotion
and maintenance of health, prevention of ill-
ness, care of persons during acute phases of
illness, and rehabilitation and restoration of
health. Are these not also the functions
of primary care as described by most
writers. . . ?[16]

Although, over the years, nursing has been
defined in specific situations according to the
functions of nurses or the clinical fields in
which they practice, or the specific job titles
they may hold, there is a thread throughout
the definitions that indicates the focus of
nursing is the health of whole human beings
in interaction with their environment—a
wholistic,* humanistic focus. The ANA 1973
Standards of Practice states, "Nursing practice is a direct service, goal-directed, and

---

*The term "wholistic" seems to have been coined to
refer to care related to the "whole" patient, physical
and psychosocial. "Holistic" now generally refers to
paranormal healing, an aspect of which is described in
the Krieger article listed in the bibliography. However,
usage is not consistent and "holistic" is used by some
authors in the sense of "wholistic."

adaptable to the needs of the individual, family, and community during health and illness. Professional practitioners of nursing bear primary responsibility and accountability for the nursing care clients/patients receive.''

Finally, a major professional statement declares:

> Unless the potential for nursing's contribution to the health and well-being of people is fully integrated from the planning stage through implementation and evaluation of health care, it will not be possible to deliver quality health services.
>
> Nursing services are the keystone of health care delivery. Nursing's contribution to health care becomes evident at the participant-planning level of determination of health systems and subsystems.
>
> Another contribution of nursing is the coordination of health services within the health system and its subsystems in order that people may have accessible movement into the system and quality comprehensive health services can be realized.
>
> The major contribution of nursing is the delivery of humanistic care to people based on personal health needs. Nursing's expertise (in addition to the traditional restorative care provided in acute care settings) is care of people with respect to health assessment, health maintenance, care of people with problems of long-term disabilities (both in and out of institutions), and the provision of coordination and continuity of health care services. . . .[17]

Nursing Functions

Nursing functions can be described in broad or specific terms. For instance, classically, the common elements have included maintaining or restoring normal life function, observing and reporting signs of actual or potential change in a patient's status, assessing his/her physical and emotional state and immediate environment, formulating and carrying out a plan for the provision of nursing care based on a medical regimen including administration of medications and treatments and interpretation of treatment and rehabilitative regimens, counseling families in relation to other health-related services, and

teaching. The nurse practitioner role adds diagnosing and treating common illnesses. Of course, some nurses still see the nurse more as a manager of nursing care than as a face-to-face clinical practitioner—in other words, responsible for nursing care, supervising and coordinating the work of others, but not personally giving care. However, in recent years, there has been a return to a clinical emphasis.

The evolving role of the nurse is a particular focus of attention. One example is the description of functions delineated by a group of independent nurse practitioners, which specifically indicates differences between medical and nursing practice and stresses concern with the whole person and his reaction to illness rather than the disease itself.[18] In one study nursing educators projected evolving functions as data gathering, including history taking and assessment; nursing diagnosis (and some aspects of medical diagnosis); nursing intervention; evaluation, including evaluation of nursing team performance and evaluation of community resources; and administration, including carrying twenty-four-hour responsibility for nursing care.[19]

In defining functions that should be common to all nurses, Schlotfeldt identifies the following:

1. Interviewing to obtain accurate health histories.
2. Examining, with use of all senses and technological aids, to ascertain the health status of persons served.
3. Evaluating to draw valid inferences concerning individuals' health assets and potentials.
4. Referring to physicians and dentists those persons whose health status indicates the need for differential diagnoses and the institution of therapies.
5. Referring to other helping professionals those persons who need assistance with problems that fall within the province of clergymen, social workers, homemakers, lawyers, and others.
6. Caring for persons during periods of their dependence, to include:

a. *compensating for deficits of those unable to maintain normal functions and to execute their prescribed therapies;*

b. *sustaining and supporting persons while reinforcing the natural, developmental, and reparative processes available to human beings in their quest for wholeness, function, comfort, and self-fulfillment;*

c. *teaching and guiding persons in their pursuit of optimal wellness;*

d. *motivating persons toward active, knowledgeable involvement in seeking health and in executing their needed therapies.*

7. *Collaborating with other health professionals and with persons served in planning and executing programs of health care and diagnostic and treatment services.*

8. *Evaluating in concert with consumers, other providers, and policy-makers the efficacy of the health care system and planning for its continuous improvement.* [20]

The degree of expertise with which a nurse carries out these functions depends on his/her level of knowledge and skills, but the profession has the responsibility of setting standards for its practitioners. In its *1973 Standards of Nursing Practice* (see Chapter 10), the ANA incorporated and ordered standards in a nursing process sequence.

The Nursing Process

Yura and Walsh state that the term *nursing process* was not prevalent in the nursing literature until the mid-1960s, with limited mention in the 1950s.[21] Orlando was one of the earliest authors to use the term,[22] but it was slow to be adopted. In the next few years, models of the activities in which nurses engaged were developed, and in 1967, a faculty group at The Catholic University of America specifically identified the phases of the nursing process as assessing, planning, implementing, and evaluating.[23] The nursing process is described as "an orderly, systematic manner of determining the client's problems, making plans to solve them, initiating the plan, or assigning others to implement it, and evaluating the extent to which the plan was effective in resolving the problems identified."[24]

At this point, there is considerable information in the nursing literature about the use of the nursing process, and many schools of nursing use it as a framework for teaching.

Nursing Theories, Concepts, and Models

As nursing has developed in professionalism, nursing scholars have developed theories of nursing, and the science of nursing is coming of age. A theoretical base of practice defines nursing's uniqueness; that is, it has a science of its own and is not simply an extension of another profession. In scientific inquiry, observations of seemingly unrelated phenomena are organized into intelligible systems that show relationships among the phenomena and a linking of truths.[25] "Nursing research describes, understands, and predicts the life process of man, supporting the probability that nursing can intervene effectively to promote the maximum health of the well and ill in individuals and social groups."[26] Nursing theory is the umbrella encompassing the concepts.

A number of conceptual models and theories upon which nursing curricula are now based have been developed.

The *behavioral system model* is generally credited to Dorothy Johnson. This theory views nursing's client as one or more behavioral systems in interaction with the environment. Nursing's goal of action is to maintain or restore the person's behavioral system balance and stability or to help the person achieve a more optimum level of functioning (balance) when this is possible and desirable.[27]

The *adaptation model* developed by Sister Callista Roy[28] includes the concepts that man is a biopsychosocial being; man is in constant interaction with a changing environment; to cope with a changing world, man uses both innate and acquired mechanisms, which are biological, psychological, and social in origin; health and illness are one inevitable dimension of man's life; to respond positively to environmental changes, man must adapt; man's adaptation is a function of the stimuli to which he is exposed and his adaptation level; man's adaptation level is such that it comprises a zone which indicates the range of stimulation that will lead to a positive response. (If the stimulus is within the zone, the person responds positively. If, however, the stimulus is outside the zone, the person cannot make a positive response); man has four modes of adaptation: physiological needs, self-concept, role function, and interdependence relations. The nurse's role is assessment, diagnosis, and intervention.

Roy states that assessment includes plotting the point on the health-illness continuum at which a patient currently rests, evaluating factors which influence him, and judging how effective his coping mechanisms are in a specific situation. Intervention, she describes as changing the person's response potential by bringing the stimuli within a zone where a positive response is possible.

Martha Roger's *Science of Unitary Man* includes a complex series of principles: helicy, resonancy, and complementarity, called principles of homeodynamics. An early Rogers publication describes the basic postulates of the theory and a schematic interpretation of man in the universe, depicting man moving through time and space as an integral part of an expanding universe, from the infinite past to the infinite future, which implies man's movement toward potential states of maximum well-being.[29]

Humanistic nursing practice theory, conceived by Josephine Patterson and Loretta Zderad, proposes that nurses consciously and deliberately approach nursing as an existential experience. Then, they reflect on the experience and phenomenologically describe the calls they receive, their responses, and what they come to know from their presence in the nursing situation. It is believed that compilation and complementary syntheses of these phenomenological descriptions over time will build and make explicit a science of nursing.[30]

The *general theory of nursing,* formulated by Dorothea Orem, is constituted from three related theories: the theory of self-care as explanatory of the actions that individuals "personally initiate and perform on their own behalf in maintaining" their own human functioning, health, and well-being (the theory also extends to care of dependent family members); the theory of deficits for engagement in self-care or care of dependents when the deficit is attributed to health state or health care requirements as explanatory of why individuals or groups can be helped through nursing; and the theory that nursing systems are the end products created and made by nurses through their endeavors in nursing practice situations. A nursing system is conceptualized as a hierarchy of three interlocking systems, a social system arising from the contractual relation of the nurse(s) to the person(s) under care; an interpersonal system arising from the interactions of these persons; and a technological system constituted from the self-connecting links among (1) the nurse's power to provide nursing to others, (2) the power of the nurse's patient or client to care for self or dependents, and (3) the totality of the care actions required now or in the future. The general theory of nursing is seen as useful in explaining all instances in which individuals or groups could objectively benefit from nursing and all instances in which nursing is provided to concrete and particular individuals and groups.[31]

Finally, Myra Levine lists four conservation *principles of nursing* that have as a postulate the unity and integrity of the individual. Nursing intervention is based on the principles of conservation of energy, structural integrity, personal integrity, and social integrity. She believes that the holistic approach to nursing care depends upon recognition of the integrated response of the individual arising from the internal environment and the interaction that occurs with the external environment.[32]

Nursing Diagnosis

The ability to make a *nursing* diagnosis and to prescribe *nursing* actions are basic to the development of nursing science.

Provision of nursing care is a problem-solving process. The nurse first gathers data about her patient, then identifies the problem. An approach to the problem is selected and carried out. Finally, the results of this approach, in terms of consequences for the patient, are evaluated. By using this process the nurse can individualize her care and be accountable for providing a scientifically based service. Nursing diagnosis is the title given to the stage of identifying the problem.[33]

A diagnostic taxonomy (a set of classifications which are ordered and arranged on the basis of a single principle or set of principles) has been in the development stage for several years and will serve as a major communication tool among nurses. It could also facilitate public understanding of what nurses do; just as physicians can pinpoint what they do in relation to treating diseases, nurses can point out nursing diagnosis as the patient problems they try to resolve.

The growth of nursing diagnosis and nursing theories have been major developments in nursing in the last twenty years. Imperative now is continued and strengthened clinical research to develop and refine these nursing theories that can serve as guides for nursing practice and as measurements of the extent to which nursing action attains its goals in terms of patient behavior.

Legal Definition of Nursing

No discussion of nursing as a profession would be complete without considering the legal definition of nursing that regulates the nurse's practice. These definitions vary from state to state, and the nursing practice acts in which they are embodied are currently in an overwhelming stage of transition. One of the major purposes of the changes was to bring these definitions into line with the current and anticipated expansion of nursing practice, although the need to meet other demands of social change was also a factor. Therefore, the model definition of nursing developed by the American Nurses' Association in the early 1950s was no longer totally appropriate. The urgency felt by the profession to clarify and legitimatize these new dimensions of nursing practice, which were being threatened by obsolete licensure laws, precipitated action on the state level, before another model law was developed by ANA in 1976. By 1978, almost all states had enacted updated laws or were in the process of considering such action. In 1979, a special committee of the ANA Congress for Nursing Practice completed "Suggested State Legislation for a Nursing Practice Act." The components of licensure laws, with emphasis on nursing and nurses' scope of practice, is given full attention in Chapter 20. However, in the context of this chapter it is probably useful to look at how *profession* is used in nurse licensure laws.

The first licensure laws used the term *registered nurses*. There were, of course, only trained and untrained nurses, and getting acceptance of standards for the registered nurse was difficult enough. By 1955, most nursing licensure laws were using a variation of the ANA model law, which began,

The practice of professional nursing means the performance for compensation of any act in the observation, care, and counsel of the ill, injured, or infirm, or in the maintenance of health or prevention of illness of others, or in the supervision and teaching of other personnel, or the administration of medications and treatments as prescribed by a licensed physician or dentist; requiring substantial specialized judgment and skill and based on knowledge and application of the principles of biological, physical, and social science. (The foregoing shall not be deemed to include acts of diagnosis or prescription of therapeutic or corrective measures.)

The definition distinguished between independent acts that the nurse might perform, but also identified certain dependent acts and prohibited diagnosis and treatment (not preceded by the word medical). At about the same time, practical nurse licensure was gaining momentum, and the model definitions used the term *practical nursing.*

The practice of practical nursing means the performance for compensation of selected acts in the care of the ill, injured, or infirm under the direction of a registered professional nurse or a licensed physician or a licensed dentist; and not requiring the substantial specialized skill, judgment, and knowledge required in professional nursing.

Thus, there was a clear distinction as to independence between the two types of nurses, which seemed to serve the purposes of the time. The 1976 ANA model law, recommending one nursing practice law with provisions for licensing practitioners of nursing, uses the terms *registered nurse* and *practical/ vocational nurse.*

The practice of nursing as performed by a registered nurse is a process in which substantial specialized knowledge derived from the biological, physical, and behavioral sciences is applied to the care, treatment, counsel, and health teaching of persons who are experiencing changes in the normal health processes; or who require assistance in the maintenance of health or the management of illness, injury, or infirmity, or in the achievement of a dignified death; and such additional acts as are recognized by the nursing profession as proper to be performed by a registered nurse.

Practical/vocational nursing means the performance under the supervision of a registered nurse of those services required in observing and caring for the ill, injured, or infirm, in promoting preventive measures in community health, in acting to safeguard life and health, in administering treatment and medication prescribed by a physician or dentist, or in performing other acts not requiring the skill, judgment, and knowledge of a registered nurse.

The latter definition differentiates between the independence of the RN's functions and the dependence of the LPN/LVN. It also places the responsibility for what the RN can legally do in the hands of the nursing profes-

sion, always considered a hallmark of professionalism.

The 1979 definition speaks of professional services for the registered nurse and technical services for the practical (vocational) nurse, probably as a manifestation of the professional/technical differentiation presented in the 1965 ANA position paper and reaffirmed by the House of Delegates in 1978. Direct accountability to the public is also a part of the definition; again differentiation between the two types of nurses is made. In the commentary section, it was noted that the definition should recognize "the singular element that distinguishes the nurse from other nursing personnel—the breadth and depth of educational preparation that justify entrusting overall responsibility for nursing services to the judgment of the registered nurse."

The practice of nursing means the performance for compensation of professional services requiring substantial specialized knowledge of the biological, physical, behavioral, psychological, and sociological sciences and of nursing theory as the basis for assessment, diagnosis, planning, intervention, and evaluation in the promotion and maintenance of health, the casefinding and management of illness, injury, or infirmity, the restoration of optimum function, or the achievement of a dignified death. Nursing practice includes but is not limited to administration, teaching, counseling, supervision, delegation, and evaluation of practice and execution of the medical regimen, including the administration of medications and treatments prescribed by any person authorized by state law to prescribe. Each registered nurse is directly accountable and responsible to the consumer for the quality of nursing care rendered.

The practice of practical (vocational) nursing means the performance for compensation of technical services requiring basic knowledge of the biological, physical, behavioral, psychological, and sociological sciences and of nursing procedures. These services are performed under the supervision of a registered nurse and utilize standardized procedures leading to predictable outcomes in the observation and care of the ill, injured and infirm, in the maintenance of health, in action to safeguard life and health, and in the administration of medications and treatments prescribed by any person authorized by state law to prescribe.

The licensure laws currently in effect continue to make a distinction between an RN and LPN/LVN; most still use the terms *professional* and *practical/vocational*, not *technical*. This lack of consistency among states may cause some confusion, but it probably also reflects the political climate within each state. New York, for instance, has for several years introduced legislation that will, by 1985, require a baccalaureate degree for registered professional nurse status and an associate degree for the registered associate nurse, eliminating the current practical nurse title. A few other states are moving in this direction, but no such law has yet been passed. The greatest resistance has come from diploma and AD nurses and educators in those programs. Graduates from those programs consider themselves professionals and feel that even with the grandfather clause in the proposed laws, they will be downgraded. Unfortunately, the tensions between opposing groups on this issue are creating destructive intraprofessional conflict.

Nursing a Profession?

Even the most enthusiastic nurse cannot say that nursing has completely fulfilled all the criteria of professionalism. It is the only health profession in which most practitioners are educated at less than a baccalaureate level. Yet, obviously, progress is being made: the body of nursing knowledge is evolving and pertinent research is being done to a growing extent; new emphasis is being put on the intellectual, judgmental aspects of nursing and the assumption of individual responsibility; nursing education is gradually moving into institutions of higher learning; the nursing organizations have, through the years, established policies and standards of practice. Although nurses as employees do not always have control over their functions, they can and should, and some changes are

occurring. Finally, nursing always has attracted individuals with a service motive, but many nurses still do not see nursing as a lifework.

Do these discrepancies mean that nursing should discard the professional connotation? Hardly. Most professions have moved through various transitional stages. But there's more to professionalism than rhetoric.

A scathing indictment of nurses who "want the name but not the game" might serve as a warning.

> *Too small a percentage of nurses have "bought" professionalism as a way of life. The larger segment "mouth" the philosophy, go through the outward rituals, all the while digging deeper ruts from which to be extracted later by another "concerned" generation of truly professional nurses. These are the nurses who find status in the status quo. They are not progressive; they have just transferred their hard-core traditionalism to other settings, and labeled it progress. These are the nurses who demand professional recognition from others, but are reluctant to assume professional responsibilities. They may get caught up in the intellectual ferment around them, but they are not seriously engaged in the professional dialogue. They may be troubled about nursing's professional role, but for self-serving reasons. To the observer, there is serious imbalance between their professional commitment and their personal ambitions. They court professionalism but balk at the price. They command higher salaries, but avoid spending their own money on professional growth . . . if they can use someone else's, namely, their employer's or the government's. Professionalism as a way of life implies responsibility and commitment.*[34]

Thus, at what point nursing achieves complete professionalism will depend to a large extent on the goals and consequent action of its practitioners.

REFERENCES

1. Sam Schulman, "Basic Functional Roles in Nursing: Mother Surrogate and

Healer," in *Patients, Physicians and Illness: Behavioral Sciences and Medicine*, Jaco, E. G. (ed.) (Glencoe, Ill.: The Free Press, 1963), p. 532.

2. Marlene Kramer, *Reality Shock: Why Nurses Leave Nursing* (St. Louis: C. V. Mosby Company, 1974), p. 21.

3. Carol Garant, "The Process of Effecting Change in Nursing," *Nurs. Forum* 17(2):158 (1978).

4. Norah Mackenzie, "The Professional Ethic," *Intl. Nurs. Rev.*, 13:60–61 (July/Aug. 1966).

5. Byron Buick-Constable, "The Professionalism Spectre," *Intl. Nurs. Rev.*, 16(2):133–144 (1969).

6. Mary Gamer, "The Ideology of Professionalism," *Nurs. Outlook*, 27:108 (Feb. 1979).

7. Thelma Ingles, "What is Good Nursing?" *Am. J. Nurs.*, 59:1246 (Sept. 1959).

8. Sister M. Olivia Gowan, *Proceedings of the Workshop on Administration of College Programs in Nursing, June 12–24, 1944* (Washington, D.C.: Catholic University of America Press, 1946), p. 10.

9. Barbara MacDonald, "This I Believe . . . Nursing's Many Meanings," *Nurs. Outlook*, 14:56–57 (July 1966).

10. Virginia Henderson, *ICN Basic Principles of Nursing Care* (London: International Council of Nurses, 1961). Expanded in Henderson's *The Nature of Nursing* (New York: Macmillan Publishing Co., Inc., 1967).

11. Rozella Schlotfeldt, "The Professional Doctorate: Rationale and Characteristics," *Nurs. Outlook*, 26:303 (May 1978).

12. Martha Rogers, "Doctoral Education in Nursing," *Nurs. Forum*, 5:77 (1966).

13. "The Nurse Practitioner Question," *Am. J. Nurs.*, 74:2188 (Dec. 1974).

14. Ingeborg Mauksch, "Critical Issues of the Nurse Practitioner Movement," *Nurse Practitioner*, 3:15 (Nov./Dec. 1978).

15. "Extending the Scope of Nursing Practice," *Nurs. Outlook*, 20:46–52 (Jan. 1972).

16. Claire Fagin, "Primary Care As An Academic Discipline," *Nurs. Outlook*, 26:753 (Dec. 1978).

17. "Nursing's Contribution and Commit-ment." Joint Statement of American Association of Colleges of Nursing, American Nurses' Association and National League for Nursing, 1973.

18. "Independent Practitioners Define Nursing Roles," *Am. Nurse*, 5:2, 9 (Nov. 1973).

19. Gertrude Torres, "Educators' Perceptions of Evolving Nursing Functions." *Nurs. Outlook*, 22:184–187 (Mar. 1974).

20. Schlotfeldt, op. cit.

21. Helen Yura and Mary Walsh, *The Nursing Process*, 2nd ed. (New York: Appleton-Century-Crofts, 1973), p. 19.

22. Ida Jean Orlando, *The Dynamic Nurse-Patient Relationship* (New York: G. P. Putnam's Sons, 1961), p. 26.

23. Yura and Walsh, op. cit., p. 21.

24. Ibid., p. 23.

25. Faye Abdellah, "The Nature of Nursing Science, Conference on the Nature of Science in Nursing," *Nurs. Res.* 18:390–393 (1969).

26. Kathleen Andreoli and Carol Thompson, "The Nature of Science in Nursing," *Image* 9:35–36 (June 1977).

27. Judy Grubbs, "An Interpretation of the Johnson Behavioral System Model for Nursing Practice," in Riehl and Roy, eds., *Conceptual Models for Nursing Practice* (New York: Appleton-Century-Crofts, 1974), pp. 160–167.

28. Sister Callista Roy, "Adaptation: A Conceptual Framework for Nursing," *Nurs. Outlook*, 18:42–45 (Mar. 1970).

29. Martha Rogers, *Educational Revolution in Nursing* (New York: Macmillan Publishing Co., Inc., 1961) pp. 18–21.

30. Josephine Paterson and Loretta Zderad, *Humanistic Nursing* (New York: John Wiley & Sons, Inc., 1976), p. 3.

31. Dorothy Orem, *Nursing: Concepts of Practice* (New York: McGraw-Hill Book Company, 1971).

32. Myra Levine, "The Four Conservation Principles of Nursing," *Nurs. Forum*, 6:45–59 (1967).

33. Sister Callista Roy, "A Diagnostic Classification System for Nursing," *Nurs. Outlook*, 23:91 (Feb. 1975).

34. Alice Clarke, "Candidly Speaking: On *Nursing Forum* and Professionalism," *Nurs. Forum*, 7(1):12 (1968).

BIBLIOGRAPHY

Abdellah, Faye G., et al. *Patient-Centered Approaches to Nursing.* New York: Macmillan Publishing Co., Inc., 1960. Based on concepts of eleven patient problems which nurses meet. Application to education and practice. A classic upon which many nursing curricula were based.

Abdellah, Faye G., et al. *New Directions in Patient-Centered Nursing.* New York: Macmillan Publishing Co., Inc., 1973. A broad picture of delivery of health services, education, and research as related to nursing. Particularly interesting are the coverage of new trends in health care services, the crisis in health care, and research.

Auld, Margaret, and Linda Birum, Eds. *The Challenge of Nursing.* St. Louis: C. V. Mosby Company, 1973. A book of readings that explores, among other things, the processes and concepts utilized by nurses assisting an individual to meet his health needs.

Aydelotte, Myrtle. "Issues of Professional Nursing: The Need for Clinical Excellence." *Nurs. Forum,* 7:72–86. In presenting her case, author also includes excellent background material on how nursing is seen (or not seen).

Bates, Barbara. "Doctor and Nurse: Changing Roles and Relationships." *N. Eng. J. Med.,* **283** (July 16, 1970), 129–134. An MD co-director of a nurse practitioner program delineates differences between new nursing roles and those of MD and PA. Well done. Almost identical article found in *AORN. J.* (Jan. 1972), pp. 53–62 and *Nurs. Dig.* (Oct. 1974), pp. 70–78.

Brown, Esther Lucile. *Nursing Reconsidered: A Study of Change,* Part 1. Philadelphia: J. B. Lippincott Company, 1970. Description of some of the significant changes that have occurred in nursing practice. Includes nursing in hospitals, extended-care facilities, and institutions for care of the aged. Stresses changing roles of the nurse.

Brown, Esther Lucile. *Nursing Reconsidered: A Study of Change,* Part 2. Philadelphia: J. B. Lippincott Company, 1971. Reports on current developments in community nursing practice; many examples of agencies that have made innovative changes. Offers recommendations for nursing's participation in planning and delivery of health services.

Chaska, Norma, Ed. *The Nursing Profession: Views Through the Mist.* New York: McGraw Hill Book Company, 1978. An unusually interesting and pertinent series of essays, many by nurse sociologists on crucial aspects of the nursing profession. Includes sections on professionalism, nursing research, theory development, nursing diagnosis, and nursing functions.

Ciske, Daren. "Primary Nursing: An Organization That Promotes Professional Practice," *J. Nurs. Admin.,* **4** (Jan.-Feb. 1974), 28–31. Description of a one-to-one assignment model in a small hospital nursing unit, with decision making decentralized to the nurse who knows the patient best.

Coladarci, Arthur P. "What About that Word Profession?" *Am. J. Nurs.,* **63** (Oct. 1963), 116–118. To overcome shortcomings of existing definitions of *profession,* the author proposes the use of "action dimensions" of service occupations: degree to which actions are socially consequential; degree to which actions are complex; degree to which the consumer is capable of evaluating the appropriateness and effectiveness of actions. Excellent references.

Donaldson, Sue, and Dorothy Crowley. "The Discipline of Nursing." *Nurs. Outlook,* **26** (Feb. 1978), 113–120. Stresses need for nursing research to focus on the nursing perspective. Defines relationship of professional discipline to practice.

Fuller, Sarah. "Holistic Man and the Science and Practice of Nursing." *Nurs. Outlook,* **26** (Nov. 1978), 700–704. Author suggests that knowledge and concepts essential to nursing are already defined by the nature of human beings.

Gamer, Mary. "The Ideology of Professionalism." *Nurs. Outlook,* **27** (Feb. 1979), 108–111. Author describes conflicts over future goals for nursing which impose strains on the ideology of professionalism.

Gebbie, Kristine, and Mary Ann Lavin. "Classifying Nursing Diagnoses," *Am. J. Nurs.,* **74** (Feb. 1974), 250–253. The authors, reporting on a national conference on classification of nursing diagnoses, indicate that such classification is also a systematic description of nursing. A tentative list of nursing diagnoses is given.

Hadley, Betty Jo. "Current Concepts of Wellness and Illness: Their Relevance for Nursing," *Image,* **6** (2) (1974), 21–27. A look at these concepts and their relevance to nursing. Detailed bibliography.

Henderson, Virginia. *The Nature of Nursing.* New York: Macmillan Publishing Co., Inc., 1966. This distinguished nurse, whose definition of nursing appears within this chapter, elaborates her concepts and describes the development of her own philosophy in this small book.

Henriques, Charles, Vincent Virgadamo, and Mildred Kahane. "Performance of Adult Health Appraisal Examinations Utilizing Nurse Practitioners-Physician Teams and Paramedical Personnel," *Am. J. Pub. Health*, **64** (Jan. 1974), 47–53. The use of medical nurse practitioners in a successful screening examination program is discussed, including selection, training, and activities.

Hershey, Nathan. "Scope of Nursing Practice," *Am. J. Nurs.*, **66** (Jan. 1966), 117–120. Introduces the concepts of a "spectrum of health care services" and component analysis of techniques, to aid in clarifying what constitutes the definable area of practice of members of a given health profession.

Hopping, Betty. "Professionalism and Unionism: Conflicting Ideologies." *Nurs. Forum*, **15** (4) (1976), 372–383. In describing the opposing values of professionalism and unionism, author questions which nursing must use to gain power.

Jahoda, Marie. "Nursing as a Profession." *Int. Nurs. Rev.*, **8** (May–June 1961), 10–21. A social psychologist of international reputation presents in considerable detail the nursing profession's challenge and chore in protecting its members and at the same time meeting the needs of patients and the community. Still pertinent.

Kellams, Samuel. "Ideals of a Profession: The Case of Nursing." *Image*, **9** (June 1977), 30–31. Non-nurse educator points out that nursing's claim to autonomy ultimately rests on building a unique expertise.

Keller, Marjorie. "The Effect of Sexual Stereotyping on the Development of Nursing Theory," *Am. J. Nurs.*, **79** (Sept. 1979), 1584–1586. Interesting concept.

Kelly, Lucie. "End Paper: Not Bad, Nursing." *Nurs. Outlook*, **26** (Apr. 1978), 275. Nursing has advanced more than many professions in what it has accomplished.

Krieger, Dolores. "Therapeutic Touch: The Imprimatur of Nursing," *Am. J. Nurs.*, **75** (May, 1975), 784–787. Author describes her research on healing by therapeutic touch.

Leininger, Madeleine. "Scholars, Scholarships, and Nursing Scholarship," *Image*, **6** (2) (1974), 5–14. A nurse educator explores the meaning of scholarship for nurses.

Lewis, Edith. "The Professionally Uncommitted." *Nurs. Outlook*, **27** (May, 1979), 323. Excellent editorial noting lack of participation of most nurses in the professional organization and thus not part of professional decision-making.

MacDonald, Barbara D. "Nursing's Many Meanings," *Nurs. Outlook*, **14** (July 1966), 56–57. A new baccalaureate graduate expresses her beliefs about nursing, beliefs that are probably shared by many other nurses. Nursing means technical skill, caring for individuals, understanding and supporting, "being there," teaching, hard work, and a reciprocal receiving and giving process.

Miller, Lynn. "An Explanation of Therapeutic Touch, Using the Science of Unitary Man," *Nurs. Forum*, **18** (10) 1979, 278–287. Describes therapeutic touch, gives historical background and relates it to Rogers' theory of nursing.

Murphy, Juanita, Ed. *Theoretical Issues in Professional Nursing*. New York: Appleton-Century-Crofts, 1971. Book of essays by various writers of which all but two are nurses, exploring the various theoretical concepts upon which nursing might be based.

Murphy, Juanita. "Role Expansion and Role Extension—Some Conceptual Differences," *Nurs. Forum*, **9** (Fall 1970), 381–389. A careful delineation of the differences between expanding and extending the nurse's role. This position has been taken by a number of nurse leaders who feel that nursing should not go the route of extending.

Roy, Sister Callista. "A Diagnostic Classification System for Nursing." *Nurs. Outlook*, **23** (Feb. 1975), 90–93. Delineates the associated philosophy, rationale, and proposed methodology for deriving such a system.

Safier, Gwendolyn. *Contemporary Nursing Leader, An Oral History*. New York: McGraw Hill Book Company, 1977. A fascinating series of interviews with seventeen living nursing leaders, including their concepts of nursing.

Stevens, Barbara. *Nursing Theory—Analysis, Application, Evaluation*. Boston: Little, Brown and Company, 1979. Good overview of the various theories, clearly described and related to education, administration and clerical practice.

Extensive references on the legal definition of nursing are given in the bibliography of Chapter 20. For more information on nursing theories and professionalism, the list of references at the end of Chapter 9 will provide a good starting point; all are pertinent and informative. Also the first two issues of *Advances in Nursing Science* (Oct. 1978 and January 1979) are devoted to "Practice Oriented Theory." The seventy-fifth anniversary issue of *AJN* (Oct. 1975) has articles on various modes of care.

Professional Ethics and Accountability

A code of ethics is considered an essential characteristic of a profession, providing one means whereby professional standards may be established, maintained, and improved. It indicates the profession's acceptance of the trust and responsibility with which society has invested it. With the increased complexity of health care and what seems to be a changing morality in the world at large, understanding and adherence to such a code is more important than ever for nurses and others in the health professions.

MORALS AND ETHICS*:
A DIFFERENTIATION

There is a tendency to use the words *moral* and *ethical* interchangeably in the literature of the health professions. However, in the last few years, the need to differentiate between the two terms has become more evident, perhaps because the complexity of modern health care and the always-changing

*The term *ethics* will be used in this chapter, although *bioethics* is becoming popular in some of the literature. Frequently, bioethics seems to be used synonymously with medical ethics, and there are experts in the field of ethics who find its meaning unclear.

societal mores often create conflicting tensions in those who face a moral-ethical dilemma.

Kohlberg, structuring a theory of moral development, used the term *stages* for individual phases of moral thinking. In the 0, or premoral, stage, the individual does not understand the rules or feel a sense of obligation to them, acting only to experience that which is pleasant (good) or avoiding that which is painful (bad). In the Preconventional Level, stages 1 and 2, the individual's moral reasoning is based on reward and punishment from those in authority. In the Conventional Level, stages 3 and 4, the expectations of the social group (family, community, nation) are supported and maintained. In the Postconventional level, stages 5 and 6, the individual considers universal moral principles, which supersede the authority of groups. Kohlberg believes that most American adults function at stages 3 to 5, but moral maturity is gained at stage 6, when the individual makes up his/her own mind about what is right and wrong.[1] Although the term *moral* is used in this analysis, there are those who interpret stage 6 as a "universal, ethical principle orientation" because:

At this stage, morality is based on decisions

170

of conscience, made in accordance with self-chosen principles of justice, which are comprehensive, universal, and consistent. These principles are abstract and ethical, rather than concrete moral rules.[2]

Taking the viewpoint that moral values are usually based on religious beliefs, but also agreeing that an individual's ethics are based on self-examination, Maurice and Warrick state:

Ethical philosophy is the reflective analysis and evaluation of the goodness or badness of human conduct. Moral theology is the prescription decreed by divine authority regulating human conduct. Both ethics and morals indicate that goodness is that which leads to amity, wholesomeness, ease, peace, and well-being. Badness leads to the opposite. In short, goodness leads to happiness and order; badness to unhappiness and chaos. The difference, therefore, is the means to the end. Ethics deals with evaluation and responsibility whereas rules and obedience characterize morals.[3]

Churchill puts it more simply:

Morality is generally defined as behavior according to custom or tradition. Ethics, by contrast, is the free, rational assessment of courses of actions in relation to precepts, rules, conduct. . . . To be ethical a person must take the additional step of exercising critical, rational judgment in his decisions.[4]

The whole issue of ethics versus morals may seem to be a purely philosophical issue; however, given the differentiation described, the code of ethics of professional nurses may mandate action that goes beyond what their immediate associates see as necessary. It is also possible that individuals must struggle with what seems to be a conflict between ethical behavior and personal religious beliefs. Even so, it may not be so difficult to make ethical decisions when there seems to be a fairly clear-cut good/bad choice, but modern science has created situations for which most people, including nurses and doctors, have not been prepared. Thus, it would not be difficult for a nurse to decide not to deliberately harm a patient, and not a great prob-

lem to give a patient an uncomfortable treatment if it would improve his condition. It is not so easy to decide whether to agree to continued resuscitation on a brain-dead patient or to sustain life in a badly deformed, brain-damaged newborn, who will require lifetime custodial care paid for by society. Although a code of ethics, per se, may not resolve those problems, it should at least give the practitioners guidelines for behavior in such a way that the rights of patients and the public are preserved, as well as to tell the public what behavior it has a right to expect from the professional practitioner.

NURSING CODES OF ETHICS

Although Isabel Hampton Robb wrote a book on ethics and nursing practice at the turn of the century, and there were columns on ethics in nursing journals, a formal code was not evident in early American nursing. In the early nursing literature, ethics appears to have been defined as *Christian morality.* There is some feeling that this was due in part to the authoritarian milieu in which nursing existed. Nursing education valued obedience, submission to rules, social etiquette, and loyalty to the physician, instead of judgment, responsibility, and humanitarianism. What might have been a substitute for an ethical code, Lystra Gretter's Florence Nightingale Pledge, quoted in chapter 3, illustrates the mixture of contemporary morality, ethics, and loyalty expected in 1893.* It also appears to be based on the Hippocratic Oath associated with physicians and supposedly drawn up at the time of Hippocrates to express the commitments of the healing practitioners. Nurses may be familiar with some of that oath's precepts:

---

*In 1935, Mrs. Gretter revised the last paragraph of the pledge to read, "With loyalty will I aid the physician in his work, and as a 'missioner of health' I will dedicate myself to devoted service to human welfare." The 1935 version is copyrighted by the Alumnae Association, Harper Hospital School of Nursing, Detroit, Mich.; the original is not copyrighted.

The regimen that I adopt shall be for the benefit of my patients according to my ability and judgment. . . . I will give no deadly drug to any. . . . Whatsoever things I see or hear concerning the life of men, in my attendance on the sick or even apart therefrom, which ought not to be noised abroad, I will keep silence thereon, counting such things to be as sacred secrets.

The Nightingale Pledge is still recited or sung (as the Nightingale Hymn) by some graduating students of nursing as the Hippocratic Oath is recited by some graduating physicians, but their respective codes of ethics have changed, as they should.

After several years of trying to decide between a pledge of conduct and a statement on the ideals of the nursing profession, in 1926, ANA's relatively new Committee on Ethical Standards presented to the ANA house of delegates a suggested code of ethics. The purpose was not to provide specific rules of conduct, but to create an awareness of ethical considerations. The code is a realistic reflection of the times, and comparison with succeeding codes illustrates that although certain basic precepts of ethical behavior may persist, codes are altered by the demands of the times and changing concepts of an emerging profession by the professionals. For instance, in the next decade, nurses' ethical concerns encompassed such diverse topics as uniform requirements and outlining diabetic diets to a patient in the absence of a physician.[5] In 1940, a "Tentative Code," published in *AJN*, was not much different from the 1926 version. Even the more modern and first official Code for Nurses (1950) has been revised a number of times (1956, 1960, 1968, and 1976) and shows the influence of societal changes. For instance, the 1950 Code emphasized respect for the religious beliefs of patients; then, with the civil rights movement, the same statement was broadened to include "race, creed, color, or status"; and currently it stresses human dignity and the "uniqueness of the client unrestricted by considerations of social or economic status, personal attributes, or the

nature of health problems." There is also decreasing emphasis on relationships with physicians and professional etiquette. The focus is on protection of the patient/client, and in this sense, represents a change to a real ethical code.

The 1976 version of the Code, with interpretive statements, was developed by an ad hoc committee of the ANA's Congress for Nursing Practice and is available from the American Nurses' Association. The interpretive statements are especially valuable because they not only enlarge upon and explain the code in more detail, but also provide more focus and direction on how the nurse can carry out the code. Particularly important is the first statement, which sets the tone of the nurse/client relationship as partners:

Whenever possible, clients should be fully involved in the planning and implementation of their own health care. Each client has the moral right to determine what will be done with his/her person. . . .

Key areas in the interpretations deal with the nurse as patient advocate, nurse participation in political decision making and public affairs, and nurse involvement in advertising of products. Nurse accountability is a major issue and is considered important enough to require a separate statement; the code now has eleven instead of ten statements.

RESEARCH AND ETHICS

When the ANA Code was revised in 1968, the major change was the addition of a statement on the responsibilities of a nurse in research activities. Specific guidelines were delineated in the ANA publication *The Nurse in Research: ANA Guidelines on Ethical Values.*[7] The increasing participation of nurses in medical research as well as nurse-initiated research made this a timely statement. Certain points received emphasis: those implicit in the nurse's responsibility for rendering quality care, such as the pro-

First ANA Suggested Code of Ethics (1926)

THE RELATION OF THE NURSE TO THE PATIENT

The nurse should bring to the care of the patient all of the knowledge, skill, and devotion which she may possess. To do this, she must appreciate the relationship of the patient to his family and to his community.

Therefore the nurse must broaden her thoughtful consideration of the patient so that it will include his whole family and his friends, for only in surroundings harmonious and peaceful for the patient can the nurse give her utmost of skill, devotion and knowledge, which shall include the safeguarding of the health of those about the patient and the protection of property.

THE RELATION OF THE NURSE TO THE MEDICAL PROFESSION

The term "medicine" should be understood to refer to scientific medicine and the desirable relationship between the two should be one of mutual respect. The nurse should be fully informed on the provisions of the medical practice act of her own state in order that she may not unconsciously support quackery and actual infringement of the law. The key to the situation lies in the mutuality of aim of medicine and nursing; the aims, to cure and prevent disease and promote positive health, are identical; the technics of the two are different and neither profession can secure complete results without the other. The nurse should respect the physician as the person legally and professionally responsible for the medical and surgical treatment of the sick. She should endeavor to give such intelligent and skilled nursing service that she will be looked upon as a co-worker of the doctor in the whole field of health.

Under no circumstances, except in emergency, is the nurse justified in instituting treatment.

THE RELATION OF THE NURSE TO THE ALLIED PROFESSIONS

The health of the public has come to demand many services other than nursing. Without the closest interrelation of workers and appreciation of the ethical standards of all groups, and a clear understanding of the limitations of her own group, the best results in building positive health in the community cannot be obtained.

RELATION OF NURSE TO NURSE

The "Golden Rule" embodies all that could be written in many pages on the relation of nurse to nurse. This should be one of fine loyalty, of appreciation for work conscientiously done, and of respect for positions of authority. On the other hand, loyalty to the motive which inspires nursing should make the nurse fearless to bring to light any serious violation to the ideals herein expressed; the larger loyalty is that to the community, for loyalty to an ideal is higher than any personal loyalty.

RELATION OF THE NURSE TO HER PROFESSION

The nurse has a definite responsibility to her profession as a whole. The contribution of individual service is not enough. She should, in addition, give a reasonable portion of her time to the furtherance of such advancements of the profession as are only possible through action of the group as a whole. This involves attendance at meetings and the acquisition of information, at least sufficient for intelligent participation in such matters as organization and legislation.

The supreme responsibility of the nurse in relation to her profession is to keep alight that spiritual flame which has illumined the work of the great nurses of all time.

tection of the individual's rights in relation to privacy, self-determination, conservation of personal resources, freedom from arbitrary hurt and intrinsic risk of injury, and the special rights of minors and incompetent persons. The nurse is expected to participate in a research or experimental activity only with the assurance that the project has the official sanction of a legally constituted research committee or other appropriate authority within the institutional or agency settings, and he or she must have sufficient knowledge of the research design to allow participation in an informed, effective, and ethical fash-

AMERICAN NURSES ASSOCIATION
CODE FOR NURSES (1976)
Preamble

The Code for Nurses is based upon belief about the nature of individuals, nursing, health, and society. Recipients and providers of nursing services are viewed as individuals and groups who possess basic rights and responsibilities, and whose values and circumstances command respect at all times. Nursing encompasses the promotion and restoration of health, the prevention of illness, and the alleviation of suffering. The statements of the Code and their interpretation provide guidance for conduct and relationships in carrying out nursing responsibilities consistent with the ethical obligations of the profession and quality in nursing care.

1. The nurse provides services with respect for human dignity and the uniqueness of the client unrestricted by considerations of social or economic status, personal attributes, or the nature of health problems.
2. The nurse safeguards the client's right to privacy by judiciously protecting information of a confidential nature.
3. The nurse acts to safeguard the client and the public when health care and safety are affected by the incompetent, unethical, or illegal practice of any person.
4. The nurse assumes responsibility and accountability for individual nursing judgments and actions.
5. The nurse maintains competence in nursing.
6. The nurse exercises informed judgment and uses individual competence and qualifications as criteria in seeking consultation, accepting responsibilities, and delegating nursing activities to others.
7. The nurse participates in activities that contribute to the ongoing development of the profession's body of knowledge.
8. The nurse participates in the profession's efforts to implement and improve standards of nursing.
9. The nurse participates in the profession's efforts to establish and maintain conditions of employment conducive to high quality nursing care.
10. The nurse participates in the profession's effort to protect the public from misinformation and misrepresentation and to maintain the integrity of nursing.
11. The nurse collaborates with members of the health professions and other citizens in promoting community and national efforts to meet the health needs of the public.

ion. If the nurse sees conflicts or questions related to the well-being and safety of the patient, this concern must be voiced to the appropriate person in the institution. At all times, nurses remain responsible for their own acts and judgments. These guidelines not only give specifics in research ethics, in which any nurse might be involved, but provide a basis for discussion on the whole issue of human research.

A more recent ANA statement on the ethical issues of research is *Human Rights Guidelines for Nurses in Clinical and Other Research* (1975), developed by two nurse researchers and accepted as a position state-

ment on human rights for nurses engaged in various kinds of research.*

THE ICN CODE FOR NURSES

In 1933, the International Council of Nurses established an Ethics of Nursing Committee to study the method of teaching ethics in nursing, to survey activities by national organizations relative to ethics, and to

---

*The legal/ethical rights of human subjects in research are discussed in more detail in Chapter 22.

collect data on ethical problems. From this evolved an ICN Code of Nursing Ethics which, after a long delay partially caused by World War II, was adopted in 1953 at a Grand Council meeting in Brazil. As might be expected, there was major emphasis on nurses, not the nursing profession. Nurses were expected to recognize the limitations as well as the responsibilities of their roles, especially when it came to obeying doctors' orders. With slight revisions in 1965 at Frankfurt, the code was retitled, the Code of Ethics as Applied to Nursing, underlining the commonalities in all codes. Finally, at the 1973 meeting in Mexico City, the Council of National Representatives accepted some drastic revisions. Considerably shorter than the 1965 code, many of the statements appear to be combined and reworded in the new code. It was presented to the ICN congress as an effort to ''enunciate concepts that would be clear, concise, universal, broad enough to be useful to nurses in many cultures but able also to stand the tests of time and social change.'' A striking change is one that makes explicit the nurse's responsibility and accountability for nursing care, deleting statements in the 1965 code that abrogated the nurse's judgment and personal responsibility and showed dependency on the physician that nurses worldwide no longer see as appropriate.

International Council of Nurses

Code for Nurses—1973
Ethical Concepts Applied to Nursing
   The fundamental responsibility of the nurse is fourfold: to promote health, to prevent illness, to restore health and to alleviate suffering.
   The need for nursing is universal. Inherent in nursing is respect for life, dignity and rights of man. It is unrestricted by considerations of nationality, race, creed, colour, age, sex, politics or social status.
   Nurses render health services to the individual, the family and the community and

coordinate their services with those of related groups.

NURSES AND PEOPLE
   The nurse's primary responsibility is to those people who require nursing care.
   The nurse, in providing care, respects the beliefs, values and customs of the individual.
   The nurse holds in confidence personal information and uses judgment in sharing this information.

NURSES AND PRACTICE
   The nurse carries personal responsibility for nursing practice and for maintaining competence by continual learning.
   The nurse maintains the highest standards of nursing care possible within the reality of a specific situation.
   The nurse uses judgment in relation to individual competence when accepting and delegating responsibilities.
   The nurse when acting in a professional capacity should at all times maintain standards of personal conduct that would reflect credit upon the profession.

NURSES AND SOCIETY
   The nurse shares with other citizens the responsibility for initiating and supporting action to meet the health and social needs of the public.

NURSES AND CO-WORKERS
   The nurse sustains a cooperative relationship with co-workers in nursing and other fields.
   The nurse takes appropriate action to safeguard the individual when his care is endangered by a co-worker or any other person.

NURSES AND THE PROFESSION
   The nurse plays the major role in determining and implementing desirable standards of nursing practice and nursing education.
   The nurse is active in developing a core of professional knowledge.
   The nurse, acting through the professional organization, participates in establishing and maintaining equitable social and economic working conditions in nursing.

IMPLEMENTATION OF THE NURSING CODE

The ANA Code of Ethics, like other professional codes, has no legal force, as opposed to the licensure law, promulgated by the State Board of Nursing (not the nurses' association). However, the requirements of the Code often exceed, but are never less than, the requirements of the law. Violations of the law may, of course, subject the nurse to civil or criminal penalties. Violations of the Code should be reported to constituent associations of ANA which may reprimand, censure, suspend, or expel ANA members. Most states have a procedure for considering reported violations that also gives the accused due process. Even if the nurse is not an ANA member, an ethical violation, at the least, results in the loss of respect of one's colleagues and the public, which is a serious sanction. All nurses, whether or not they are ANA members, should be familiar with the profession's ethical code, for they have a professional obligation to uphold and adhere to the Code and ensure that nursing colleagues do likewise.

Implementation of the Code is at two levels. Nurses may be involved in resolving ethical issues on a broad policy level, participating with other groups in decision making to formulate guidelines or laws. But, the more common situation is ethical decision making in daily practice, on a one-to-one basis, on issues that are probably not a matter of life and death but must be resolved on the spot by the nurse who faces them. As Levine wrote,

> Much of the emphasis on ethical issues in health care has been on life and death situations, dealing particularly with the definition of death and the distribution of limited life-sustaining resources. But there are overlooked ethical challenges in the mundane, everyday routine activities of professional practice, and these have gone largely unexamined.
> Ethical behavior is NOT the display of one's moral rectitude in times of crises. It is the day-by-day expression of one's commitment to other persons and the ways in which

human beings relate to one another in their daily interactions.[8]

The Code, and particularly the interpretations, are useful as guidelines here, but nurses must recognize that in specific incidents, reaction will be both intellectual and emotional and strongly influenced by the nurse's cultural background, education, and experience. Bergman has presented a problem-solving format to help resolve ethical conflicts, but notes that the nurse must also weigh personal beliefs, the customs and mores of the persons involved, and legal aspects.[9]

A nine-step procedure, developed in a course on medical ethics, may also be useful in helping nurses to make ethical decisions and to think through their own ethical beliefs. These steps are as follows:

1. *Identify the health problem. This clearly must be at least brought to light, if not agreed upon, before any decision can be made.*
2. *Identify the ethical problem.*
3. *State who's involved in making the decision (the nurse, the doctor, the patient, the patient's family).*
4. *Identify your role. (Quite possibly, your role may not require a decision at all.)*
5. *Consider as many possible alternative decisions as you can.*
6. *Consider the long- and short-range consequences of each alternative decision.*
7. *Reach your decision.*
8. *Consider how this decision fits in with your general philosophy of patient care.*
9. *Follow the situation until you can see the actual results of your decision, and use this information to help in making future decisions.[10]*

In using this system, it is helpful to refer to the ANA Code of Ethics so that the philosophical concept is more clearly related to the reality situation.

OTHER CODES OF ETHICS

It is generally conceded that medicine was the first profession in the United States to adopt a code of ethics. As a matter of interest and comparison, the most recent code drawn up by the American Medical Association is presented, with permission of that organization. Presumably, nurses and physicians working in close relationship can cooperate more intelligently and harmoniously if each is aware of the other's ethical standards determining professional conduct, as well as the impact of social pressures on those standards. The latter point is particularly pertinent when comparing the old AMA "Principles of Medical Ethics," in effect from 1957 to 1974, with the new set adopted by the AMA House of Delegates in 1980. A public statement said that the new code reflected many recent changes in scientific knowledge, methods of practice, medical education and social attitudes. Nevertheless, there was some speculation that the liberalization of the code was due to outside pressures: the greater impact of governmental regulation (such as the FDA action described later) and the increasing number of suits against AMA related to restrictions advocated by the previous code. An example is old Section 3 which drew the wrath of chiropractors with its statement that physicians should not voluntarily associate professionally with anyone not practicing a method of healing founded on a scientific basis. A positive point, however, is new Section II, with its note of consumer advocacy.

AMA Principles of Medical Ethics (1980)

Preamble. *The medical profession has long subscribed to a body of ethical statements developed primarily for the benefit of the patient. As a member of this profession, a physician must recognize responsibility not only to patients, but also to society, to other health professionals, and to self. The following Principles adopted by the American Medical Association are not laws, but standards of conduct which define the essentials of honorable behavior for the physician.*

[I.] A physician shall be dedicated to providing competent medical service with compassion and respect for human dignity.

[II.] A physician shall deal honestly with patients and colleagues, and strive to expose

those physicians deficient in character or competence, or who engage in fraud or deception.

[III.] A physician shall respect the law and also recognize a responsibility to seek changes in those requirements which are contrary to the best interests of the patient.

[IV.] A physician shall respect the rights of patients, of colleagues, and of other health professionals, and shall safeguard patient confidences within the constraints of the law.

[V.] A physician shall continue to study, apply and advance scientific knowledge, make relevant information available to patients, colleagues, and the public, obtain consultation, and use the talents of other health professionals when indicated.

[VI.] A physician shall, in the provision of appropriate patient care, except in emergencies, be free to choose whom to serve, with whom to associate, and the environment in which to provide medical services.

[VII.] A physician shall recognize a responsibility to participate in activities contributing to an improved community.

Other professional groups also have ethical codes; law, pharmacy, veterinary medicine, and education were among the first. However, in the last ten years, an interesting phenomenon has occurred: ethics has become fashionable, and codes of ethics have been adopted by organizations representing business and industry. In surveying approximately 1,800 fraternal, professional, trade, and special interest associations in 1972, Smith found that 350 had codes and another 10 per cent were developing them. Although this may seem rather a sparse number, apparently it is about twice the number found twenty-five years previously.[11] Both business journals and the popular literature have been commenting on business and industry's burgeoning acceptance of the need for ethical behavior (code or no code). Possibly the new outlook is at least partly a reaction to political and other scandals involving "respectable" people. Legislators, stimulated by public pressure, have increasingly incorporated aspects of ethical behavior into legislation, with legal penalties for violations. Professionals, however, bear a basic responsibility more visible than that of other groups, for the public has granted them certain privileges, with certain expectations in return.

> The public expects ethical practice and conduct from professional men, and it is angered by violations of standards which it assumes ordinarily control practice. Each violation diminishes trust. Without trust, a profession would perish.[12]

Professionals today also need to look at their ethical codes in terms of whether they are focused on the consumer or are more inclined to emphasize professional etiquette —relationships within or across professional lines. For instance, the AMA has omitted in the new code the phrase, "He should not solicit patients," is interpreted by the AMA as prohibiting advertising, which, it said, might subject the public to charlatans with cut-rate fees. On the other hand, the Federal Trade Commission in 1978 cited prohibition of advertising as restraint of trade that does not allow the consumer full, informed choice. And if the advertising M.D. is really a charlatan, why not expose him according to the precepts of the code? Therefore, advertising by professionals has been legalized and is becoming more common, although still considered unethical by some. (The ANA code says advertising should be through means that are in dignified form, such as professional cards, listings in reputable directories, or professional publications.)

A similar point in the ethics/etiquette debate could be made about the ninth statement in the Code for Nurses, which implies support of collective bargaining actions. Although improved conditions of employment might also improve nursing care, one does not necessarily follow the other in terms of protecting the patient. It *does* protect the nurse from charges of unethical conduct.

It is perhaps the influence of changing times that self-serving aspects of ethical codes have diminished considerably over the last few years and recent revisions of most codes are beginning to show more concern

for protecting society than for protecting the profession.

ETHICAL ISSUES AND DILEMMAS IN NURSING

The major ethical issues for those in the health professions today are often identified as the quality of life versus the sanctity of life; the right to live versus the right to die; informed consent; confidentiality; rights of children; unethical behavior of other practitioners; role conflict (who's responsible?); and the allocation of scarce resources (who shall live?). Increasingly, these issues have become subjects of legislation or court decisions (as discussed in Section 5), but even this does not lessen the potential conflict in which nurses may find themselves. Not only must they confront the distinct possibility that their personal value systems might be different from that of the profession, but they are also caught in the value systems of their employing institutions.* In the first situation, they must come to terms with their responsibility to the patient or client, regardless of their personal beliefs. For instance, today nurses are faced constantly with deciding their roles in euthanasia or abortion. The decision for action may not be easy. When it comes to ending the life of a terminally ill patient or participating in an abortion, the nurse may choose not to participate if the action is against his or her moral principles. But what of care to responding, reacting patients? There are documented reports of both physicians and nurses showing pointed indifference and/or actual mental or physical cruelty to women with induced abortions.[13] This type of behavior can hardly be tolerated, but it is possible that in this and other situations the nurse needs some help beyond personal resources.[14] (Both ANA and some of the specialty nursing organizations have issued statements on some of the

---

*A survey on nurses' attitudes and/or action in specific, everyday situations is discussed in Chapter 11.

controversial ethical situations, such as abortion.)

But suppose the nurse does respond to both the ethical and legal responsibilities, such as being sure that a patient has given an *informed* consent before a particular kind of treatment. What if this comes into conflict with what the doctor or the hospital sees as a limit to the nurse's role (for example, the doctor decides whether the patient knows enough to make an informed decision)? Will the nurse's job be in jeopardy? Will she/he be subtly punished? What if the nurse reports unethical or illegal behavior on the part of another practitioner? Again, what happens? And who provides backup support? Nursing administration? Nursing peers? And what of dealing with nurses or doctors who are incompetents, drug abusers, or alcoholics, both in ethical and legal problems? Does the profession protect the co-professional or the public? Unlike personal ethical conflicts, these are real dilemmas that may have serious economic repercussions for the nurse, and it is quite possible that a nurse cannot resolve them alone. Instead, nursing must develop a support system for individual nurses who experience conflict in the employment setting with respect to implementation of the Code of Ethics, and the precepts of the Code must be widely publicized so that not only nurses, but the public and others in health care understand the ethical basis of nursing practice.

ACCOUNTABILITY

As nurses seek changes in their nursing practice acts to allow them to practice more independently in order to give optimum services to the public, the issue of the nurse's accountability to the public for the quality of nursing care rendered acquires new significance.

In the dictionary the term *accountable* means "answerable." One nursing definition is, "the responsibility for the services one provides or makes available,"[15] but taking

the meaning a step further, it can also mean that an individual may be liable to the extent that the actions taken are consistent with the responsibilities for which he or she contracted.[16]

Other disciplines besides nursing accept the concept of accountability. A definition applicable to nursing states:

> *Accountability . . . means that an agent, public or private, entering into a contractual agreement to perform a service will be held answerable for performing according to agreed-upon terms, within an established time period, and with stipulated use of resources and performance standards. This definition of accountability requires that the parties to the contract keep clear and complete records and that this information will be available for outside review. It also suggests penalties and rewards; accountability without redress or incentive is mere rhetoric.*[17]

Regardless of which definition one chooses, the facts are plain; the nurse as contractor offering his or her services is responsible for the quality of those services. To whom is a key question.

Accountability of the nurse to the public is a legal fact, because the entire purpose of licensure is to protect the public, and the licensing board has the right and responsibility to discipline incompetent and unethical practitioners. However, the law does not identify quality of performance; it only guarantees minimum safe practice. In most cases such accountability is only implicit in the law, but the Washington State Nursing Practice Act, developed by the state nurses' association makes it explicit: "The registered nurse is directly accountable and responsible to the individual consumer for the quality of nursing care rendered." In 1979 the ANA included a similar statement in a suggested nurse licensure law.

Besides the law, a second area of accountability is to the group with whom the nurse is professionally associated, usually the employing agency, but also another power source, the physician. One limited study pointed out that many nurses, the majority of physicians, and even patients see the nurse as being accountable to the physician or the employing agency. Of those nurses who did not agree, half felt that they were accountable to the profession of nursing and the others first to themselves and then to the public.[18] Observers in the health field would probably tend to agree that these findings are not atypical. In part, the attitude of those with this opinion might well be attributed to two factors: that nurses are primarily employees (and the American work ethic seems to say that the worker is responsible to the employer who pays his salary rather than the consumer whom he presumably serves) and the long-held nurse-as-doctor's-hand-maiden concept. In the hospital bureaucracy, it has been noted, nurses have been socialized by the system to the realization that "keeping things running" is one of the major criteria for judging effectiveness. For those who maintain that therefore professional nursing cannot be carried on in today's hospitals, there remains one question: whose responsibility is it if not that of the professional nurse? For that matter, a professional nurse employed as such has a responsibility to patient as client, physician as colleague, and agency as employer to perform effectively in that role. Beyond these groups, the nurse, as part of a profession, is also accountable to that group, responsible to practice according to the profession's standards.

The concept of accountability is not new in nursing, although the term is gaining a new popularity in all aspects of health care. The publicity given to the publication of the American Hospital Association's Patient's Bill of Rights (see Chapter 22), which if adopted by a hospital could be interpreted as an informal contract between patient and hospital, gives some indication of the degree of interest the public has in their rights as patients. Small wonder! As a rule, a patient once admitted to a hospital seems to lose all rights. Stripped of his clothes and personal belongings, limited by rules he does not com-

prehend (and for which no one gives reasons), poked and prodded, observed and directed by dozens of unknown individuals who never introduce themselves, patients, with some logic, have likened their hospital stay to being in prison. Recognizing these needs, the National League for Nursing in 1959 drafted an early version of a patient's bill of rights from a nursing viewpoint.[19] It began with the basic assumptions that

Nursing care encompasses health promotion, the care and prevention of disease or disability, and rehabilitation, and involves teaching, counseling and emotional support as well as the care of illness.

Nursing care is an integral part of total health care and is planned and administered in combination with related medical, educational, and welfare services.

Nursing personnel respect the individuality, dignity, and rights of every person, regardless of race, color, creed, national origin, social or economic status.

It concluded:

The patient has a right to expect:
1. *That he will receive the nursing care necessary to help him regain or maintain his maximum degree of health.*
2. *That the nursing personnel who care for him are qualified, through education, experience and personality, to carry out the services for which they are responsible.*
3. *That the nursing personnel caring for him will be sensitive to his feelings and responsive to his needs.*
4. *That, within the limits determined by his doctor, the patient and his family will be taught about his illness so that the patient can help himself, and his family can understand and help him.*
5. *That plans will be made with him and his family, or if necessary for him, so that if possible, continuing nursing and other necessary services will be available to him throughout the period of his need. These plans will involve the use of all appropriate personal and community resources.*
6. *That nursing personnel will assist in keeping adequate records and reports and will treat with confidence all personal matters*

that relate to the patient.

7. That efforts will be made by nursing personnel to adjust the surroundings of the patient so as to help him maintain or recover his health.

These excerpts from the original document are included to point out one way in which some very basic nursing responsibilities could be presented to the patient, remembering that the patient has traditionally been kept unaware of what he might expect of nursing care. And although these "rights" may seem rather elementary, they clearly relate to the nursing code of ethics, which describes very specific areas of accountability. Certainly the requirement of competency, current and continuing, is basic to any practice and is also particularly timely today.

Another NLN committee developed a new document on patient's rights in 1977.

Nursing's Role in Patients' Rights

NLN believes the following are patients' rights which nurses have a responsibility to uphold:

* People have the right to health care that is accessible and that meets professional standards, regardless of the setting.
* Patients have the right to courteous and individualized health care that is equitable, humane, and given without discrimination as to race, color, creed, sex, national origin, source of payment, or ethical or political beliefs.
* Patients have the right to information about their diagnosis, prognosis, and treatment—including alternatives to care and risks involved—in terms they and their families can readily understand, so that they can give their informed consent.
* Patients have the legal right to informed participation in all decisions concerning their health care.
* Patients have the right to information about the qualifications, names, and titles of personnel responsible for providing their health care.
* Patients have the right to refuse observation by those not directly involved in their care.

* Patients have the right to privacy during interview, examination, and treatment.
* Patients have the right to privacy in communicating and visiting with persons of their choice.
* Patients have the right to refuse treatments, medications, or participation in research and experimentation, without punitive action being taken against them.
* Patients have the right to coordination and continuity of health care.
* Patients have the right to appropriate instruction or education from health care personnel so that they can achieve an optimal level of wellness and an understanding of their basic health needs.
* Patients have the right to confidentiality of all records (except as otherwise provided for by law or third-party payer contracts) and all communications, written or oral, between patients and health care providers.

The dimensions of professional nursing practice have been discussed in Chapter 9, and it is implicit that these will continue to evolve. If these are the elements of accountable practice, in what way can it be determined that they are being carried out effectively? For some time nursing has tended to avoid evaluation because of the lack of precise means of measuring nurse-patient interaction. Abdellah suggests that evaluating the professional qualifications and competencies of the personnel providing care and evaluating the effect on the consumer are some of the ways in which measurement can be approached.[20] Within the last few years the use of peer evaluation has been stressed as a tool for evaluation. The American Nurses' Association has defined peer review as "the process by which registered nurses, actively engaged in the practice of nursing, appraise the quality of nursing care in a given situation in accordance with established standards of nursing practice.[21]

Four major purposes for peer review were given: (1) to evaluate the quality and quantity of nursing care; (2) to determine the strengths and weaknesses of nursing care;

(3) to provide evidence to utilize as the basis of recommendations for new or altered policies and procedures to improve nursing care; and (4) to identify those areas where practice patterns indicate more knowledge is needed.[22] Although the standards set for peer review are generally those determined by nursing in the setting where the evaluation is done, the ANA Standards of Practice,[23] made more explicit for evaluating purposes, are frequently considered a logical starting point.

There are a number of ways in which peer review is carried out, but primarily the review involves a concurrent evaluation of nursing care plans, charts, and other written evidence of nursing care along with observations and interviews with patients, or a retroactive study of the documents related to nursing care. The details of some of these approaches can be found in the references cited at the end of the chapter. To be sure, one technique or another can be taught. The heart of the issue, as it relates to accountability, is the acceptance and utilization of the total concept of peer evaluation. Passos lists some of the problems:

1. *Facing the issue of trust.*
2. *Relating professional standards, developed by peers to the policies and procedures which govern settings where nurses practice.*
3. *Closing the gap between actual practice and the boundaries of practice as defined in nursing practice acts.*
4. *The confidentiality of recipient data, which must be dealt with in peer review in any type of "audit" procedure.*
5. *Helping nurses to accept the* lack *of anonymity of their performances—individuals must be identifiable if one of the uses to which we must put evaluation is the judgment of the level of accountability of nurse practitioners in the setting.*
6. *Cost analyzing nursing contributions at different levels of quality.*[24]

She concludes:

If we cannot find solutions for the problems of how accountability is to be mani- *fested, monitored, regulated and controlled, how will we know that a nurse behaving in a particular way in a given situation is performing with the professionalism for which she is accountable? If we fail to concern ourselves with the means by which manifest nurse behavior can be monitored and regulated, then there is no point in talking about the attribute. . . . Our dilemma in trying to trace this attribute within the nursing process is due in part to the fact that nursing is a social process in which human beings are continually interacting with other human beings in ways that are imperfectly measurable or predictable.*[25]

There are other ways of documenting accountability, such as the activities of the American Nurses' Association in regard to continuing education and certification (Chapters 20 and 25). But in the long run, professional accountability is a personal responsibility and the individual nurse must assume it. When pressure increased to substitute institutional licensure for individual licensure, nursing constantly maintained that the strength of high-quality nursing care lay in the individual responsibility and accountability of the nurse, which is a part of individual professional licensure. If nurses believe this and believe as well in their profession and its contributions to health care, they will show themselves proudly accountable.

REFERENCES

1. Lawrence Kohlberg and Elliot Turiel, "Moral Development and Moral Education," in *Psychology and Education*, ed. by G. Lesser (Chicago: Scott, Foresman and Company, 1971) as described in Ruth Bindler, "Moral Development in Nursing Education," *Image*, 9:18–20 (Feb. 1977).
2. Rosemary Krowczyk and Elizabeth Kudzma, "Ethics: A Matter of Moral Development," *Nurs. Outlook*, 26:255 (Apr. 1978).
3. Shirley Maurice and Louise Warrick, "Ethics and Morals in Nursing," *MCN*, 2:343 (Nov.-Dec. 1977).
4. Larry Churchill, "Ethical Issues of a

Profession in Transition," *Am. J. Nurs,* **77:**873 (May 1977).

5. Lyndia Flanagan, *One Strong Voice* (Kansas City, Mo.: Am. Nurses' Assn., 1976), pp. 88–91.

6. William McGlothlin, *Patterns of Professional Education* (New York: G. P. Putnam's Sons, 1960), p. 211.

7. "The Nurse in Research: ANA Guidelines on Ethical Values," *Am. J. Nurs.,* **68:**1504–1507 (July 1968).

8. Myra Levine, "Nursing Ethics and the Ethical Nurse," *Am. J. Nurs,* **77:**846 (May 1977).

9. Rebecca Bergman, "Ethics-Concepts and Practice," *Intern'l. Nurs. Rev.,* **20**(5):141 (1973).

10. Mary Murphy and James Murphy, "Making Ethical Decisions Systematically," *Nurs. 76,* **6:**CG13 (May 1976).

11. Robert H. Smith, "New Directions for Ethical Codes," *Assoc. and Society Manager,* **7:**124 (Dec.-Jan. 1974).

12. William McGlothlin, *Patterns of Professional Education* (New York: G. P. Putnam's Sons, 1960), p. 211.

13. Rothlyn Zahourek, "Therapeutic Abortion and Cultural Shock," *Nurs. Forum,* **10:**8–17 (Winter 1971).

14. W. F. Chan and J. F. McDermott, Jr., "Abortions and Acute Identity Crisis in Nurses," *Am. J. Psychiat.,* **128:**952–957 (Feb. 1972).

15. Michigan Nurses' Association, *Position on Nursing Practice* (East Lansing: Michigan Nurses' Association, 1971), p. 4.

16. Joyce Passos, "Accountability: Myth or Mandate," *J. Nurs. Admin,* **3:**16 (May/June 1973).

17. Myron Lieberman, *Accountability: Review of Literature and Recommendations for Implementation* (Raleigh: North Carolina Department of Public Instruction, Divisions of Planning, Research, and Development, May 1972), p. 2.

18. Minerva Applegate, "A Pilot Study for Determining Relationships Between Members of the Medical and Nursing Profession," (unpublished paper, Teachers College, Columbia University, May 1973).

19. National League for Nursing, *What People Can Expect of Modern Nursing Service* (New York: National League for Nursing, 1959).

20. Faye Abdellah et al. *New Directions in Patient-Centered Nursing* (New York: Macmillan Publishing Co., Inc., 1973), p. 24.

21. "Peer Review Guidelines Proposed," *Am. Nurse,* **5:**1,5 (July 1973).

22. Ibid.

23. American Nurses' Association, *Standards of Nursing Practice* (Kansas City, Mo.: The American Nurses' Association, 1973).

24. Passos, op. cit., p. 21.

25. Ibid., p. 21.

BIBLIOGRAPHY

ETHICS

B., Elaine, Clare M., June S., and Janet A. "Helping the Nurse Who Misuses Drugs," *Am. J. Nurs.,* **74** (Sept. 1974) 1665–1671. Stories of nurse drug users.

Beebe, Joyce, and Henry Thompson. "A Paradigm of Ethics for the Maternal Child Nurse," *MCN,* **4** (May/June 1979) 141–147; 184. Nurse midwife and minister discuss a specific case in which ethics, morals, and patient's rights apply. Excellent. Good references.

Bandman, Elsie. "The Dilemma of Life and Death: Should We Let Them Die?" *Nurs. Forum,* **17**(2) (1978), 118–132. Analysis of situations in which nurse may or may not be in a decision-making position as to whether patients live or die.

Bergman, Rebecca. "Ethics-Concepts and Practice," *Int. Nurs. Rev.,* **20** (Sept.-Oct. 1973) 140–141 ff. The author describes how the ICN Code came to be revised and discusses the relevance of ethics to nursing today.

Bermosk, Loretta, and Raymond Corsini. *Critical Incidents in Nursing* (Philadelphia: W. B. Saunders Company, 1973). Thirty-eight nurses relate incidents about their practice in which there was a serious problem or controversial issue. Experienced, knowledgeable people discuss the issues each saw as important. A number are related to power, autonomy, and ethics.

Curtin, Leah. "Nursing Ethics: Theories and

Pragmatics." *Nurs. Forum* **17** (1) (1978) 4–11. Director of the National Center for Nursing Ethics suggests how nurses might manage ethical dilemmas, giving examples of actual situations.

Curtin, Leah. "A Proposed Model for Critical Ethical Analysis," *Nurs. Forum* **17**(1) (1978) 12–17. Another proposed model to help nurses in ethical conflicts.

Davis, Ann, and Mila Aroskar. *Ethical Dilemmas and Nursing Practice* (New York: Appleton-Century-Crofts, 1979). Primarily a collection of essays reflecting authors' views on a variety of ethical issues and their impact on nursing. Includes case studies.

Derbyshire, Robert C. "Medical Ethics and Discipline," *JAMA,* **228:** (Apr. 1, 1974), 59–62. The effectiveness of disciplinary agencies and some of the problems and concerns of medical ethics are discussed.

Donahue, M. Patricia. "The Nurse—A Patient Advocate?" *Nurs. Forum,* **17**(2) (1978) 143–151. Explores the role of nurse as patient advocate. Stresses need to understand issues involved in human rights, nurses' rights, accountability, responsibility, and risk-taking.

Doreck, Rachel. "Policing Members' Ethics," *Assoc. and Society Manager,* **9** (Apr.-May 1976), 31–33ff. Interesting look at how various organizations carry out their ethical codes.

Downs, Florence. "Ethical Inquiry in Nursing Research," *Nurs. Forum,* **6** (Winter 1967), 12–20. A nurse-researcher raises issues about ethical standards that should prevail in nursing research, particularly in relation to human subjects.

Jacobsen, Sharon. "Ethical Issues in Experimentation with Human Subjects," *Nurs. Forum,* **12** (Winter 1973), 58–71. Author discusses philosophical background of human experimentation, the social psychology of the experiment, deception in human experimentation, and safeguards for ethical practice in research.

Krawczk, Rosemary, and Elizabeth Kudzma. "Ethics: A Matter of Moral Development," *Nurs. Outlook,* **26** (Apr. 1978), 254–257. Seminar method for helping students in ethical development is described. Good information on ethical theory.

Lipp, Martin, et al. "Marijuana Use by Nurses and Nursing Students," *Am. J. Nurs.,* **71** (Dec. 1971), 2339–2341. A detailed survey shows significant uses of marijuana by nursing students, regardless of legal and professional consequences.

Maurice, Shirley, and Louise Warrick. "Ethics and Morals in Nursing," *MCN,* **2:** 343–347 (Nov.-Dec. 1977). A well-thought-out differentiation between morals and ethics.

Pellegrino, Edmund D. "Nursing and Medicine: Ethical Implications in Changing Practice," *Am. J. Nurs.,* **64:**110–112 (Sept. 1964). To adapt to constantly changing trends in patient care, nurses and physicians must cooperatively examine and change patterns of practice. The criteria of patient welfare, which is the core of ethical codes, remains, but the "etiquette" provisions in present codes may require some alteration.

Perspectives on the Code For Nurses (Kansas City, Mo.: ANA, 1978). Papers given at 1976 ANA convention relate code to education, practice, and research, as well as an interesting historical overview on the code.

"Reader Response to Ethical Inquiry in Nursing Research," *Nurs. Forum,* **6:**163–178 (Spring 1967). Three nurses engaged in research present differing points of view on Down's article.

Robb, Isabel Hampton. *Nursing Ethics.* Cleveland: E. C. Koeckert, 1922. This text may not be available in every nursing school library, but it is included here as one example of the several books on ethics that were published prior to 1930, when great emphasis was placed on ethics for the professional nurse. Practical, inspirational, and applicable today, it is also delightful reading.

Silva, Mary. "Science, Ethics and Nursing," *Am. J. Nurs.,* **74:**2004–2007 (Nov. 1974). Review of scientific advances that have created new ethical dilemmas for nurses. Guidance on ways to cope with this.

Smith, Robert H. "New Directions for Ethical Codes," *Assoc. and Society Manager,* **7:**124–128 (Dec.-Jan. 1974). Describes basic considerations for developing ethical codes.

Tancredi, Lawrence. *Ethics of Health Care* (Washington, D.C.: National Academy of Sciences, 1974). Essays and responding commentaries on ethics in health in such areas as government decision making, consumer evaluation, professional values, care of the chronically ill and aged.

Tate, Barbara. *The Nurse's Dilemma* (Geneva: ICN; AJN Co. in New York), 1977. Using ICN Code as a frame of reference, describes incidents of ethical concern from various countries.

Yarling, Roland. "Ethical Analysis of Nursing Problems: The Scope of Nursing Practice in Disclosing the Truth to Terminal Patients," Part I, *Supervisor Nurse*, 9 (May 1978), 40–50; Part II, *Supervisor Nurse*, 9 (June 1978) 28–34. Analysis of a case in considerable detail, including moral and legal issues, medical issues, rights and obligations of a nurse. Extensive reading list.

See also *Am. J. Nurs.*, May 1977, for special section on ethics, pp. 845–876. Excellent. Also: *Nursing 74*, September and October (1974) issues for survey of ethical problems; *Sup. Nurse* Aug. 1979 has heavy emphasis on the ethics and management of cardiac-pulmonary resuscitation, particularly in a critical-care unit. Also interesting are the letters to the editor responding to an editorial on the subject in the April 1979 issue. Entire issue of *Nurs. Cl. of N. Am.* (Mar. 1979) is devoted to bioethical issues.

ACCOUNTABILITY

Bloch, Doris. "Criteria, Standards, Norms—Crucial Terms in Quality Assurance," *J. Nurs. Admin.*, 7:20–30. Definitions of major terms and delineation through use of hypothetical model.

Corn, Florence, and Kathleen Magill. "The Nursing Care Audit—A Tool For Peer Review," *Sup. Nurse*, 5 (Feb. 1974), 20–23 ff. One hospital's specific plan for nursing audit is described, with samples of the forms used.

Felton, Geraldine et al. "Pathway to Accountability; Implementation of a Quality Assurance Program." *J. Nurs. Admin.*, 6 (Jan. 1976) 20–24. Analyzes the experiences of a large nursing service with deliberate planning for change to improve and assure high quality nursing care.

Flynn, Beverly and Dixie Ray. "Quality Assurance in Community Health Nursing." *Nurs. Outlook*, 27 (Oct. 1979), 650–653. Survey of selected community health nursing agencies reveals that there are a number of programs in quality assurance: some problems are noted.

Gold, Harold, et al. "Peer Review—A Working Experiment," *Nurs. Outlook*, 21 (Oct. 1973), 634–636. This peer review of clinical specialists showed unsatisfactory results in that there appeared inadequate ability or desire to evaluate in any negative fahion. The writers conclude

that this might be caused by lack of personal security and lack of criteria for specialized nursing, and they make recommendations.

Hoover, Julie, and Marie Zimmer. "Nursing Quality Assurance: the Wisconsin System," *Nurs. Outlook*, 26 (Apr. 1978), 242–248. Detailed discussion of an evaluation system that defines population groups broadly, using fewer criteria.

Lohmann, Grace. "A Statewide System of Record Audit," *Nurs. Outlook*, 25 (May 1977), 330–332. Nursing care audit system for small rural home care agencies.

Maas, Meridean. "Nurse Autonomy and Accountability in Organized Nursing Services," *Nurs. Forum*, 12 (Summer 1973), 237–257. An analysis of nurse autonomy and accountability as a necessary means for improving patient care, using a long-term care facility as an example.

Marram, Gwen. "Patients' Evaluation of Their Care: Importance to the Nurse," *Nurs. Outlook*, 21 (May 1973), 322–324. A study indicates that patient evaluation is important to the nurse, probably because of professional ideology; however, basically patients' evaluations have no real influence on the hospital system or quality of care.

Mullins, Anna et al. "Peer Review: A Model for Professional Accountability," *J. Nurs. Admin.* 9 (Dec. 1979) 25–30. Describes implementation of peer review process for the classification, promotion, and ongoing evaluation of professional nurses.

Nehring, Virginia, and Barbara Geach. "Patients' Evaluation of Their Care: Why They Don't Complain," *Nurs. Outlook*, 21 (May 1973) 317–321. The reluctance of patients to complain about the quality of care is found to be related to their fear of reprisal and lack of understanding of questionnaires used. Researchers find that nurses tend to be resentful and suspicious of evaluation efforts, but that there is a serious need for patient input and changes in care.

Passos, Joyce. "Accountability: Myth or Mandate?" *J. Nurs. Admin.*, 3 (May-June 1973), 19–22. Nurses must agree to whom and for what they are accountable. Mechanisms for documentation and peer review are identified as critical needs.

Passos, Joyce. "Accountability: The Long Road Back to Professional Practice." *J. NYSNA.* 7 (Dec. 1976) 27–38. Historical background is useful. Shows relationship of professionalism and accountability. Good list of references.

Phaneuf, Maria. "Quality Assurance: A Nursing View," *Hospitals* **47** (Oct. 16, 1973), 62–68. A number of instruments for evaluation of patient care are reviewed and the problems and potentials of such evaluations are explored.

Phaneuf, Maria. "The Nursing Audit for Evaluation of Patient Care," *Nurs. Outlook,* **14** (June 1966), 51–54. An early article by this expert on nursing audits describes one approach—the appraisal of patient records.

Plan for Implementation of the Standards of Nursing Practice (Kansas City, Mo.: ANA, 1975). Includes historical perspective, rationale for implementation, structural standards and models.

Ramey, Irene. "Setting Standards and Evaluating Care," *J. Nurs. Admin.,* **3** (May-June 1973), 27–35. The development of philosophies, objectives, and standards of an evaluation tool that includes the intellectual and interpersonal aspects of professional nursing is given. A specific example illustrates.

Ramphal, Marjorie. "Peer Review," *Am. J. Nurs.,* **74** (Jan. 1974), 63–67. The need for nurses to participate in regulation of their practice in order to maintain standards and the problems involved are discussed.

See also various issues of *Journal of Nursing Administration,* which frequently carries articles on quality assurance. The entire issue of Spring 1977 is devoted to quality assurance and peer review.

11

Profile of the Modern Nurse

Studying the actual and perceived characteristics of nurses was part of the vocational image research done by social scientists in the 1940s and 1950s, and a great deal of data is available. In recent years these kinds of studies have been carried out by nurses, particularly in relation to personality characteristics and attitudes. Unfortunately, most of the latter are small studies by graduate students with considerable limitation in scope. Thus, comparisons are difficult, particularly in the personality studies for which a large number of instruments are available. For demographic data, there is a greater likelihood of national samples, and in these the difficulty lies in the inconsistency of study components from year to year. Overall, however, the studies and surveys are thought-provoking and present an interesting overview of the practitioners of nursing today. The heterogeneity of nursing is quickly evident, for today's nursing work force will include men and women who might have graduated forty-five years ago, as well as new graduates. Therefore, their attitudes and perhaps their behavior have been affected by concepts that span that time period.

There are also differences between the image and the reality. This has always been

true. When Dickens wrote about the slovenly Sairey Gamp, there were dedicated women functioning as nurses. Even the British newspapers' glowing reports of Florence Nightingale as the gentle lady with the lamp overlooked her tough and efficient administrative stance, which had a large part in providing better care for soldiers in the Crimea. Nevertheless, Simmons, who has summarized a large number of these studies, notes that these role images operate as forces in the social milieu to promote or impede progress in nursing.[1]

This chapter, in building a profile of the modern nurse (and student), will deal with five major entities: the nurse as seen by the public, demographic data, personality characteristics of nurses, nursing attitudes, and minority groups in nursing. Obviously, it is necessary to present only a synopsis of the available data, but both the references and the bibliography will provide useful follow-up.

THE IMAGE OF NURSING

As might be expected, the public derives its image of the nurse from a variety of sources: from personal acquaintance, con-

187

tact in an illness situation, or the public communications media—books, magazines, newspapers, radio, and television.

Personal acquaintance almost always introduces the factors of like or dislike, with little relation to, or knowledge of, professional performance. The emotionalism involved if the contact is during illness is inevitable, because neither patient nor family and friends can be objective then. The media vary the image according to whether an article is intended as a sensational exposé, a factual review, or entertainment. There is also some indication that an individual's social status has an effect on his perception of the nurse. The public has traditionally held two extreme images of the nurse (whom they tend to see as female). One portrays her as humanitarian, altruistic, more or less competent, and endowed with sympathy, compassion, and an exceptional ability to gain rapport. The other portrays her as a professional, well-trained, technically efficient, cool-headed and able, and relatively independent.[2] In the last twenty-five years, the concept of nurse as manager, removed from patient care, has been added, and more recently, the nurse as super-nurse.

In Birdwhistell's 1947 study[3] and Deutscher's 1955 study,[4] both in the Midwest, the upper class looked down on nursing, whereas the lower class considered it "the noblest of professions" and both men and women agreed that they would like their daughters to be nurses, in part because they could make good marriages and give their husbands and the children the advantage of their acquired knowledge. In social status (Birdwhistell) the upper class saw the nurse as somewhat higher than the hairdresser, but considerably lower than the social worker—a skilled menial who would be tipped. The middle class placed the nurse higher than the stenographer, but lower than a secretary, someone who works before marriage, a widow, divorcee, or career woman (someone who cannot get a husband or is a neglectful wife). Middle-class women felt that their own daughters should go to college where they would meet "people of their own class." All three classes considered the nurse "faster" or "freer" in sexual matters than women in other occupations. Surprisingly, a later study of nurse self-images showed that nurses' recognition of the last image was common, but they also felt that the public saw them as hard-working women with considerable technical knowledge and skill and generally devoted to their duty to patients.

In 1961 Friedson presented somewhat similar findings. The nurse was considered most helpful by the lower class and praised for her teaching, counseling, and knowledge, but the upper class felt that she had little to offer.[5] Other social scientists agreed that, in general, the public did not see the nurse as a professional.

Although the early studies may appear totally out of date, remnants of these attitudes persist. One sociologist reports that the public is generally favorable toward nursing as an institution or profession within the general society and considers it prestigious and altruistic, but that in the hospital setting the image of the nurse is still associated with the performance of menial tasks; the nurse is an efficient and competent drudge who is an extension of the doctor's right hand. This sociologist feels that, in general, the image may be static, rooted in conditions pertaining five, ten, or twenty years ago, and that the nursing profession should make a serious effort to correct the image[6].

At best, as a more recent survey indicates, a considerable degree of confusion about nursing exists.[7] Although a vast majority of the public surveyed identified nursing as a profession, there was almost no support for nursing autonomy, and most thought nurses functioned best as assistants, not colleagues, of the doctor. The better educated, more affluent respondents were more inclined to support nurses' expanded role, collegiality, and autonomy (although the latter percentage was quite low). On the other hand, they were least likely to want a daughter to become a nurse, and very few in any category, especially men, wanted a son to do so. Yet the adjectives most used about nurses were: responsible, knowledgeable, caring, competent, skilled, efficient, neat, dedicated, and kind.

An examination of differences in occupational prestige as seen by physicians, graduate business students, and patients presents still another insight. As compared with a variety of physician specialists and others in the health field, patients rated the RNs above some physicians, the director of nursing, the hospital administrator, and all other health professionals; physicians rated all nurses above other health professions or occupations except dentistry, as did graduate students. The most important criterion stated by all three groups was "degree of skill." A number of questions were raised as to how much the prestige rating was influenced by personal contact and how much by reputation or image.[8] In Maryland, for instance, where a 1979 poll to determine how citizens rated the various professions resulted in nursing being at the top of the list, nurses were active in political and community affairs and quite visible as productive, respected professionals.* There is no doubt that some misconceptions result from contact with various uniformed health workers in hospitals, not always clearly identified as to whether they are aides, PNs, or RNs. (In the 1979 *RN* magazine survey, most people identified a nurse by white cap and uniform). But another major influence is the media. Interviews and researched articles or programs generally portray the nurse in a reasonably accurate way. As a rule, however, in fiction, the media have not, and still do not, correct a distorted image. Comic strips, novels, and television tend to portray the nurse (almost always female) either as a very sweet and/or sexy young girl, playing obedient handmaiden to the doctors, or as a tough, starched older woman, efficient and brusque. The popularity of medically oriented television series in the 1970s was supposedly a reflection of the public's intense interest in the

---

*As reported by *AJN* December, 1979.

field. But the images of the nurses portrayed have been no more accurate, and even nursing advisers to the shows seldom get the script changed. On the screen, Nurse Rached in the award-winning movie *One Flew Over the Cuckoo's Nest*, which was also a book and a play, was probably thoroughly hated by millions of people. An equal number may have leered at the nurses in the British hospital comedy series, or "MASH," or even in the various pornographic films where nurses are portrayed primarily as sex objects.[9,10]

Still, in the last few years, one of the best-selling nonfiction books was *Nurse*, which gives an accurate description of nursing practice in a hospital. A Broadway hit focused on the struggle of a woman overcoming a stroke, and the critics commented repeatedly on the sensitivity and support of the nurse as an important ingredient in the patient's improvement. With the President's veto of the Nurse Training Act in late 1978, newspapers across the country ran articles, columns, and political cartoons indicating disapproval of the veto. There are also an increasing number of newspaper and magazine articles on the changing role of the nurse, particularly in relation to the nurse midwife and nurse practitioner. It is a fact that a number of the latter were suggested or encouraged by nurses who recognized the importance of nurses' visibility as professionals.

Accuracy in the portrayal of nurses in the entertainment media will probably always be difficult, because the concern is entertainment, not truth. Inaccurate portrayal could probably be claimed by most occupations. Yet, some minority groups through concerted action have had some impact, as have women's groups, through complaints or boycotts. At the least, the inaccuracies have been brought to light. However, nurses will also recognize some of the nurse figures in the media, even if exaggerated. Are there not nurses, like Rached, who do not question detrimental practices, or who are dominating, prejudiced, rigid, even cruel, in their practice? Eliminating them might be an important phase in changing the public image, for then fiction will not imitate fact.

The Deutscher study also revealed that physicians tended to place nurses slightly below teachers but above social workers in occupational ratings (but thought nurses more humanitarian than teachers). On checking a scale of saint, Sunday school teacher, housewife, waitress, or "loose woman," to choose the term which to them most resembled a nurse, the majority chose the morally neutral category of housewife. (The next highest categories were saint and Sunday school teacher.) Another interesting point is that older physicians generally rated nurses more favorably on all questions than did younger physicians. This was also true of another study, where, in addition, physicians objected to professionalization of nurses.[11]

If physicians' current image of the nursing *profession* can be equated with their image of the nurse, it is clear that their perceptions are as confused as they were a hundred years ago. (See Chapters 3 and 4.) Now, as then, there are physicians and leaders in organized medicine who see and applaud the changes in nursing toward full professionalism; others find this trend either threatening, incongruent with what they think a nurse's role should be, or not as desirable as the "good old days."[12] One popular magazine, which also considered the misconceptions about nursing unfortunate, presented an accurate picture of the modern nurse. However, the interviews with physicians revealed that there has been little change in physicians' attitudes toward nurses.[13]

Supporting this contention is another survey by a nursing journal.[14] The vast majority of physicians surveyed saw nurses as their assistants and gave extremely limited definitions of nursing. Younger physicians were more inclined to think that nurses needed BSNs, encouraged expanded roles and favored (to a minor degree) giving nurses more responsibility. The clinical expertise of nurses, as defined by physicians, was praised by most. Although this survey presents some interesting viewpoints, it should be remembered that the kinds of questions asked frequently create a particular slant to such polls. For instance, another physician survey published in another journal within the same time frame seemed to contradict not only the findings of the other survey, but nurses' concepts of physicians' attitudes.[15]

A final comment might be made about the patient's image of an ideal nurse. Individuals, particularly when writing as former patients, have indicated that they wanted to be treated as human beings—wanted the nurse to be kind, friendly, pleasant, courteous, considerate, smiling, concerned, and reassuring. They are often not concerned with her competence but simply trust her to be safe. In one study "tender touch" was cited as the nurse's most important trait. A composite picture of the ideal nurse image as described in interviews with patients and nonpatients in a 1960 study revealed:

> She is qualified to the degree of being proficient. That is to say, she really knows her job. It's most important for her to understand me; that is, she can put herself into my shoes, experience some of my problems. While she is performing her work she expresses a sort of gentleness and friendliness. She is well-informed in other than her major role responsibilities. She is congenial with others, even though I am her primary concern. She appears to be happy. I don't mean that she is "bubbling over," but she is a person who seems to be enjoying life. Whenever I need her most, she is right there supporting me. I want to be able to really talk to her, and I expect her to be able to express herself well. Sometimes, even before I become uncomfortable, she will anticipate my needs and make me comfortable. When she performs a function she takes time to explain the "whys" and "hows" of it. She is always clean and well-groomed; and finally, I guess I do want her to feel sorry for me at certain times.[16]

The RN magazine survey and other public feedback gives some evidence that patients may not feel too differently today.[17,18]

DEMOGRAPHIC DATA

The Statistics Department of the American Nurses' Association, under contract with the Division of Nursing DHEW, probably maintains the most current general demographic data on registered nurses. The 1979 report (which reflects 1977 data) shows that there are a little more than 1,400,000 RNs; 98 percent of them are female. Approximately 92 percent are white; 2.5 percent, black; 2.1 percent, Asian; and 1.4 percent, Hispanic. More than 72 percent are married and almost 14 percent have never been married. More than 30 percent are in the twenty-five to thirty-four year age group, and the next highest percentage are the thirty-five to forty-four-year-old group; the next, forty-four to fifty-five. Almost 75 percent of all registered nurses are employed in nursing, but about 30 percent work only part time. Of these working nurses, not quite 70 percent are staff nurses, about 21 percent are somewhere in the administrative track, 5 percent are teachers, and less than 3 percent identify themselves as nurse practitioners or clinical specialists. It is estimated that a little more than 60 percent of employed nurses work in hospitals, the next largest per cent (about 6 to 8 percent each) in nursing homes, public health and physicians' offices, followed by student health, nursing education, private duty, and occupational health. Roughly 78 percent of all nurses have less than a baccalaureate degree of any kind (67 percent diploma); about 4 percent have a master's degree; and a little more than 2,000 nurses (approximately 0.2 percent have a doctorate.

Probably the most comprehensive current study of nurses that includes more specific details is the longterm longitudinal NLN Nursing Careers study, begun in 1962, which was designed to obtain definitive biographical characteristics of nursing students, their occupational goals, and their reasons for choice of nursing as a career. Later, HEW supported extension of the study to include students who entered associate degree, diploma, and baccalaureate RN programs in 1965 and 1967. In all, the sample consisted of some 800 participating nursing programs and 45,000 students. Data continue to be gathered, but the first major report was published in 1972 and supplies comprehensive data on nurses practicing today.[19]

Almost all students admitted to all three programs were women. The highest percentage of men (4.5 per cent) occurred in an associate degree program in 1967. Most students were native born. Most entering students were eighteen or nineteen, but those in associate degree programs were usually older, only a little more than 50 per cent being under twenty. Approximately one fourth of the AD students were or had been married, compared to 4 per cent in the other programs. More than a third of the married students in AD programs reported having three or more children, compared to one fifth of the married diploma students.

More than 95 per cent of all students entering diploma programs, 92 per cent in baccalaureate, and 90 per cent in AD programs were white. The number of blacks entering baccalaureate programs increased slightly in 1967, but decreased in AD programs. Never was there the proportional ethnic distribution of white and black equal to the United States census data (around 11 per cent black). Most students indicated affiliation with a Christian religion. Higher porportions of students entering diploma programs were Catholic, possibly because a number of Catholic groups continue to operate diploma schools, so that if a student wishes a religiously affiliated school, the diploma program would be readily available. The oldest child, usually a daughter, entered nursing in all programs in higher proportion than other siblings.

More than 60 per cent of entering baccalaureate students were in the top fourth of their high school class; almost half of the diploma students, and more than a third of the AD. The great majority of all students came from communities of less than 50,000, and more than 75 percent were attending nursing schools in their home state. The only geographic mobility was seen in baccalaureate students, of whom one fifth left their home state.

Some of the students in all programs had attended a nursing school before, this being most prevalent, about 17 per cent, in AD programs. Between 30 and 40 per cent of these had attended a practical nursing school or were already practical nurses; a smaller percentage had gone to diploma and baccalaureate programs.

Generally, both parents were living and native born. Fathers of AD and diploma students were predominantly sales or clerical workers or had a skilled trade. For baccalaureate students, "sales or clerical worker" was also a frequent category, but professional or semiprofessional ranked second, followed by skilled workers. Only among diploma students did semiskilled or unskilled make up 12 per cent or more of the total group.

Fathers of baccalaureate students had twelve and "sixteen or more" years of education most frequently; diploma and AD students twelve years, but a considerable number reported eight years or less education. Most employed mothers in all groups were sales or clerical workers; only in the baccalaureate group were service-type positions, usually schoolteachers, recorded. About 4 to 9 percent of the students' mothers were nurses, the most in the baccalaureate group. Essentially, students came from families within the $5,000 to $9,999 or $10,000 to $14,999 category. Students in all three programs received some financial assistance, those in baccalaureate programs requiring most (up to 41 percent).

The predominant reason for entering nursing, given by all students, was "to help others." About a third of each group said that they had chosen nursing because it is a good, desirable, respected, worthwhile, or rewarding profession. Around 15 percent thought nursing would provide good economic secur-

ity, and a number felt that it was one field in which a woman could always find employment. Previous employment or volunteer work in the health field influenced a small percentage of the students, and a slightly smaller percentage (between 5 and 10 percent) mentioned nursing as a calling or vocation, or implied some religious influence. Up to 20 percent simply stated that they had "always wanted to be a nurse." Most frequently mentioned as having influenced the student to enter nursing were members of the family, a friend, or acquaintance, whose occupation was not mentioned. If the occupation of the helpful person was mentioned, it most frequently was nursing. These factors are quite similar to those found in a smaller study.[20]

Students also answered open-ended questions as to the nursing program they had elected to enter. Of the baccalaureate students, most wished both college and nursing and also felt that with baccalaureate educations they would have a better nursing career. Associate degree students selected their programs primarily because of the program length, and secondly for financial reasons. Reasons for selecting the diploma program were evenly divided between the belief that it would give them a better education and the length. In all cases, most students chose their specific school because they believed it was a good school and the location was convenient.

Essentially all students felt that they would do general nursing in hospitals after graduation, and almost all planned to work after marriage. Approximately 40 to 50 percent of the AD and diploma students were planning more education after graduation; the baccalaureate students were almost equally divided among "yes," "no," and "undecided" answers.[21]

One follow-up of the Nurse Career Pattern Study (1975) focused on graduation and withdrawal from nursing programs.[22]* The rates of graduation from nursing education programs appeared to differ according to program; 53.6 percent baccalaureate, 60.6

percent associate degree, 69.7 percent diploma. These rates are considered somewhat higher than those of other students in two- and four-year colleges, but nursing students also differ biographically from those students. Three biographical variables seemed to be related to graduation and withdrawal in all three programs: ethnic group identification, family incomes as reported at the beginning of the study, and high school academic standing. Nonwhite students and those in the bottom half of their high school class were less likely to graduate. Family background had a differing effect in the various programs. Other noteworthy findings: older married students had higher graduation rates in AD programs, but this finding was reversed for diploma and baccalaureate programs. Roman Catholic students in diploma and baccalaureate programs graduated in larger proportions than those with other or no stated religious preference; a larger percentage of men withdrew. Most students withdrew in the first year of the program; the major reason for withdrawal was scholastic failure, followed by "no longer interested" (mostly baccalaureate), marriage, personal/family problems (especially married and formerly married students), and financial problems. A number of withdrawing students indicated continuing interest in the nursing field; some entered other programs or took nursing-related jobs, and others said they hoped to return to nursing education programs later. The report discusses in considerable detail other demographic/biographic variables.

The subjects of the Nursing Career Pattern Study were followed at one, five, ten and fifteen years after graduation. A comparison of the AD, diploma, and BS graduates ten years after graduation presents some interesting similarities and differences. At that point, only between 9 to 11 per cent had remained single. Of the married, or formerly

*Some of these data are also found in the first Career Pattern Report cited previously.

married (about 6 percent), only between 11 and 13 percent reported having no children; between 65 and 68 percent had two or more children. Evidently, having small children affected the nurses' working patterns. Whereas about 90 percent were working one year after graduation, this dropped at the five-year and again at the ten-year mark to 60 percent (BS), 64 percent (diploma), 67.5 percent (AD). The reasons most frequently given were home responsibilities, children, and no financial need to work, as well as difficulty in getting suitable hours. The older, married AD student, who had been the most likely to complete the program, also tended to remain in the work force longer. The numbers of the married women working part time increased with the years and appeared to be directly related to child care. Most of the single and formerly married were still working full time in nursing. Only a little more than 3 percent of the diploma nurses were working in non-nursing positions, but double that number of baccalaureate nurses had changed fields, about half to other professions. Positions held by the nurses ten years after graduation covered almost every field of nursing, but more than 60 percent of the AD and diploma nurses remained in hospital nursing, as opposed to 42 percent of the baccalaureate. The next largest percentage of AD nurses were employed (7 percent and under) in doctor's or dentist's offices, public health agencies, and nursing homes; baccalaureate nurses (15 to 16 percent) in schools of nursing, community health agencies, and public or private schools. Except if they were working part time, only about 30 percent of AD and diploma and 24 percent of the BS nurses remained in staff positions. In each group there were teachers, head nurses, and supervisors. In contrast to both AD and diploma graduates, baccalaureate nurses were most likely to be teachers and least likely to be head nurses.

AD nurses were most likely (84.6 percent) to have worked in two or more states, diploma nurses least (43 percent). All groups found it easier to get the type of position they wanted prior to 1970. The two major reasons cited concerning difficulty after that period were unavailability of desired hours or clinical field. (This probably changed during the nursing shortage of the late 1970s.) Twenty-four per cent of the AD graduates completed baccalaureate programs, slightly more than half in nursing; about 6 percent completed master's degrees. About 10 percent of the diploma graduates received baccalaureate degrees, 7 percent in nursing. Eighteen per cent of the baccalaureate graduates completed master's degrees, primarily in nursing; another 7 percent had completed or were enrolled in nurse-practitioner certificate programs. More than 80 percent of all the graduates indicated that their expectations of satisfaction with nursing had been met, but only about 60 percent felt that salary and working conditions met their expectations; all of these figures were remarkably consistent from the first through tenth years.[23]

These studies are all available on microfiche, but useful summaries have been briefly reported in *NLN Data Digest* in 1976, 1978, and 1979. A final report on the Career Pattern Study (1979–1980) gives an in-depth analysis and comparison of those who entered nursing in 1962, 1965, and 1967.

One other RN survey of interest was commissioned by the ANA in late 1978 in relation to their own members. The sample was considered representative of nurses in terms of general demographic data, but may or may not reflect the attitudes of all nurses. Among other things, the poll showed that politically, ANA members were about evenly split in supporting the Republican and Democratic parties, and that 91 percent were registered to vote. In relation to two major political/feminist issues, 73 percent supported and 22 percent opposed ratification of the equal rights amendment, and 61 percent believed that the decision about abortion should be left to the woman; only 9 percent opposed abortion in general, although 28 percent opposed federal funding. Generally, they also supported the concept of collective bargaining.*

PERSONALITY CHARACTERISTICS OF NURSES

Studies of personality characteristics of nurses either relate to the total population from samples of nurses with various backgrounds in various types of nursing programs geographically distributed (or a determination of consistency in this heterogeneous sampling), or individual studies, usually relatively small, of students in the different nursing programs or of nurses working in various specialties. Which personality traits are studied depends both on the overall purpose of the researcher and the type of test used. A much-quoted study using the Edwards Personal Preference Schedule (EPPS) is on the personality characteristics of heterogeneous groups of nursing students as compared to female college students.[24] Considered most striking was that these studies indicated nurses had a greater need for deference (need to conform to custom) and less need for dominance (need to supervise and direct action of others) than the college students. Six of the seven studies indicated that nursing students have a greater need for endurance (need to complete a job undertaken) and a lesser need for autonomy (need to be independent of others in making decisions). Also generally indicated was a greater need for order (need to have things organized). There was some further indication that nurses had more need for abasement (need to give in and avoid fights) and nurturance (need to help others) and a lesser need for exhibition (need to be the center of attraction), affiliation (need to form strong attachments), and change (need to do new things). One interpretation made by the author was that these personality characteristics are encouraged by head nurses and supervisors

*As reported in *AJN* July, 1979.

and are perhaps acquired as a matter of survival on the future work scene. He questioned whether the more aggressive, independent, dominant, original thinkers have been forced out of nursing programs. There was some objection to Costello's report by nurses who felt it was extremely negative,[25] but he defended it strongly.[26] One of the critics of the study later summarized updated data, and some variations were found.[27] Among the more interesting findings is that after five years of work experience, nurses had significantly higher scores on the "autonomy" and "order" scales and lower scores (less need) in "change" and "abasement."[28] Differences between sophomore students in 1962, 1965, and 1968 were also noted, with the latter considerably more autonomous and less likely to conform to custom. Changes from sophomore to senior years showed increased autonomy and aggression, and decreased deference, abasement, and dominance scores,[29] changes perhaps paralleling changes in the students' contemporaries. However, the author also concluded as a result of these and many more studies that nurses had a number of characteristics that inhibited therapeutic effectiveness in patient relationships.[30]

The danger in taking any study as a single answer to nursing personalities is illustrated by the work of several psychologists using the same tests on two different samples of students. In the first, which involved a mixed group of students and RNs, the nurses were found to be lacking assertiveness and competitive striving as compared with dietitians and dietetic interns. The author felt that having passive traits, nurses could perhaps be more empathic and compassionate with patients.[31] The other psychologists, using the same test on a group of sophomore baccalaureate student nurses, found this group more hostile and aggressive, and relatively more disturbed in their interpersonal relationships with their parents, compared to normative data for women. They saw some of these results as interfering with nursing practice.[32]

Besides the obvious difficulty of comparing the nurse groups to two separate and different groups, the nurses themselves were not like groups. A study such as Costello's, using the same test for various groups of nurses and determining commonalities, probably gives better information, although continual updating of these data is necessary.

These two studies also pointed out some differences between baccalaureate and other students, always an area of interest. One such study done with a limited sample in the West revealed no statistically significant difference in intelligence, leadership potential, responsibility, emotional stability, or sociability. The major difference was that baccalaureate students saw the ideal nursing situation as more professional than the real situation, and diploma and associate degree students saw the ideal situation as more traditional than the real situation.[33] However, other studies have shown differences among students with different educational experiences.

Evidence of the current concern as to whether women nursing students are success-oriented is seen in recent studies.[34] In one, it was found that 53 per cent of the baccalaureate female nursing students studied seemed to accept the academically successful female, but 47 per cent were ambivalent about the compatibility of intellectual attainment and social acceptance. They were seen as apparently having a more pronounced occupational orientation than women in the general college programs. Is this still a question of the doctor-nurse, male-female syndrome? A review of the literature indicates that sex role identity was an important variable in the process of professional socialization. Female nurses with masculine and feminine role identities had a higher total image of nursing and were more professionally oriented than those with a highly feminine sex identity (more likely to be diploma students).

Studies have also been done on personality characteristics of nurses in special areas of nursing. Two of these studies cited differences between nurses studying to be teachers and those studying to be supervisors. The first were found to be higher in "psychological mindedness, tender-minded sensitivity and need for reflectiveness"[35] as well as being "charming, warm, insightful persons with a wide range of interests and high personal aspirations." Prospective supervisors were judged to be "overly sensitive, moralistic, somewhat rebellious persons who avoid close interpersonal relationships, lack verbal facility, and do not have a clearly formulated personal philosophy.[36] Another study compared registered nurses in graduate school studying in various specialties. In characteristics determined as "warmth, has capacity for close relationships," those ranking first were in maternal-child nursing and least in psychiatric nursing; for "hostility towards others," psychiatric nursing ranked first and public health last; for "tends to project own feelings and own motivations on others," rankings were psychiatric nursing first and public health nursing last. Psychiatric nursing majors were found to be more independent than all other groups, but all others ranked higher on maturity and personal warmth.[37]

Staff psychiatric nurses, as opposed to other nurses, seem to have a more positive belief in themselves, more self-confidence, perseverance, independence, and determination. (They also have a higher separation and divorce rate.)[38]

Studies of various kinds have been done on nurse practitioners because this is a relatively new role. One seems to be typical of the findings: that in the EPPS, nurse practitioners score higher on autonomy, dominance, change, exhibition, and heterosexuality.[39] However, it should be remembered that the results may vary according to the comparison group. One further example of the studies done in special areas of nursing presents a profile of the coronary care nurse that includes both demographic and personality characteristics. The conclusion was that although many socioeconomic factors were held in common with other nurses, CCU nurses entered this field because more responsibility and challenge were offered and because they could enhance their knowledge and introduce new ideas. The other nurses showed a patient- or self-centered orientation.[40] It is to be expected that such personality studies will continue and provide new data for study. However, all of these studies, although of considerable interest, should be regarded with some caution. The lack of consistent findings creates some questions of overall usefulness, although the heterogeneity of nurses is undoubtedly a key factor in their diverse results.[41]

ATTITUDES OF NURSES

One kind of research on nurses that has been done continually explores their attitudes about nursing in general, work situations, and reactions toward certain kinds of patients. The finding of the NLN study previously cited, indicating that individuals entered nursing because they "wanted to help others," has been consistent over the years. Therefore, because it is evident that a number of students left nursing before completing the program, or did not work in nursing after graduation, and because nurses have also been accused of some indifference to quality care, the basic question as to why arises. A number of writers have cited "disillusionment with nursing" as a major reason why nurses leave jobs or nursing itself. Yet, further investigation seems to show that the disillusionment, for graduates as for students, is more related to the practice setting than to the practice. Whether the study is almost twenty years old[42] or one of the many new studies, nurses still appear to find their greatest satisfaction in relation to patient care. Many are discouraged because they cannot give the comprehensive care that they believe in, but are forced into functional and bureaucratic work patterns that do not give primary attention to the patient's total care.[43] Although there are in nursing, as there are in any profession, some who are primarily interested in a job or in earning money—the utilizer, migrant, or appliance nurse (one who works only long enough to buy a new home appliance)—the majority of nurses still apparently have some of the same motivations with which they entered nursing.

Changing the situations and circumstances that cause disillusionment and consequent loss of high quality care is a key priority for nursing today. This might be illustrated by a series of surveys done by a popular nursing journal. Recognizing that usually only those with reasonably strong feelings answer a questionnaire printed in a journal, it is particularly interesting that about 10,000 nurses replied. Some of the key points that emerged in the quality of care survey[44,45] follow:

> *Ninety-two percent believed that the overall quality of care patients received was good to excellent.*
> *Ninety-six percent believed they were competent or moderately competent to deliver quality nursing care.*
> *Seventy-seven percent rated the performance of their co-workers as good to excellent in physical care, with lesser ratings in rehabilitation, psychological support, patient education, and discharge planning.*
> *Eighty-one percent believed that physicians with whom they worked gave good physical care, but their psychological care was rated poor to fair by 77 percent.*
> *Eighteen percent said they had encountered a situation where a nurse had accidentally caused a patient's death; 42 percent had seen death caused by a doctor.*

A response that attracted newspaper headlines was that 38 percent of the nurses said that they would not choose to be a patient in the hospital where they worked. Nurses also had firm opinions on what caused patient care to be poor—primarily, inadequate staffing, too many nondirect nursing activities, inadequate budget, inadequate support from nursing administration, and interdepartmental hospital politics.

In the study on job satisfaction a year and a half later,[46,47,48] the three major dissatis-factions were unsafe practices, which included incompetent nurses and doctors; overcrowding and dangerous understaffing; poor leadership, with ineffective nursing service administrators and indifferent, authoritarian hospital administrators; and communication breakdown both to and from administration. Nevertheless, 79 percent of nurses found their jobs satisfying (about the same as those in the NLN study). Nurses in administration, education, community health, industry, and schools of nursing were most satisfied. (Studies of nurse practitioners show that they are also very satisfied with their jobs.) In terms of clinical areas, the most satisfied were emergency room nurses, and the least, psychiatric nurses. Four out of five nurses in hospitals believed that they worked in situations in which they were unable to take care of patients as well as they could or should.

A number of other interesting findings related to opinions about working hours, physical working conditions, and morale. What was cited overwhelmingly as the most important consideration of both men and women in looking for a job was opportunity for professional growth; supportive nursing administration was also high on the list. The least important for women were fringe benefits, and for men, choice of hours or shifts. The fact that a 1974 study listed both salary and fringe benefits as high on the list of influential factors in seeking a workplace[49] may indicate that in the few intervening years these had improved enough to be generally satisfactory or that in any one region they tended to be competitive in like agencies.

The ambivalence of nurses in relation to job satisfaction and dissatisfaction may also be reflected in another of the magazine samples taken among subscribers.[50] The "average nurse" answering this questionnaire was a married staff nurse in her mid-twenties, working in a community hospital in an urban center, and earning $8,000 to $12,000 a year. She was not a union member but did belong to her professional organization. These nurses were ambivalent about joining unions, but the majority either approved or agreed that "someone should represent nurses, but not unions." Their major reasons for the need to organize were to make management listen, gain increased wages, gain more fringe benefits, and gain more say in the quality of patient care.

The differences in findings in this survey and others points out the difficulty in determining how accurately any survey reflects the voice of nursing. At the least, it is important to consider how the sample was selected, who responded, and how questions were worded. This is particularly true when the survey is done by a journal, for, inevitably, one purpose must be to attract and hold readers. One example is a survey done by a journal whose editorial stance is directed toward the nondegree staff nurse. The survey was presumably aimed at finding how nurses felt about the entry into practice issue.[51] Unfortunately, the questions tended to slant toward expected answers—that most nurses in that readership did not agree with the ANA position that entry into professional practice should be at the baccalaureate level. In general, that was the answer that emerged; however, because of the unclear questions, the poll cannot be viewed as definitive, despite the editor's insistence. For instance, to the question, "What would make you professional?" 47.8 percent answered bachelor's degree, 42.8 percent diploma degree, 16.8 percent associate degree, and 19.1 percent equivalency exam. It appeared that almost everyone supported his/her own program, and a few more opted for the baccalaureate. Yet, at another point, most agreed that advanced education was desirable. In the long run, the only clear result of the poll was that it showed many of the nurses who responded had a somewhat confused picture of what the ANA position really was—a situation that caused considerable emotionalism, because their inaccurate interpretation was that nurses without baccalaureate degrees would find both their status and their jobs threatened. That alone, of course, does present one aspect of nursing attitudes at the time.

Other studies receiving considerable attention today investigate students' or RNs' attitudes toward certain types of patients, for example, geriatric, alcoholic, or mentally ill patients; those who have abortions; or those in certain socioeconomic and ethnic groups.[52,53] The purpose is primarily to determine what these attitudes are and why, how they affect patient care, and how to encourage or change particular attitudes. What may be surprising is that nurses do not react much differently from middle-class, white lay people in their attitudes about patients who are poor, alcoholic, mentally disturbed, have what are considered socially undesirable diseases, or come from certain ethnic groups. One study of several years ago also showed that registered nurses are much more conservative on matters relating to human sexuality than are nursing students, female medical students, or female graduate students.[54] It is to be expected that as new, more diverse students become graduates, many of these attitudes will change. However, the American culture must also be considered; foreign nurses have different attitudes on many of these points.[55]

MINORITY GROUPS IN NURSING

Studies done on the general population of nursing students and graduates are inevitably influenced by the fact that the majority of nurses are both women and white. There is increasing interest in the minority groups in nursing, usually minority in terms of race, or ethnic group, such as black, American Indian, Spanish-speaking, foreign-trained nurses, and also including the male minority.

Of the studies now existing, there is some concentration on blacks, and questions usually focus on why they do or do not enter nursing, why there is such a large proportion who do not complete nursing education programs, and possible answers to these problems. Reasons given that explain why many of the racial and ethnic minorities, who are often also considered socioeconomically deprived, do not enter nursing include lack of role models, lack of understanding of what nursing is, lack of proper counseling, and inability to qualify because of poor academic records.[56] A summary of some of these studies and others as they relate to blacks is presented in one study that concentrates on methods of retaining these students.[57] A specific group of disadvantaged black baccalaureate students given special prenursing counseling and guidance, academic help, and orientation to nursing were compared to all disadvantaged students in the NLN Career Pattern Study (all programs) who did not have such concentrated attention. (Actually most of the latter were white.) It was found that the first group had a lower drop-out rate, and fewer of those who did withdraw did so because of disenchantment with nursing or academic failure. It was concluded that such help is a key factor in retention, although most of the students did not need all aspects of the remediation programs. It was considered meaningful that underachievers in high school who successfully completed the nursing programs had been given academic, personal, and financial assistance, a fact that might have implications for student selection on the basis of test scores and high school grades. An interesting fact emerged concerning students who became RNs: both study groups indicated dissatisfaction with their working conditions—not salary. It was recommended that a follow-up study determine the reasons for dissatisfaction.

A 1977 HEW study on health manpower presented additional information on black women entering collegiate nursing.[58] (Almost no black men showed interest in the field.) About one in ten aspiring nurses in 1974 was a black woman, frequently from a severely disadvantaged background, in terms of both education and economics. Black women students tended to be older than white students and almost two in five were financially independent of their parents, more than any other group of females interested in health careers. They also expressed major concern about their ability to pay for their college education, but few received scholarship aid or sought loans. Therefore, it is not surprising that most enrolled in two-year colleges. Although unsure of their academic and mathematical ability, black women who planned to become nurses, as their white counterparts, rated themselves high on public speaking, writing, leadership, popularity, intellectual and social self-confidence, motivation, and physical attractiveness, and they set a high priority on helping others. They seemed to have a wider range of interests and were more concerned with future financial success and less in raising a family.

Nursing recruitment for all ethnic minorities has gradually increased, stimulated particularly by HEW special project grants available since 1965. Included were one RN program on an Indian reservation and one geared especially to Mexican-Americans. By the late 1970s, nursing programs reported to the NLN an enrollment of between 3.2 and 6.7 percent black students, primarily AD and BS, and between 0.8 and 2.1 percent students with Hispanic backgrounds, primarily in AD programs. About 1 percent were Oriental or American Indian. In all cases, larger percentages of the minority students entered practical nurse programs. Data are not complete because some schools refuse to answer questions about minorities, but it appears that, except for Oriental and American Indians, minority enrollment declined in the late 1970s.

Because there is a feeling that the needs of some of these groups are not being met by existing organizations, there is an increase in formation of both local and national organizations by the various ethnic minorities. Nevertheless, if negative job discrimination is present, it probably is less likely to show in salaries. For instance, black nurses, on the average, earn more than their white nurse peers, but they also tend to work in larger cities where salaries are higher.

Men have been neglected as potential sources of nurse power, although male nurses have existed almost as long as female nurses. By 1910 about 7 per cent of all student and graduate nurses were men, but in succeeding years the percentage declined until by 1940 it had dropped to 2 per cent. Most men were graduates of hospital schools connected with mental institutions; there were few schools for men connected with general hospitals and few coeducational ones.*

Men suffered the same discrimination within nursing that women have in male-dominated fields, although this was not always the fault of nursing. For instance, men nurses were kept in the enlisted ranks in the regular armed services until 1966, when with the continuous pressure of the ANA, commissions were finally available to them in the Regular Nurse Corps. During World War II, men nursing students were not exempt from the draft, although the need for nurses was critical. Therefore nursing enrollment for men dropped drastically to less than 200. After the war, enrollment began to climb slowly until, in the 1971–1972 academic year, a total of 5,170 men, about 6 per cent, were admitted to basic RN programs, nearly twice the proportion of the previous three years, and 2,751 to PN programs (more than in any other type of program). Of the RN programs, most men were enrolled in associate degree programs and the fewest in diploma programs. Graduation figures for men were also higher: In the next years, the percentage of men enrolled remained at about 5 per cent in RN programs and 4 per cent in PN programs as did the percentage in the work force (2 percent).

The increase in enrollment may be attributed in part to the Nurse Training Act of 1971, which called for identification and recruitment of "individuals with a potential for education or training in the nursing profession." Two interesting programs that developed at that time were an AD program in Texas aimed toward discharged medical corpsmen and an evening diploma program in New York for retiring policemen and firemen. Completion rates have been considerably higher than those for other types of nursing schools, but then the major reasons given by many men for entering the field are job availability, security, and mobility, as well as working conditions and salary. (Interest in people is also a factor.)

Men obviously look at nursing as a career. In comparison with women, more are employed in nursing after graduation, and of these, some 60 percent work full time. Like women, they are most likely to be employed in hospitals; their second choice, 11 percent, is the military. Only one third hold staff level positions in hospitals, which may be related to their greater tendency to work full time and also the desire to move into better-paying administrative positions. Some female nurses, particularly those who are younger, perceive employer discrimination in favor of the males, but DHEW figures on beginning employment show close relationships between salaries of males and females. The greatest percentage level difference (4 percent) is at the $10,000 and above range, but as with the black nurses, there may be some relationship to job choice in large urban centers. Some surveys and studies show that overall women nurses recognize that men nurses are accepted by both patients and physicians and believe that they can make a valuable contribution to nursing.[59] Discrimination has been given visibility primarily in assignment of private duty nurses.[60] The opposite stance, that men nurses will dominate the higher echelons of nursing, is also voiced, even in other countries.[61,62] Studies (many using small samples) of the attitudes, values, personality characteristics, and concerns of men who choose nursing as a career show varied results, often related to geography and the time of the study.[63,69]

Comparison of several studies seemed to indicate that more recent students were less likely to come into nursing to increase social

---

*See Chapter 3.

and economic status, because their parents were already in a middle-class or higher socioeconomic level. It seems that men are influenced into nursing through previous contacts or work in the health field. Their families seldom encourage them, but usually do not object. Men report that although friends are generally supportive, they get negative reactions from other classmates and strangers, who show a tendency to view them as homosexuals. These attitudes created some role strain for the men, as did women in authority, which has been described as status contradiction and prestige loss. Students voiced opposing opinions that they were spoiled and favored by women in these positions or that they were discriminated against or at least treated differently from women students; some noted no differences. Small studies in personality have reported such varying data as: men nurses have more empathy than women nurses or any non-nursing college student; men and women in nursing were more likely to have similar attitudes and personalities than those outside nursing; and men maintain the high social values necessary to the nursing profession, at the same time bringing their own critical, rational, and empirical interests to the field.

Areas of nursing preferred by men differed in the baccalaureate and other programs. The first preferred surgical nursing, intensive or coronary care, and nursing education. Diploma and AD men preferred administration, anesthesia, psychiatry, operating room, and teaching. All men generally listed specialties requiring technical competence and responsibility; they also wanted higher salaries and status. Again, this picture is constantly changing. In one small baccalaureate study, not one man student indicated interest in either anesthesia or administration. In another, the concern was in choosing a field in which role conflict would be lessened, such as those not requiring personal physical care or a uniform. There is some indication that men nurses also show interest in physician's assistant and nurse practitioner roles.

Obviously, there is no one profile of the modern nurse, particularly in these dynamic times. However, the information obtained from these various studies reveals more about the practitioners of nursing. An oft-quoted but unidentified statement defines nurses as a "migrating mass of maidens meditating matrimony." That may still be true in some cases, but it tells only a small part of the nursing story.

REFERENCES

1. Leo Simmons and Virginia Henderson, *Nursing Research—A Survey and Assessment* (New York: Appleton-Century-Crofts, 1964), p. 172.
2. Lucie Young, "A Frame of Reference for Nursing Education" (unpublished Ph.D. dissertation, School of Education, University of Pittsburgh, 1965), p. 127.
3. Simmons and Henderson, op. cit., pp. 175–181.
4. Irwin Deutscher, *A Study of the Registered Nurse in a Metropolitan Community* (Kansas City, Mo.: Community Studies Inc., 1957), as reported in Simmons and Henderson, op. cit., pp. 179–184.
5. Eliot Friedson, *Patients' Views of Medical Practice* (New York: Russell Sage Foundation, 1961).
6. Hansi Pollak, "Community Attitudes," *Int. Nurs. Rev.*, **14:**37–38 (Jan.-Feb. 1967).
7. Anthony Lee, "How Nurses Rate With the Public," *RN* **42:**25–39 (June 1979).
8. Stephen Shortell, "Occupational Prestige Differences Within the Medical and Allied Health Professions," *Soc. Sci. and Med.*, **8:**1–9 (1974).
9. See bibliography: Beletz, Greenleaf, Hott, Richter, Wheelock.
10. "Oh Nurse, Your Image Is Showing," *Am. Nurse*, **6:**4 (May 1974).
11. T. Ford and D. Stephenson, *Institutional Nurses: Roles, Relationships and Attitudes in Three Alabama Hospitals* (Alabama: University of Alabama Press, 1954), as reported in Simmons and Henderson, op. cit., pp. 176–177.
12. See bibliography: Ambrose, Hoekelman, Kalisch.

13. Trucia Krushner, "The Nursing Profession—Condition: Critical," *Ms* (August 1973), pp. 72–77, 100–102.

14. Anthony Lee, "How Nurses Rate with MDs: Still the Handmaiden," *RN,* 42:20–30 (July, 1979).

15. Loy Wiley, "What Doctors *Really* Think of Nursing—and Nurses," *Nurs. 79,* **9:** 73–77 (Aug., 1979).

16. Jane Holliday, "An Ideal Image of the Professional Nurse with a Method for Formulating a Composite Ideal Image" (unpublished Ed.D. dissertation, Teachers College, Columbia University, 1960).

17. Robert Veninga, "Communications: A Patient's Eye View," *Am. J. Nurs.,* **73:**320–322 (Feb. 1973).

18. A Measure of Self Worth," *Am. J. Nurs.,* **74:**635 (Apr. 1974).

19. Lucille Knopf, *From Student to RN* (Bethesda, Md.: Department of Health, Education, and Welfare, 1972).

20. Joe Taylor and Frances Richter, "What Motivates Students into Nursing?" *Hospitals,* 213:59–61 (Jan. 1, 1969).

21. Knopf, op. cit., pp. 7–17.

22. Lucille Knopf, *Graduation and Withdrawal from RN Programs* (Bethesda, Md.: Department of Health, Education and Welfare, 1975).

23. "Nurse Career Pattern Study: Baccalaureate Degree Nurses Ten Years After Graduation," *NLN Data Digest* (Mar. 1979).

24. C. G. Costello, "Attitudes of Nurses to Nursing," *Can. Nurse,* **63:**42–44 (June 1969).

25. E. Kemp and J. Peitchinis, "Nurses' Attitudes: Fact or Fallacy," *Can. Nurse,* **64:**51–53 (Feb. 1968).

26. "Dr. Costello Asnwers His Critics," *Can. Nurse,* **64:**54 (Feb. 1968).

27. Jacquelyn Peitchinis, "Therapeutic Effectiveness of Counseling by Nursing Personnel," *Nurs. Res.,* **21:**138–148 (Mar.-Apr. 1972).

28. Ibid., p. 181.

29. Ibid., p. 142.

30. Ibid., p. 144.

31. Sidney Cleveland, "Is There a Typical Nursing Personality?" *RN* (Dec. 1965), pp. 46–51.

32. Lewis Bernstein, Eugene Turrell, and Richard Dana, "Motivation for Nursing," *Nurs. Res.,* 14:222–226 (Summer 1965).

33. Mary Ann Richards, "A Study of Differences in Psychological Characteristics of Students Graduating from Three Types of Basic Nursing Programs," *Nurs. Res.,* **21:**258–261 (May-June 1972).

34. See bibliography: Pender, Stromberg.

35. Lois Graham, "Differential Characteristics of Graduate Students Preparing for Teaching or Supervision in Two Clinical Specialites, *Nurs. Res.,* **16:**184 (Spring 1967).

36. Doris Miller, "Characteristics of Graduate Students Preparing for Teaching or Supervision in a Nursing Specialty," *Nurs. Res.,* **15:**168–171 (Spring 1966).

37. Doris Miller, "Characteristics of Graduate Students in Four Clinical Nursing Specialities," *Nurs. Res.,* **14:**106–113 (Spring 1965).

38. Sylvester R. Mloff, "Personality Correlates of a Psychiatric Nurse," *J. Psych. Nurs.,* **14:**19–23 (Feb. 1976).

39. Martha Strum White, "Psychological Characteristics of the Nurse Practitioner," *Nurs. Outlook,* **23:**160–166 (Mar. 1975).

40. Elsa Kelberg, "Coronary Care Nurse Profile," *Nurs. Res.,* **21:**34 (Jan.-Feb. 1972).

41. Barbara Lewis and Cary Cooper, "Personality Measurement Among Nurses: A Review," *Int. J. Nurs. Stud.,* **13:**209–229 (1976).

42. Simmons, op. cit., pp. 182–196.

43. Marlene Kramer, *Reality Shock: Why Nurses Leave Nursing.* St. Louis: C. V. Mosby Company 1974.

44. G. Ray Funkhouser, "Quality of Care, Part I," *Nurs. 76,* **6:**22–31 (Dec. 1976).

45. G. Ray Funkhouser, "Quality of Care, Part II," *Nurs. 77,* **7:**27–33 (Jan. 1977).

46. Marjorie Godfrey, "Job Satisfaction, Part I," *Nurs. 78,* **8:**89–102 (Apr. 1978).

47. Marjorie Godfrey, "Job Satisfaction, Part 2," *Nurs. 78,* **8:**105–120 (May 1978).

48. Marjorie Godfrey, "Job Satisfaction, Part 3," *Nurs. 78* **8:**81–95, (June 1978).

49. Marjorie Godfrey, "Your Fringe Benefits: How Much Are They Really Worth?" *Nurs. 75,* **5:**73–75ff. (Jan. 1975).

50. Marjorie Godfrey, "Someone Should

Represent Nurses,'' *Nurs. 76*, **2:**73–90 (June 1976).

51. Anthony Lee, ''No!'' *RN* **42:**83–93 (Jan. 1979).

52. See bibliography: Blaylock, Brinton, Cornish, Gillis, Gunter, Larson, Minehan, Moody, Nelson, Richek, Rickelman, Schmid, and *Nurs. 74* survey.

53. See bibliogrpahy in Chapter 10 on abortion attitudes.

54. Harold Lief and Tyana Payne, ''Sexuality—Knowledge and Attitudes,'' *Am J Nurs, 75:*2026–2029 (Nov. 1975).

55. Lois Davitz, et al., ''Foreign and American Nurses: Reactions and Interactions,'' *Nurs. Outlook*, **24:**237–242 (Apr. 1976).

56. See Bibliography: Miller, Winder.

57. M. Elizabeth Carnegie, *Disadvantaged Students in RN Programs* (New York: National League for Nursing, 1974).

58. *Freshmen Interested in Nursing and Allied Health Professions: A Summary Report*, DHEW Publication No. HRA 77–46, 1977.

59. Myron D. Fottles, ''Attitudes of Female Nurses Toward Male Nurses,'' *J. Health and Soc. Behav.*, 17:98–110 (June 1976).

60. Bruce Nortell, ''Leading Cases—Male Nurse and Sex Discrimination,'' *JAMA*, **237:**1610–1611 (Apr. 11, 1977).

61. Rita Austin, ''Sex and Gender in the Future of Nursing, Part 1,'' *Nurs. Times*, **73:**113–116 (Aug. 1977).

62. Rita Austin, ''Sex and Gender in the Future of Nursing, Part 2,'' *Nurs. Times*, **73:**117–119 (Sept. 19, 1977).

63. Patricia Bush, ''The Male Nurse: A Challenge to Traditional Role Identities,'' *Nurs. Forum*, 15:390–405 (1976).

64. Bonnie J. Garvin, ''Values of Male Nursing Students,'' *Nurs. Research*, **25:**352–357 (Sept./Oct. 1976).

65. Malcolm Macdonald, ''How Do Men and Women Students Rate in Empathy?'' *Am. J. Nurs.*, **77:**998 (June 1977).

66. Hal Rogness, ''A Student Surveys His Classmates,'' *Nurs. Outlook*, **24:**303–305 (May 1976).

67. Adrian Schoenmaker, ''Nursing's Dilemma: Male Versus Female Admission Choice,'' *Nurs. Forum*, **15:**406–412 (1976).

68. Adrian Schoenmaker and David Radosevich, ''Conflict Between Expectations and Reality,'' *Nurs. Outlook*, **24:**298–303 (May 1976).

69. Arthur Williams, ''Characteristics of Male Baccalaureate Students Who Selected Nursing as a Career,'' *Nurs. Res.*, **22:**520–524 (Nov.–Dec. 1073).

BIBLIOGRAPHY

Adams, Jerry, and Lilyan Klein. ''Students in Nursing School: Considerations in Assessing Personality Characteristics,'' *Nurs. Res.*, **19** (Jan.–Feb. 1970) 362–366. Notes differences in nursing students in later classes—possibly because of like changes in students' contemporaries.

Alexander, Judith. ''How the Public Perceives Nurses and Their Education,'' *Nurs. Outlook*, **27** (Oct. 1979), 654–656. Survey in South Carolina indicates that majority of public thought nurses should have baccalaureate.

Ambrose, David M. ''Physicians and Nurses Rank Importance of Nursing Activities.'' *Hospitals*, **51** (Nov. 1977) 115–118. Nursing activities, ranked by each, show almost completely different priorities and concepts of nurse role.

Bailey, June, and Karen Claus. ''Comparative Analysis of the Personality Structure of Nursing Students,'' *Nurs. Res.*, **18** (July-August 1969), 320–326. Shows similar findings as those in Costello studies.

Bates, Barbara, and Robert W. Chamberlin. ''Physician Leadership as Perceived by Nurses,'' *Nurs. Res.*, **19** (Nov./Dec. 1970), 534–539. Nurses have some reservations on quality and type of leadership.

Beletz, Elaine. ''Is Nursing's Public Image Up to Date?'' *Nurs. Outlook*, **22** (July 1974), 432–435. A small survey of hospital patients points out that the public still seems unaware of changes in nursing practice.

Blaylock, J. M. ''Characteristics of Nurses and of Medical-Surgical Patients to Whom They React Positively and Negatively: A Synopsis of Findings,'' in *Eighth Nursing Research Conference*, Albuquerque, N. M. Mar. 15–17, 1972, pp. 113–122. New York: American Nurses' Association, 1972. Findings indicated that some nurses reacted negatively to patients who did not conform to their wishes and expectations and tended to approve conforming, mannerly persons.

Brinton, Diana. "Value Differences Between Nurses and Low-Income Families," *Nurs. Res.*, **21** (Jan.–Feb. 1972), 46–52. Concepts of priority and importance of health differed little between nurses and low-income mothers in the study, but nurses were not aware of the mother's health care values. Other data in relation to values of mothers and their keeping appointments are given.

Brown, J. S., Y. B. Swift, and M. L. Oberman. "Baccalaureate Students' Images of Nursing: A Replication," *Nurs. Res.*, **23** (Jan–Feb. 1974) 53–59. A study done earlier in California was replicated in Oregon, and it was found that both sets of students held similar views of nursing and of professional occupational values. Although some changes occurred in a year of study, neither achieved great consensus regarding what they believed characterized nursing.

Brown, R. G. and R. W. Stones. "Personality and Intelligence Characteristics of Male Nurses," *Int. J. Nurs. Stud.*, **9** (Aug. 1972), 167–176. In study of 500 men in nursing programs in England, the men were found to be more extroverted than the female entrants and were less neurotic than established norms for the personality test given.

Carnegie, Mary Elizabeth. *Disadvantaged Students in RN Programs.* New York: National League for Nursing, 1973. A comparative study of school completion records of two groups of socioeconomically disadvantaged students in programs leading to RN licensure. Demographic data.

Cleland, Virginia, et al. "Social and Psychological Influences on Employment of Married Nurses," *Nurs. Res*, **25** (Mar./Apr. 1976), 90–97. Study of 2,000 married nurses and their work patterns. Recommendations made for changing these.

Cornish, R. D., and M. V. Miller. "Attitudes of Registered Nurses Toward the Alcoholic." *J. Psychiatr. Nurs.*, **14** (Dec. 1976) 19–22. Found that nurses' attitudes were negative toward patients identified as alcoholics. Case study format used.

Elms, Roslyn and Jean Moorehead. "Will the 'Real' Nurse Please Stand Up: The Stereotype vs Reality," *Nurs. Forum* **16**(2) (1977) 112–127. Compares real nurses with stereotypes.

Ezrati, Janet Bostrom. "Midwifery in the Media," *J. Nurse-Midwifery*, **22** (Summer 1977), 35–38. Reviews and analyzes public image of midwifery over last fifty years.

Felton, Jean, and Iva Pleasant. "Men in Occupational Health Nursing," *Occup. Health Nurs.*, **18** (Jan. 1970), 9–18. A study of the role of men in occupational health nursing presents data concerning number, education, salary.

Gilbert, Marie. "Personality Profiles and Leadership Potential of Medical-Surgical and Psychiatric Nursing Graduate Students." *Nurs. Res*, **25** (Mar./Apr. 1975), 125–130. Explores one method of measuring leadership potential as related to personality traits and how personality characteristics relate to choice of speciality area.

Gillis, Marion, Sr. "Attitudes of Nursing Personnel Toward the Aged." *Nurs. Res.*, **22** (Nov.–Dec. 1973), 517–520. RNs, LPNs, and aides in five nursing homes and a hospital were studied to determine differences in attitudes toward the aged in relation to age, education, length of employment, and type of agency.

Godfrey, Marjorie. "Your Fringe Benefits: How Much Are They Really Worth?" *Nurs. 75*, **5** (Jan. 1975), 73–75ff. Survey of various hospitals and what they provided in fringe benefits at that time.

Greenberg, Emily, and Burton Levine. "Role Strain in Men Nurses." *Nurs. Forum*, **10** (Fall 1971), 417–430. A small study of men nurses to determine if they are affected by discrimination. Although bias against men was not found to be great, they do suffer from role strain and seek areas of specialization to minimize it.

Greenleaf, Nancy P. "Coming to Terms With Nurse Rached." *Sup. Nurse*, **7** (June 1976), 48–50. Thoughtful article that explores nurses' image of themselves and the myths embodied by Nurse Rached.

Gunter, Laurie. "Students' Attitudes Toward Geriatric Nursing." *Nurs. Outlook*, **19** (July 1971), 466–469. This study indicated that students had a considerable number of sterotypes regarding the aged. Although a course and experience changed this, their negative attitudes did not change.

Hoekelman, Robert. "Nurse-Physician Relationships." *Am. J. Nurs.*, **75** (July 1975), 1150–1152. Collegial relationships are hampered by sexism, educational differentials, misunderstandings of each other's role, and basic dishonesty in interaction.

Hott, Jacqueline. "Updating Cherry Ames." *Am. J. Nurs.*, **77** (Oct. 1977), 1581–1583. Interview with the author of this popular juvenile series, with amusing suggestions for a new updated version.

Hutcheson, J. D., Jr., et al. "Toward Reducing Attrition in Baccalaureate Degree Nursing Programs: An Exploratory Study." *Nurs. Res.*, **22** (Nov.–Dec. 1973), 530–533. It appeared that the only apparent meaningful variables in drop-outs were in relation to clinical performance and relationships with teachers.

Jones, Carolyn. "Why Associate Degree Nursing Students Persist." *Nurs. Res.*, **24** (Jan./Feb. 1975), 57–59. Small study of personality factors of AD students who remained in nursing programs.

Kalisch, Beatrice, and Philip Kalisch. "An Analysis of the Sources of Physician and Nurse Conflict." *JONA*, **7** (Jan. 1977), 51–57. Vast differences in roles and how each perceives the other's role, as well as overlapping of functions, create serious problems in collegiality.

Knopf, Lucille. *From Student to RN.* DHEW Pub. No. (NIH) 72–130. Washington, D.C.: U.S. Government Printing Office, 1972. The first report of the Nurse Career-Pattern Study. Contains demographic data of students in all kinds of nursing programs.

Krall, Vita. "Personality Factors in Nursing School Success and Failure." *RN,* **19** (May–June 1970), 265–268. Lack of success, in this study of diploma students, appears to be because of academic problems and inadequate self-concept.

Kramer, Marlene. "Role Conceptions of Baccalaureate Nurses and Success in Hospital Nursing." *Nurs. Res.*, **19** (Sept.–Oct. 1970), 428–438. Report on beginning of long-term study on 220 collegiate nurses to determine whether success or failure is result of professional or bureaucratic orientation.

Larson, Sister Paula. "Nurse Perceptions of Patient Characteristics." *Nurs. Res.*, **26** (Nov./Dec. 1977), 416–421. Nurses were found to stereotype lower-class patients as dependent, passive, unintelligent, lazy, careless, uninformed, unsuccessful. Patients with less acceptable illnesses were viewed more negatively than those with more acceptable illnesses.

Lee, Anthony. "Nursing's Shopworn Image: How It Hurts—and Helps." *RN,* **42** (Aug. 1979), 42–47. Compares attitudes of physicians and the public about nursing and makes suggestions to nurse about updating nursing's image.

Lee, Gerald. "A Male Nurse in OB." *Imprint.* **20** (Dec. 1973), 18, 19ff. A man nursing student discusses the reactions of patients, families, and the students to a male nursing student in the obstetrical unit.

Marram, Gwen. "Patients' Evaluation of Nursing Performance." *Nurs. Res.*, **22** (Mar.–Apr. 1973), 153–157. In a study of the importance to nurses of patient evaluation, it was found that nurses were more likely to consider the evaluation sound if the task evaluated was one visible to the patient.

May, W. T., and Robert Ilardi. "Change and Stability of Values in Collegiate Nursing Students." *Nurs. Res.*, **19** (July–August 1970), 359–365. This study compared nursing students to a similar study ten years earlier. Results indicate some changes that seem to parallel more general changes in students' contemporaries.

"Men in Nursing." *RN* **36** (Aug. 1973), 33–43. Series of articles covering statistical review of increase of men in nursing, career goals, change of image, reasons for increase.

Miller, Michael. "On Blacks Entering Nursing." *Nurs. Forum,* **11** (Summer 1972), 248–263. Review of some of literature related to blacks entering nursing and report of study of 331 freshman nursing students in the South. Reasons for entering nursing, selection of school, background, and other data were studied.

Minehan, Paula. "Nurse Role Conception." *Nurs. Res.*, **26** (Sep./Oct. 1977), 374–378. Evaluation of the Corwin Bureaucratic, Professional and Service-Traditional Scales, often used in the 1950s to study nurses' concepts of their roles, are questioned as to usefulness with different types of students entering nursing.

Moody, P. M. "Attitudes of Cynicism and Humanitarianism in Nursing Students and Staff Nurses." *J. Nurs. Ed.,* **12** (Aug. 1973) 9–13. It was concluded in this study that although there was some loss of humanitarianism during the educational program, this reasserts itself after nurses enter practice.

Moses, Evelyn and Aleda Roth. "Nursepower: What Do Statistics Reveal about the Nation's Nurses?" *Am. J. Nurs.*, **79** (Oct. 1979), 1745–1756. An abbreviated version of the ANA 1977 National Sample Survey of Registered Nurses.

Muhlenkamp, A. F., and J. L. Parsons. "Characteristics of Nurses: An Overview of Recent

Research Published in a Nursing Research Periodical." *J. Vocational Behav.*, **2** (July 1972), 261–273. Review of forty-eight research studies (1960–1970) on nurses' characteristics. Indications are that characteristics are generally consistent with the female stereotype, but as this stereotype is discarded by individuals, changes are predicted.

Nelson, B. K. "The Unpopular Patient." *Mod. Hosp.*, **121** (Aug. 1973), 70–72. One study indicates that nurses do not like patients who are unpleasant, long-term, mentally ill, dying, and hypochondriacs.

Nichols, Glennadee. "Important, Satisfying, and Dissatisfying Aspects of Nurse Jobs." *Sup. Nurse* 5 (Jan. 1974) 10–15. Perceptions of young nurses. Rated as most important in job were independence in making professional decisions, type of clinical work, assignment according to preference, opportunity to voice opinions, and working relationships with co-workers.

——. "Nursing Ethics: What Are Your Personal and Professional Standards?" *Nurs. 74*, **4** (Sept. 1974), 34–44.

——. "Nursing Ethics: The Admirable Professional Standards of Nurses-Part 2." *Nurs. 74*, **4** (Oct. 1974), 56–66. Survey asking readers to respond to specific, everyday ethical questions. Interesting.

O'Neill, M. F. "A Study of Baccalaureate Student Values." *Nurs. Res.*, **22** (Sept.–Oct. 1973) 437–443. In this study significant differences were found between nursing student values and value norms of the general female college population and those in other curricular fields, as well as differences among students in the various schools studied.

Peitchines, Jacquelyn. "Therapeutic Effectiveness of Counseling by Nursing Personnel: Review of the Literature." *Nurs. Res.*, **21** (Mar.–Apr. 1972), 138–148. Although the author draws certain conclusions in relation to nurses' counseling effectiveness, the greater value of this article is the review of studies on personality traits of nursing and the extremely comprehensive bibliography on the subject.

Pender, Nola. "Students Who Choose Nursing: Are They Success Oriented?" *Nurs. Forum*, **10** (1971) 64–71. In this study, a very slight majority of baccalaureate nursing students appeared to accept the academically successful female; almost half were ambivalent about the compatibility of intellectual attainment and social acceptance.

Popoff, David. "What Are Your Feelings About Death and Dying—Part I." *Nurs. 75* **5** (Aug. 1975) 15–24.

Popoff, David. "What Are Your Feelings About Death and Dying—Part II." *Nurs. 75*, **5** (Oct. 1975), 39–50. Interesting responses by nurses on the subject.

Richek, H. G. "A Note on Prejudice on Prospective Professional Helpers." *Nurs. Res.*, **19** (Mar.–Apr. 1970), 172–175. A small study of nursing and social work students found nursing students more prejudiced toward blacks, but both showed prejudiced attitudes.

Richek, H. G., and Tempie Nichols. "Personality and Cognitive Characteristics of Prenursing Majors." *Nurs. Res.*, **22** (Sept.–Oct. 1973), 443–448. Out of 300 female college freshmen, those opting for nursing were compared to those selecting related fields on personality-attitudinal and cognitive variables.

Richter, Laurelton, and Elizabeth Richter. "Nurses in Fiction." *Am. J. Nurs.*, **74** (July 1974), 1280–1281. A look at the fiction about nurses and nursing to which young women are exposed, showing how inaccurate a picture it portrays.

Rickelman, Bonnie. "Characteristics of Nurses and of Psychiatric Patients to Whom They React Postively and Negatively," in *Eighth Nursing Research Conference*, Albuquerque, N.M., Mar 15–17, 1972, pp. 123–131. New York: American Nurses' Association, 1972. Traits of liked patients are listed. It is suggested that nurses seek the type of relationship that supports the nurse rather than the patient.

Roth, Aleda et al. *1977 National Survey of Registered Nurses*. Kansas City, Mo: Am. Nurses' Assn. 1979. Extensive data on nurses.

Schmid, Nancy, and Donald Schmid. "Nursing Students' Attitudes Toward Alcoholics." *Nurs. Res.*, **22** (May–June 1973) 246–248. This study concluded that nursing students have a less accepting attitude toward alcoholics than toward the physically disabled, and these attitudes remained stable.

Stromberg, Marilyn. "Relationship of Sex Role Identity to Occupational Image of Female Nursing Students." *Nurs. Res.*, **25** (Sept./Oct. 1976), 363–369. A relationship between sex role identity and image of nursing was found to exist, with the student's image of nursing more in harmony with the image advanced by the profession, when sex role identity was more masculine. Extensive references.

"Times Are Changing—Men Seen on the Nursing Front." *Imprint*, **17** (May 1970), 3–5. Reactions of men students to nursing are reviewed, including benefits to health care and problems encountered.

Wheelock, Alan. "The Tarnished Image." *Nurs. Outlook* **24** (Aug. 1976), 509–510. Describes how nurses are pictured in movies, including pornographic films.

Williams, Reg Arthur. "Characteristics of Male Baccalaureate Students Who Selected Nursing as a Career." *Nurs. Res.*, **22** (Nov.–Dec. 1973), 520–525. In this study of men students in Western baccalaureate nursing programs, demographic data are reported as well as preferred areas of practice and interest in other health fields.

Winder, Alvin. "Why Young Black Women Don't Enter Nursing." *Nurs. Forum*, **10** (Winter 1971) 56–63. The author concludes that lack of role models is a major reason and makes some suggestions for improving recruitment and retention of black students.

Wolff, Ilse S. "As Others See Us." *Nurs. Outlook*, **2** (Aug. 1954), 408–412. Discussion of the image of the nurse in fiction as a reflection of popular ideas about the nursing profession. Stimulating and disconcerting reading.

See also references at end of Chapter 11, the surveys of nursing opinion done periodically by *Nursing*, the latest *Facts About Nursing* (ANA), annual review of nursing education programs published by NLN, and various DHHS publications that give data about nursing.

NURSING EDUCATION
AND
RESEARCH

12

Major Issues and Trends in Nursing Education

Unlike most professions, nursing has a variety of programs for entry into the profession (also called basic, preservice, or generic education). This situation confuses the public, some nurses, and employers, who are not sure how nurses graduating from these programs differ in background and the level of performance that can be expected. The three major educational routes that lead to RN licensure are the diploma programs operated by hospitals, the baccalaureate degree programs offered by four-year colleges and universities, and the associate degree programs usually offered by junior (or community) colleges. A master's degree program for beginning practitioners is also available at a few colleges, and a professional doctorate in one. These admit students with baccalaureate or higher degrees in a field other than nursing.

Although at one time diploma schools educated the largest number of nurses (more than 72 per cent of the total number of schools in 1964 were diploma), the movement of nursing programs into institutions of higher learning has been consistent. Between 1968 and 1972, associate degree (AD) programs increased by 211 to 541, baccalaureate programs increased by 58 to 293, and di-

ploma programs decreased by 84 to 543. By 1979, according to National League for Nursing records, there were 688 AD programs, 368 baccalaureate programs, and 333 diploma programs.

The pattern, then, has been for an increase in all collegiate programs and a decrease in diploma programs. However, a zero growth rate in admissions, which had been predicted, occurred in 1977. In 1978, there was a slight drop in total admissions (only the AD programs increased), and this was expected to continue. The continued closing of diploma schools and slow increase in numbers of other kinds of nursing education programs was also expected. However, such unpredictable factors as the sudden shortage of practicing nurses, as occurred in 1979, or the amount of federal aid to schools or students often change the picture.

There are certain similarities that all basic nursing programs share, in part because all are affected by the same societal changes.

1. Nursing education is becoming more expensive, and financial support is less available for school and student. The inflationary costs affecting society and education also affect nursing programs and

210

the institutions in which they are located. Moreover, the better the preparation of the teachers and the quality of other resources and facilities, the more costly the program. Both state and federal governments have been tightening the financial reins on programs, often apparently indifferent to the effect on quality or student needs. Therefore, although there is verbal encouragement for faculty to develop innovative programs, funds are seldom available for this purpose. Tuition seldom, if ever, covers the cost of the program, but, even so, it has been rising consistently. Students are finding it more and more difficult to receive scholarships, loans, and grants, particularly with the great cutback in federal funds beginning in 1972. Also, both because of cost and social trends, fewer students live in dormitories, and those who do, pay for room and board.

2. The student population is more heterogeneous. Few, if any, schools now refuse to admit or keep married students with or without families. Often, leave is granted for childbirth. It is not unusual to have a grandparent in a class, as more mature individuals look for a new or better career. The tight job market in many fields brings to nursing individuals with degrees and, sometimes, careers in related or unrelated fields. As noted in Chapter 11, in the last decade all programs include more men and other minority groups, by a small but definite percentage. In all cases, the diploma programs admit the lowest percentage of these groups.

3. Educational programs are generally more flexible. Educational trends in this direction plus the admission of a very mixed student body, including aides, LPNs or RNs seeking advanced education have required a second look at proficiency and equivalency testing, self-paced learning, and new techniques in teaching.

4. In many ways, educational programs tend to copy each other, or are subject to the same waves of educational faddism and jargon. For instance, whereas once most curricula were based on the same standard clinical and supportive courses, the "integrated" curriculum became popular in the 1950s. In addition, most now subscribe to models and theoretical frameworks as the basis for curriculum development.

5. State approval is required and national accreditation is available for all basic programs. Every school of professional nursing, in all three categories as well as practical nurse programs, must meet the standards of the legally constituted body in each state authorized to regulate nursing education and practice within that state. These are usually called state boards of nursing or given some similar title. Without the approval of these boards, a school cannot really operate, because the graduates would not be eligible to take the licensing examination. In addition, many schools of nursing also seek accreditation by the National League for Nursing. Accreditation by the League is a voluntary matter, not required by law. Increasing numbers of schools seek it, however, because it represents nationally determined standards of excellence and may affect eligibility for outside funding.

6. Faculty and clinical facilities are in short supply. Faculty with the recommended doctoral degree for baccalaureate and graduate programs and master's degree for the other programs are increasing, but the goal has not been met, particularly at the doctoral level. Clinical facilities are at a premium. Most schools, including diploma programs, use a variety of facilities, and in a large city, several schools may be using one specialty hospital or clinical area (particularly obstetrics and pediatrics) for student experience. In rural areas, distance, small hospitals, and fewer patients are problems. Community health resources are at a premium.

Schools are also searching for new types of clinical experiences with various ethnic groups.

7. There is a slow, but perceptible trend toward involving students in curriculum development, some policy making, and program evaluation. Again, the social trends, but also the maturity of students and their demands to have a part in the educational program, are making some inroads on total faculty and administrative control of schools.

8. All nursing students have learning experiences in clinical settings, as selected by their faculty. Somewhere a myth arose through the years that only practical nurse and diploma students gave "real" patient care in their educational programs, that AD students barely saw patients, and that baccalaureate students prepared only for teaching and administration. The amount of time spent in the clinical area may differ among programs within a particular credential as much as among the different types. The educational focus should be different, but in all good programs students care for selected patients in order to gain certain skills and knowledge according to their program's objectives.

9. It is generally agreed that the standards by which nursing education programs are judged should include criteria involving the institution itself (financial support, other support services, a review process for quality); students (selection, retention, evaluation, participation in identifying and evaluating program goals); faculty (preparation, research and publication efforts, development and evaluation of program and selves, participation in governance); programs (objectives communicated, satisfactory learning opportunities provided, relationships with service institutions identified, evaluation done); facilities and resources (funds, support services, facilities specific to program); organization and administration (functions so as to enhance goals of program).

EXTERNAL CONSTRAINTS ON NURSING EDUCATION

Nursing education, like other educational fields, is strongly affected by external constraints over which it has limited, or no, control.[1] To constrain means to compel, oblige, force, or restrain. Nursing education is the object of multiple constraints: those imposed as a part of the system of higher education, those imposed by the responsibilities of a health profession to the public, and those imposed by a more or less cohesive group of practitioners who are, in essence, employers, employees, colleagues, change agents, and even critical consumers. That the constraints imposed by those groups may well be in conflict with each other only puts added pressure on nursing education. Nevertheless, it should not be assumed that the results of these constraints are necessarily bad; in fact, they often hasten what is long overdue.

The effects of the national economy are not limited to increased costs of the program and increased tuition. Double-digit inflation and the tremendous increase in the cost of living have made nursing as a profession "where you can always get a job" attractive not only to other careerists whose field is in decline, but also to second-career housewives. On the other hand, the fact that more temporarily retired nurses are likely to work more coupled with the general inability of anyone to guess accurately the nurse manpower needs even in the next decade leaves schools in a quandry as to how many students they should admit. New limitations to federal and state funding for both schools and students put another brake on expansion, or perhaps, more accurately, point the direction of new programs. For instance, nurse practitioner programs are increasing in part because that is what is being funded. Any specialty, such as oncology, psychiatry, even preparation for administration or teaching, seems to expand or contract according to funding availability. Moreover, the content of the curriculum may be influenced by the federal guidelines required if federal funds are accepted. Student makeup is also involved; with funds for recruiting and retaining minorities, the numbers were increased. The survival of entire programs may be at stake; nursing schools have been closed because a board of directors decided they were not economically feasible to operate. Nevertheless, a tight money market has also resulted in a creative sharing of resources and in regional planning for nursing education.

Naturally, professional education is influenced by the knowledge explosion and technological advances in its area. For nursing, this demands that practitioners keep updated, as is discussed later, and raises multiple questions of curriculum content. Should nurses be educated as generalists or specialists? At what educational level? For primary, secondary, or tertiary care? For acute or long-term care? At what level? If new graduates are expected to practice at a minimum safe and effective level, what is the minimum content that should be in all curricula? If something new is added, should something else be dropped, or should there be less taught about everything? Are there more effective ways for students to learn, such as independent, self-paced learning? The increase in knowledge also puts more pressure on the profession to create and/or expand a knowledge base for nursing. How then to enlarge the miniscule number of nurses with doctoral education and research interests? These questions are being answered in a variety of ways by nurse educators, but they will continue to recur.

There are a number of social movements that affect nursing education. One noted previously is the recognition of students' rights. Another is renewed emphasis on the American belief in upward mobility. Moving to advanced education in nursing for either PNs or RNs has generally not been easy; most believe that unnecessary obstacles have been placed in their way. Pressure by organized minority groups and unions, as well as the studies and edicts of national commissions and state and federal governments

have all been important factors in developing more flexible educational patterns. The public's legitimate demand for competent practitioners has also focused more attention on continuing education. In addition, changes in the delivery of health care services, which may involve both new techniques (space medicine, organ transplants) and new or newly emphasized settings (maternity centers, neighborhood health centers), clients (teen-agers, elderly), health attitudes (prevention, self-care), or other concerns (environmental health, iatrogenic disease), as well as the changing role of other professionals and paraprofessional health workers all affect nursing education.

Finally, there are the constraints placed on nursing education by the profession, the organizations that represent it, and its various practitioners. These can create more strain than external pressures because, unfortunately, there is no common nursing voice, so the demands are often conflicting. One key example is the lack of agreement between nursing education and nursing service about the utilization of the graduates of the three kinds of programs. Another is the difference in philosophy as to whether professional nursing education can be a series of steps that builds on previous experience and education, or whether professional education is so different from technical education that it requires an almost totally fresh start. Still another concerns whether graduate education must be primarily clinical. Even though both state board approval and accreditation are fairly well controlled by nurses and affect educational programs, agreement prevails neither at a state or national level. Most devastating of all is the bitter divisiveness caused by the issue of entry into practice.

ENTRY INTO PRACTICE

With at least three types of basic educational programs evolving in nursing, the uncertainty of both the public and the profession as to the differences among these practitioners has appeared to escalate. To add to the confusion, graduates of all of these programs are eligible to take the same licensing examination and have the same cut-off point for passing. There have been arguments that no one could expect the public and employers to differentiate among nursing graduates when they are all designated as RNs on licensure. Often, all kinds of nurses are employed in the same capacity, with the same assignments, same expectations, and same salary. Are they all professional nurses? If so, what justification is there for three separate types of educational programs?

An important function of ANA is that of setting standards and policies for nursing education. A major action was taken in 1965, when, through the Committee on Education, ANA took the position that nursing education should take place within the general educational system. Reaction to the position paper* was decidedly mixed. Although this very same concept had been enunciated by leaders in nursing almost since the profession's inception, reiterated through the years, and accepted as a goal by the 1960 House of Delegates, many nurses misunderstood the paper's intent and considered it a threat. Probably the greatest area of misinterpretation lay in the separation of nursing education and practice into professional, technical, and assisting components. Minimum preparation for professional nursing practice was designated at the baccalaureate level, technical nursing practice at the associate degree level, and education for assistants in health service occupations was to be in short, intensive preservice programs in vocational education settings, rather than in on-the-job training. Obviously omitted were both diploma school education and practical nurse education. A large number of hospital-based diploma graduates, students, faculty,

*Correctly titled: "Educational Preparation for Nurse Practitioners and Assistants to Nurses—A Position Paper."

and hospital administrators saw the omission as both degradation, particularly because the term *professional* was reserved for the baccalaureate nurse, and as a move to eliminate diploma education, which at the time comprised the largest number of nursing education programs in existence. Cooler heads recognized that the trend for nursing education had been toward inclusion in educational institutions for the past ten years, and that it would be totally unrealistic and undesirable to eliminate this large segment of nursing education precipitously. Later both ANA and NLN statements advocated careful community planning for phasing diploma programs into institutions of higher learning. It was also pointed out that as practical nursing programs improved and increased their course content, their program length was coming close to that of the associate degree program. Nevertheless, the storm raged for more than fifteen years, although repeated attempts were made to clarify the content and intent of the document. It was felt that ANA suffered a membership loss through the alienation of some diploma nurses. As expected, social and economic trends gradually brought about many of the changes suggested by the position paper, and the definitions of professional and technical nurse were widely used in the literature (although there was no major indication that employers were assigning nurses according to technical or professional responsibilities). In June 1973, in what some considered a belated effort to placate diploma nurses and assure them of their importance to ANA, but what ANA identified as a move to encourage unity in the profession, a "Statement on Diploma Graduates" was issued. In essence, the statement asked all units of ANA to give special attention to the needs and interests of diploma graduates, particularly in relation to continuing education and upward mobility. In addition, a task force was appointed "to examine the contemporary relevance of the terms 'professional' and 'technical' to distinguish basic preparation for nursing practice and to recognize all registered nurses as professionals."[2] Although there appeared to be no major reaction from diploma nurses about this statement, some nurses considered it a step backward, because it appeared to aim at tentative rejection of the concept that professional nursing was different from technical nursing.[3]

In February 1974, the Commission on Nursing Education approved a report on the contemporary relevance of the terms *professional* and *technical.* Meanwhile, the NLN's associate degree group rejected the term *technical,* but others continued to use it.

In 1976, the New York State Nurses' Association's voting body overwhelmingly approved introduction of a "1985 Proposal" in the 1977 legislative session. Although variations of the proposal evolved over the next few years, basically the purpose was to establish licensure for two kinds of nursing. The professional nurse would require a baccalaureate degree, and the other, whose title tended to change because of various objections, would require an associate degree. The target date for full implementation was 1985; currently licensed nurses would be covered by the traditional grandfather clause, which would allow them to retain their current title and status (RN). The bill did not pass at that time but was consistently reintroduced each legislative session, with some changes. Some time later, the Ohio Nurses' Association introduced similar legislation, also without success. Immediately, the "1985 Proposal" became a term symbolizing designation of baccalaureate education as the entry level into *professional* nursing and a rallying point for nurses who opposed this change. And there was, and is, considerable opposition, primarily from diploma and AD nurses and faculty, some hospital administrators, and some physicians. Nursing organizations were formed whose major focus was opposition to such proposals. Nevertheless, an increasing number of state nurses' organizations, primarily made up of diploma nurses, voted in convention to work toward

the goal of baccalaureate education for professional nursing. In 1978, the ANA House of Delegates passed such a resolution, as did the National Student Nurses' Association. The ANA resolution had emerged from an ANA-sponsored "Entry into Practice" conference held earlier that year. The 400 or so participants included representatives from various nurses' associations, the federal government, all types of schools of nursing, and administrators and staff nurses from all types of employment settings. The papers and the recommendations of group discussions have been published.[4] The major recommendations supported the concept of two categories or types of practitioners in nursing (although they could not agree on titles), that competencies be developed for those levels, and that career mobility opportunities be increased, including the use of innovative and flexible educational programs. All of these were incorporated into resolutions that the ANA House of Delegates also approved in 1978.

Entry into practice and its inevitable corollary, changes in nurse licensure, continue to be a major issue in nursing; almost all state nurses' associations have taken a stand or are in the process of doing so, as are other nursing organizations. Most state nurses' associations tend to favor it as a necessary and inevitable step in the development of nursing, but the California Nurses' Association was the first to support entry at a lesser academic level with a clear career ladder plan in mind. Many specialty organizations are supporting the "1985 Proposal," but the NLN in 1979 made a statement supporting all four pathways into nursing, including practical nursing. One of its major activities is accreditation of all those programs. Again, as expected, the National Federation of Licensed Practical Nurses has taken the stand that the LPN/LVN title and "profession" be retained. Obviously, the issue is highly divisive. There are those who think that the system should stay as it is,[5] others who opt for changing the baccalaureate nurse's title and license to indicate advanced preparation,[6] and a few who are projecting to the time when a professional nurse doctorate, like the MD and DDS of physicians and dentists, will be the entry level to the profession.[7]

Some natural fears of nonbaccalaureate nurses are to be expected: that they will lose status and job opportunities despite the grandfather clause and that those who desire baccalaureate education will find it too expensive, unavailable, or rigidly repetitive. As to the first, there is already some selectiveness and has been; in the latter, there is slow, but definite progress. In all probability, the issue will not be quickly resolved, but inevitable societal and professional changes, such as the decrease in diploma schools and the expectations of professional practice (nursing is the only health profession for which entry is less than a baccalaureate) will be major factors in the final outcome. Still, there are problems that must be resolved and data obtained (for example, will cost limit access to professional nursing? Will such a plan improve patient care?).[8] Because nursing as a profession loses power every time its practitioners erupt into battles of internal dissension, it is imperative that nurses work together toward a satisfactory conclusion soon, a conclusion that includes appreciation and respect for all competent nurses and focuses on providing the best possible nursing care to the public.[9]

OPEN CURRICULUM PRACTICES

One of the key developments in nursing education is the implementation of the open curriculum concept, which the NLN defines as a system "which incorporates an educational approach designed to accommodate the learning needs and career goals of students by providing flexible opportunities for entry into and exit from the educational program, and by capitalizing on their previous relevant education and experiences."[10]

This concept has emerged only gradually. Nurse educators most aware of social and economic trends and sympathetic to the goals of those struggling for upward mobility gradually began to plan and implement programs to meet these needs over a period of time; too many others ignored the signs of disillusionment among those seeking further education in nursing. Both poor and ethnic minorities, often guided into lower-level nursing positions, and the middle-class nurses who had chosen diploma or associate degree education, as well as service corpsmen returning from active duty became increasingly irritated at the difficulty of moving into other levels of nursing programs. All became increasingly hostile toward a system that offered no credit for previous study and experience, or, at most, recognized a few transferable liberal arts courses. Unions in some hospitals included in their contracts provisions for organized programs of education for non-professionals. Other health workers turned to the legislatures. The result was evident in such states as California, which enacted laws to force schools of nursing to give credit to prospective students with previous health experience,[11] and in recommendations of the federal government.[12,13]

Soon it became evident that nursing programs at all levels were responding to some degree to the mandate for more flexibility. An NLN survey in 1971 showed that approximately 1,500 programs from the total of about 2,700 practical, diploma, associate degree, and baccalaureate programs in nursing provided some aspect of educational mobility. Today, there are many more.[14] At the least, they accept transfer credit as a means of advanced placement. More innovative programs have designed new methods for measurement of knowledge and competency or have developed entirely new programs. The NLN Open Curriculum Project,[15] which followed the NLN statement of support for open curriculum, produced many such examples and resulted in the publishing of the *Directory of Career Mobility Opportunities in Nursing Education* in 1973.

There are a variety of approaches for

providing flexibility in nursing education.[16] The ladder approach, which provides direct articulation between programs, is used to move from nursing assistant to practical nurse to AD or diploma nurse to baccalaureate nurse, with any combinations in between. For some, this means the ability to begin at a basic level and move one step at a time to the highest achievable level. For others, it means one can aim at a particular level, but be able to exit at distinct points, become licensed, and earn a living if necessity or circumstances dictate. A number of baccalaureate programs are also being developed that enroll only RNs into the upper division, accepting past nursing education as the lower division to be built on.

There are, of course, those nurse educators who do not agree that the "ladder" is a viable concept. They believe that each program in nursing has its own basis, content, and goals, that one cannot be based on another, and that the ladder tends to denigrate the role of workers at each level, implying the necessity to move upward.[17,18] There is similar resistance to programs that provide a core of courses for movement into other health occupations. One solution seems to be the utilization of standardized and teacher-made tests to measure the individual's knowledge, according to a clear delineation of the achievement expectations of the program.[19] There are a number of standardized tests available in both the liberal arts and nursing, but there is still some question as to how to test for clinical competency. Methods used include use of videotapes, simulated experiences, practicums, and minicourses in the clinical setting.

An exciting approach is to allow students to proceed through a course at their own pace through testing, self-study, and use of media.[20] A number of schools are experimenting with self-pacing and self-learning and reports indicate that students find it stimulating and satisfying.

Other ways of giving more opportunities for students are to offer courses more frequently, during evening hours, weekends, and in summer, to allow part-time study, and to have class sessions off the main campus in areas convenient to students living in communities not easily accessible to the main campus. This latter is sometimes considered a form of external degree or "university without walls."

However, the N.Y. State Regents External Degree is an example of open curriculum that moves far beyond this simple concept. The purpose of the program is to meet the needs of those individuals who choose to learn on their own, whether through individual study, job experience, travel, or other forms of life experience. It is open to all applicants, without regard to age, residence, or methods of preparation. The program's philosophy is that what a person knows is more important than where or how he learned it. The entire program is based on testing. In 1971 an associate degree in nursing was included in the program, developed by a committee of noted associate degree educators.[21] In late 1974 work on this first external degree in nursing was completed, including tests for clinical competency. Applicants are not eligible to take the clinical performance examination, given in actual patient care settings, until all the clinical paper and pencil exams are passed. Enrolled in the External Degree Program, as of September 1975, were students ranging from eighteen to seventy years old from forty-two states besides New York; 60 percent were LPNs, 11 percent aides or orderlies, and 7 percent RNs seeking academic degrees. Not only did those taking the licensing exam exceed national norms for all kinds of students, but their employers expressed great satisfaction with their performance.[22] The program is now NLN-accredited.

The baccalaureate program for the external degree was completed in 1979 and is expected to provide additional opportunity for nurses seeking a bachelor's degree in nursing. Information may be obtained by writing to Regents External Degrees BSN, 99 Washington Avenue, Albany, New York 12230. Although there are some educators who oppose the external degree on philosophical grounds,[23] it is expected that studies conducted relative to the program will provide data of significance to other states contemplating external degree programs that include nursing. Such data may also help educational programs seeking more effective techniques for proficiency and equivalency testing.

In 1976, as part of the NLN Open Curriculum Project, 1,765 programs (including PN programs) that had designated themselves as following some sort of open curriculum practices, were invited to participate in a survey. The 34 percent who responded were roughly proportionate to all types of open curriculum programs and were a good representation of all sizes of enrollment. They provided valuable information about the type of practices, planning methods, special resources, benefits and difficulties, evaluation methods, and self-estimates of program success.[24] As the authors noted, if the "1985 Proposal" becomes reality, the necessity for upward mobility becomes even more essential. Of greatest importance in these changes in education is the fact that individuals will have greater opportunities to continue formal education, if they desire, and both nursing and society will benefit.

DOES NURSING EDUCATION PREPARE COMPETENT PRACTITIONERS?

From the time that the last diploma program gave up the apprenticeship approach to nursing education, there have been accusations that the new graduates of modern nursing programs are not competent. Further investigation usually shows that new graduates are not as technically skillful or as able to assume responsibility for a large group of patients as the nurses with whom they are compared—the diploma graduates of yesterday. (Most of those doing the comparing were once the product of those times.) Nevertheless, the criticisms are understandable. For the director of nursing with tightening fiscal

constraints, a lengthy orientation and in-service program is a strain on the budget; for the staff nurse and supervisor, someone who requires extra help or supervision on the usual short-staffed unit is a temporary impediment.

For some unknown reason, useful communication between nursing education and nursing service is erratic at best and nonexistent at worst. In some areas, joint appointments of faculty and clinicians enables each to contribute to the goals of the other, but this practice is largely limited to medical centers and university programs. Other productive steps are joint planning for experiences during the student's educational program or in an internship and opportunities for faculty to practice during weekends, summers, or sabbaticals. Unfortunately, however, although there seems to be little disagreement on the qualities, knowledge, and skills nurses need, there is almost no agreement on how much of each and what level of competency is needed at graduation.

Although graduates from all three types of programs are the targets of employer disapproval, the diploma graduate, whose program is focused on the hospital and who frequently stays at the hospital, may find adjustment a little easier. Associate degree graduates who have been practical nurses and have had experience in caring for many patients are also somewhat immune from criticisms about slow adjustment. However, because most graduates today do not have these backgrounds, how justified are the criticisms? How differently do the graduates of the RN programs perform?

There is a question, first of all, as to whether the various kinds of programs actually prepare different kinds of practitioners. Nurse educators say they do, but often the statements of philosophy and objectives or the NLN competency statements, described in Chapter 13, have obvious areas of overlap. Moreover, at least one study[25] indicates that there is a lack of clarity in how heads of AD and BS programs see their type of program as differing from the other. Specifically, most programs did not seem to adhere to the differences spelled out in the literature. For instance, many of the AD program directors thought their graduates had as broad a judgment base as the baccalaureate nurse, and many prepared these nurses for administrative functions without the necessary educational base. On the other hand, this is probably a matter of catching up with reality, because so many employers give AD nurses responsibilities for which they are not prepared. But should the teacher then educate the employer instead of re-educating the student?

The nursing literature abounds with articles on content and methods; nurse educators are most certainly concerned about preparing the best possible practitioner. There is concern that new graduates be competent to give both physical and psychological/emotional care. Just how much of this is best taught in a clinical setting is a point of controversy. How much of what kind of clinical experience prepares nurses best? It has been suggested that additional emphasis be given to the physical care needed because of the patients' pathophysiological problems.[26] There is also some indication that students need practice in basic technical skills, which some schools deal with by encouraging additional self-study in labs. In others, a concentrated period of time in one or two clinical areas at the end of the program eases students into the work situation and allows them to integrate their clinical knowledge and skills over a continuum of time and to learn to organize the care of larger groups of patients, setting appropriate priorities. Certain programs also have cooperative arrangements with clinical facilities to allow students a paid work-study period in the summer, or specific academic terms in which they work full time while supervised in practice.[27] Clerkships, preceptorships, field placements, or clinical electives are other options. There are mixed feelings about whether working as an aide or ward clerk is helpful because of the limited legal scope of practice and the possibility that students are subtly forced into assuming more responsibility than is legal.

As to differences in practice among diploma, AD, and BS nurses, this is difficult to determine because most studies have been done by graduate students. Not only are the numbers small and the studies seldom replicated, but what is being measured is usually different from study to study. If success in state boards is considered a criterion for competency, the results are no more definitive; differences *within* each type of program are greater than those *among* the programs.[28] However, in 1979, the members of an NLN Task Force on Competencies of Graduates of Nursing Programs, after reviewing the literature and analyzing statements of the NLN educational councils about each of their programs,* concluded that there *were* differences in the competencies (defined as minimal expectations of new graduates) in education, practice, and accountability. The common core of all was seen as nursing theory and the nursing process, although the latter varied in depth and breadth. A chart comparing expectations of the graduates clearly showed the ambiguity of the statements of competency and some amazing omissions. For instance, specific competencies as communicator, patient teacher, and manager of patient care were identified only by the AD statement. It was also noted that other differences occurred in the practice role in terms of structured/unstructured settings and focus of care. Another difference was in accountability, which increased with amount and type of education and experience.[29] But, aside from this, one of the most bitter arguments in nursing education is whether baccalaureate or diploma nursing provides the "best" education for professional nursing. In a thought-provoking article, Ramphal maintains that a potentially profession-destroying tragedy is that the strengths traditionally characteristic of diploma education and the strengths of collegiate education are so often seen as either/or

---

*See Chapter 13.

propositions.[30] At times, clinical competence is misequated with "sheer technical competence that is fundamentally anti-intellectual, anti-conceptual and anti-theoretical." But emphasis on the conceptual part of nursing "divorced from a base in practice, runs the risk of triviality, at best, and solipsistic pseudointellectualism, at worst." Another option was suggested.

An ideal professional nursing education program seems conceivable which would combine strengths characteristic of each type of program at its best: 1) a program in which the talents of faculty combine the capabilities of clinicians who either are continuing in practice or frequently return to practice and who are not content with current practice but are actively engaged in improving it; 2) a program in which the faculty as a group is also endowed, not only with intellectual command of relevant theories and concepts, but in which some, at least, are actively engaged in theory development through research, particularly clinical research; 3) a program in which students' understanding of theories and concepts is enriched through clinical teaching by instructors able to help them gain intellectual command of theory through practice; and 4) a program in which at least some clinical practice provides an opportunity for students to experience continuity and accountability in order to develop clinical judgment—that is, the weighing of alternatives in decision making necessary for responsible professional practice.[31]

One could add to this a vital ingredient that is possibly best taught by role models if it is not already a part of the individual nurse's makeup—the quality of humankindness, the caring aspect of nursing which, although it cannot substitute for knowledge, skills, and competency, is indispensable. Without it, there is no nursing care.

PREPARATION OF FACULTY AND EDUCATIONAL ADMINISTRATORS

The quality of teachers in any educational program and the leadership of the program's director are key factors in the overall quality of the program. They develop and implement the curriculum, usually select the students, and provide a milieu in which learning is either a chore or a joy, or something in between.

Teaching a clinical subject is not the same as teaching a course in liberal arts; teachers must not only know the theoretical concepts, but should also be competent practitioners and role models. Should they also know how to teach? How to evaluate? These questions are arising in other practice disciplines because for years practicing clinicians have been the teachers, whether or not they were able to communicate their knowledge to students adequately. The problem in nursing is twofold. Because of trends and opportunities in graduate education, there are nursing faculty who have learned curriculum and teaching skills, but shy away from actual patient care because they feel inadequate, and there are newly minted clinicians with graduate degrees who have difficulty communicating their how-how. Expanding knowledge and new nursing roles also combine to create the situation in which experienced teachers who have been competent in their field must continually acquire new skills, such as physical assessment skills.

Currently, graduate education seems to be focused on both a clinical major and a functional minor (teaching or administration, primarily). However, the programs also seem to be geared to specialty areas or separated into acute care (episodic) or primary care. How well are these teachers prepared for integrated curricula or for the AD programs in which teaching at a specialty level is a luxury? And is there a place for a nurse with a non-nursing master's?

A serious problem is that the majority of teachers of nursing do not meet the academic requirements for their positions. This means that a large number of students are being taught by faculty with no more education than they themselves are receiving. The scarcity of qualified faculty also tends to lead to academic inbreeding, which has serious implications for high-quality education.[32] In 1976, about 12 percent of nurse faculty had less than a baccalaureate degree and most taught in diploma and practical nurse programs; 36 percent had baccalaureates and most also taught in these programs; 48 percent had master's degrees and most of them taught in AD or baccalaureate/graduate programs; about 4 percent had doctorates, almost all of whom taught in baccalaureate or graduate programs. Yet, the education for all university faculty is usually a minimum of a doctorate, and it is generally agreed that all other teachers of nursing programs should have at least a master's. The lack of appropriate credentials, regardless of the teacher's individual qualifications, puts nursing faculty at a distinct disadvantage in a university setting. Frequently, they are not considered true colleagues (a problem they also have when dealing with physicians in the clinical setting), and they have difficulty in competition for higher rank, tenure, or appointment on committees. There are those who believe these factors help create problems in their relationships with students, causing an inclination to be repressive.[33]

However, acquiring a doctorate is not without its problems. There are still relatively few programs in nursing that award doctorates, and most faculty have a doctorate in education. This seems appropriate. However, if faculty should also do research in their field, how does such a doctorate prepare for clinical research? Is a doctorate in a related science preferable? (Lack of faculty research and failure to utilize research findings in teaching are other major criticisms of nursing education.) With the scarcity of doctoral nurses, the type of degree has not yet become a serious issue, but it is tending in that direction.

The issue of preparation for the decanal role has received some attention in the last few years. Usually, the dean of a baccalaureate and a higher-degree program is expected to hold a doctoral degree. However, few are prepared to assume the academic and administrative role that is mandated. One national survey shows that the doctoral degrees held by deans include PhDs in nursing and other disciplines, as well as professional degrees in education and health administration.[34] Very few have had educational programs specifically designed for the decanal role; few are available. Recommendations have been made for both continuing education on the job or preservice preparation for careers in educational administration that include an internship, guided by a mentor.

ACCREDITATION

The major accrediting organization for all nursing programs is the National League for Nursing.* The issues involved relate in part to the accrediting process and in part to who should do the accrediting.[35] In the first major HEW report (1971) that examined all forms of health manpower credentialing, accreditation is defined as "the process by which an agency or organization evaluates and recognizes an institution or program of study as meeting certain predetermined criteria or standards."[36] As noted previously, educational accreditation is a voluntary process, but it presumably indicates excellence in program and resources and therefore attracts students and faculty. Most of all, it opens the door for crucial federal funding.

Concern about the accreditation of health education programs led to a major Study of Accreditation of Selected Health Education Programs (SASHEP), the report of which was released in 1972. Sponsored by the American Medical Association, the Association of Schools of Allied Health Professions, and the National Commission of Accrediting, the SASHEP report proved as controversial as the accrediting system. In essence, it concluded that

Problems of accountability, structural deficiencies, pressures for expansion and increased levels of financial support, and the absence of objective scientific validation of accrediting standards and procedures have converged to undermine the potential effectiveness, social value, and public credibility

*The history and process is described in Chapter 26.

in many health fields. Heavy social reliance on accreditation as a manpower credentialing mechanism has tended to focus increased public attention on the shortcomings of accreditation. . . .[37]

The SASHEP working papers and reports thoroughly explore such issues as the expense of accreditation to colleges and universities with multiple health profession or occupation programs, particularly indirect costs in faculty and administrative time for preparation and materials; the inconsistency in the criteria and approach of each discipline; the rigidity of some accreditation boards that discourage innovation; the discontent of allied health groups controlled by the "parent discipline"; the lack of public representation on accrediting bodies; and, most of all, the lack of scientific development and validation of accreditation criteria.

Although nursing was obviously not one of the groups for whom the report was directly intended, some of SASHEP's criticisms of the accreditation system apply just as much to the long-established NLN accreditation process. The fact that ANA is now operating an accreditation system for continuing education and that some of these programs are also being accredited by NLN and approved by other nursing groups is bound to cause further intraprofessional conflict.

In addition, there has been increased governmental activity on the accreditation issue. The Federal Trade Commission (FTC) has raised a "restraint of trade" question when an organization both accredits the educational programs and then provides a certification mechanism for the graduates of that program. Two long-standing examples are the American College of Nurse Midwives and the American Association of Nurse Anesthetists, both of which have been the sole accreditors of the educational programs in their respective specialties and also the sole certifiers of the practitioners.* Because in many states a nurse cannot practice that spe-

cialty without certification and certification exams are not open to those who did not attend an accredited program (except in rare special circumstances), the FTC maintains that such total control over practice may lead to restraint of trade. As ANA accredits short-term nurse practitioner programs and also increases its certification programs for entry into the specialty, the same charge may be leveled.

Perhaps the new manifestation of an old disagreement is the most important issue to be resolved in nursing. Should ANA or NLN control the accreditation of all nursing education programs? Although most nursing leaders are members of both organizations, they appear to be somewhat schizophrenic when it comes to making a choice. There are philosophical issues: should the "real" all-nurse professional organization set educational standards and accredit programs, or is the NLN, which was given that responsibility at the reorganization of the major nursing organizations in 1952, to continue? (Now, both organizations publish educational standards, which are interesting to compare.) There is also an obvious matter of control and income. Much NLN income is derived from activities related to accreditation: agency membership, consulting, and the accreditation process.

There are also those who say that some programs, such as those espousing ladder concepts, have not been accredited because they were not in harmony with the philosophy of the accrediting board or of NLN staff members, although they met the basic guidelines of accreditation: a school shall be evaluated in relation to its own statement of philosophy, objectives, and its overall strengths and weaknesses, and accredited if its strengths are greater than its weaknesses. Whether there is any truth in this accusation or whether the programs were not of a satisfactory quality was an ongoing dispute in the 1970s and probably one reason for a new surge of interest in the possibility of an ANA accreditation program. The summary statement on accreditation from the Credentialing Study, briefly described in Chapter 5, was:

*Both organizations have now separated out these activities from overt association control (see Chapter 27).

Accreditation is the process by which a voluntary, non-governmental agency or organization appraises and grants accredited status to institutions and/or programs or services which meet predetermined structure, process, and outcome criteria. Its purposes are to evaluate the performance of a service or educational program and to provide to various publics information upon which to base decisions about the utilization of the institutions, programs, services, and/or graduates. Periodic assessment is an integral part of the accreditation process in order to ensure continual acceptable performance. Accreditation is conducted by agencies which have been recognized or approved by an organized peer group of agencies as having integrity and consistency in their practices.[38]

At the same time, the committee recommended that all education programs and organized nursing services seek accreditation and that definitions and standards be established by the professional society (ANA). The process of accreditation was to be one of the functions of a credentialing center, seen as a federation of organizations that could conceivably include the NLN and other organizations that accredit nursing programs. However, the NLN, which refused to participate in the credentialing study, also rejected the final report. Just what impact this report will have on nursing credentialing is still to be determined. However, unless some of the problems of accreditation are solved, it will continue to be a major issue, and its real usefulness may be clouded by dispute.

Other Issues

There are a number of other issues in nursing education, such as those related to continuing education. What kind of continuing education do nurses need? Who decides? Who is best qualified to provide it? Who should pay? Should it be mandatory for relicensure? Who is responsible for seeing that it is available to all nurses? Will it improve practice?*

Other issues relate to recruitment and retention of minority students who may or may not fall into the "disadvantaged" category; legal aspects of admission and student and faculty rights (Chapter 22); what kind and how much preparation is needed for specific clinical areas, such as operating room nursing, public health nursing, and occupational health nursing; the kind of education for RNs entering baccalaureate programs (basically the same as for the generic student? advanced? specialized?), and intradisciplinary education (should PN and various RN students learn together?).Interdisciplinary education has also been a point of discussion for some time, with relatively little action taken. There has been minimal experimentation with the concept of core courses from which individual students could move to various health professional programs, as well as certain shared courses when students are already enrolled in separate programs. One approach that takes considerable planning but has shown some good results places professional students in working teams to provide coordinated care for patients (usually in a home or a clinic).

As nursing education continues to be more complex, as does society, new issues will emerge as others are resolved. The danger lies in nonresolution of long-term issues that are professionally divisive and potentially detrimental to the public's welfare.

REFERENCES

1. Lucie Kelly, "External Constraints on Nursing Education," in *Current Perspectives in Nursing Education: The Changing Scene,* ed. by Janet Williamson (St. Louis: C. V. Mosby Company, 1978), pp. 9–19.
2. "Statement on Diploma Graduates," *Am. Nurse,* 5:5 (June 1973).
3. Dorothy Sheahan, "The Hospital School Graduate—Can the Birthright Be Restored?" *Nurs. Forum,* 12:260–279 (Fall 1973).
4. American Nurses' Association, *Entry Into Practice: Proceedings of the National Conference,* Feb. 13–14, 1978 (Kansas City, Mo.: The Association, 1978).

*See Chapter 13 for further discussion.

5. See the survey reported in *RN* in 1979: January, pp. 83–93; February, pp. 39–46; March, pp. 52–58 present arguments against the "1985 Proposal." April, pp. 64–76, concludes that it is inevitable and necessary but requires careful planning.

6. Erline McGriff and Laura Simms, "Two New York Nurses Debate the NYSNA 1985 Proposal," *Am. J. Nurs., 76:930–935 (June 1976).

7. Rozella Schlotfeldt, "The Professional Doctorate: Rationale and Characteristics," *Nurs. Outlook,* **26**:302–311 (May 1978).

8. Andrew Dolan, "The New York State Nurses' Association 1985 Proposal: Who Needs It?" *J. of Health, Politics, Policy and Law,* 2(4):508–530 (Winter 1978).

9. Lucie Kelly, "End Paper: Me-Politics and Nursing," *Nurs. Outlook,* **27**:303 (Apr. 1979).

10. Carrie Lenburg and Walter Johnson, "Career Mobility Through Nursing Education," *Nurs. Outlook,* **22**:266 (Apr. 1974).

11. Lucie Kelly, "Nursing Practice Acts," *Am. J. Nurs.,* **74**:1312–1313 (July 1974).

12. Department of Health, Education, and Welfare, *Report on Licensure and Related Health Personnel Credentialing* (Washington, D.C.: The Department, 1971), pp. 74–75.

13. DHEW, *Credentialing Health Manpower* (Washington, D.C.: The Department, 1977), pp. 16–17.

14. Lenburg and Johnson, op. cit., p. 266.

15. Ibid., pp. 265–269.

16. Lucie Kelly, "Open Curriculum: What and Why," *Am. J. Nurs.* **74**:2232–2238 (Dec. 1974).

17. Thelma Ingles and Mildred Montag, "Debate: Ladder Concept in Nursing Education, Pro-Con," *Nurs. Outlook,* **19**:726–730 (Nov. 1971).

18. Margaret Shetland, "This I Believe—About Career Ladders, New Careers, and Nursing Education," *Nurs. Outlook,* **18**:32–35 (Sept. 1970).

19. Mildred Katzell, "Evaluation for Educational Mobility," *Nurs. Outlook,* **21**:453–456 (July 1973).

20. Dorothy Corona, "College Education Tailor-made for Registered Nurses," *Am. J. Nurs.,* **74**:1312–1313 (July 1974).

21. Dolores Wozniak, "External Degrees in Nursing," *Am. J. Nurs.,* **73**:1014–1018 (June 1973).

22. Carrie Lenburg, "The External Degree in Nursing: The Promise Fulfilled," *Nurs. Outlook,* **24**:422–429 (July 1976).

23. Sister Dorothy Sheahan, "Degree, Yes—Education, No," *Nurs. Outlook* **22**:22–26 (Jan. 1974).

24. Lucille Notter and Marguerite Robey, "Open Curriculum Practices," *Nurs. Outlook,* **27**:116–121 (Feb. 1979).

25. Mary Kohnke, "Do Nursing Educators Practice What Is Preached?" *Am. J. Nurs.,* **73**:1571–1575 (Sept. 1973).

26. Sister Patricia Miller, "Clinical Knowledge: A Needed Curriculum Emphasis," *Nurs. Outlook,* **23**:222–224 (Apr. 1975).

27. Joann Crancer, et al., "Clinical Practicum Before Graduation," *Nurs. Outlook,* **23**:99–102 (Feb. 1975).

28. Eileen A. McQuaid and Michael Kane, "How Do Graduates of Different Types of Programs Perform on State Boards?" *Am. J. Nurs.,* **79**:305–308 (Feb. 1979).

29. *Working Paper of the NLN Task Force on Competencies of Graduates of Nursing Programs.* (New York: National League for Nursing, 1979).

30. Marjorie Ramphal, "Rethinking Diploma School and Collegiate Education," *Nurs. Outlook,* **26**:768–771 (Dec. 1978).

31. Ibid., p. 770.

32. Michael Miller, "Academic Inbreeding in Nursing," *Nurs. Outlook,* **25**:172–177 (March 1977).

33. Thetis Group and Joan Roberts, "Exorcising the Ghosts of the Crimea," *Nurs. Outlook,* **22**:368–372 (June 1974).

34. Sister Bernadette Armiger, "The Educational Crisis in the Preparation of Deans," *Nurs. Outlook,* **24**:164–168 (Mar. 1976).

35. Lucie Young Kelly, "Credentialing of Health Care Personnel," *Nurs. Outlook,* **25**:568 (Sept. 1977).

36. DHEW, *Report on Licensure and Related Health Personnel Credentialing* (Washington, D.C.: U.S. Government Printing Office, 1971), p. 7.

37. *Study of Accreditation of Selected Health Educational Programs Commission Report* (Washington, D.C.: National Commission on Accrediting, 1972), pp. 15–16.

38. *The Study of Credentialing in Nursing: A New Approach, The Report of the Committee* (Kansas City, Mo.: American Nurses' Assn., Jan. 1979), p. 89.

BIBLIOGRAPHY

Berry, Charles, and E. J. Drummond. "The Place of the Humanities in Nursing Education." *Nurs. Outlook,* **18** (Sept. 1970), 30–31. These educators argue that liberal education is essential for the nurse to assume a full professional role and give their reasons, in terms of changing roles.

Boyle, Rena. "Articulation: From Associate Degree Through Masters." *Nurs. Outlook,* **20** (Oct. 1972), 670–672. An early "open curriculum" program that allows the student to progress through these levels, but also terminate at the end of any program.

Brodie, Donald, and Robert Heaney. "Need for Reform in Health Professions Accrediting." *Science,* **201** (Aug. 1978), 589–593. A multiprofessional mechanism is offered as a means of reforming health professions' accrediting. Good reference list.

Bullough, Bonnie, and Vern Bullough. "A Career Ladder in Nursing." *Am. J. Nurs.,* **71** (Oct. 1971), 1938–1943. Supports concept of career ladder, but cites some of the obstacles. Historical background given.

Chamings, Patricia, and James Teevan. "Comparison of Expected Competencies of Baccalaureate and Associate Degree Graduates in Nursing." *Image,* **11** (Feb. 1979), 16–21. Report of a small study indicates that expectations of BS and AD faculty differed regarding student competencies.

Christman, Luther. "The Practitioner-Teacher." *Nurse Educator,* **4** (Mar./Apr. 1979), 8–15. Describes the practitioner-teacher model which maintains teachers' full professional role of service, education, and research.

Cobin, Joan, et al. "A Five-Level Articulated Program." *Nurs. Outlook,* **24** (May 1976), 309–312. Eight-school consortium in California enables continuous progression from nurses' aide to the doctoral level.

Cooper, Vickie, Paula Balber, and Judy Ackerholt. "Nursing Education: Teach the Woman to Know Her Place." *Imprint,* **18** (Jan.–Feb. 1971) 10–11 ff. Three nursing students give their concepts of recruitment for nursing education and comment on some of the inconsistencies in nursing education programs in relation to attitudes reinforced by faculty.

Crancer, Joann, et al. "Clinical Practicum Before Graduation." *Nurs. Outlook,* **23** (Feb. 1975), 99–102. Describes six-week clinical experience that eases AD students into role of the staff nurse.

de Tornyay, Rheba. "Changing Student Relationships, Roles, and Responsibilities." *Nurs. Outlook,* **25** (Mar. 1977), 188–193. Today's students, more distrustful and demanding, and less malleable, require different faculty response and relationships.

de Tornyay, Rheba, and Millie Russell. "Helping the High-Risk Student Achieve." *Nurs. Outlook,* **26** (Sept. 1978), 576–580. Extra help in learning to cope with new situations and responsibilities aids educationally disadvantaged students.

Dickey, Frank. "Accreditation—What About the Public?" *Nurs. Outlook,* **19** (Oct. 1971), 668–669. The executive director of the National Commission on Accrediting cites the need for accountability to the public, with the need to consider the relevance of accrediting criteria to the quality of the product of the educational programs.

Diers, Donna. "A Combined Basic-Graduate Program for College Graduates." *Nurs. Outlook,* **24** (Feb. 1976), 92–98. Description of Yale program which offers both basic nursing and clinical specialization.

Fagin, Claire, Margaret McClure, and Rozella Schlotfeldt. "Can We Bring Order Out of the Chaos of Nursing Education?" *Am. J. Nurs.,* **76** (Jan. 1976), 98–107. Three nursing leaders give their suggestions for eliminating the ambiguity between what we say nurses do and what they really do.

Gray, Judith, et al. "Do Graduates of Technical and Professional Nursing Programs Differ in Practice?" *Nurs. Res.,* **26** (Sept./Oct. 1977), 368–373. Small study of one school shows certain differences. Good reference list of earlier studies.

Group, Thetis, and Joan Roberts. "Exorcising the Ghosts of the Crimea." *Nurs. Outlook,* **22** (June 1974), 368–372. The prevailing milieu in nursing education is found to be, all too often, authoritarian, male-dominated, and militaristic. The plight of faculty and students is described, with some suggestions for solutions.

Harvey, Lillian. "Educational Problems of Minority Nurses." *Nurs. Outlook,* **18** (Sept. 1970),

48–50. A black educator discusses some of the diverse problems of black students in advanced programs, including previous educational deficits, ethnic differences, and loneliness, and makes suggestions for how the students may be helped.

Hillsmith, Katherine. "From RN to BSN: Student Perceptions." *Nurs. Outlook,* 26 (Feb. 1978), 98–102. Controversial article notes discrepancy between RNs' intellectual and emotional acceptance of BSN as criterion for professional nursing.

Katzell, Mildred. "Evaluation for Educational Mobility." *Nurs. Outlook,* 21 (July 1973), 453–456. Means by which nursing programs evaluate previous knowledge and experience of entering students.

Katzell, Mildred. "Upward Mobility in Nursing." *Nurs. Outlook,* 18 (Sept. 1970), 36–39. A testing specialist discusses open curriculum, including how tests can be used for advanced placement, and criteria to determine a test's effectiveness.

Kohnke, Mary. "Do Nursing Educators Practice What Is Preached?" *Am. J. Nurs.,* 73 (Sept. 1973), 1571–1578. Nursing educator looks at baccalaureate and AD nursing programs and sees that the differences described in the literature appear to blur or disappear in the actual situation.

Laverdier, Rita. "An Accelerated Nursing Curriculum." *Nurs. Outlook,* 21 (Aug. 1973), 524–526. Description of a means for accelerating RNs through a baccalaureate program by examinations, program planning, and independent study.

Leininger, Madeleine. "This I Believe—About Interdisciplinary Health Education for the Future." *Nurs. Outlook,* 19 (Dec. 1971), 787–791. A thought-provoking challenge to develop innovative programs.

Lenburg, Carrie, ed. *Open Learning and Career Mobility in Nursing* (St. Louis, Mo.: C. V. Mosby Company, 1975). Describes various types of open curriculum models as well as background, issues, and problems.

MacPhail, Jannetta. "Promoting Collaboration Between Education and Service." *Nurse Educator,* 1 (Sept./Oct. 1976), 19–22. Describes methods such as joint appointments of various types.

Mason, Elizabeth, and John Parascandola. "Preparing Tomorrow's Health Care Team." *Nurs. Outlook,* 20 (Nov. 1972), 728–731. Description of interdisciplinary program that helps health professional students to function interprofessionally. Includes evaluation and future plans.

Mauksch, Ingeborg. "Let's Listen to the Students." *Nurs. Outlook,* 20 (Feb. 1972), 103–107. Urges faculty to allow students to become involved in the educational process to help them become selfdirecting, creative, and socially responsive practitioners.

Mullane, Mary Kelly. "Changing Faculty Relationships, Roles, and Responsibilities." *Nurs. Outlook,* 25 (Feb. 1977), 120–123. Nursing leader reiterates need for nursing faculty to achieve integration into general faculty circles in order to maintain nursing's acceptance in universities.

Nahm, Helen. "What We Have Learned in Thirty Years of Accrediting Nursing Schools," in *Converting Threats Into Challenges—Adaptations in Baccalaureate and Graduate Education in Nursing* (New York: NLN, 1975). An excellent historical overview of accreditation, as well as some goals for the future.

Nyquist, Ewald. "The External Degree Program and Nursing." *Nurs. Outlook,* 21 (June 1973), 372–377. Description of the background, purposes, and proposed implementation of New York State's external degree in nursing by the N.Y. Commissioner of Education who initiated the external degree concept in the state.

Pierik, M. Madaline. "Joint Appointments: Collaboration for Better Patient Care." *Nurs. Outlook,* 21 (Sept. 1973), 576–579. Report of a university setting where nursing education and nursing service share joint appointments and work together for mutual benefit.

Raderman, Rhoda, and D. V. Allen. "Registered Nurse Students in a Baccalaureate Program: Factors Associated with Completion." *Nurs. Res.,* 23 (Jan.–Feb. 1974), 71–73. This small study indicates that significant factors related to completion or withdrawal of RNs are overall grade point average in the program, scores on standardized tests, and type of initial nursing program.

Ramphal, Marjorie. "Rethinking Diploma School and Collegiate Education." *Nurs. Outlook,* 78 (Dec. 1978), 768–771. Thoughtful comparison of the major concepts of the two types of program with excellent recommendation.

Roy, Ann. "The Placement Process." *Nurse Educator,* 4 (Jan./Feb. 1979), 14–18. Describes a nontraditional approach to meeting the individual learning needs of RN students in a BS program.

Schlotfeldt, Rozella. "Nursing in the University Community." *Nurs. Forum,* **5** (1966), 22–27, No. 1. Present and future faculty members of university nursing schools must expand their research activities, upgrade their academic preparation, and create new roles and relationships in health and other disciplines if they are to assume their responsibilities as full members of the university community.

Schmiedel, Edna. "One Rung at a Time—Up the Career Ladder." *Nurs. Outlook,* **21** (June 1973), 400–403. A practical nurse tells of her move through AD, baccalaureate, and graduate nursing education, problems, and successes.

Selden, William. "Health Occupations Credentialing: Three Views." A report on SASHEP reprinted from *Am. Voc. J* (Feb. 1973), in *Nurs. Digest,* **1** (Sept. 1973), 33–48. Some controversial viewpoints are expressed relating to the accreditation process and institutional credentialing. Informative in general, and also brings out key points of the Study of Accreditation of Selected Health Educational Progress report.

Sheahan, Sister Dorothy. "Degree, Yes—Education, No." *Nurs. Outlook,* **22** (Jan. 1974), 22–26. A denunciation of the New York external degree program in nursing, citing particularly lack of socialization to nursing by these RNs.

Shetland, Margaret. "This I Believe—About Career Ladders, New Careers and Nursing Education." *Nurs. Outlook,* **18** (Sept. 1970), 30–35. A nursing dean disagrees with the career ladder concept, citing as some reasons that each type of nursing program must be built on its own base, which differs from another, and that there should be dignity and satisfaction at whatever level an individual functions.

Simmons, Sandra. "A University Extension Program for RNs" *Nurs. Outlook,* **20** (Dec. 1972), 798–801. In one university, a plan was developed to enable RNs to obtain a BS degree totally off campus. Need, program design, facilities, and problems are discussed.

Soules, H. Maxine. "Professional Advancement and Salary Differentials Among Baccalaureate, Diploma, and Associate Degree Nurses." *Nurs. Forum,* **17** (1978), 184–201. Survey shows that all nurses are placed in similar positions and promoted primarily on the basis of longevity.

Steinbaum, Barbara, and Grace O'Neill. "Part-Time Evening Nursing Program." *Nurs. Outlook,* **20** (Feb. 1972), 124–125. A flexible program allows any student with high school or equivalent to enter this AD program in nursing given in the evenings. Students are varied and special counseling is offered.

Styles, Margretta, and Holly Wilson. "The Third Resolution." *Nurs. Outlook,* **27** (Jan. 1979), 44–47. Description of a new educational program (AD to master's degree), developed in response to ANA resolution urging opportunities for RN career mobility.

Tanner, Libby, and Ethel Soulary. "Interprofessional Student Health Teams." *Nurs. Outlook,* **20** (Feb. 1972), 111–115. Describes interdisciplinary education project in which students of nursing, medicine, and social work worked together as a health team. Problems are noted with suggested solutions. References are included on other interdisciplinary projects.

USDHEW. *The Decanal Role in Baccalaureate and Higher Degree Colleges of Nursing.* (Bethesda, Md.: The Department, 1975.) Papers given at a conference of deans about the roles, responsibilities, and opportunities of nursing deans.

Wood, Lucille. "Proposal: A Career Plan for Nursing." *Am. J. Nurs.,* **73** (May 1973), 832–835. The writer, who has done a lengthy study on career ladder education, discusses her proposal, a five-stage approach from an entering curriculum with beginning skills to preparation of nurse researchers.

Wooley, Alma. "From RN to BSN: Faculty Perceptions." *Nurs. Outlook,* **26** (Feb. 1978), 103–108. A companion to the Hillsmith article showing how faculty can deal with anxieties, tension, and resistance of RNs in collegiate programs.

Wozniak, Dolores. "External Degrees in Nursing." *Am. J. Nurs.,* **73** (June 1973), 1014–1018. An examination of the New York State external degree for nursing, giving more specifics than the overview in Nyquist's article.

Wu, Ruth. "Granting Credit for Previous Learning." *Nurs. Outlook,* **26** (Nov. 1978), 707–712. Describes how one California college uses transfer of credit in a career mobility program.

Young, Kenneth. "Issues in Accreditation." *Nurs. Outlook,* **24** (Oct. 1976), 622–624. Reviews problems in accreditation, but also supports concept as way to maintain quality.

See also: references at end of chapter and references and bibliography of other chapters on related topics—ANA, NLN, credentialing, programs in nursing education; entire issue of *Imprint* (Apr. 1979), special focus on nursing education; Feb. 1976 issue of *Nursing Outlook* (Nursing: A Career for College Graduates); the ANA *Standards for Nursing Education,* the NLN Criteria for Accreditation, and ANA's *A Case for Baccalaureate Preparation in Nursing* (1979). The news section of *AJN* carries news items monthly on progress and problems of the entry into practice debate (for instance, a special report on state action in April, 1978). *American Nurse* also carries such news items as well as editiorials and articles on the subject.

13

Programs in Nursing Education

Educational preparation for licensure as a registered nurse takes place primarily in diploma programs, associate degree (AD) programs, and baccalaureate (BSN) programs. As noted in Chapter 12, the numbers have been shifting, with a decrease in diploma programs and an increase in AD and BSN programs. This chapter gives an overview of these educational modes as well as graduate education and continuing education. Open curriculum is discussed in Chapter 12.

DIPLOMA PROGRAMS

The diploma, or hospital, school of nursing was the first type of nursing school in this country. Prior to the opening of the first hospital schools in the late 1800s, there was no formal preparation for nursing. But after Florence Nightingale established the first school of nursing at St. Thomas's Hospital, England, in 1860, the idea spread quickly to the United States.

Hospitals, of course, welcomed the idea of training schools because, in the early years, such schools represented an almost free supply of nursepower. In the early years, and with some outstanding exceptions, the edu-

cation offered was largely of the apprenticeship type; there was some theory and formal classroom work, but for the most part students learned by doing, providing the major part of the nursing care for the hospitals' patients in the process.

This is no longer true. Today, in order to meet standards set in each state for operation of a nursing school and to prepare students to pass the licensing examinations, diploma schools must offer their students a truly educational program, not just an apprenticeship. Hospitals conducting such schools employ a full-time nurse faculty, offer students a balanced mixture of course work (in nursing and related subjects in the physical and social sciences) and supervised practice, and look to their graduate nursing staff, not their students, to provide the nursing service needed by patients. The educational program has been generally three years in length, although most of these schools have now adopted a shortened program. Upon satisfactory completion of the program, the student is awarded a diploma by the school. This diploma, it should be understood, is not an academic degree. In fact, because neither hospitals nor nursing programs based in hospitals are legally considered educational institutions in the main-stream of education, *no* academic credit can be given for any courses given by the school's faculty. For this and economic and educational reasons, large numbers of diploma schools enter into cooperative relations with colleges or universities for educational courses and/or services. It is not uncommon for diploma students to take their physical and social science courses and, occasionally, liberal arts courses at a college. If these courses are part of the general offerings of the college, college credit is granted, and the credit is usually transferable if the nursing student decides to transfer to a college or continue in advanced education. (If the course is tailored to nursing only, it is often not transferable to an advanced nursing program, but is sometimes counted as an elective.) The school usually provides all other necessary educational resources, facilities, and services to students and faculty, such as libraries, classrooms, audio-visual materials, and practice laboratories. At one time, it was taken for granted that students would be housed, and the school had dormitory and recreational space, as well as educational facilities in a separate building. Although the physical setup may still be thus arranged, such housing must now be paid for and may also be used by others educated in or involved with the hospital. The primary clinical facility is the hospital, although the school may contract with other hospitals or agencies for additional educational experiences. Advocates of diploma education usually say that early and substantial experiences with patients seem to foster a strong identification with nursing, particularly hospital nursing, and thus graduates are expected to adjust to the employee role without difficulty.

Admission requirements to diploma schools usually call for a college preparatory curriculum in high school, with standing in the upper half, third, or quarter (depending on the school) of the graduating class. Personal characteristics and health are also assessed.

There are a variety of concepts of what the diploma graduate is or should be. A statement approved by the NLN Council of Diploma Programs in 1978 is reprinted with permission.

Role and Competencies of Graduates of Diploma Programs in Nursing

NURSING
The graduate of the diploma program in nursing is eligible to seek licensure as a registered nurse and to function as a .beginning practitioner in acute, intermediate, long-term, and ambulatory health care facilities. In order to fulfill such roles, graduates should demonstrate the following competencies:*

ASSESSMENT
* *Establishes a data base through a nursing history, including a psychosocial and physical assessment.*
* *Utilizes knowledge of the etiology, pathophysiology, usual course, and prognosis for the prevalent illnesses and health problems.*
* *Establishes priorities when providing nursing care for one or more patients.*
* *Recognizes the significance of nonverbal communication.*

PLANNING
* *Formulates a written plan of nursing care based on the assessment of patient needs.*
* *Includes in the nursing care plan the effects of the family or significant others, life experiences, and social-cultural background.*
* *Involves the patient, family, and significant others in the development of the nursing plan of care.*
* *Incorporates the learning needs of the patient and family into an individualized plan of care.*
* *Applies principles of organization and management in utilizing the knowledge and skills of other nursing personnel.*

IMPLEMENTATION
* *Meets the health needs of individuals and families.*

---

*Competency, as used in this document, is the ability to apply in practice situations the essential principles and techniques of nursing and to apply those concepts, skills, and attitudes required of all nurses to fulfill their role, regardless of specific position or responsibility.

- *Utilizes concepts, scientific facts and principles when providing nursing care.*
- *Performs technical nursing procedures.*
- *Initiates appropriate intervention when environmental and safety hazards exist.*
- *Initiates preventive, habilitative, and rehabilitative nursing measures, according to the needs demonstrated by patients and families.*
- *Performs independent nursing measures and/or seeks assistance from other members of the health team in response to the changing needs of patients.*
- *Collaborates with physicians and members of other disciplines to provide health care.*
- *Documents nursing interventions and patient responses.*
- *Utilizes effective verbal and written communication.*
- *Communicates pertinent information related to the patient through established channels.*
- *Assists the physician in implementing the medical plan of care.*
- *Applies knowledge of individual and group behavior in establishing interpersonal relationships.*
- *Teaches individuals and groups to achieve and maintain an optimum level of wellness.*
- *Utilizes the services of community agencies for continuity of patient care.*
- *Protects the rights of patients and families.*

EVALUATION
- *Evaluates the effectiveness of nursing care and takes appropriate action.*
- *Initiates and cooperates in efforts to improve nursing practice.*

Diploma school graduates constitute the greatest bulk of the practicing nurses today. In 1964, more than 88 percent of the 582,000 employed nurses were diploma school graduates. However, with the drop in the number of diploma schools, this percentage had changed to 67 percent in 1977. The percentage *educated* in diploma schools was almost 75 percent, but about 7 percent of those had received BSNs.

The perceptible shift away from diploma school preparation for nursing can be explained (in an oversimplified way) by three factors: (1) some hospitals are terminating their schools, either because of the expense involved in maintaining a quality program and the objections of third-party payors, such as insurance companies and the government, to having the cost of nursing education absorbed in the patient's bill, or because of difficulty in meeting professional standards, particularly employing qualified faculty, who are in short supply for all programs; (2) increasing numbers of high school graduates are seeking some kind of collegiate education; and (3) the nursing profession is more and more committed to the belief that preparation for nursing, as for all other professions, should take place in institutions of higher education rather than in hospital-controlled programs because hospitals are primarily service institutions rather than educational institutions.

These social and educational trends will probably continue, but it is expected that diploma programs will be on the scene for some time, and the quality programs will continue to prepare quality graduates. The vast majority of current diploma programs are NLN-accredited, and many of the schools that dissolved or were "phased into" associate degree or baccalaureate programs were also accredited. The National Commission study recommended that strong, vital schools be encouraged to seek regional accreditation and degree-granting status, but only a few have done so. Another recommendation, that other hospital schools move to effect interinstitutional arrangements with collegiate institutions, has been acted upon more readily.[1]

Hospitals tend to continue as the clinical laboratories for other nursing education programs. In the communities where associate or baccalaureate degree programs are interested in opening nursing programs, there is often joint planning over a period of years for the new programs to evolve as the diploma program closed—a "phasing-in" process. Prospective candidates for the diploma program might be directed to the new program, sometimes qualified diploma faculty is employed by the college, and frequently arrangements are made to use space in the hospital previously occupied by the diploma school (although the faculty and the program are basically located at the campus). The major purpose of such a move is to provide for continuity in the output of nurses to meet the needs of the community.

The good diploma school has met these needs well for many years.

ASSOCIATE DEGREE PROGRAMS

By far the greatest increase, in both numbers of programs and students enrolled in them, has been in the associate degree programs in nursing that are two years in length and offered by junior or community colleges (occasionally four-year colleges). They are relative newcomers on the nursing education scene. The first three programs of this type were started in 1952; by 1965 there were more than 130 such programs, and in 1978, there were 677 AD programs graduating more than 37,000 students each year. More than half of these schools are NLN-accredited, and most of the others are accredited by regional accrediting groups as part of their college's accreditation.

The associate degree program is the first nursing education program developed under a systematic plan and with carefully controlled experimentation. In her doctoral dissertation, published as a book in 1951, Mildred Montag conceived of a nursing technician, with nursing functions less in scope than those of the professional nurse and broader than those of the practical nurse. This nurse was intended to provide care to patients in the part of the continuum of care that calls for intermediate functions requiring skill and some judgment—a bedside nurse, not intended to assume administrative responsibilities. Montag listed the functions as (1) to assist in the planning of nursing care for patients, (2) to give general nursing care with supervision, and (3) to assist in the evaluation of the nursing care

given.[2] The emerging community college, preparing other kinds of technicians, was seen as a suitable setting for this education, putting nursing education in the mainstream of education and placing the burden of cost on the public in general instead of on the patient. The curriculum was to be an integrated one, half general education and half nursing, with careful selection of educational and clinical experiences.[3] An associate degree would be awarded at the end of two years. The program was considered to be terminal and not a first step toward the baccalaureate.

At the end of 1951, the five-year Cooperative Research Project in Junior and Community College Education for Nursing was funded, and seven junior colleges and one hospital school were selected to participate in the project; each had complete autonomy in the development and conduct of its pilot program, but had free access to consultation from the project staff (see Chapter 5).

The results of the project showed that AD nursing technicians could carry on the intended nursing functions, that the program could be suitably set up in community colleges, with the use of clinical facilities in the community without charge or student service, and that the program attracted students. The success of the experiment plus the rapid growth of community colleges combined to give impetus to these new programs.*

Over the years, as Montag predicted, the AD curricula have varied and changed: for instance, when college policies permit, there is a tendency to put a heavier emphasis and more time on the nursing subjects and clinical experiences, sometimes through the addition of summer sessions. Some programs are also adding team leadership and managerial principles because their graduates are put in positions requiring these skills.

---

*For an excellent, brief overview of the history, development, and achievements of the AD programs, see Alice Rines, "Associate Degree Education: History, Development, and Rationale," *Nursing Outlook,* **25**: 496–501 (Aug. 1977).

There are changes in philosophy as to what the technical nurse is and does. In one study, associate degree deans agreed that the knowledge base of the AD program was narrow in scope, the judgment area was as broad as that of the professional nurse, and the responsibilities were similar. They agreed that the technical nurse worked under the supervision of the professional nurse but should be considered a collaborator with professionals. Some did not see the program as terminal, seeing a difference in amount rather than kind of *professional* education.[4] The entire concept of the AD nursing program as terminal has changed over the last twenty years, along with general societal and educational concepts of *terminal*. Obviously, no educational program should be terminal in the sense that graduates cannot continue their education toward another degree. Whether or not they get full or only partial credit for their previous education depends on the philosophy and policies of the baccalaureate program they select. Nevertheless, what should be emphasized is that the AD nurse need not continue *formal* education to hold a valuable place in the health care system. (Continuing education is a responsibility of all.)

Because the catalogs of most AD nursing programs declare that they are preparing for technical nursing practice, the description of technical practice as differentiated from professional practice in the controversial ANA position paper on nursing education may be helpful:

> *Technical nursing practice is carrying out nursing measures as well as medically delegated techniques with a high degree of skill, using principles from an ever-expanding body of science. It is understanding the physics of machines as well as the physiologic reactions of patients. It is using all treatment modalities with knowledge and precision.*
>
> *Technical nursing practice is evaluating patients' immediate physical and emotional reactions to therapy and taking measures to alleviate distress. It is knowing when to act and when to seek more expert guidance.*
>
> *Technical nursing practice involves working with professional nurse practitioners and others in planning the day-to-day care of patients. It is supervising other workers in the technical aspects of care.*
>
> *Technical nursing practice is unlimited in depth but limited in scope. Its complexity and extent are tremendous. It must be rendered under the direction of professional nurse practitioners, by persons who are selected with care and educated within the system of higher education; only thus can the safety of patients be assured. Education for this practice requires attention to scientific laws and principles with emphasis on skill. It is education which is technically oriented and scientifically founded, but not primarily concerned with evolving theory.[5]*

Whether or not the term *technical* will continue to be used is not clear. The concept of a technical worker, honored in other fields, has not been fully accepted in nursing, possibly because it is considered a step down from the professional label that has been attached to all nurses through licensing definitions and common usage over the years. Montag, noting the difficulty of choosing an appropriate term for the new type of proposed nurse, said, "It is also probable that the term 'nursing technician' will not satisfy forever, but it is proposed as one which indicates more accurately the person who has semi-professional preparation and whose functions are predominantly technical."[6]

The use of the term was rejected by the NLN Council of Associate Degree Programs in a 1974 action which noted that "technical" as applied to nursing practice was not fully understood or accepted. It was also rejected by the National Student Nurses' Association as connoting a less qualified non-professional. Even ANA sometimes seems to shy away from specifically designating the other-than-professional nurse as technical, although the 1979 model practice act does use the term.

More important than the name are the role and functions of the associate degree nurse. Because of nursing shortages, lack of understanding of the abilities and preparation of

Competencies of the Associate Degree Nurse on Entry into Practice

ASSUMPTIONS BASIC TO THE SCOPE OF PRACTICE

The practice of graduates of associate degree nursing programs:

- Is directed toward clients who need information or support to maintain health.
- Is directed toward clients who are in need of medical diagnostic evaluation and/or are experiencing acute or chronic illness.
- Is directed toward clients' responses to common, well-defined health problems.
- Includes the formulation of a nursing diagnosis.
- Consists of nursing interventions selected from established nursing protocols where probable outcomes are predictable.
- Is concerned with individual clients and is given with consideration of the person's relationship within a family, group, and community.
- Includes the safe performance of nursing skills that require cognitive, psychomotor, and affective capabilities.
- May be in any structured care setting but primarily occurs within acute-and extended-care facilities.
- Is guided directly or indirectly by a more experienced registered nurse.
- Includes the direction of peers or other workers in nursing in selected aspects of care within the scope of practice of associate degree nursing.
- Involves an understanding of the roles and responsibilities of self and other workers within the employment setting.

ROLES OF PRACTICE

Five interrelated roles have been defined for graduates of the associate degree nursing program based upon the above assumptions underlying the scope of practice. These roles are: provider of care, client teacher, communicator, manager of client care, and member within the profession of nursing. In each of these roles, decisions and practice are determined on the basis of knowledge and skills, the nursing process, and established protocols of the setting.

ROLE AS A PROVIDER OF CARE—As a provider of nursing care, the associate degree nursing graduate uses the nursing process to formulate and maintain individualized nursing care plans by:

Assessing

- Collects and contributes to a data base (physiological, emotional, sociological, cultural, psychological, and spiritual needs) from available resources (e.g., client, family, medical records, and other health team members).
- Identifies and documents changes in health status which interfere with the client's ability to meet basic needs (e.g., oxygen, nutrition, elimination, activity, safety, rest and sleep, and psychosocial well-being).
- Establishes a nursing diagnosis based on client needs.

Planning

- Develops individualized nursing care plans based upon the nursing diagnosis and plans intervention that follows established nursing protocols.
- Identifies needs and establishes priorities for care with recognition of client's level of development and needs, and with consideration of client's relationship within a family, group, and community.
- Participates with clients, families, significant others, and members of the nursing team to establish long- and short-range client goals.
- Identifies criteria for evaluation of individualized nursing care plans.

Implementing

- Carries out individualized plans of care according to priority of needs and established nursing protocols.
- Participates in the prescribed medical regime by preparing, assisting, and providing follow-up care to clients undergoing diagnostic and/or therapeutic procedures.
- Uses nursing knowledge and skills and protocols to assure an environment conducive to optimum restoration and maintenance of the client's normal abilities to meet basic needs.
  - Maintains and promotes respiratory function (e.g., oxygen therapy, positioning, etc.).
  - Maintains and promotes nutritional status (e.g., dietary regimes, supplemental therapy, intravenous infusions, etc.).
  - Maintains and promotes elimination (e.g., bowel and bladder regimes, forcing fluids, enemas, etc.).
  - Maintains and promotes a balance of activity, rest, and sleep (e.g., planned activities of daily living, environmental adjustment, exercises, sensory stimuli, assistive devices, etc.).
  - Maintains an environment which supports physiological functioning, comfort, and relief of pain.
  - Maintains and promotes all aspects of hygiene.
  - Maintains and promotes physical safety (e.g., implementation of medical and surgical aseptic techniques, etc.).
  - Maintains and promotes psychological safety through consideration of each individual's worth and dignity and applies nursing measures which assist in reducing common developmental and situational stress.
  - Measures basic physiological functioning and reports significant findings (e.g., vital signs, fluid intake and output).
  - Administers prescribed medications safely.
- Intervenes in situations where:
  - Basic life support systems are threatened (e.g., cardiopulmonary resuscitation, obstructive airway maneuver).
  - Untoward physiological or psychological reactions are probable.
  - Changes in normal behavior patterns have occurred.
- Participates in established institutional emergency plans.

Evaluating

- Uses established criteria for evaluation of individualized nursing care.
- Participates with clients, families, significant others, and members of the nursing team in the evaluation of established long- and short-range client goals.
- Identifies alternate methods of meeting client's needs, modifies plans of care as necessary, and documents changes.

ROLE AS A COMMUNICATOR—As a communicator, the associate degree nursing graduate:

- Assesses verbal and non-verbal communication of clients, families, and significant others based upon knowledge and techniques of interpersonal communication.
- Uses lines of authority and communication within the work setting.
- Uses communication skills as a method of data collection, nursing intervention, and evaluation of care.
- Communicates and records assessments, nursing care plans, interventions, and evaluations accurately and promptly.
- Establishes and maintains effective communication with clients, families, significant others, and health team members.
- Communicates client's needs through the appropriate use of referrals.
- Evaluates effectiveness of one's own communication with clients, colleagues, and others.

ROLE AS A CLIENT TEACHER—As a teacher of clients who need information or support to maintain health, the associate degree nursing graduate:

- Assesses situations in which clients need information or support to maintain health.
- Develops short-range teaching plans based upon long- and short-range goals for individual clients.
- Implements teaching plans that are specific to the client's level of development and knowledge.
- Supports and reinforces the teaching plans of other health professionals.
- Evaluates the effectiveness of client's learning.

ROLE AS A MANAGER OF CLIENT CARE—As a manager of nursing care for a group of clients with common, well-defined health problems in structured settings, the associate degree nursing graduate:

- Assesses and sets nursing care priorities.
- With guidance, provides client care utilizing resources and other nursing personnel commensurate with their educational preparation and experience.
- Seeks guidance to assist other nursing personnel to develop skills in giving nursing care.

ROLE AS A MEMBER WITHIN THE PROFESSION OF NURSING—As a member within the profession of nursing, the associate degree nursing graduate:

- Is accountable for his or her nursing practice.
- Practices within the profession's ethical and legal framework.
- Assumes responsibility for self-development and uses resources for continued learning.
- Consults with a more experienced registered nurse when client's problems are not within the scope of practice.
- Participates within a structured role in research (e.g., data collection).
- Works within the policies of the employee or employing institution.
- Recognizes policies and nursing protocols that may impede client care and works within the organizational framework to initiate change.

---

technical nurses, a tendency to use the diploma nurse of previous years as a standard, and general traditionalized concepts of nursing roles, employers of nurses have often not used AD nurses, even though employed as staff nurses, in the manner that best utilized their preparation. AD nurses have been placed quickly as team leaders and charge nurses, positions in which they were not intended to function.

In 1978, the NLN Council of Associate Degree Programs published a statement on the "Competencies of the Associate Degree Nurse on Entry into Practice." The assumptions basic to the scope of practice are particularly interesting because they clarify the kind of client and setting in which the AD nurse can function. The statement is reprinted with permission.

Like other RNs, AD nurses are accountable for their own practice and are expected to function ethically and legally. In addition, the NLN Council made a point of saying that although these nurses work within the policies of an employing institution, they would also work within the organizational framework to initiate change in policies or nursing protocols that might impede client care. There has been some complaint that AD nurses are not proficient in some technical skills, cannot handle large patient loads, and are slow to assume full staff nurse responsibilities and activities.[7,8] The reaction of some AD educators to these complaints, which has been to lengthen the program by adding clinical time or pseudointernships, has, in turn, been criticized by others who say this perverts the AD educational philosophy, which emphasizes an integrated curriculum and carefully selected learning experiences, enhanced by backup practice laboratories and student conferences.[9,10] Many educators also believe that the AD students' request for additional clinical experience is probably no more frequent than that of other students, reacting to criticisms that new graduates are not instant, seasoned practitioners. Almost everyone agrees that AD graduates have a good grasp of basic nursing theory, have inquiring minds, and are self-directed in finding out what they don't know. It is also generally agreed that a good orientation program is the key to satisfactory acclimation to the work setting. Certainly there are nurse administrators who see the AD graduate, properly utilized, as an asset to nursing service.[11,12] One point on which nursing in general agrees is that the AD nurse is here to stay and makes a vital contribution to health care.

BACCALAUREATE DEGREE
PROGRAMS

The first baccalaureate program in nursing was established in 1909 under the control of the University of Minnesota, through the efforts of Dr. Richard Olding Beard. Since then, these programs have become an increasingly important part of nursing education.

The individual enrolled in a baccalaureate degree program in nursing obtains both a college education culminating in a bachelor's degree and preparation for licensure and practice as a registered professional nurse.

The program considered by the ANA as minimum preparation for professional nursing is usually four academic years in length (in a few instances, five) and sometimes a summer session. Unless the college is tax-supported, with minimal tuition fees, baccalaureate nursing education is usually more expensive for students than other basic programs.

The baccalaureate degree program includes three types of courses—general education and the liberal arts, the sciences germane to and related to nursing, and nursing courses. In some programs, the student is not admitted to the nursing major and therefore has no nursing courses per se, until the conclusion of the first two years of college study. In other programs, nursing content is integrated throughout the entire four years.

As in the other nursing programs, the baccalaureate program has both theoretical content and clinical experience. One difference lies in that for the baccalaureate student, the courses in the physical and social sciences will have greater depth and breadth, inasmuch as they are given on a college level. The students majoring in nursing take the regular college courses in the sciences and humanities. And because the only difference between them and the other students in the college is the subject in which they are majoring (nursing instead of history or English literature, for instance), they must meet the same admission requirements and maintain the same academic level as all other students. The nursing program is an integral part of the college or university as a whole.

A statement on the "Characteristics of Baccalaureate Education in Nursing" was developed by the NLN Council of Baccalaureate and Higher Degree Programs in 1978 and is reprinted with permission.

The baccalaureate program in nursing, which is offered by a senior college or university, provides students with an opportunity to acquire: (1) knowledge of the theory* and practice of nursing; (2) competency in selecting, synthesizing, and applying relevant information from various disciplines; (3) ability to assess client needs and provide nursing interventions; (4) ability to provide care for groups of clients; (5) ability to work with and through others; (6) ability to evaluate current practices and try new approaches; (7) competency in collaborating with members of other health disciplines and with consumers; (8) an understanding of the research process and its contribution to nursing practice; (9) knowledge of the broad function the nursing profession is expected to perform in society; and (10) a foundation for graduate study in nursing.

Nurses are prepared as generalists at the baccalaureate level to provide within the health care system** a comprehensive service of assessing, promoting, and maintaining the health of individuals and groups. These nurses are prepared to: (1) be accountable for their own nursing practice; (2) accept responsibility for the provision of nursing care

---

*Throughout this statement, theory is used in the universal sense as it applies to all disciplines.

**The health care system includes social, cultural, economic, and political components. It can be conceptualized from an individual perspective of nurse and client/family to the broad, national health care scene. For the most part, the graduates of baccalaureate programs in nursing work within the local health care system although fully aware of the regional and national health care scenes. The master's graduates in nursing are proficient in working within the local health care system and have learned to extend their influence and effectiveness to and through the regional and national levels.

through others; (3) accept the advocacy role in relation to clients; and (4) develop methods of working collaboratively with other health professionals. They will practice in a variety of health care settings—hospital, home, and community—and emphasize comprehensive health care, including prevention, health promotion, and rehabilitation services; health counseling and education; and care in acute and long-term illness.

Baccalaureate nursing programs are conceptually organized to be consistent with the stated philosophy and objectives of the parent institution and the unit in nursing. These programs provide the general and professional education essential for understanding and respecting people, various cultures, and environments; for acquiring and utilizing nursing theory upon which nursing practice is based; and for promoting self-understanding, personal fulfillment, and motivation for continued learning. The structure of the baccalaureate degree program in nursing follows the same pattern as that of baccalaureate education in general. It is characterized by a liberal education at the lower division level, on which is built the upper division major. In baccalaureate nursing education, the lower division consists of foundational courses drawn primarily from the scientific and humanistic disciplines inherent in liberal learning. The major in nursing is built upon this lower division general education base and is concentrated at the upper division level. Upper division studies include courses that complement the nursing component or increase the depth of general education.

Consistent with the foregoing characteristics and directly related to the "Criteria for the Appraisal of Baccalaureate and Higher Degree Programs in Nursing," the graduate of the baccalaureate program in nursing is able to:

- *Utilize nursing theory in making decisions on nursing practice.*
- *Use nursing practice as a means of gathering data for refining and extending that practice.*
- *Synthesize theoretical and empirical knowledge from the physical and behavioral sciences and humanities with nursing theory and practice.*
- *Assess health status and health potential;*

plan, implement, and evaluate nursing care of individuals, families and communities.
- *Improve service to the client by continually evaluating the effectiveness of nursing intervention and revising it accordingly.*
- *Accept individual responsibility and accountability for the choice of nursing intervention and its outcome.*
- *Evaluate research for the applicability of its findings to nursing actions.*
- *Utilize leadership skills through involvement with others in meeting health needs and nursing goals.*
- *Collaborate with colleagues and citizens on the interdisciplinary health team to promote the health and welfare of people.*
- *Participate in identifying and effecting needed change to improve delivery within specific health care systems.*
- *Participate in identifying community and societal health needs and in designing nursing roles to meet these needs.*

The most notable differences between baccalaureate education and that of the other basic nursing programs are related to liberal education, development of intellectual skills, and the addition of public health, teaching, and management skills. Baccalaureate nurses have the opportunity to become liberally educated in their programs. Almost all programs allow free electives in the humanities and many allow electives in the sciences and nursing courses. Students are able to participate in the cultural and social activities throughout their whole program and develop relationships with professors and students in other disciplines. Although technical skills are essential to nursing, learning activities that assist students to develop skills in recognizing and solving problems, applying general principles to particular situations, and establishing a basis for making sound judgments are also given emphasis. This enables the nurse to function more easily when a familiar situation takes an unexpected turn or when it is necessary to deal with an unfamiliar situation. The baccalaureate program is the only basic program offering both theory and practice in public health nursing. There are also courses in administrative and teaching principles. Both these skills are clearly necessary when the baccalaureate nurse functions as team leader, coordinating, planning, and directing the activities of other nursing personnel or as primary nurse. It is on the basis of such backgrounds that the roles of a baccalaureate nurse are sometimes described as those of a practitioner engaged in direct patient care, teacher, leader, collaborator, and student (an inquiring person).[13] Of great impact is the early preparation of the baccalaureate nurse as nurse practitioner in primary care (see Chapter 15), which is a newer manifestation of all of these roles.

On completion of the program, most BSN graduates select hospitals as their first place of employment, but then often turn to public health nursing. However, in the last few years, those hospitals that have primary nursing, which gives nurses individual responsibility for a group of patients, seem to have been more able to attract and retain baccalaureate nurses. Those with long-term plans for teaching, administration, or clinical specialization continue into graduate study, usually preceded by some experience. As might be expected, BSN graduates are more likely to complete a graduate degree than their diploma or AD counterparts.

According to a 1977 ANA survey, almost 12 percent of all nurses were studying for a post-RN degree. Of these, about one quarter were seeking master's or higher degrees, but almost 68 percent were studying for a baccalaureate. The number of RNs enrolled in baccalaureate programs has increased steadily. The 6 percent enrolled in AD programs were diploma RNs seeking the AD as a step toward the baccalaureate; almost 10 percent of the diploma nurses seeking degrees were enrolled in these programs.[14] Some RNs, because of circumstances, desire, or lack of counseling, choose non-nursing majors, which generally precludes their acceptance in a graduate program in nursing. In most nursing programs, RNs receive some credit and/or advanced standing for their previous education through challenging examinations, but the program and degree are the same as

for the generic students. Frequently, courses and clinical experiences are individualized to meet RNs' needs and goals. A noticeable trend is admission of students with baccalaureate or advanced degrees in fields other than nursing. These students, of course, receive a second baccalaureate. Depending on how many of their previous courses satisfy the BSN requirements, their program may consist primarily of the upper division major nursing courses. A few baccalaureate programs have been especially designed for the baccalaureate graduate, and no others are admitted. However, there are other alternatives for these second-careerists.

OTHER GENERIC EDUCATIONAL PROGRAMS FOR RN LICENSURE

A number of years ago, several nursing education programs, such as Yale and Western Reserve University, admitted only baccalaureate graduates and granted a master's degree in nursing as the basic educational credential. Today, there is a resurgence of interest in such programs. Some prepare for a generalist role, others, for a specialty as clinical specialist or nurse practitioner. Depending on the school's philosophy and other factors, the student may take the licensing examination before completion of the master's if the state law permits it. (Not included in this discussion is the ladder concept, in which a student may get a license after completion of an AD or baccalaureate and then continue directly to the master's degree.)

The first program for a professional doctorate (ND) for college graduates was at Case-Western Reserve in 1979. It was designed for "liberally educated men and women who are gifted intellectually, willing to invest themselves in a rigorous, demanding, rewarding program of study, and committed to a sustained professional career."[15] As described, the program, if adopted by others, should be located only in universities with health science centers preparing several types of health professionals. Because such universities also offer advanced graduate education, the ND students would be prepared in an academic climate of scholarship and research. Faculty are to be prepared at the highest level of scholarship, with some engaged in teaching and research and others, jointly appointed, master's-prepared clinicians engaged in clinical practice, teaching, and some aspect of research. The curriculum would prepare the ND graduates to become proficient in delivery of primary, episodic, and long-term nursing care, and to enable them to evaluate their own practice and that of their assistants, being accountable for the outcomes of all nursing practice. Graduates of this program would continue graduate study in a specialization and/or a functional area such as teaching or administration. As is true of medical students whose professional degree is a doctorate, they might also obtain a master's or Ph.D. concurrently with the first doctorate. This innovative approach, seen as a major step toward the emergence of nursing as a full-fledged profession, will be under close scrutiny for some years to come.

GRADUATE EDUCATION

Graduate education in nursing, of a kind, can be traced back to the first decades of the twentieth century. However, there was considerable confusion in those early years in that what was called graduate education was actually education *for graduate nurses* beyond their basic program. The first program concentrated on public health nursing and preparation for teaching and supervision.[16] As late as 1951 it was finally recognized that there was little differentiation between the programs leading to a baccalaureate degree and those leading to a master's; the master's was found to be little more than a symbol that the nurse had previously earned a bachelor's degree. This led to a series of recommendations to place graduate education for nurses on the same basis as that in other disciplines.[17] In the following years, graduate programs *for practice* in public health nursing, teaching, and education were developed, but in 1952 there were only 1,449 nurses who had completed programs for advanced nursing practice, teaching, supervision, and administration, a figure aptly described by the League as "microscopic" compared with the nation's needs.[18] By 1962, nurses with graduate preparation had increased to 11,500 out of the 550,000 nurses in practice at that time. The Surgeon General's Report, citing the need for teachers, nurse administrators, and others requiring advanced education, called for a doubling of baccalaureate graduates and a tripling of master's and doctor's degrees by 1970.[19]

Even with the federal traineeships, scholarships, and loans that followed the report, that goal was not achieved. In 1972, there were approximately 25,000 nurses (out of 778,470) with master's degrees (not all in nursing).[20] About 1,000 had doctoral degrees. By 1977, the number of nurses holding master's degrees or doctorates increased to 4.7 percent of the total number of nurses, as opposed to 3.3 percent in 1972.[21] About 2,000 held doctoral degrees, most of which were not from a school of nursing.

Today, the purpose of master's education is to prepare professional nursing leaders in the areas of clinical specialization, teaching, and administration. Nurses with these special skills and knowledge are desperately required now and will be for the foreseeable future.

Perhaps because so much of the emphasis in graduate programs over the years had been on attaining functional skills in teaching and administration, with little attention given to clinical knowledge and skills, a 1969 ANA statement on graduate education proclaimed that the "major purpose of graduate education should be the preparation of nurse clinicians capable of improving nursing care through the advancement of nursing service and theory."[22] However, it soon became evident that nurses in education and administration did indeed need the functional skills required in these fields. Almost ten years later, a new statement focused on "the preparation of highly competent individuals who can function in diverse roles, such as clinical nurse generalists or specialists, researchers, theoreticians, teachers, administrators, consultants, public policy makers, system managers, and colleagues on multidisciplinary teams . . . prepared through master's, doctoral, and postdoctoral programs in nursing that subscribe to clearly defined standards of scholarship."[23] Nontraditional graduate programs, such as those previously described, were also encouraged because they "can provide for significant contributions to the advancement of scholarship in nursing."[24] Other nontraditional approaches, such as interinstitutional exchange programs, consortium arrangements, and satellite and off-campus programs, were also cited as innovative and approved "in concert with beliefs about pluralism, diversity, and flexibility in graduate education."[25]

It is interesting to note that programs in *nursing* are specified, presumably signalling that master's and doctoral degrees in other fields, without a nursing component, are not encouraged. A 1979 NLN statement also emphasizes expansion of nursing knowledge: "Individuals prepared at the master's level in nursing improve nursing and health care through their expert practice, and through the advancement of theory in nursing." Acquisition of research skills is considered essential. In general, master's education in nursing includes concentrated study of a specific area of nursing, introduction to research methods, and independent study of a nursing problem, using research techniques. The latter is called a master's thesis, project, or study. Most NLN-accredited master's programs offer study of a clinical area, such as medical-surgical nursing, maternal-child nursing, community health nursing, or psychiatric nursing with advanced experience, based on a theoretical framework developed by that faculty and including relevant advanced courses in the natural and social sciences. The depth of clinical study varies

in relation to whether the nurse plans to become a clinical specialist or nurse practitioner or wishes to concentrate on a functional area such as teaching, administration, or consultation, for which other appropriate courses will also be offered. Increasingly, a practicum (planned, guided learning experiences in a practice setting that allow a student to function within the role) is being recommended for the functional as well as the clinical areas, but they vary greatly from program to program, from one day a week for a semester to almost a year's full-time residency.

Master's degree education in nursing has been described as providing students with an opportunity to:

> *(1) acquire advanced knowledge from the sciences and the humanities to support advanced nursing practice and role development; (2) expand their knowledge of nursing theory as a basis for advanced nursing practice; (3) develop expertise in a specialized area of clinical nursing practice; (4) acquire the knowledge and skills related to a specific functional role in nursing; (5) acquire initial competence in conducting research; (6) plan and initiate change in the health care system and in the practice and delivery of health care; (7) further develop and implement leadership strategies for the betterment of health care; (8) actively engage in collaborative relationships with others for the purpose of improving health care; and (9) acquire a foundation for doctoral study.*[26]

Graduate programs in nursing vary in admission requirements, organization of curriculum, length of program, and costs. Admission usually requires RN licensure, graduation from an approved (or accredited) baccalaureate program with an upper division major in nursing,* a satisfactory grade point average, achievement on selected tests, and, sometimes, nursing experience. Part-time study is available in some programs, but often certain courses must be taken in sequence, and at least some full-

---

*Some programs will admit a few nurses without BSNs and assist them in making up deficiencies.

time study may be required. It should be remembered that not all graduate programs offer all the possible majors; there is even limitation on the number of clinical majors available. An NLN pamphlet, "Master's Education in Nursing, Route to Opportunities in Contemporary Nursing," presents an overall view of all accredited nursing master's programs, including curricula offered, admission requirements, availability of part-time study, length of program, approximate cost, and availability of housing.

Although some nurses choose to obtain graduate degrees outside the field of nursing, advanced positions in nursing usually require a nursing degree, preferably with advanced clinical content and experience.* Currently, there are some seventy universities with accredited nursing master's programs in the United States, which obviously means that a program is not necessarily easily accessible to all nurses who seek graduate education. Nevertheless, selection of a suitable graduate program is essential, and nurses should carefully review catalogs to determine which programs meet their career goals.

Nurses with master's degrees are expected to assume leadership positions in one way or another, both in terms of the profession and public service. A renewed recognition of the importance of interdisciplinary collaboration is also worth noting:

> The leadership strategies developed and implemented for the betterment of health care encompass the range of activities needed to influence both nursing education and nursing practice constructively. Furthermore, these strategies are designed to promote the personal and professional investment of self and to employ professional standards and ethical conduct. The leadership strategies emanate from a broad theoretical base and enable the leader to prescribe, decide, influence, and facilitate changes for nursing and health. The direction and scope of leadership are directly related to one's field of operation and to the publics served. The roles of change agent and consumer advocate are also affected through the selection and implementation of a broad range of appropriate strategies.
>
> The interdisciplinary collaboration role of the graduate of a master's program is characterized by initiation and interpretation. Master's-prepared nurses utilize newly acquired functional role skills to design, initiate, and assume a leadership role as well as a collaborative role. They take an active part in delineating the goals and standards of the group and in designing the mode and terms of operation. One of the major responsibilities of a master's graduate in nursing is to interpret the role and function of nurses to others.[27]

The first American nurse to earn a doctorate received her PhD in psychology and counseling in 1927. In 1973, the American Nurses' Foundation provided specific individual information about 1,019 nurses with doctoral degrees in the world, of whom 964 were in the United States.[28] For the first time, doctoral nurses in the United States had also been identified by sex and race: forty-six black, eleven Oriental, and one Egyptian; twenty-five were men, including three blacks.*

Until 1946, when two of the forty-six colleges and universities offering advanced programs in nursing also initiated doctoral education for nurses, nurses who desired doctoral studies had to attend programs outside of nursing. By 1969, some twenty-five different doctoral degrees were being awarded to nurses, including the Doctor of Nursing (DN), Doctor of Nursing Science (DNS or DNSc), Doctor of Nursing Education (DNEd), and Doctor of Public Health Nursing (DPHN), as well as Doctor of Philosophy (PhD), and Doctor of Education (EdD) with majors in another field and minors in nursing, or one of these degrees in another discipline, related or not.

There is still disagreement, and some con-

---

*The exception may be graduates from schools of public health, who have had programs in public health nursing and/or administration that do not include clinical components per se.

*New data about doctoral nurses were in the process of preparation by ANF in 1980.

fusion, in nursing circles as to the kind of education and degree a nurse should get in a doctoral program. The first definitive statement on doctoral education in nursing was made by the NLN in 1955, the same year that the HEW Division of Nursing activated the Predoctoral and Postdoctoral Nursing Research Fellowship Program in order to assist nurses to qualify for doctoral study in a discipline outside nursing and to encourage the preparation of research personnel. At that time, the NLN committee considering graduate programs made certain assumptions about the doctoral degree:

> *(1) the doctorate should not be a third professional degree in nursing but should be based upon a second professional degree and constitute new and enlarged experience in relevant intellectual disciplines and scholarly research in the application of such disciplines to nursing; (2) the degree could be interdisciplinary, possibly in the social sciences, biological sciences, and education; (3) in those institutions not permitting interdisciplinary doctorates, the degree should be awarded in a single discipline such as sociology, biology, and the like.*[29]

By 1960, then, the major activity in doctoral education for nurses focused on establishing collaborative arrangements with other disciplines in a university through which nurses could receive doctoral degrees. Only four institutions offered doctoral programs in which an area of nursing, teaching, or administration in nursing was the focus of study.[30] In 1963, the Nurse Scientist Graduate Training Grants Program was initiated by HEW and new attention was given to doctoral study. The national nursing organizations and universities held a number of programs and conferences to discuss philosophical bases and explore trends affecting doctoral study. The "appropriate" doctoral degree for nurses has been a matter of debate. Some nursing leaders favor granting a PhD in nursing with a minor in a relevant discipline. Others have felt that although the nursing PhD is an ultimate goal, nursing science is not sufficiently developed to make

this practical immediately. Instead they suggest either a PhD in some other discipline with a minor in nursing or a strictly professional degree such as the DNS. It is believed that a nurse with an academic degree (PhD) in a cognate discipline could help to generate knowledge, and the nurse with the professional degree (EdD or DNSc) would apply this new knowledge.[31]

The following varied principles concerning doctoral education for nursing are most often stated:

> 1. *The doctoral program should be pursued in an established discipline such as the natural, biological, or behavioral sciences with or without a minor in nursing.*
> 2. *A program culminating in a PhD with a major in nursing should give candidates a theoretical base of pure research in nursing.*
> 3. *Programs leading to a professional degree, e.g., DNSc, should prepare the graduate for scholarly practice of nursing as a clinical specialist or nurse therapist.*
> 4. *Doctoral programs in health care administration, public health, and education should be open to nurses who wish to prepare for such relevant fields of practice.*[32]

The Nurse Scientist Program, federally funded, gave considerable impetus to the first principle, and in 1973 there were nine institutions with formal programs for the nurse-scientist. With discontinuation of federal funds, these programs were essentially nonexistent a few years later. There are also strong proponents of the second principle by those who firmly believe that "nursing is characterized by an organized body of abstract knowledge specific to nursing . . . not a summation of facts and principles drawn from other sources," and who feel that nursing's future as a learned profession and its yet unrealized potential for human service are dependent largely to the extent that scholarly education through doctoral study is made explicit.[33] The concern of others is that practitioners of nursing use concepts from related disciplines to develop, test, and apply nursing theory and conduct research contributing to nursing knowledge and practice. And finally, there are those who feel that administrators in education and nursing services would find degrees in relevant fields most valuable. Nurses have moved in all these directions; as of 1971, 47 per cent held degrees in the behavioral sciences; 34 per cent in education; 8 per cent in behavioral sciences; 6 per cent in nursing; 2 per cent in public health; and about 3 per cent in other fields.[34]

The ANA statement on doctoral programs takes a relatively broad view:

> Doctoral programs of study are designed to prepare nurses as theoreticians, scholars, researchers, administrators, health policy teachers, planners, and clinicians. Now and in the future, doctoral programs should be directed toward the formulation and testing of theories; the creation of research designs, methods, and tools to study nursing and health problems; and the development of scientific and humanistic knowledge appropriate to the care of man in health and illness.[35]

Although there are still many nurses enrolled in non-nursing doctoral programs, the pendulum may have swung toward doctoral degrees in nursing in the last few years. A 1976 survey pinpointed thirty-five established or proposed doctoral programs in nursing (excluding the nurse scientist programs). The specific degrees included EdD, PhD, DNS, DNSc, and ND, with areas of study in all major specialites in nursing as well as nursing education and administration. The growth is phenomenal, considering that in 1974 there were only seven such programs.[36]

Nevertheless, there are two major deterrents to program development: qualified faculty and adequate finances. The glut of PhDs in other fields has discouraged funding for doctoral education of all kinds, and the general reluctance of the federal government to continue financing nursing education is beginning to extend to graduate education. (Almost all doctoral programs have some federal funding (soft money); hard money

from state or institution is generally at a no-growth level at this time.)

The characteristics of high-quality nursing doctoral programs have been described as:

1. Well-prepared faculty holding earned doctorates, with the majority holding a doctoral degree in nursing.
2. Evidence of research and scholarly productivity of faculty.
3. Maintenance of a learning climate conducive to intellectual curiosity, advancement of clinical knowledge, and identification of researchable problems.
4. Evidence of continuous, active, productive, quality-based research in the parent institution.
5. Selection of students who are intellectually capable and professionally committed to nursing and the health care of all people.
6. Philosophical and financial accountability of the parent institution to support a doctoral program in nursing and make university resources available for the conduct of the program.
7. Consideration of regional and national resources to enhance program offerings, assure quality, and augment areas of faculty expertise.
8. Provision for evaluation of the doctoral program and the impact of graduates.[37]

These make clear the need for appropriate faculty and resources.*

Although the role of doctoral nurses is still not clearly understood by many lay people and even some other disciplines, nursing leaders see an urgency in increasing this too small pool of scholars, because the shortage is expected to remain acute into at least the mid-1980s. Their role is well described by one:

> . . . doctoral programs in nursing must be designed to prepare highly knowledgeable and competent researchers, clinicians, teachers, and administrators for academic and

---

*A relatively recent phenomenom is the external doctorate described extensively by Brower (see bibliography).

service settings. As doctoral programs increase in number, it is important that they maintain commitments to highly disciplined modes of thought, quality research work, and demonstrated skills in writing and leadership. If doctoral education for nurses maintains such commitments, the critical leadership crises in nursing would be mitigated; leadership, new scientific and humanistic thrusts will take their place in nursing history. Nurses who are graduates of doctoral programs should have a scientific and humanistic grasp of general and special problems of nursing, and should be prepared to challenge past modes of thought and to risk new kinds of nursing practices.[38]

PROGRAMS FOR PRACTICAL NURSES

Professional nurses work closely with practical nurses (PNs) in all branches of hospital and public health nursing. Moreover, in the last few years, an increasing number of practical nurses have been entering RN programs at either a beginning or advanced level. It is helpful, therefore, to be informed about the educational preparation of a practical nurse, as well as the basic RN programs.

Practical nurses (called vocational nurses in Texas and California) fall into three general groups: (1) those whose only teacher has been experience and who are not licensed to practice (this type of practical nurse is gradually disappearing from the scene); (2) those with experience but no formal education who have taken state-approved courses to qualify them to take state board examinations and become licensed, or who have been licensed through a grandfather clause; and (3) those who have graduated from approved schools of practical nursing and, by passing state board examinations, have become licensed in the state or states in which they practice. There are also a few who were enrolled in RN programs and were permitted by their state law to take the PN examination after a certain number of courses. The large majority of LPNs are licensed by examina-

tion. Practical/vocational nurses are usually educated in one-year programs in vocational schools, hospitals, or community colleges. Academic credits are awarded by the colleges. In 1978, there were 1,329 practical nurse programs, which admitted about 61,000 students, a slight increase from the previous academic year.[39] The growth rate of both programs and numbers of students had been increasing steadily over the years, but appears to have leveled off and perhaps decrease. PN education has been heavily supported by the federal government for some time. The desire for licensed practical nurses to continue to RN status is manifested by their increased admission (and graduation) from RN programs. For some years, PN programs have seemed to attract more blacks, more men, and more older students than any other type of nursing program. However, many of these potential students, if qualified, now seem to choose AD or baccalaureate programs.

Legitimate practical nurse programs must be approved by the appropriate state nursing authority and may also be accredited by either NLN or the National Association for Practical Nurse Education and Service (NAPNES). Upon graduation, the student is eligible to take the licensing examination to become a licensed practical nurse (LPN) or a licensed vocational nurse (LVN). The licensing law is not mandatory in all states, but all nursing organizations support mandatory licensure. Many PNs are still licensed by waiver, having taken no licensing examination, but becoming licensed through the usual grandfather clause in effect when laws become mandatory. Although they can be legally employed, employers with a choice usually prefer graudates from an approved school who have been licensed by examination.

PN programs emphasize technical skills and direct patient care, but a (usually) simple background of the physical and social sciences is often integrated in the program. Clinical experience is provided in one or more hospitals. The number of skills taught seems to increase each year, probably because of employers' demands.

There is some trend to make a PN program the first year of a two-year associate degree program. A student may exit at the end of the year, become licensed and work, or become licensed and not work and continue into the second year, becoming eligible for the RN examination. Some RN programs, particularly associate degree, will give some or total credit for the PN program (often only if the PN has also passed the licensing examination). In PN programs, most teachers have only a baccalaureate degree or less, but NLN recommends preparation for the broad scope of nursing and preparation in teaching. As in all areas of health care, there is a need for continuing education programs. Employers frequently offer courses, reviews, or inservice programs for giving medications and performing new treatments, but the two practical nursing organizations and NLN have provided total programs on care of geriatric patients, psychiatric patients, and others. There are also numerous continuing education programs geared particularly toward the LPN licensed by waiver.

The LPN works in hospitals, doctors' offices, extended care units, nursing homes, private homes, and other health facilities, including to some extent, community health agencies.

In 1980, the National Federation of Licensed Practical Nurses (NFLPN) substituted for its long standing "Statement of Functions and Qualifications," a new document "Nursing Practice Standards for the Licensed Practical/Vocational Nurse." The preface notes that these standards are applicable in any practice setting and that, since the scope of licensed practical nursing has extended into specialized nursing services, these are included in the document. In addition, a code of ethical practice and conduct is presented, and the need for continuing education is emphasized in the standards.

Key statements from this statement are presented below, with permission of NFLPN.

Definition

Practical/Vocational nursing means the performance for compensation of authorized acts of nursing which utilize specialized knowledge and skills and which meet the health needs of people in a variety of settings under the direction of qualified health professionals.

Scope

Practical/Vocational nursing comprises the common core of nursing and, therefore, is a valid entry into the nursing profession.

Opportunities exist for practicing in a milieu where different professions unite their particular skills in a team effort for one common objective—to preserve or improve an individual patient's functioning.

Opportunities also exist for upward mobility within the profession through formal education and for lateral expansion of knowledge and expertise through both formal and informal education.

Practice

1. *Shall accept assigned responsibilities as an accountable member of the health care team.*
2. *Shall function within the limits of educational preparation and experience as related to the assigned duties.*
3. *Shall function with other members of the health care team in promoting and maintaining health, preventing disease and disability, caring for and rehabilitating individuals who are experiencing altered health state.*
4. *Shall know and utilize the nursing process in planning, implementing, and evaluating health services and nursing care to the individual patient or group.*
   a. *Planning: The planning of nursing includes:*
      * *assessment of health status of the individual patient, the family and community groups*
      * *an analysis of the information gained from assessment*
      * *the identification of health goals*

b. *Implementation: The plan for nursing care is implemented to achieve the stated goals.*
   - *observing, recording and reporting significant changes which require intervention or different goals*
   - *applying of nursing knowledge and skills to promote and maintain health, to prevent disease and disability and to optimize functional capabilities of an individual patient ·*
   - *assisting the patient and family with activities of daily living and encouraging self-care as appropriate*
   - *carrying out therapeutic regimens prescribed by a physician or other qualified health care providers.*
c. *Evaluation: The plan for nursing care and its implementations are evaluated to measure the progress toward the stated goals and will include appropriate persons and/or groups to determine:*
   - *the relevancy of current goals in relation to the progress of the individual patient, the family and community*
   - *the involvement of the recipients of care in the evaluation process*
   - *the quality of the nursing action in the implementation of the plan*
   - *a re-ordering of priorities or new goal setting in the care plan*
5. *Shall participate in peer review and other evaluative processes.*
6. *Shall participate in the development of policies concerning the health and nursing needs of society and in the roles and functions of the LP/VN.*

Because, unfortunately, PNs are often pressed to perform functions beyond the level of their education (such as charge nursing and certain specialty practice) there is an increasing movement by PNs to "be paid for what we do, not what we are." The overall situation is causing great concern for all nurses.

Continuing Education

It is generally agreed that professional practitioners of any kind must continue to learn because they are accountable to the public for a high quality of service—a service impossible to maintain if pertinent aspects of the tremendous flow of new knowledge are not integrated and used.

A thought-provoking model of the fleeting hold professionals have on knowledge gained in their educational programs was described some years ago in a library journal and will now be discussed.

Assuming that the professional life of an individual (in this example, a physician) is forty years, the amount of clinically applicable knowledge available in mid-career should be 100 percent. However, the body of knowledge available at the time of the educational program is only about half, leaving 50 percent useful. It is only possible to teach a fraction of this knowledge in any educational program, leaving 20 percent useful. Of this, a small part is erroneous, leaving 19 percent useful. Not all that is taught is learned, leaving 16 percent useful. Much of what is learned is forgotten within a few years, leaving 8 percent useful; some of what is learned is never used because of specialization, leaving 5 percent useful. Much of what is learned becomes obsolete in 20 years, leaving 3 percent of useful knowledge gained in the professional's basic educational program.[40]

While the precision of the figures can obviously be challenged, the message is clear, even in nonquantitative terms: ongoing learning (continuing education) is necessary if a professional is to function effectively.

For nurses, specifically, the need for continuing education is primarily to keep them abreast of changes in nursing roles and functions, acquire new knowledge and skills (and/or renew that which has been lost), and modify attitudes and understanding. To achieve these goals, various approaches to continuing education can be utilized, such as: formal academic studies that might lead to a degree; short-term courses or programs given by institutions of higher learning, not necessarily providing academic credit; and independent or informal study carried on by the practitioner, utilizing opportunities made available through professional organizations and employing agencies. It should be made clear that continuing one's education does not mean that enrollment in a formal academic, degree-granting program is necessary, although it might well be a reasonable route for a nurse who has specific career goals. On the other hand, neither does achievement of the highest academic degree mean an end to continued learning.

One statement of philosophy, probably not too different from that developed by other groups, is useful in delineating the scope of continuing education:

> Continuing education in nursing consists of planned, organized learning experiences designed to augment the knowledge, skills, and attitudes of registered nurses for the enhancement of nursing practice, education, administration, and research, to the end of improving health care to the public. Defined broadly, continuing education is a lifelong learning process that builds on and modifies previously acquired knowledge, skills, and attitudes. The structure and content of continuing education must be flexible in order to meet the nursing practice needs and career goals of nursing personnel.[41]

A number of states have, in the last decade, enacted legislation requiring evidence of continuing education (CE) for relicensure of nurses (and of certain other professional and occupational groups), and formalized programs have been increasing. They are given under the auspices of educational institutions, professional organizations, and commercial for-profit groups, but most now seek some sort of recognition or accreditation so that their programs will be acknowledged by licensing boards as legitimate sources of continuing education. Most also use the Continuing Education Unit (CEU), nationally accepted for unit measurement of all kinds of CE programs. (Ten contact hours equal one unit.)

Both the ANA and NLN and their constituent organizations have been engaged in planning and implementing a voluntary system of continuing education for nurses. The ICN has urged its members to take the lead in initiating, promoting, or further developing a national system of continuing nursing education. The ANA has set both standards and guidelines. The latter includes such points as working with other organizations, employees, and educational systems to provide continuing education to nurses, but a major focus is development of Continuing Education Approval and Recognition Programs (CEARP) or Continuing Education Recognition Programs (CERP). Almost all state nurses' organizations (SNAs), except in those states where CE is mandatory, now have some form of CERP program. Generally, their purpose is to record and/or recognize nurses' voluntary participation in Continuing Education and approve CE offerings. Contact hours, or CEUs, or recognition points (one point is equal to one contact hour) are the time measurements used. Depending on how extensive the recording services are, a fee may be charged to the nurse. When the SNA also has an accreditation or approval program for the offerings, the CE provider inevitably pays a fee.[42] The ANA accreditation program, with its regional accrediting committees, is a separate entity and provides the learner, employer, state board, or other interested consumer some assurance that the accredited program has met certain standards. To meet the criteria, the provider group usually must include information about its educational resources, qualifications of the teachers, objectives, outline, and evaluation techniques to be used for each program. Continuing education programs of the schools accredited by the NLN are usually included in the total accreditation, but some also seek ANA CE accreditation.

Whether or not CE is mandatory, more nurses seem to be actively attending formal programs of all kinds. How much CE improves practice is still an arguable question, for measurement of direct results is seldom practical. However, it has been shown that the motivation of the learner and the opportunity to apply what is learned are key factors.

Although in-service programs are not always accepted for legal CE requirements, most employers make such programs available (or mandatory) for improvement of nursing practice. Because such programs can be quite costly, there is increased interest in providing educationally sound programs, directed toward meeting specific practice goals and building in an evaluation mechanism.[43] In some cases, evidence of CE is a job requirement or necessity for promotion. Opportunities and funds to attend programs are part of some collective bargaining agreements. However, nurses, especially if they consider themselves professionals, should be prepared to pay for their own continuing education.

One of the greatest thrusts in continuing education in the last ten years has been the nurse practitioner programs. When the first program was begun at the University of Colorado in 1965, it was as continuing education. Until recently, a majority of the almost 200 programs either were or began in that mode. They ranged for some time from on-the-job training to organized programs of a year or more, culminating in a certificate. Those funded by HEW must be at least a year in length, according to governmental guidelines. The first semiformal approval mechanism was a joint statement of the ANA and the American Academy of Pediatrics, which issued guidelines in 1972. However, later there was some disagreement on the degree of physician control, and by 1974, the ANA had developed accreditation guidelines for continuing education that were specific to the various types of nurse practitioner programs. Although there is a definite trend toward master's degree education for nurse practitioners, it is expected that the continuing education programs will not be completely phased out for some time.

Is continuing education readily available to most nurses? Despite some justifiable complaints that formal programs are not always available in certain geographic areas, there are many ways for nurses of all educational levels to continue their professional development. Examples of self-directed learning activities include self-guided, focused reading, independent learning projects, individual scientific research, informal investigation of a specific nursing problem, correspondence courses, self-contained learning packages using various media, directed reading, computer-assisted instruction, programmed instruction, study tours, and group work projects.* The first nursing journal, to have developed self-learning programs that include evaluation, for a minimal fee, was the *AJN*. There have also been other innovative ways in which nurses are offered learning opportunities, such as through mobile vans, television, telephone systems, as well as increased regional programs by nursing organizations.

The opportunities for continuing education in nursing are considerably greater than they were some years ago. What kind of continuing education a nurse chooses will remain, to a large extent, an individual decision. However, the necessity to be currently competent is both a legal and ethical requirement for any professional. Equally important, nursing cannot advance unless all nurses accept the responsibility of lifelong learning.

REFERENCES

1. Jerome Lysaught, *An Abstract for Action* (New York: McGraw-Hill Book Company, 1970), p. 109.
2. Mildred Montag, *The Education of Nursing Technicians* (New York: G. P. Putman's Sons, 1951), p. 70.
3. Ibid., pp. 94–100.
4. Mary Kohnke, ''Do Nursing Educators

---

*The ANA pamphlet, ''Self-Directed Continuing Education,'' cited in the references, provides additional detail on how to manage self-learning.

Practice What Is Preached?" *Am. J. Nurs.*, **73**:1572 (Sept. 1973).

5. American Nurses' Association, *Educational Preparation for Nurse Practitioners and Assistants to Nursing: A Position Paper* (New York: The Association, 1965), pp. 7–8.

6. Montag, op. cit., p. 73.

7. Lynne Beverly and Mary Junker, "The AD Nurse: Prepared To Be Prepared," *Nurs. Outlook*, **25**:514–518 (Aug. 1977).

8. Julian Cicatiello, "Expectations of the Associate Degree Graduate: A Director of Nursing's Point of View," *J. Nurs. Ed.*, **13**:22–25 (Apr. 1974).

9. Peggy Bensman, "Have We Lost Sight of the AD Philosophy?" *Nurs. Outlook*, **25**:511–513 (Aug. 1977).

10. Betty W. Martin and Dorothy Jean McAdory, "Are AD Clinical Experiences Adequate?" *Nurs. Outlook*, **25**:502–505 (Aug. 1977).

11. Marjorie Cantor, "Associate Degree: Education for What?" *J. Nurs. Ed.*, **13**:26–31 (Apr. 1974).

12. Rachel Rotkovitch, "The AD Nurse: A Nursing Service Perspective," *Nurs. Outlook*, **24**:234–236 (Apr. 1976).

13. *The Graduate of Baccalaureate Degree Nursing Programs*, The Association (Boulder, Colo.: Western Interstate Commission for Higher Education, 1968).

14. Aleda Roth, et al., *1977 National Sample Survey of Registered Nurses: A Report on the Nurse Population and Factors Affecting Their Supply* (Kansas City, Mo.: ANA, 1978), pp. 86–87.

15. Rozella Schlotfeldt, "The Professional Doctorate: Rationale and Characteristics," *Nurs. Outlook*, **26**:309 (May 1978).

16. Mary Roberts, *American Nursing* (New York: Macmillan Publishing Co., Inc., 1954), pp. 182–183.

17. Ibid., pp. 533–534.

18. Ibid., pp. 535–536.

19. Department of Health, Education, and Welfare, *Toward Quality in Nursing. Report of the Surgeon General's Consultant Group on Nursing* (Washington, D.C.: The Department, 1963), p. 22.

20. *Facts About Nursing, '72–'73*, op. cit., p. 10, 39.

21. Roth, op. cit., p. 79.

22. American Nurses' Association, *Statement on Graduate Education in Nursing* (New York: The Association, 1969).

23. American Nurses' Association, *Statement on Graduate Education in Nursing* (Kansas City, Mo.: The Association, 1978), p. v.

24. Ibid., p. 4.

25. Ibid.

26. "Characteristics of Graduate Education in Nursing Leading to the Master's Degree," *Nurs. Outlook*, **27**:206 (March 1979).

27. Ibid.

28. American Nurses' Foundation. *International Directory of Nurses with Doctoral Degrees* (New York: The Foundation, 1973).

29. Report of Committee to Formulate Guiding Principles for the Administration and Organization of Master's Programs in Nursing, in *Proceedings of the Meetings of Representatives of Graduate Programs in Nursing* (May 1955) (mimeo).

30. Jean Campbell, "Post-master's Education in Nursing," *Nurs. Outlook*, **9**:554 (Sept. 1961).

31. Department of Health, Education, and Welfare, *Future Directions of Doctoral Education for Nurses*, Report of a Conference (Bethesda, Md.: The Department, 1971), pp. 6–8.

32. Council of Baccalaureate and Higher Degree Programs, *Memo to Members* (New York: National League for Nursing, Feb. 1973), p. 2.

33. Martha Rogers, "Doctoral Education in Nursing," *Nurs. Forum*, **5**:69–74 (Spring 1966).

34. Susan Taylor et al., "Nurses with Earned Doctoral Degrees," *Nurs. Res.*, **20**:415–427 (Sept.-Oct. 1971).

35. American Nurses' Association, *Statement on Graduate Education in Nursing*, 1978, op. cit., p. 3.

36. U. S. Department of Health, Education and Welfare, *The Doctorally Prepared Nurse* (Bethesda, Md.: The Department, 1976), pp. 17, 33–37.

37. American Nurses' Association, (1978) op. cit., pp. 3 and 4.

38. *The Doctorally Prepared Nurse,* op. cit., p. 5.
39. "Educational Preparation for Nursing—1977," *Nurs. Outlook,* **26**:568 (Sept. 1978).
40. Kelly West, "Influences of the Scholar," *Bulletin of the Med. Lib. Assn.,* **56**:43 (Jan. 1968).
41. *Self-Directed Continuing Education in Nursing,* (Kansas City, Mo.: American Nurses' Association, 1978), p. v.
42. "The Status of Continuing Education: Voluntary and Mandatory," *Am. J. Nurs.,* **77**:410–416 (Mar. 1977).
43. Dorothy del Bueno, "No More Wednesday Matinees," *Nurs. Outlook,* **24**:359–361.

BIBLIOGRAPHY

Allen, Virginia. *Community College Nursing Education.* New York: John Wiley & Sons, Inc., 1971. This book documents the development of an AD program, including historical development, recruitment, qualifications, and responsibilities of nurse faculty, information on student preparation, curriculum, educational resources, and a follow-up of the graduates with evaluation of their state board achievement and job responsibilities.

American Nurses' Association. *Reference Sources for Research and Continuing Education in Nursing.* Kansas City, Mo.: The Association, 1977. Papers given at a conference. Useful information.

Bates, Barbara, and Joan Lynaugh. "Teaching Physical Assessment." *Nurs. Outlook,* **23** (May 1975), 297–302. NP and MD who teach nurse practitioners note that this cannot be done in haphazard fashion.

Berry, Charles, and E. J. Drummond. "The Place of the Humanities in Nursing Education," *Nurs. Outlook,* **18** (Sept. 1970) 30–31. These educators argue that liberal education is essential for the nurse to assume a full professional role and give their reasons, in terms of changing roles.

Blair, Eunice. "Needed: Nursing Administration Leaders." *Nurs. Outlook,* **24** (Sept. 1976), 550–554. Describes graduate program synthesizing clinical nursing knowledge with management theory and skills.

Bliss, Ann, and Eva Cohen, Eds. *The New Health Professionals.* Germantown, Md.: Aspen Systems Corp., 1977. Has sections on education of nurse practitioners, including HEW training guidelines.

Brower, H. Terri. "The External Doctorate," *Nurs. Outlook,* **27** (Sept. 1979), 594–599. Explores the nature and characteristics of nontraditional doctoral education, including pros and cons.

Bullough, Bonnie. "The Associate Degree: Beginning or End?" *Nurs. Outlook,* **27** (May 1979), 324–328. Describes program in which AD nurse may advance to BSN program and attitudes of students about such an educational approach.

Cleland, Virginia. "Developing a Doctoral Program." *Nurs. Outlook,* **24** (Oct. 1976), 631–635. Guidelines for determining kind of doctoral program to be developed, as well as needed resources.

Cooper, Signe. "A Brief History of Continuing Education in Nursing in the United States." *J. Contin. Educ. Nurs.,* **4** (May–June 1973), 5–13. An expert in continuing education reviews the key points in the history of nursing continuing education.

Cooper, Signe. "Continuing Education: Yesterday and Today." *Nurse Educator,* **3** (Jan./Feb. 1978), 25–29. Gives some historical background, but emphasizes current concerns in continuing education.

del Bueno, Dorothy. "How To Get Your Money's Worth Out of Continuing Education." *RN,* **41** (Apr. 1978), 37–42. Expert in continuing education presents guidelines and general information for nurses seeking continuing education.

Donley, Sr. Rosemary, et al. "Graduate Education for Practice Realities." *Nurs. Outlook,* **21** (Oct. 1973), 646–649. This study reports preferences of a small sample of nurses with graduate degrees on what would have been their choice of program as related to their current jobs. Specific kinds of courses were considered desirable, as well as preparation in both a functional and clinical area.

Downs, Florence. "Doctoral Education in Nursing: Future Directions." *Nurs. Outlook,* **26** (Jan. 1978), 56–61. Describes problems such as limited funds and increased admissions, as well as need for differentiation among doctoral degrees.

Haferkorn, Virginia. "Continuing Education for the Specialty Nurse." *Nurs. Outlook,* **23** (Apr.

1975), 245–247. Description of continuing education program for coronary care nurses that might be used as a prototype for similar programs.

Howell, Farley. "Employer's Evaluations of New Graduates." *Nurs. Outlook,* **26** (July 1978), 448–451. Hospital director of nursing in one state compared the graduates of the three basic RN programs.

Knafl, Kathleen. "How Real Is the Practicum for Nurse Practitioner Students?" *Nurs. Outlook,* **27** (Feb. 1979), 131–135. Points out the importance of extensive clinical experiences in nurse practitioner program.

Lynaugh, Joan, and Barbara Bates. "Clinical Practicum in Ambulatory Care." *Nurs. Outlook,* **23** (July 1975), 444–448. Companion to the May article describing teaching sites and methodology.

Miller, Michael, and Beverly Flynn. *Current Perspectives In Nursing: Social Issues and Trends.* St. Louis: C. V. Mosby Company, 1977. Includes issues in nursing education such as graduate preparation in community health.

Montag, Mildred. *Community College Education for Nursing.* New York: McGraw-Hill Book Company, 1959. Report of the "experiment in technical education for nursing," the study of the original AD nursing programs. Includes organization, curriculum, and evaluation.

Montag, Mildred. *The Education of Nursing Technicians.* New York: G. P. Putnam's Sons, 1951. The original concept of AD nursing is described in this classic book, including background, public needs, educational program.

Montag, Mildred. *Evaluation of Graduates of Associate Degree Programs.* New York: Teachers College Press, 1972. A report of the second evaluation of AD programs, using the same or nearly the same evaluation tools used in first evaluation. Includes demographic data, performance on licensing exams, areas of employment, and evaluation of graduates by employers. Readable and interesting.

Newman, Margaret. "The Professional Doctorate: A Position Paper." *Nurs. Outlook,* **23** (Nov. 1975), 704–706. Makes argument for different pattern of nursing education, with doctorate as base for professional education.

O'Connor, Andrea. "Reasons Nurses Participate in Continuing Education," *Nurs. Res.* **28** (Nov. Dec. 1979), 354–359. Identifies motivational orientations of these nurses. Chief factor: maintaining currency.

O'Brien, Margaret, et al. "Expanding the Public Health Nurse's Role in Child Care." *Nurs. Outlook,* **23** (June 1975), 369–373. An example of continuing education for preparation of nurse practitioners.

Siegal, Hildegarde. "Master's Preparation for Joint Practice." *Nurs. Outlook,* **27** (Jan. 1979), 57–60. A graduate education program for nurse practitioners that helps students to work independently and interdependently with MDs in primary care settings.

Smoyak, Shirley. "Specialization in Nursing: From Then to Now." *Nurs. Outlook,* **24** (Nov. 1976), 676–681. Gives historical perspective to clinical specialist education.

Stokinger, Mary, and Janet Wallinder. "A Graduate Practicum in Health Planning." *Nurs. Outlook,* **27** (Mar. 1979), 202–205. Master's students serve as health planners within a health systems agency.

Styles, Margretta. "Continuing Education in Nursing: One Hope for Professional Coherence." *Nurse Educator,* **1** (July/August 1976), 6–9. Looks at how continuing education can serve as an organizing and cohesive force in nursing.

Styles, Margretta. "The Third Resolution." *Nurs. Outlook,* **27** (Jan. 1979), 44–47. Describes new AD-MS program.

Taylor, Susan, et al. "Nurses with Earned Doctoral Degrees." *Nurs. Res.,* **20** (Sept.–Oct. 1971), 415–427. The authors provide data on nurses who earned doctorates prior to 1971, particularly related to employment and types of degrees.

Wilson, Holly, and Shirley Chater. "Graduate Education: Challenge to the Status Quo." *Nurs. Outlook,* **21** (July 1973), 440–443. Young authors opt for creativity in graduate programs to help nurses deal with unknown tomorrows. Thoughtful and interesting.

Ziemer, Mary. "Sounding Board: Just What Is Simple Nursing?" *Nurs. Outlook,* **27** (May 1979), 344–345. Thoughtful consideration of old nursing education concept that suggests education should move from simple to complex.

See also references at end of Chapter 13; *Nursing Administration Quarterly,* Vol 2 (winter 1978)—entire issue devoted to continuing education; Vol. 3, No. 3 and 4 (1979)—entire issue devoted to nursing education from nursing administration standpoint; *Nursing Outlook,* Oct. 1975—almost entire issue is devoted to articles on graduate education; *Nursing Outlook* (Aug. 1977), for ''Focus on Associate Degree Nursing'' articles; and *Nursing Outlook* (Oct. 1978), which has major articles on community health nursing. The various publications of ANA and NLN include standards, guidelines, and statements on various aspects of nursing education; publication catalogs are published each year. Especially important among the ANA publications (not cited in text) are. *Standards for Nursing Education* (1975), *Statement in Flexible Patterns of Nursing Education* (1978), *A Case for Baccalaureate Preparation in Nursing* (1979). In 1979, the NLN initiated the *NLN Nursing Data Book*, a compilation of statistics result-

ing from the several periodic surveys conducted by its Division of Research. The NLN statements on education quoted in this chapter can be found in *Nursing Outlook* as follows: July 1978, pp. 457–458 (AD); Aug. 1978, p. 520 (diploma); Jan. 1979, p. 51 (baccalaureate); Mar. 1979, p. 206 (master's). The *Journal of Continuing Education* is devoted entirely to that topic and contains many useful articles, and Elda Popiel's *Nursing and the Process of Continuing Education,* 2d ed. St. Louis: C. V. Mosby Company 1977, presents many facets of continuing education as seen by various experts in the field. Note also ANA's *Directory of Nurses with Doctoral Degrees, 1980.*

Nursing Research: Status, Problems, Issues

HISTORICAL OVERVIEW

Like so many beginnings in nursing, research in nursing probably had its start with Florence Nightingale, who made detailed reports on observations of both medical and nursing matters during the Crimean War, documented the evidence, and pointed out significant data, which resulted in reform. After that, there was no other published research by nurses in the early periods of nursing. This was partly because it became an apprenticeship occupation in the United States and because in the Victorian era, females were encouraged to leave intellectual initiative to males, and nurses often epitomized Victorian females. However, nurses gradually gained more education, moved into universities, and formed a professional organization.

Early studies that might be called a form of research were primarily for the improvement of nursing education and nursing service, because the early leaders were almost always responsible for both those areas and there were obvious knowledge gaps. (At a time when medicine was only semiscientific, it is natural that nurses, scientifically untrained, would not attempt to establish a sci-

entific base for nursing.) But there was an attempt to gather data about nursing. One of the first, if not the first, study of American nursing education was Adelaide Nutting's survey of the field, published in 1906. Lillian Wald's school nursing project in New York was probably the first demonstration project reported in the *American Journal of Nursing* (by Dock in 1902). Wald herself wrote *House on Henry Street* in 1915, about that innovative experiment in public health nursing.* Other studies followed. In 1909 an ANA committee initiated a series of studies of public health. In 1912 Adelaide Nutting's survey of nursing education was published by the U.S. Bureau of Education, followed by the first major study of nursing, the 1923 Goldmark Report. These and succeeding studies made by the Committee on the Grading of Nursing Schools, described in Chapter 5, greatly influenced the direction of nursing, and to some degree, nursing research. Although most of these studies focused on the nurse rather than nursing care, some of the nurse-teachers in universities did experiment with nursing techniques. In the late 1920s and 1930s, a few fellowships were granted to

---

*See Chapters 3 and 4 for further details.

nurses in graduate programs who showed aptitude for research, and by 1930, nursing leadership recognized the value of research and attempted to foster it. However, few were in positions to become involved in problems of patient care, and the nurses closest to the patient did not see themselves in a research role.[1]

Notter,[2] as well as Simmons and Henderson, cite a handful of nurses who did minor studies related to clinical nursing, most often of nursing procedures, in the 1920s and 1930s. But while medical research was plunging ahead and finding new answers to disease, research in nursing and about nursing was still related to the image, role, and functions of the nurse and was done as often as not by social scientists rather than nurses. Still, there was support by nurses of some of this research, such as the five-year ANA-initiated study of nursing functions, which yielded much useful data.[3,4] By 1970, ANA had also established a Commission on Nursing Research, and in 1972 a Council of Nurse Researchers was started.

The growth of the university schools of nursing had a definite effect on nursing research, as better-prepared faculty and students became involved in studies, sometimes a particular school concentrating on particular problems. Some universities also developed research centers, such as the Institute of Research and Service in Nursing Education at Teachers College in 1953, and Wayne State's Center for Health Research in 1969. This trend continued through the 1970s. In addition, the launching of *Nursing Research* in 1952 and the publication of several texts in nursing research at about the same time drew nursing closer to professionalism. The sponsorship of research by national health agencies and services, which emphasized the patient and patient care, may also have been a turning point toward clinical research. The American Nurses' Foundation was established by ANA specifically to further nursing research by conducting and supporting projects, as it still does today.

As might be expected, federal interest in nursing research was highly influential in its development. In 1955, a Research Grant and Fellowship Branch was set up in the Division of Nursing Resources of the U.S. Public Health Service, providing funds that enabled many nurses to complete their doctoral studies, as well as funds for other research, faculty development, workshops, and the nurse scientist programs.[5] A Department of Nursing was also established in the Walter Reed Institute (1957).

In 1963 the surgeon general's report noted that research is one of the obligations of society and urged increased government funding because with the rapidly changing patterns of medical care organization, the need for nursing research had outstripped resources available for studies of nursing care. "The potential contributions of nursing research to better patient care are so impressive that universities, hospitals, and other health agencies should receive all possible encouragement to conduct appropriate studies."[6] Even so, funds were not available in large amounts, and progress in the development of clinical nursing research was slow. Seven years later, the National Commission for the Study of Nursing and Nursing Education (NCSNNE) expressed dismay that so little research had been done on the actual effects of nursing intervention and care; the profession had few definitive guides for the improvement of practice. The kinds of clinical studies done by nurses were cited as major contributions to health, and it was urged that funds for nursing research be increased. Although funds were increased for a time, continued cutbacks in federal funds soon created a major problem in nursing research as well as in education. Still, nurses have been forging ahead in nursing research, particularly clinical research, seeking funds from foundations as well as the government.*

_____

*1977 was the twenty-fifth anniversary of *Nursing Research*, and that entire year's issues have articles on the historical development of research in nursing.

WHY NURSING RESEARCH?

Schlotfeldt's definition of the term *research* is useful: all systematic inquiry designed for the purpose of advancing knowledge.[7] Research of one kind or another has been responsible for the major advances in most fields, has resulted in modern technology, and has had a dramatic effect on medicine. The notion that much of the science of nursing is derived from medicine or the social sciences probably evolved because nursing did borrow many of its concepts and practice patterns from other disciplines. Some nurses began to recognize that many of these concepts had not been tested or tested recently and certainly had not been tested in relation to nursing practice. Others began to wonder what in nursing care made that critical difference in patient outcome. What was the impact of nursing care, and how could it affect health care, and how could it affect health care of the future? The NCSNNE believed that the answer lay in nursing research.

> *This commission believes it is essential for the future of health care in this country to begin a systematic evaluation of the impact of nursing care. We advocate the development of objective criteria such as measurable improvement in patient condition, evidence of early discharge or return to employment, reduced incidence of readmission to care facilities, and lowered rates of communicable disease. We do not suggest for a moment that nursing is wholly responsible for these or any other factors in the qualitative measurement of health care. We do believe, however, that nursing represents an important independent variable in our total health system. As such, we must learn how we can utilize nurses— more effectively, more efficiently, and more economically.*[8]

From another point of view, this kind of research was also necessary to determine just what nurses should be taught—the underlying theory or theories of nursing. Practice disciplines have always needed to develop their own bodies of verified knowledge and to evaluate that knowledge in practice, both for survival as a profession and for the well-being of their clients. Thus, it has been constantly reiterated by nursing leaders and scholars in the last few decades that the primary tasks of nursing research are development and refinement of nursing theories that serve as guides to nursing practice and can be organized into a body of scientific nursing knowledge, and finding a valid means for measuring the extent to which nursing action attains its goals in terms of patient behavior.

WHAT IS RESEARCH?

Notter makes a useful comparison of problem solving related to patient care (sometimes also described as the nursing process) and scientific inquiries.[9] Although both go through such steps as (1) identifying a problem, (2) analyzing its various aspects, (3) collecting facts or data, (4) determining action on the basis of analysis of the data, and (5) evaluating the result, in scientific inquiry step 4 includes developing a hypothesis, as well as setting up a study design or method. After the analysis and evaluation of data in terms of the hypothesis, the findings of the research are reported. These steps may be relatively simple or very complex; they may involve laboratory equipment, human experimentation, or neither. Research may be designated as *basic,* the establishment of new knowledge or theory that is not immediately applicable, or *applied,* the attempt to solve a practical problem. Either way, the same steps are taken.

There are several types of research, and nurses may be involved in any of them, or more than one. *Historical* or *documentary* research provides not only a record of the past, but because history tends to repeat itself, its study can prevent mistakes and help point new directions. Real historical research requires study of original records or documents (primary sources) to prevent distortion that comes with interpretation by succeeding historians. Historical research is having a new resurgence in nursing. Not only are the past and its human figures being studied on the basis of new hypotheses, but there is interest in preserving the ideas and attitudes of contemporary nursing leaders—while they are still alive. One good example of a technique being used is the oral history, which involves audiotaped or videotaped interviews that may also be published, such as Gwendolyn Safier's *Contemporary American Leaders in Nursing, An Oral History* (New York: McGraw-Hill Book Company, 1977). (Also available for short-term loan are videocassettes in the Sigma Theta Tau Distinguished Leaders in Nursing Series.)*

Descriptive research describes what exists and analyzes the findings in terms of their significance. The purpose may be simply to get information such as ANA's *1977 National Sample Survey of Registered Nurses,* which reports on the nurse population and factors affecting their supply, or to gather facts that might be later used as a basis of a hypothesis of another type of study. Various techniques can be used: interviews, observations, case studies, or literature review. The studies can be both clinical and nonclinical.

In *experimental* research, the researcher manipulates the situation in some way to test a hypothesis. Preferably, one controlled setting or group in which certain factors or variables are held constant, and an experimental setting or group in which one or more variables are manipulated are used and the results compared. Such studies might be done in a laboratory, using animals, chemical or biological substances, or people. If the study involves human beings, whether in a standard laboratory, in a clinical setting, or in the field (the subject's home, school, workplace), the ethical principles and/or laws related to human experimentation must be observed. There are, of course, ethical principles that apply to all types of research.

PROBLEMS AND ISSUES

Besides the basic fact that there are not enough nurses prepared to do research, and that those that are do not always choose to do so, there are a number of other problems and issues related to nursing research.* One of the major problems is utilization of nursing research. Unfortunately, nursing has a history of ignoring the results or recommendations of research, or at least, delaying action. For instance, early recommendations from studies of nursing education about educational preparation of nurses are only now coming to fruition, after about a seventy-five-year time lag. But here, at least, social and economic factors may have been contributors to such slow action. What about utilization of *clinical* findings?

Gortner and others have categorized practice-related research as studies: (1) building a science of practice (systematic identification of health problems and health needs of patients and relationships between nursing and patients), (2) refining the "artistry of practice" (laboratory and field studies on what nurses do), (3) concerned with descriptive, analytical, and experimental studies of physical and social environments in which nurses and their clients interact, (4) aiming to develop methodology or measurement tools, and (5) dealing directly with application of research findings to the field through replication on a small or large scale.[10] The extensive examples given show that there is useful practical application, but that often the results go no further than reporting at a research conference. For example, an author investigating the extent to which just one research finding was used by eighty-seven nurses, concluded, "A clear picture e-

---

*Further information is available from Sigma Theta Tau (see Chapter 27).

*The important issues of ethics and patients' rights in research are presented in Chapters 10 and 22.

merged: the practitioner either was totally unaware of the research literature relative to her practice, or if she was aware of it, was unable to relate to it or utilize it. There was an apparent isolation of research from practice."[11] This author also noted that most practicing nurses neither subscribe to nor understand nursing research journals, that because they are not researchers, they are not invited to (or interested in) research conferences, and that the researchers and practitioners tend to be in two different settings—universities and service agencies—with limited contact. These findings do not differ much from those of others exploring this dilemma. In a survey of 215 nurses, most of whom were involved in direct patient care, the obstacles most frequently cited related to use of research findings were reading and understanding the report, relevance of findings for practical situations, inability to find research findings, suggestions too costly or time-consuming to implement, resistance to change in the workplace, and rewards for using nursing research were not worthwhile.[12]

Oddly enough, another problem in nursing research is indiscriminate or unthinking application of nursing research findings. Nurses who become aware of research that seems to be pertinent to their field tend to use it without appropriate evaluation or validation. In some cases, this happens because most nurses currently practicing have not been taught to evaluate the quality of research, although guidelines are available in the literature. Moreover, there is a gap in providing guidelines for applying research to individuals' practice settings. To do so, the consumer (of research) must first make a critical validation of the study, that is, question each step of the author's assumptions, findings, and conclusions. If the conclusions are weak, tentative, or contradicted by others, convincing others to apply the research becomes a problem. If the settings or subjects are too different from the consumer's practice environment, the findings may not make a useful transition. If there are too

many constraints in the practice environment, the attempt to implement the findings may require considerable groundwork. Nevertheless, assuming that the study is valid, even indirect application on the cognitive level has useful dimensions in expanding nurses' theory base and making them alert to other studies that might be more directly applicable.[13]

The quality of nursing research is sometimes raised as a problem or issue. Much, probably most, of the research in the past twenty years has been done as part of the requirements for a master's or doctoral degree. Although it may be of satisfactory quality, it is almost always limited in scope, both because of monetary and time constraints. There are those who say that master's degree research particularly tends to be somewhat superficial, and even shoddy, lacking little more purpose than to complete the degree, with almost no follow-up or replication likely. This may be true, particularly in schools that have limited numbers of faculty prepared in research techniques. Those qualified may be overextended and others, whose own research experience is limited, may assume some of the responsibilities.

Because education and scholarship are frequently equated, why do so few nursing faculty engage in research, research in which their students might also participate? There are a number of reasons given: most nursing faculty are not educationally qualified for university positions; their high number of student contact hours allows little time for individual research; they are not as clinically competent as they should be or do not have access to clinical facilities that permit clinical research; there is little research money available externally and lack of institutional support, as well; most nurse faculty are women, and studies have shown that women prefer to teach rather than do scholarly research. Whatever the reason or combination of reasons, there is increased pressure for nursing faculty to do research, particularly clinical research, in the area in which they teach. If teachers selected a particular problem to study over time, replication, now lacking, would be possible. If several teachers and/or other researchers studied clusters of problems, whether through consortia or cooperative groups of faculty and nursing service, nursing would have a more solid and extensive theory base. Then, too, peer evaluation and long-term experience would undoubtedly strengthen research skills.

The controversy of who should engage in what kind of research seems rather foolish in light of the need. There are proponents of "pure" or basic research, who feel that nursing needs a scientific base before practice can be studied. The separation is artificial. Basic research can be a foundation for applied clinical research but, given the unanswered questions in nursing care, there is no reason that there should not be research of both kinds, the abstract and the pragmatic. Equally pointless is the scientist/practitioner dichotomy. Probably all good nurses should have some configuration of practice, education, and research skills, because all are part of nursing's role. Clinicians who do not know, understand, or care about research are missing a source of knowledge that will enhance their practice; an investigator without sound clinical knowledge is not fully prepared. Currently, most practicing nurses who may see a need to know about research findings do not see themselves as involved in the process. Although most nurse-researchers are happy to have staff nurses help gather data for them, some are reluctant to teach, encourage, or assist them in research development on the grounds that they lack sufficient education and background. Others believe that there are various levels of research and that opportunity to carry out a simple study based on a felt need can stimulate interest and further learning in research. With the slow, but definite, increase of nurse researchers in service agencies, the opportunity to foster a research mentality among nurses is considerably greater than even a decade ago.

Communication of nursing research has been of concern because without communication, there can be no replication, application, utilization, or evaluation by others. In the last few years, means of reporting research and participating in peer review have increased considerably. As late as 1977, *Nursing Research* was the only journal in the United States devoted exclusively to reporting nursing research, but since that time several others have come on the scene. Because they are "refereed" journals, that is, the articles are reviewed and approved by a panel of experts before publication, presumably the methodology, content, and analysis have been scrutinized by others in research and found appropriate. This may or may not be true of research articles in other nursing or non-nursing journals, but here, too, such articles are increasing in number, although they are not necessarily presented in as much detail.

Carnegie[14] lists other major avenues of reporting research: the federal government, state, regional, and national organizations, foundations, universities, and health agencies, all of which might be responsible for publication of newsletters, abstracts, reports, articles, monographs, books, and conferences, seminars, programs (with proceedings), as well as publishing houses that produce various indexes. *Dissertation Abstracts International* carries abstracts of all doctoral dissertations, complete xerographic copies of which can be purchased through the publisher, University Microfilms, Ann Arbor, Michigan. In addition, there are individual and university libraries, governmental and private networks of health science libraries, and professional association libraries which use computer-based retrieval service techniques to prepare bibliographies on requested topics. An updated list of reference works for nurses, developed by the Interagency Council on Library Resources for Nursing, is periodically found in *Nursing Outlook* under the title, "Reference Sources for Nursing." A new information resource, the first computerized Nursing Information Center, is now operational through the efforts of the Division of Nursing in HHS.[15]

One final problem should be mentioned. For various reasons, such as that nursing's image does not include a scholarly component, many other disciplines and the public are not aware of what nursing research is done or even that there is such a thing. Not only does that tend to place nursing at a less than professional level, but it also limits the opportunities of nurses to "sell" nursing research as worthy of support. Medicine has multimillion dollar research grants, but nursing still must struggle for acceptance and funding. Thus, the need to make nursing research visible, to show the contribution it has and can make to health care, is vital.

Nurses are gradually becoming more interested in and sophisticated about research. Many basic nursing programs are including aspects of research, ranging from reading assignments to critical evaluation of statistics and basic research techniques. All good graduate nursing programs emphasize research and encourage or require research projects related to some aspect of nursing science or practice. Faculty and administration of educational programs have developed strategies for integrating research into the faculty work load.[16] A survey of schools given federal funds for research shows that a vital factor in success is the commitment of both faculty and institution to research.[17]

Nurses need not be in a student or faculty role to participate in research. There are, and may always be, nurses who are part of medical or interdisciplinary research teams. Most commonly, these nurses gather, report, and record data, a task for which they are specifically trained. There is seldom any utilization of nursing knowledge or application to nursing care. Nevertheless, there are now other teams involved in *nursing* research. Such group arrangements have been described as a team in one institution doing a particular study; separate studies of different aspects of one problem; replication in several settings; or a single study carried out simultaneously in several settings.[18]

Nurses can always raise questions about their own practice and patient responses, which can be communicated to a researcher, if the nurses do not have the necessary knowledge and skills. At the very least, nurses are obligated to become aware of appropriate current research in their own clinical field, so that they maintain competence. In fact, the frequent publication of various kinds of research in the public media would soon leave nurses less knowledgeable than the general public if nurses ignore the impact of research. Participation in national research conferences sponsored by HHS and/or nursing organizations allows for both exchange of ideas and critiques of research. But before the results of research can be utilized for improvement of practice, the "average" nurse as well as the researcher must be drawn into involvement, becoming acquainted with pertinent studies, learning to make some judgment of which research is valid, beginning to test theories in the clinical setting, and adding his or her own contributions. In addition, with the development of new nursing roles, there is a definite need for research in these areas, something that was frequently neglected previously when nurses took on added responsibilities.[19]

There are all levels of research, which is basically a planned, systematic attempt to answer a question or solve a problem; there is no reason why a questioning nurse, committed to improvement of nursing care and equipped with the basic tools needed, cannot help provide some of the answers. In essence, research is a vital part of the role of nursing and nursing education.

REFERENCES

1. Leo Simmons and Virginia Henderson, *Nursing Research—A Survey and Assessment* (New York: Appleton-Century-Crofts, 1964), pp. 7–24.

2. Lucille Notter, *Essentials of Nursing Research*, 2nd ed. (New York: Springer Publishing Co., Inc., 1978), pp. 9–10.

3. American Nurses' Association, *Nurses Invest in Patient Care* (New York: The Association, 1956).

4 .Everett Hughes, et al. *Twenty Thousand Nurses Tell Their Story* (Philadelphia: J. B. Lippincott Company, 1958).

5. Faye Abdellah, "Overview of Nursing Research 1955–1968," (Part I). *Nursing Research*, **19:** 6–17, Jan/Feb. 1970; (Part II). *Nursing Research*, **19:**151–162, Mar./Apr. 1970; (Part III). *Nursing Research*, **19:**239–252, May/June 1970.

6. DHEW, *Toward Quality in Nursing*, Report of the Surgeon General's Consultant Group on Nursing (Washington, D.C.: The Department, 1963), pp. 51–53.

7. Rozella Schlotfeldt, "Research in Nursing and Research Training for Nurses: Retrospect and Prospect." *Nursing Research*, **24:**177 (May/June 1975).

8. Jerome Lysaught, *An Abstract for Action.* (New York: McGraw Hill Book Company, 1970), p. 85.

9. Notter, op. cit., pp. 20–23.

10. Susan Gortner et al., "Contribution of Nursing Research to Nursing Practice." *J. Nurs. Admin.*, **6:**23–27 (Mar./Apr. 1976).

11. Shake Ketefian, "Application of Selected Nursing Research Findings Into Nursing Practice: A Pilot Study," *Nursing Research*, **24:**89–92 (Mar./Apr. 1975).

12. Jean Miller and Susan Messenger, "Obstacles to Applying Nursing Research Findings," *Am. J. Nurs.*, **78:**632–634 (Apr. 1978).

13. Cheryl Stetler and Gwen Marram, "Evaluating Research Findings for Applicability in Practice," *Nurs. Outlook*, **24:**559–563 (Sept. 1976).

14. M. Elizabeth Carnegie, "Avenues for Reporting Research," Editorial, *Nursing Research*, **26:**83 (Mar./Apr. 1977).

15. Virginia Saba and Kathleen Skapik, "Nursing Information Center," *Am. J. Nurs.*, **79:**86–87 (Jan. 1979).

16. Jacqueline Fawcett, "Integrating Research into the Faculty Workload," *Nurs. Outlook*, **27:**259–262, (Apr. 1979).

17. Marjorie Batey, *Research Development in University Schools of Nursing* (Hyattsville, Md.: DHEW, 1978).

18. Carol Lindeman and Janette Krueger, "Increasing the Quality, Quantity and Use of Nursing Research," *Nurs. Outlook*, **25:**450–454 (July 1977).

19. Carolyn Williams, "Nurse Practitioner Research: Some Neglected Issues," *Nurs. Outlook*, **23:**172–177 (Mar. 1975).

BIBLIOGRAPHY

Abdellah, Faye, and Eugene Levine. *Better Patient Care Through Nursing Research*, 2nd ed. New York: Macmillan Publishing Co., Inc., 1979. Two experienced researchers present basic concepts of research in nursing, including how-to-do-it aids, an overview of history and trends. Excellent references.

Benoliel, Jeanne. "The Interaction Between Theory and Research." *Nurs. Outlook*, **25** (Feb. 1977), 108–113. Researcher describes continual interchange necessary between nursing practice, theory development, and scientific investigation. Extensive reference list.

Brand, Karen, and Ida Martinson. "Evolution of a Nursing Research Center." *Nurs. Outlook*, **24** (Nov. 1976), 704–707. How faculty strengthened the research dimension of their school, from philosophy to grant award to evaluation.

Christy, Teresa. "The Methodology of Historical Research: A Brief Introduction." *Nursing Research*, **24** (May-June 1975), 189–192. Nurse historian describes three essential steps in production of written historical work. Also reading suggestions for those interested in historiography.

Cleland, Virginia. "Developing a Doctoral Program." *Nurs. Outlook*, **24** (Oct. 1976), 631–635. Interesting point-by-point discussion of how this program was initiated.

Crawford, Gretchen, et al. "Evolving Issues in Theory Development." *Nurs. Outlook*, **24** (May 1979), 346–351. Discussion of theory issues: whether nursing science is basic or applied, unified or pluralistic; paths to knowledge development. Extensive bibliography.

Cruise, Robert and Patricia Cruise. "Research for Practicing Nurses." *Sup. Nurse*, **10** (Oct. 1979), 52–55. Help for nurses who can and should be doing research.

Diers, Donna. "Finding Clinical Problems for Study." *J. Nurs. Admin.*, **1** (Nov./Dec. 1971), 15–18. Guidelines for selecting profitable research problems (often based on discrepancies in practice) are suggested.

Diers, Donna, *Research in Nursing Practice*, Philadelphia: J. B. Lippincott Co., 1979. Although not intended for the beginning student in research, enthusiasm for research pervades book. Especially good chapter on evaluating and writing research. Excellent and extensive references.

Diers, Donna and Susan Molde. "Some Conceptual and Methodological Issues in Nurse Practitioner Research," *Res. in Nurs. and Health* **2** (June 1979) 73–84. Review of selected literature to identify these issues. Implications for increasing rigor of research in primary care identified.

Downs, Florence. "Research in Nursing: The Genie in Florence Nightingale's Lamp." *Nurs. Forum*, **12** (Winter 1973), 48–57. The author encourages clinical nursing research to answer some of the many questions that need to be examined, gives examples of practical problems and encouragement to overcome them.

Downs, Florence, and Juanita Fleming. *Issues in Nursing Research*. New York: Appleton-Century-Crofts, 1979. Seven contributors discuss research issues related to education, support, clinical versus theoretical research, human subjects, conceptual frameworks, as well as an overview of history and trends.

Downs, Florence, and Margaret Newman. *A Source Book of Nursing Research*, 2nd ed. Philadelphia: F. A. Davis Co., 1977. Twenty-two contributors present studies that are models and may be critiqued by readers. Introduction presents critique technique.

Fleming, Juanita, and Jean Hayter. "Reading Research Reports Critically." *Nurs. Outlook*, **22** (Mar. 1974), 172–174. A guide for nurses and students on how to look critically and knowledgeably at research studies and findings.

Gortner, Susan. "Research for a Practice Profession." *Nursing Research*, **24** (May/June 1975), 193–197. Discusses developments in nursing research in clinical practice.

Gudmundsen, Anne. "The Conduct of Inquiry Into Nursing." *Nurs. Forum*, **18** (1979), 52–59. Philosophical discussion on how theoretical base of nursing can become known: methods of tenacity, authority, intuition, and science.

Notes that latter is the only method allowing for self-correction.

Jacox, Ada. "Nursing Research and the Clinician." *Nurs. Outlook*, **22** (June 1974), 382–385. Cites importance of clinical practitioners' sharing significant problems for study and carrying out the necessary research, the problems involved in such activities, and suggested solutions.

Kalisch, Beatrice. "Creativity and Nursing Research." *Nurs. Outlook*, **23** (May 1975), 314–319. Concludes that creative research requires innovative individual, with enhancing education and administrative support.

Reference Sources for Research and Continuing Education in Nursing. Kanses City, Mo.: American Nurses' Association, 1977. Papers given at an ANA program present detailed information on resources.

Ludemann, Ruth. "The Paradoxical Nature of Nursing Research." *Image*, **11** (Feb. 1979), 2–8. Looks at ways in which the value of research can be incorporated into nurses' professional thinking.

Notter, Lucille. 'The Case for Nursing Research." *Nurs. Outlook*, **23**:760–763. Noted researcher discusses some of the problems and potential solutions in nursing research. Good reference list.

Nuckolls, Katherine. "Nursing Research: Good for What?" *Nurs. Forum*, **11** (Fall 1972), 374–384. To determine how to improve nursing services through research, the author discusses the question of whether changes are needed, whether they are effective, and the needed follow-up.

Polit, Denise, and Bernadette Hungler. *Nursing Research: Principles and Methods*. Philadelphia: J. B. Lippincott Co., 1978. A comprehensive text that brings a nursing approach to application of research to nursing problems. Intended for graduate students.

Roy, Sister Callista. "Relating Nursing Theory to Education: A New Era." *Nurse Educator*, **4** (Mar./Apr. 1979), 16–21. A nurse theoretician assesses relationship between nursing theory and nursing education, and need for education to use and develop nursing theory.

Simmons, Leo, and Virginia Henderson. *Nursing Research: A Survey and Assessment*. New York: Appleton-Century-Crofts, 1964. Primarily a review and assessment of research in selected areas of nursing, with reference to many important historical and educational studies.

Taylor, Susan. "Bibliography on Nursing Research, 1950–1974." *Nursing Research,* **24** (May/June 1975), 207–225. A bibliography of 1,004 items of information published in English from 1950–1974 in twenty-two broad categories. Includes all types of publications. Invaluable.

Verhonick, Phyllis, Ed. *Nursing Research.* Boston: Little, Brown and Company, 1975. Ten contributing authors, all experienced researchers, present fruitful approaches to nursing research.

Werley, Harriet. "Research in Nursing as an Input to Educational Programs." *J. Nurs. Educ.,* **11** (Nov. 1972), 29–38. The author encourages preparation and participation of nursing students in nursing research, stressing the need for early orientation to research as a commitment in professional nursing.

Werley, Harriet. "This I Believe—About Clinical Nursing Research." *Nursing Outlook,* **20** (Nov. 1972), 718–722. A nurse researcher presents some background on nursing research efforts and cites problems, progress, and needs.

Werley, Harriet, and Fredericka Shea. "The First Center for Research in Nursing: Its Development, Accomplishments and Problems." *Nurs.*

Res., **22** (May/June 1973), 217–231. Useful both from historical perspective and as model for other centers.

See also references at end of Chapter 14, as well as references and bibliographies of Chapters 5, 9, 10, 22 and 29, all of which have components relating to nursing research. Several other books that present overviews of the profession by expert contributing authors have chapters or sections about or related to research issues, problems, trends, or techniques: Chaska, Norma, ed. *The Nursing Profession: Views Through the Mist.* New York: McGraw-Hill Book Company, 1978, pp. 155–223; Miller, Michael, and Beverly Flynn. *Current Perspectives in Nursing: Social Issues and Trends.* St. Louis: C. V. Mosby Company, 1977, pp. 3–53; Williamson, Janet. *Current Perspectives in Nursing Education: The Changing Scene.* St. Louis, Mo.: C. V. Mosby Company, 1978, pp. 62–110. The first two issues of *Advances in Nursing Science* focus entirely on practice-oriented nursing theory (Oct. 1978 and Jan. 1979). It is also useful to become acquainted with the books on nursing research and all the nursing research journals. The latter frequently have abstracts of research as well as detailed articles. The Summer, 1978 issue of *Nursing Administration Quarterly* is devoted to the impact of research on patient care, as is most of *Image* Oct. 1979.

THE PRACTICE OF NURSING

Areas of Nursing Practice

One of the most exciting aspects of nursing is the variety of career opportunities available. Nurses, as generalists or specialists, work in almost every place where health care is given, and new types of positions or modes of practice seem to arise yearly. In part, this is in response to external social and scientific changes; for instance, shifts in the makeup of the population, new demands for health care, discovery of new treatments for disease conditions, recognition of health hazards, and health legislation. In part, these roles for nurses have emerged because nurses saw a gap in health care and stepped in (nurse practitioner; nurse epidemiologist) or simply formalized a role that they had always filled (nurse thanatologist).

Usually, further education is required to practice competently in specialized areas. Sometimes, this is part of on-the-job training, but frequently it requires formal or other continuing education. Practice in areas of clinical specialization will vary to some extent according to the site of practice and the level and degree of specialization. For instance, in a small community hospital, a nurse may work comfortably on a maternity unit, giving care to both mothers and babies; in a tertiary care setting, perinatal nurse spe-cialists, psychiatric nurse specialists, and nurses specializing in the care of high-risk mothers may work together; in a neighborhood health center, the nurse-midwife may assume complete care of a normal mother and work with both the pediatric nurse practitioner and hospital nurses.

In addition, nurses hold many positions not directly related to patient care as consultants, administrators, teachers, editors, writers, patient care educators, executive directors of professional organizations or state boards, lobbyists, health planners, utilization review coordinators, nurse epidemiologists, sex educators, even anatomic artists, airline attendants, and legislators.

Therefore, it is difficult to find any one way to present areas of practice. In this chapter, the approach used is to first describe positions and the responsibilities and conditions of employment for each.* Certain systems (Armed Forces, Public Health Service, Veterans Administration), which may have different requirements or opportunities, and international nursing are treated separately. An overview of the various health

---

*Guidance on job seeking is given additional attention in Chapter 30.

care settings is given in Chapter 7. Kinds of specialty nursing are considered briefly, although the nurse practitioner role, because of its relative newness and its still somewhat controversial position in health care, is given more attention. Further information is available from the specialty nursing organizations, educational programs, and career articles published in various nursing journals.

In discussing conditions of employment, specific salaries are not generally given, both because they are changing rapidly in the unstable economic climate and because they vary geographically (highest in the West; lowest in the North Central and Southern states) and according to whether they are urban, rural, or suburban. Nevertheless, a 1977 ANA survey[1] listed some mean monthly salaries (includes all levels of nursing positions within each category):

Overall mean	$ 1,079
Hospitals	1,096
Nursing Home	1,025
Nursing Education	1,233
Public Health	1,079
Student Health	962
Occupational Health	1,133
Physician's Office	868
Self-employed	1,499
Federal Agency, State Board of Nursing	1,304

Other listings of current salaries are also reported periodically in many nursing journals, in federal statistics, and in the current ANA *Facts About Nursing.*

Patterns of employment have changed over the years. The largest single number of RNs is still employed in hospitals, but what was once a very popular field, private duty, has dropped considerably. In the ANA survey[2] it was estimated that of the 1,401,633 who held active licenses in that September and who were located in the United States, an estimated 978,234 (69.8 percent) were employed in nursing; about 68 percent reported full-time work and 32 percent, part-time. Of the total number employed, the fields of

nursing reported as the primary job were as follows:

Hospital	61.4%
Nursing Home	8.1%
Public Health	7.9%
Physician's Office	7.1%
Student Health	4.2%
Nursing Education	3.9%
Private Duty	2.9%
Occupational Health	2.5%
Self-employed	0.5%
Placement Service	0.4%
Other	1.0%

Of those working on a self-employed, fee-for-service basis, as a primary position, the largest percentage identified themselves as utilization review coordinators (37.7 percent), nurse anesthetists (15.9 percent), patient educators (11.8 percent), consultants (10.8 percent), and nurse practitioners (9 percent). Relatively higher proportions of nurses employed in nursing education, public health, occupational health, student health, and hospitals were working on a full-time basis in comparison to those who were in nursing homes, physicians' and dentists' offices, private duty, and self-employed.

The estimated percentage of RNs employed in nursing by type of position was as follows:

General duty/staff nurse	63.6%
Head nurse	8.7%
Instructor	4.9%
Supervisor	6.8%
Consultant	0.5%
Administrator	4.9%
Other	10.5%
Not reported	0.1%

In the "other" category, some 34,000 were in patient care coordinator positions; more than 9,000 nurse practitioners, 576 nurse midwives, and more than 8,000 clinical nurse specialists together comprised about 1.8 percent; nurse anesthetists about 1 percent, and researchers about 0.2 percent.[3] Career opportunities are presented in the following sections.

HOSPITAL NURSING

Positions described in hospital nursing include all those in which the employing agency is a hospital, whether private or voluntary, general or special, hospitals of all sizes; and hospitals operated by a city, county, state, or the federal government, no matter how much they differ in policies and procedures. The one element all hospitals have in common is that they are in existence primarily to take care of patients. The greatest differences from an employment point of view are types of responsibility, advancement opportunities, and salaries.

NONGOVERNMENTAL HOSPITALS

Nursing service positions in hospitals follow a pattern that varies principally with the size and clinical services of the hospital.

General Duty or Staff Nurse

The first-level position for professional nurses is that of general duty or staff nurse and is open to graduates of diploma, associate degree, and baccalaureate programs in nursing education. Individual assignments within this category will depend upon the hospital's needs and policies and the nurse's preferences and ability.

Staff nursing includes planning, implementing, and evaluating nursing care through assessment of patient needs; organizing, directing, supervising, teaching, and evaluating other nursing personnel; and coordinating patient care activities, often in the role of team leader. It involves working closely with the health team to accomplish the major goal of nursing—to give the best possible care to all patients.

To help attain this goal, the American Nurses' Association published, in 1973,

standards of practice applicable to all nursing situations. Additional, more specific standards are also available for medical-surgical, maternal-child, geriatric, community health, psychiatric mental health nursing practice, and a number of subspecialties. The general standards of practice, which can also be guidelines for practice, are

1. *The collection of data about the health status of the client/patient is systematic and continuous. The data are accessible, communicated, and recorded.*
2. *Nursing diagnoses are derived from health status data.*
3. *The plan of nursing care includes goals derived from the nursing diagnoses.*
4. *The plan of nursing care includes priorities and the prescribed nursing approaches or measures, to achieve the goals derived from the nursing diagnoses.*
5. *Nursing actions provide for client/patient participation in health promotion, maintenance, and restoration.*
6. *Nursing actions assist the client/patient to maximize his health capabilities.*
7. *The client's/patient's progress or lack of progress toward goal achievement is determined by the client/patient and the nurse.*
8. *The client's/patient's progress or lack of progress toward goal achievement directs reassessment, reordering of priorities, new goal setting, and revision of the plan of nursing care.*[4]

Involved in meeting these standards are literally hundreds of specific nursing tasks, some of which can be carried out by less prepared workers; it is the degree of nursing judgment needed that determines who can best help any patient.

Because the goals of the various kinds of nursing education programs differ, theoretically the responsibilities of each type of nurse should also differ in the staff nurse position. Unfortunately, the tendency is to assign all to the same kinds of tasks and responsibilities, so that viable differences are not utilized. This is so common that there is even a tendency to praise as innovative those nursing services who do delineate nursing roles and responsibilities at the staff nurse level according to educational background.

Some hospitals categorize staff nurse positions as I, II, III, and so on, depending on education, experience, and clinical proficiency. Salary increases are given at each level, and this horizontal promotion allows the nurse competent in, and preferring, bedside care to be rewarded without being forced into an administrative role. The increased utilization of clerical and non-nursing personnel to assume non-nursing tasks also frees the nurse for the patient contact for which nurses are prepared.

Three basic methods of assignment for patient care in the hospital are functional, team, and case.[5] In *functional nursing,* the emphasis is on the task; jobs are grouped for expediency and supposedly to save time. For instance, one nurse might give all medications, another all treatments; aides might give all the baths. Obviously, the care of the patient is fragmented, and the nurse soon loses any sense of "real" nursing; patients cannot be treated as individuals or given comprehensive care. Nevertheless, there is a tendency to use this approach in many hospitals, especially on shifts that are understaffed. The work gets done; there is generally little nurse or patient satisfaction.

Team nursing presumes a group of nursing personnel, usually RNs, PNs and aides working together to meet patient needs. It became popular after World War II, when the shortage of nurses was acute. For team leader, a baccalaureate degree had been suggested by the Surgeon General's Consultant Group on Nursing (1963),[6] but there are not enough baccalaureate graduates to fill these positions, and it is usual to have either a diploma or AD graduate act as team leader. Other team members are under the direction of the team leader who assigns them to certain duties or patients, according to their knowledge or skill. She/he has the major responsibility for planning care and coordinates all activities, acting as a resource person to the team. In addition, if there are few or no other RNs on the team, the team leader may perform nursing procedures requiring RN qualifications. Often, the team leader is the only nurse directly relating to the physician, but, too often, actual patient contact is infrequent or sporadic. The original concept of the team has been diluted. Planning and evaluation are seldom a team effort; conferences to discuss patient needs are irregular; and too frequently, the team leader does mostly functional nursing, doing treatments and giving medications in an endless cycle. Nevertheless, the professional nurse should expect to be part of a nursing team or, more likely, leader of this team, because most hospitals utilize some version of team nursing, at least to the extent that the registered nurse supervises and directs other nursing personnel in patient care.

Instituted in the 1970s and gaining in popularity is "primary" nursing, a somewhat confusing designation for the *case method,* where total care of the patient is assigned to one nurse, which was the traditional caregiving pattern. A major difference between primary nursing and other methods of assignment is the accountability of the nurse. The patient has a primary nurse just as she/he has a primary physician. A nurse is a *primary nurse* when responsible for the care of certain patients throughout their stay and an *associate nurse* when caring for the patients while the primary nurse is off duty. In most places, that nurse is responsible for a group of patients twenty-four hours a day, even though an associate nurse may assist or take over on other shifts. The primary nurse is in direct contact with the patient, family/significant others, and members of the health team, and plans cooperatively with them for total care and continuity. The head nurse then is chiefly in an administrative and teaching (personnel) role. Almost always the primary nurse is an RN, often baccalaureate. Sometimes the nursing team involved in primary nursing comprises all RNs, with the exception of aides who are generally limited to "hotel service," dietary tasks, and transportation. There is almost unanimous agreement that the primary nursing pattern is much more satisfying to patients, families, physicians, and nurses and that care is of a highly improved quality. Although there has been some concern over the increased cost of an all-RN staff and the more personalized care, data show that after the initial start-up time, costs are no greater and sometimes less than that of other staffing patterns.[7]

Almost half of all hospitals are still under 100 beds in size, so there may be relatively little separation of specialties with the exception of obstetrics, pediatrics, and more frequently now, psychiatric care. Even here, when there is a declining census, hospitals are beginning to cooperate by sharing such facilities. Therefore, the staff nurse is most often truly a generalist; even if he or she is assigned in a special area, rotating to other areas regularly (often because of short staffing) may be necessary. A new graduate should, with appropriate orientation and individualized in-service education, be able to function at the staff nurse level in any of these areas. Positions in the emergency room and outpatient department (which are receiving an increasing number of patient visits), operating room, rehabilitation unit, or intensive care unit may require specialized training, but newly developed settings within the hospital, such as an outpatient surgery unit[8] or "overnight" unit[9] also present new challenges in nursing care, without necessarily mandating more formalized education.

Hospitals with home care services usually require nurses to have had public health experience to function in this area. Nursing roles are changing in all of these clinical areas. In the operating room, for instance, many of the technical aspects are carried out by OR technicians, whereas the RN has overall responsibility for the safety of the patient, supervision and education of auxiliary nursing personnel, and sometimes support of the patient through pre- and postoperative visits. The increased utilization of nurse practitioners and clinical specialists, discussed later, adds another dimension to nursing care in these specialty areas. Although students usually do not have extensive experiences in the areas noted, even limited exposure may attract the nurse to certain kinds of practice. The emergency room and intensive care unit, where quick life-determining decisions must be made, independent judgments are not unusual, and tension is often high, will probably not attract the same kind of individual as the geriatric unit or rehabilitation unit, where long-term planning, teaching, and a slower pace are the norm.

Qualifications and Conditions of Employment. The basic requirement for a staff position is graduation from an approved school of nursing and nursing licensure or eligibility for licensure. If the latter, the nurse may be designated as a GN (graduate nurse) and must take and pass the licensure examinations within a specific period of time. Sometimes there is a lesser salary offered until the RN is acquired, and the new graduate may be limited to a general nursing unit, that is, not the coronary care unit or another that requires an investment of intensive in-service education. Nevertheless, in the hospital the variety of experiences are endless. Larger hospitals and those in medical centers may offer a greater variety of specialties, exotic surgery, and rare treatments, and the advantage of being in the center of hospital, medical and nursing research. Smaller hospitals may be less impersonal, are often in the nurse's own community, and provide the opportunity to be a generalist in smaller patient units (which does not necessarily mean a smaller patient load). A nurse is usually hired for a particular specialty unit (except for very small hospitals), but it is not uncommon to be asked to "float"—replace a nurse on any unit. Floating should not extend to units that require special knowledge and skill unless the nurse is so trained. In some hospitals, there are "float pools"—highly skilled nurses who never have a regular unit.

In most cases, hospital nurses will be required to rotate shifts and work on holidays. For this reason, it is possible to work part-time in most hospitals. Usually there are salary differentials for evenings and nights. Fringe benefits also vary greatly and may include health plans, retirement plans, arrangements for continuing education, holidays, sick time, and vacation time. The amount of autonomy varies considerably. Opportunities for promotion may be through clinical advancement or the managerial ladder.

Most staff nurses are interviewed and hired by the hospital's personnel department and/or the nursing service department. Another alternative is to be employed by a "Rent-a-Nurse" or temporary service company (TSC).[10] Those nurses most commonly using TSCs are nurses beyond a hospital mandatory retirement age, some new graduates, nurses enrolled in advanced educational programs, and nurses with small children who cannot work full time or all shifts. TSCs are businesses that employ nurses, and often other professional, technical, and clerical workers, paying them a salary for the hours worked, with the usual legal deductions, after billing the institution or patient/client using the worker's services. There are local and national services, and selecting a reputable one is extremely important. Job assignments may be made an hour or a week ahead, but the nurse is not obligated to take it; however, a no-show is usually dismissed. There is a great deal of flexibility and variety, but there are also disadvantages, even with a good TSC: no job security, no benefits, sometimes only the minimum rate paid by the area hospitals with no increases, and, of course, the constant reorientation to new nursing units and patients, even hospitals. It is not for the career nurse.

Clinical Nurse Specialist

The *clinical nurse specialist* (CNS), who may also be called a nurse specialist, nurse clinician, or clinical specialist, has become an increasingly important part of the nursing practice scene since the early 1960s. A clinical specialist is an expert practitioner within a specialized field of nursing, or even a sub-

specialty. There are clinical specialists in all the major clinical areas, but also some concentrating on cancer, rehabilitation, and perinatal nursing, tuberculosis, care of patients with ostomies, neurological problems, respiratory conditions, epilepsy, and many other subspecialties.

Clinical nurse specialists control, plan, and provide for the nursing care of a selected and specific group of patients comprising their case load. The patients requiring such services may be identified by the CNS who makes patient rounds or be referred by other members of the health care team, including nurses and physicians. One classic description follows:

> *The clinical specialist in nursing has more knowledge than the nurse-generalist about particular types of problems experienced by patients. This knowledge, acquired through advanced study or training, leads her to consider various alternatives in explaining a given patient situation, in predicting the future course of events, and in prescribing nursing actions. She, thus, can be more discriminating and more definitive in identifying the nature of the patient's problems and in selecting appropriate intervention.*
>
> *. . . To be effective, she must accept responsibility for all the nursing care the patient receives, in her absence as well as in her presence. . . . She must also be prepared to be accountable for her decisions, for the quality of care received and for the actions of all those who render nursing service to that patient under her directive.[11]*

Specific responsibilities include

1. *Determining the nursing care requirements of the patient (including family) through systematic assessment; establishing a nursing diagnosis; considering the findings and therapeutic plan of others on the health team; and delineating short- and long-term goals.*
2. *Making these findings available in a written record, as well as the nursing regimen to be followed.*
3. *Executing those parts of the regimen requiring the CNS's expertise, and organiz-*

ing and directing the activities of other nursing personnel involved in the care.

4. *Evaluating and revising the regimen as necessary.*

5. *Being available for consultation with the staff, but also seeking appropriate consultation from other colleagues.*

6. *Collaborating with others in developing and implementing a comprehensive plan of care for patients in his/her case load.*

7. *Ensuring continuity of care for the patient after the patient is discharged from the CNS's care.*[12]

In addition, the CNS frequently acts as role model and teacher for the nursing staff and develops or is involved in nursing research. As one nursing service consultant has said, "It is imperative that these specialists be utilized to aid nurses at all levels to increase their clinical skills and to broaden their concepts of nursing."[13] Whether or not administrative responsibilities are included depends on the setting. Originally, the intent was to give the CNS staff authority, that is, reporting directly to the chief nurse administrator and acting in an advisory capacity to the nursing staff and supervisors. However, a line position (superior-subordinate or direct vertical relations) gives administrative authority, and there have been some problems when a CNS as staff makes recommendations and the supervisor chooses not to accept them, especially in relation to personnel matters (such as an incompetent nurse), or when the CNS is seen as an outsider. There seems to be a trend now for the CNS to also assume a supervisory position focused on nursing care or to be given certain administrative authority. A clinical specialist in the traditional supervisor role of personnel management is sometimes limited in the amount of time devoted to clinical nursing.

Qualifications and Conditions of Employment. Generally, the clinical specialist is expected to have a master's degree in nursing, with emphasis on the specialty area, although some are employed in the position because of experience, clinical expertise, and possibly continuing education without any degree. Salaries are expected to be on the level of supervisor or higher, but at times these salaries are individually negotiated, depending on education, experience, and role expected by the employer. Basic fringe benefits may be the same as for other nurse employees; sometimes more vacation is offered.

Frequently, there is a great deal of flexibility in the CNSs' time. They may work no specific shift but care for the patients selected according to the patients' needs, which may mean being available evenings or nights, or, by choice, even available on call if a problem arises. (Telephone consultations with patients who develop problems or need support at home are not uncommon.) There should be time available for library research and home visits. A CNS usually has office space, preferably near the clinical units.

Although there are not nearly enough clinical specialists to meet patient needs, not all hospitals employ this kind of nurse, or they employ only a limited number of them because they believe they cannot (or do not choose to) afford the increased salary. Clinical specialists are most commonly found in large hospitals, medical centers, or certain government hospitals such as the Veterans Administration.

NURSING SERVICE ADMINISTRATION

The administrative hierarchy in hospital nursing usually consists of head nurse, supervisor, assistant or associate director of nursing, and director of nursing; the titles vary with the times and the philosophy of the hospital concerning nursing service administration.

Head Nurse

Head nurses are in charge of the clinical nursing units of a hospital, including the operating room, outpatient department, and emergency room. They may be called charge nurses, or more recently, nursing coordinators. In a hospital functioning as a line and staff organization (as most are), head nurses are responsible to the person next higher on the scale, usually the supervisor, or in a smaller hospital, the assistant director of nursing or the director. The head nurse position is the first administrative position most nurses achieve (or perhaps that of assistant head nurse, who may share some of the head nurse functions and substitute for the head nurse in his or her absence).

It is the head nurse's function to manage the nursing care and assure its quality in a relatively small area of the hospital. How this is done again depends on the philosophy of nursing service and often on the individual's personality. If a democratic philosophy of administration prevails, the staff participates in decision making both on the unit and in the entire setting. The head nurse exerts leadership in assisting the group to make decisions and coordinates the overall activities.

As the complexity of patient care increased, head nurses found themselves inundated with paper work, which limited their major role in managing nursing care. Hospital administrators began to realize that it was less expensive and more efficient to employ clerical personnel to answer phones and questions, to complete and route forms, to order and check supplies and drugs, and to perform the myriad other necessary clerical tasks that have kept the head nurse away from administration of patient care. Ward clerks, ward managers, floor managers, unit managers, service assistants, or whatever the local term is, have a wide variety of responsibilities, with some ward clerks even taught carefully to transcribe doctors' orders. Hospitals utilizing computers have been able not only to cut down on every nurse's paper work, but to add greater assurance of accurate, rapid communication interdepartmentally. Esther Lucile Brown, viewing changes in nursing, commented that there is a trend toward decentralization of

nursing authority, which means that nurses on individual units may make nursing care and other decisions without going through the nursing hierarchy. Under such circumstances, the head nurse is "expected to give far more attention than formerly to acting as consultant and teacher for staff, to following the clinical progress of the patients, and to maintaining ready communication with physicians and other health personnel." She cited one hospital where head nurses, with their desk work reduced to about one hour a day, go on medical rounds, hold conferences several times a week with their nursing staff, attend interdisciplinary patient conferences, become acquainted with the patients individually, assist with patient care, including counseling, and help staff nurses and other nursing personnel as questions or difficulties arise.[14] The head nurse may or may not make out the time schedule for the nursing staff on the unit, but does plan the patient assignments with the team leader.

In 1978, ANA delineated responsibilities for three levels of nurse administrator. The first-line level is identifiable as the head nurse level. The responsibilities included for this role are:

1. *Providing for direct nursing care services to clients.*
2. *Evaluating nursing care given and assuring appropriate documentation, guidance, and supervision of staff members.*
3. *Selecting nursing personnel for hire.*
4. *Evaluating staff, including disciplinary action and separation from service.*
5. *Providing for teaching and staff development.*
6. *Coordinating nursing care with other health services.*
7. *Participating in and involving staff in nursing research.*
8. *Providing clinical facilities and learning experiences for students.*[15]

Where there is primary nursing, there is more emphasis on personnel management and teaching in the head nurse role. Regardless of the staffing pattern, staff evaluation is a major responsibility. Considered first-line managers, head nurses control the quality of care more than anyone else and often know best how to eliminate waste, improve utilization of personnel and dollars, keep communication systems open, and provide direct leadership.

Qualifications and Conditions of Employment. Qualifications for head nurses are usually evidence of successful nursing experience and preferably a baccalaureate degree, the latter also recommended in the surgeon general's report. Currently, most head nurses have no degree, but there is a trend for RNs to seek degrees. The successful head nurse should have, besides nursing expertise, administrative ability. Unfortunately, in many hospitals, moving into administrative positions is the only mode of advancement for RNs. Because a good clinician may not be interested or able in nursing administration, such promotions are not always successful. Noting the stated problems of large groups of head nurses studied, Price recommended that personnel should not be assigned to charge responsibilities without advance orientation, that college education should be encouraged, and that effective ways of introducing personnel gradually to leadership positions should be found.[16] To some extent, the assistant head nurse position offers this training opportunity, but additional training and education are considered vital for most nurses assuming this position.[17]

Head nurses may earn between $500 and $2,000 more per year than staff nurses; other benefits may vary. Benefits acquired by staff through collective bargaining may or may not apply to the head nurse position. In most instances, the head nurse works only the day shift, but may alternate on weekends and holidays with the assistant head nurse.

Supervisor

It has been said that the role of the *nursing supervisor* is the most ill-defined in the hospital hierarchy. Because basic management principles for span of control usually specify that no more than six to eight people should report to an administrator, except for small hospitals, the supervisor usually is needed as the middle-management person. There are some hospitals that have eliminated the supervisor, at least on the day tour of duty, putting responsibility directly on the head nurse. In general, however, the supervisor is responsible for several clinical units, delineated by either location or specialty. In a small hospital, the supervisor might be responsible for all the clinical units, and in any hospital, the evening and night supervisors usually have larger areas to supervise. In most hospitals, these supervisors are the only administrative personnel available for any department after 5 P.M. Therefore, they find themselves acting as temporary hospital administrators, devoting more time to overall hospital problems than to their main responsibility, nursing care. At times they dispense drugs because no pharmacist is present, thus violating the Pharmacy Practice Act in most states. Some of the larger and/or more progressive hospitals have now arranged for an assistant administrator to be available for the general administration responsibilities, but this is still more the exception than the rule. Even when limited to nursing, the role of the supervisor often encompasses an enormous amount of responsibility and diversity: many aspects of personnel management, if not including hiring and firing; evaluation and improvement of patient care; staffing and coordination of nursing systems (policies, procedures, resources). Stevens has suggested that for better management, these areas of responsibility be divided among different supervisors responsible for each. They would then deal with head nurses only in relation to those areas.[18] Responsibilities of this middle management role as delineated by the ANA Commission on Nursing Services are as follows:

1. *Participating in nursing policy formulation and decision making.*

2. *Problem solving and supervising the delivery of nursing care.*
3. *Evaluating care provided.*
4. *Collaborating with other departments.*
5. *Coordinating staff activities.*
6. *Staffing and scheduling of personnel.*
7. *Arranging for equipment and supplies.*
8. *Recruiting and selecting personnel.*
9. *Evaluating staff for promotions and transfers, disciplinary action, and separation of service.*
10. *Providing orientation, training, and continuing education for staff.*
11. *Undertaking or facilitating research activities.*
12. *Providing and coordinating clinical learning experiences for students.* [19]

Qualifications and Conditions of Employment. Generally, supervisors have been employed after showing evidence of ability in a head nurse or other administrative position. Clinical expertise may or may not have been a factor, but an advanced degree was probably a distinct advantage (even if not in administration). Increased emphasis is being put on the combination of clinical expertise and administrative skills and at least baccalaureate degrees. In larger hospitals, master's degrees are stressed, preferably with experience and/or a nursing administration major in the educational program. Actually, the large majority of supervisors have no degree at all, although there is a trend toward enrollment in both degree programs and in continuing education programs that focus on middle-management skills.

Salaries of supervisors tend to be approximately $1,000 more a year than that of head nurses, but salaries may vary according to education and experience. Some fringe benefits, such as vacation time, may be greater. Supervisors tend to remain on one work shift, although they also work weekends and holidays. Even more than that of the head nurse, the supervisor position is considered administrative by employers. This has made it difficult for these individuals to be included in collective bargaining with other nurses. ANA has differentiated supervision of nurs-

ing care from managerial supervision in labor negotiations, and there have been NLRB rulings in that direction.

Assistant or Associate Director of Nursing

Assistant or *associate directors of nursing* work with the director of nursing in any or, occasionally, all aspects of the director's responsibility. Specific areas of responsibility may be assigned, particularly if the institution is a large one. If there is a diploma program of nursing, its head may also have the title of associate director of nursing. The assistant or associate is generally expected to have at least some of the qualifications of the director or be in the process of acquiring them. As a rule, this individual is hired by the director and thus is expected to share a harmonious philosophical approach and be compatible in the work relationship with the director. Salary is often negotiable on the same basis as that of the director, although it is, of course, usually less. Probably a great majority of the nurses assuming assistant or associate positions do so for the experience and as a step toward becoming a top nurse administrator. They do get that experience, but in a large hospital, many of their day-to-day activities are more likely to be in a direct relationship with staff and somewhat less involved in top-level hospital planning. There are opportunities to represent nursing service on hospital committees and to chair key nursing committees. A good director will relate to the associates as peers who will participate in the determination of overall nursing service, policies, and strategies. It is a highly varied position, with no set routine, but extended hours.

Director of Nursing

The *director of nursing* position is the highest in the nursing service hierarchy. The title may also be director of nursing service, superintendent of nurses, chief nurse, nurse administrator, or, if this individual is considered part of the top echelon of hospital administration, assistant administrator for nursing, vice-president for nursing, or a variation of whatever title the administrator of the hospital carries. Both nurses and others, including the ANA[20] and the American Hospital Association,[21] have endorsed such a title with the concomitant responsibilities. Nursing service is generally the largest individual department in the hospital, often employing more than half the total number of employees, affects and is affected by the functions of all other departments, and "participation and cooperation of the administrator of the department of nursing service in formulating policies and procedures is an essential element in accomplishing the administration's objective of coordinating functions among the various departments of the institution."[22] Some directors are also formally responsible for other departments in the hospital.

The last major study on directors of nursing services, done in 1968, provides some interesting data. Ages of directors of nursing ranged from twenty-one to seventy-seven years, with the median age forty-eight. Eighty-eight per cent had graduated from diploma schools; 9 per cent were basic baccalaureate graduates. Although most sought education beyond their basic program, slightly less than one third had no academic credential beyond the diploma. Around 40 per cent had master's degrees and about 27 per cent had baccalaureate degrees; at that time only two had doctorates. Only about 40 per cent had majored in nursing service administration. About 86 per cent had held the position of director less than fifteen years; most had less than ten years nursing experience.[23]

A later survey, which included nurse administrators and their assistants in all settings, including schools of nursing, showed that half (13,953) worked in hospitals. About 60 percent of the total were between the ages of forty and fifty-nine; nearly 60 percent were married; about 20 percent had a master's degree or above, and the numbers majoring in nursing administration were increasing; 37 percent had earned a baccalaureate.[24]

It is generally agreed that those in the position of chief nurse administrator must be leaders, both of the nursing personnel and also in nursing generally, so that they can also represent nursing when relating to other health disciplines. The ANA, in describing the role of the nurse administrator at the executive level, identifies that person as responsible for the nursing department and managing from the perspective of the organization as a whole, as well as responsible for the integration of nursing with other functional areas of the health care agency in the mutual achievement of organizational goals. "The nurse executive ensures that standards of nursing practice are established and implemented so that sound nursing care is provided to consumers."[25]

Unfortunately, a serious problem is that regardless of ANA and AHA recommendations, most directors are not yet part of the upper echelon of hospital administration; a surprising number neither prepare the nursing department budget nor are able to make recommendations on budgetary matters or other policy decisions.

Actually, as a matter of two extremes, nurse administrators in very small hospitals or in large medical center hospitals have few similarities in areas of responsibilities. A director of a small hospital may be a jack-of-all-trades, such as one in a thirty-bed hospital personally known to the author who scrubs in for surgery, comes in for emergency admissions, and often repairs minor plumbing problems. Because small hospitals are also usually in rural areas or small towns, management takes on a personalized dimension.[26] On the other hand, in some medical centers, directors of nursing are also assistant or associate deans or deans of collegiate nursing programs and do little direct management. Although the learning needs of these groups may differ, the list elicited by various organizations probably reflects the nurse administrator's responsibilities as well as concerns: fiscal management and budgeting, personnel management and labor relations, managing change, staffing and personal development in the managerial role.[27]

Qualifications and Conditions of Employment. The ANA Commission on Nursing Services recommended the following qualifications for the administrator of nursing services in 1969 and they are still appropriate.

> The competence of the administrator of nursing services involves an ability to facilitate and coordinate a diverse staff of nursing specialists who are making decisions about the nursing needs of individuals, families, and other social groups, and an ability to make decisions about the organization and delivery of nursing services. Two requisites for this leadership role are an understanding of the social, political, and economic influences affecting programs of health care and competence in dealing with any problems in the relationships of professional practitioners and within the complex social system in which nursing is practiced.
>
> Abilities essential to the administrative leader of a program of comprehensive nursing care are the following:
>
> 1. The ability to think and act in terms of the total system of health care and to recognize the need for adapting that system to the needs of people.
> 2. The ability to think and act in terms of the distinctive and contributory role of the nursing profession.
> 3. The ability to use pertinent knowledge and methods of working with and through people who are concerned with, or affected by, health care.
> 4. The ability to use knowledge, methods, and techniques pertinent to directing, guiding, and assisting nursing staff members in fulfilling their responsibilities for nursing services.
>
> Basic to these skills is the ability to coordinate, integrate, and reconcile the needs of nursing practitioners, and their goals for nursing service, with organizational requirements and objectives.
>
> Minimum educational qualifications for administrators of nursing services should include completion of a baccalaureate program which has prepared them for professional nursing practice, and completion of a master's degree program with a dual focus on clinical nursing practice and on administration of organized nursing services. Professional experience should have contributed and enhanced the development of the competencies described above.[28]

The 1978 statement cites only educational qualifications: a baccalaureate in nursing and either a master's or a doctoral degree in nursing administration with prior competent administrative experience.[29]

As shown earlier, these academic qualifications are not yet common, although also recommended by the Surgeon General's Report.[30] (The AHA specifies no academic credentials, but rather "sound educational and professional qualifications in administration.")[31] There is also an increasing, though not large, number of nurses with doctorates who are becoming nurse administrators, particularly in medical centers. Despite philosophic differences of opinion, there is some agreement that the nurse administrator must be clinically knowledgeable, if not proficient, and that it is helpful to have knowledge and skills in newer management techniques, including industrial engineering techniques, labor relations orientation, personnel management, financial theories and skills, systems theory, and organizational theory as well as knowledge of systems of health care delivery. Postprogram perceptorships are recommended by some.[32]

One group of top nurse administrators pinpointed some essential skills and knowledge: understanding management and administrative methodology dealing with organizational structure and systems and systems for quality assurance; having to plan for future needs; sharpening communication skills; developing political sophistication; having a sense of timing; widening knowledge about relationships within the health field; expanding awareness of the community and consumer needs.[33]

Salaries for directors of nursing are usually negotiated, but vary a great deal depending on location, size of hospital, responsibilities, and qualifications. This is a difficult, complex position with major responsibilities, frequently great pressure, and no routine forty-hour week, either in time or activities. The director is often expected to be active in community, professional, and other activities, which extend beyond working hours. In some cases, dismissal can be instant and with no reason given (particularly if there is no contract), if the director has not pleased the administration or the hospital board of directors. On the other hand, the leadership of a capable and farsighted director of nursing can create dramatic changes in the quality of nursing care and delivery of health care, and bring immense personal satisfaction and reward.

In-Service Education

A position that may be at the assistant-associate level and that is becoming an integral part of nursing service is that of *in-service education director,* also called director of staff development or in-service coordinator. At one time, the responsibility for orientation of all nursing staff, training of nonprofessional nursing staff, and in-service education programs was a fringe duty of an assistant or associate who had other major responsibilities. Rapid changes in health care, scientific and medical advancements, the great diversity in first-level staff nurse applicants, increases in ancillary nursing personnel, and concern about the continuing education of all nurses have brought the position of in-service education director and instructor into a new focus.

Although in-service education still has a major responsibility for orientation and development of new staff, it is no longer a matter of a few lectures by physicians or demonstration of new equipment. In some hospitals it is an organized, evaluated series of learning experiences based on nurses' needs, and sometimes done on the basis of self-learning.

Some of the current changes are planned programs of continuing education, based not just on the administration's concept of the learners' needs, but also on input from the learners; enlargement of in-service staff for around-the-clock teaching sessions; better-qualified teachers; the employment of knowledgeable outside speakers; the utiliza-

tion of more sophisticated teaching media; planned teaching on the clinical unit, and self-learning packages.

The responsibilities of the in-service director include the organization, planning, evaluation, and often implementation of orientation, continuing education, and training programs for the nursing service department, and, increasingly, for other hospital departments. (For instance, all interested hospital personnel might be taught the fundamentals of emergency resuscitation and external cardiac massage.) This educator must be aware of other resources available for the teaching program, but is personally responsible for the overall development of courses and programs. If there is a large in-service department, one or more in-service instructors may share with the director in the teaching programs.

Despite the fact that most in-service divisions are still within nursing, a trend to be noted is the move toward hospital-wide training and education departments, which may include continuing education programs for all health professionals and support staff, and patient education. Nurses still tend to be directors of these departments (all but those involving medicine), but master's-prepared health educators with administrative experience are beginning to be recruited.

Qualifications and Conditions of Employment. Although some in-service directors and/or instructors have no degrees, it is desirable that they have at least a baccalaureate degree, with some knowledge of teaching principles and techniques, particularly in relation to the adult learner, clinical expertise, and preferably a master's degree (especially as in-service director). They should also be able to work through and with others, with enough self-confidence to assume a staff role with little inherent authority.[34]

Because of the cost of in-service education, there is also a need to develop both strong evaluation tools and programs that meet the goals of the institutions as well as the learner.[35] Salary may depend on these qualifications and the kinds of responsibilities assumed; usually, salary and benefits are at the level of the supervisors for the in-service director, less for the instructor. Some sessions may be held in the evening or at night, but the majority of activities are usually in the day. This position is particularly attractive to nurses who are stimulated by teaching all levels of nursing personnel and who enjoy remaining in the hospital setting.

Other Positions for Nurses in Hospitals

There are a number of other employment opportunities for nurses in hospitals, although they may have only a tangential relationship to nursing and are often under a department other than nursing service. Nurses on the IV team are especially trained, and responsible, for all the intravenous infusions given to patients (outside of the operating room and delivery room). On the basis of a predetermined protocol, they may bring the appropriate intravenous solution to the bedside or obtain it on the unit, add ordered drugs, and start and/or restart the infusion. In some institutions they are also permitted to start a blood transfusion.

The nurse-epidemiologist or infection control nurse focuses on surveillance, education, and research. The surveillance aspect is designed for the reporting of infections and the establishment, over a period of time, of expected levels of infections for various areas. Patients with infections are checked and it is determined whether the infection was acquired after admission. Reports are used for epidemiologic research, and staff is educated in prevention of infection.[36] Nurses have also been trained as epidemiologists in public health agencies, where they perform similar but broader duties that involve the total community.[37]

The project director or manager in the hospital evolves from a new organizational framework in which the executive delegates individual responsibility for specific projects and activities. That person seeks information and ideas from others and develops a project approved by the executive. Usually, the project director has no staff, although when there is staff assigned temporarily, they continue to be accountable to their functional superior. Examples of projects are quality assurance, performance evaluation, or hospital construction.[38]

A challenging role is that of ombudsman, where a nurse acts as an intermediary between the patient and the hospital in an attempt to alleviate or prevent problems of the patient related to the hospital or hospitalization. Nurses are also being employed as utilization review agents.[39] This role originated with the Medicare regulation that if Medicare patients' hospital stay was prolonged beyond a necessary length of time, the cost of the additional stay was not paid. A selected nurse or nurses check patients and their records at predetermined periods to gather data for the Utilization Review Committee. A more sophisticated and newer version of the role is that of nurse coordinator with a Professional Standards Review Organization. These nurses prepare a detailed patient profile assessing the patient's need in relation to appropriate level of care, length of stay, utilization of ancillary services, and discharge planning. Using their nursing judgment and experience, they decide whether medical care is in conformance with established criteria. These data are reviewed with the medical adviser, a practicing physician, who uses the information gathered and synthesized by the nurse in his review and evaluation of deviations from established norms and criteria.[40]

Finally, new emphasis on health education in the hospital and community has resulted in the creation of a community health coordinator, who develops and/or coordinates the various aspects of patient teaching as well as the teaching of outpatients and other interested individuals in the community, on health matters. This nurse may not be a part of nursing service, and is more likely to direct the teaching program than to do the teaching personally.[41]

MUNICIPAL, COUNTY, AND STATE HOSPITALS

Municipal, county, and state hospitals are primarily intended to provide hospital accommodation for indigent citizens within prescribed political boundaries. In many instances they operate on a much broader scale and accept patients who pay part or all of their hospital bills. The fact remains, however, that these hospitals are supported principally by city, county, and state funds which come from taxpayers. This means that decisions about the amounts allocated for operating them rest in the hands of a central board, which may also allocate funds for schools, prisons, and many other institutions, all of which invariably want and need more money than they receive. Furthermore, the hospitals are usually obligated to accept all patients who come to them for treatment, even though they may be overcrowded and understaffed. This often spreads money and personnel very thin.

Many of these hospitals conduct outstanding educational programs for all categories of health personnel, and appointments to their staffs are considered highly desirable, particularly from the point of view of experience.

Nursing positions in these hospitals usually follow the same general pattern as in other hospitals. Staff nurses rarely need additional qualifications, except possibly for work in a hospital treating such specific diseases as tuberculosis or leprosy. However, in cities where a large part of the poor population comes from an ethnic group that speaks another language, nurses from that ethnic group or speaking that language are particularly welcome.

Staff nurses in a large city, county, or state hospital may find that a great deal of the nursing care is given by practical nurses and nurse's aides. The principal functions of RNs may be teaching, directing, and supervising other workers, in many instances doing very little bedside nursing themselves. They may find the patient load very heavy at times; however, there may also be more challenges and greater satisfaction here than in a comparable position in any other type of hospital, both because of the learning opportunities and the opportunity to be a change agent in providing quality care for the socially disadvantaged.

Because these hospitals are government-operated, nurses and all other staff members are eligible for the benefits given to any employee of the particular government concerned. These benefits, which are so important to one's economic security, vary throughout the country, but they often include an early retirement or pension system, not usually offered by nongovernmental institutions.

Nurses who work in a city, county, or state hospital are employees of the governing political body, not the hospital. Salary checks are issued from a central office. Salary increments are often given according to a scale based on length of employment. Nurses seeking employment in one of these hospitals may apply directly to the hospital they wish to work in or to the appropriate central agency, which will usually be located in the municipal building, county courthouse, or state house. If there is no particular preference, the central office may give information about all available positions for which the nurse is qualified and help in the selection of the one best suited.

NURSING WITH THE FEDERAL GOVERNMENT

Professional nurses interested in a career with the federal government will find opportunities in both military and non-military services. The military services include the Army, Navy, and Air Force. The Veterans

Administration is not a military service, although it is closely allied. The other principal nonmilitary federal service employing nurses is the Public Health Service (PHS).

Many nursing positions in nonmilitary federal services are for specialists in education, administration, research, or clinical areas and therefore require education and experience beyond the basic program. There are many others, however, particularly with the PHS and the Veterans Administration (VA), for which newly graduated professional nurses may qualify as soon as registered to practice. Both the PHS and the VA sometimes employ new graduates temporarily, pending registration, if the applicant has applied for or completed state board examinations.

The federal government owns and operates more than 400 hospitals in this country in which many government employees (and sometimes their dependents), veterans of the armed services, merchant seamen, American Indians, and other special groups are eligible for care without charge, regardless of their ability to pay. In addition, the federal government also operates hospitals in other countries for members of the armed services stationed in these countries.

Among the various federal agencies operating hospitals—and sometimes other health services—are the VA, the PHS, the Air Force, the Army, the Navy, and the U.S. Department of Justice (Bureau of Prisons). All these hospitals are supported financially by taxes. These hospitals usually have high standards of service, equipment, and facilities and are able to attract highly qualified personnel. Many of the country's outstanding physicians and nurses are members of their staffs. Research and teaching are integral parts of the work of a great many of the larger institutions. Although each branch of the armed services operates hospitals primarily to provide care for its own members, all branches will care for a member of any service in an emergency and until transfer is feasible. Sometimes, because of regional considerations, these patients are kept in the original hospital for the entire period of illness.

All those eligible for care in a government hospital—with the exception of prisoners and during wartime—may, if they prefer, go to a nongovernment hospital for care, but they have to pay their own bills unless authorized to make the change. In some instances it is more economical and practical for the government to pay civilian hospitals to care for members of the armed services and other federal employees than it is to operate federal hospitals in all localities or transport the patients long distances. Exceptions are also sometimes made for cases that would benefit from some special treatment facility not available in a government hospital.

Professional nurses who work in most hospitals operated by the federal government perform essentially the same functions as nurses in a civilian hospital in a comparable position. They give, teach, and direct nursing care. They coordinate the work of many health groups and plan and implement patient care in cooperation with the health team.

Nurses who work in hospitals connected with federal prisons* have somewhat different duties, of course. But their primary concern and responsibility is to keep the prisoners well and give them skilled nursing care when they are ill. In addition, nurses sometimes teach prisoners to care for themselves and each other as a form of rehabilitative therapy. For example, a woman may learn to be a nurse's aide and thus have a skill she can use when she leaves prison.[42]

The organization of nursing service within a federal hospital is similar to that of a civilian hospital, and the adaptable professional nurse would find little difficulty in adjusting to its few dissimilarities.

Qualifications and Conditions of Employment. Each branch of the federal govern-

---

*Nursing in state or municipal prisons is generally similar.

ment has set up basic qualifications for professional nurses who wish to join its ranks and has established criteria for advancement. The conditions of employment also follow a similar pattern in the several branches of the federal government nursing services.

U.S. PUBLIC HEALTH SERVICE

Founded in 1798, the U.S. Public Health Service is the federal agency specifically charged with promoting and assuring the highest level of health attainable for every individual and family. It is also responsible for collaborating with governments of other countries and with international organizations in world health activities. It is a vital force in advancing research in the health sciences, in developing public health programs, and in providing therapeutic and preventive services. The PHS offers opportunities for a variety of nursing assignments: the PHS hospitals and the Clinical Center research hospital in Bethesda, Maryland; public health and clinical nursing in the Indian Health Program; and consultation in such fields as community health, environmental health, hospital services, clinical specialties, nursing education, and nursing research. Assignments depend on the nurse's education and experience, professional aptitudes, personal and career preferences, and needs of the service.

The graduate nurse may enter the PHS either by appointment to the Commissioned Corps or the Federal Civil Service. Minimum requirements are U.S. citizenship, at least eighteen years of age, graduation from an approved school of nursing, and physical eligibility. Graduates from associate degree or diploma programs of less than thirty months are often appointed at a lower rank than other graduates; they are required to have an additional year of nursing experience to achieve the same rank as other graduates. The Commissioned Corps is a uniformed ser-

vice comprised of professionals in medical and health-related fields. Pay, allowances, and other privileges are comparable to those of officers of the armed forces. Appointments may be made at the junior assistant grade, equivalent to ensign in the Navy or second lieutenant in the Army. The top rank is surgeon general, equivalent to rear admiral and major general. Currently, two nurse members of the corps have achieved the rank of assistant surgeon general. A candidate must have a bachelor's degree from a regional college or university and, if without prior military service, must be under forty-four.

Opportunity for collegiate nursing students to become familiar with the careers in the PHS as well as to further their professional knowledge is offered through the Commissioned Officer Student Training and Extra Program (COSTEP). In the junior COSTEP a limited number of carefully selected students are commissioned as reserve officers in the corps and called to active duty for training during "free periods" of the academic year. Assignments are made in the continental United States for 31 to 120 consecutive days in any twelve-month period, in the areas of medical and hospital services, research, or public health practice. Salary and privileges are at the junior assistant health service grade and include housing, travel, and medical care. After satisfactory performance, a COSTEP officer may be retained in the Inactive Reserve Commissioned Corps of the PHS while continuing college education. Upon completing professional education, the officer may request active status and retain his or her commission. If active duty is not desired, the commission is terminated. In the senior COSTEP, collegiate nursing students are placed on active duty during their final year with all benefits plus tuition and fees. Persons selected for this program are obligated for an additional two years of service. To be eligible, students must have completed two years of a baccalaureate program, expect to return to college after each COSTEP assignment, and be otherwise eligible for appointment to the Commissioned Corps.

The civil service system is considered the basic mode of federal employment and comprises a range of professional and nonprofessional personnel. A civil service examination is not required for RNs before appointment because they have passed the state board examinations. There is opportunity for advancement through a well-defined merit system. Nurses employed under civil service in PHS do not have Social Security benefits. They are eligible for retirement benefits, which they may receive upon resignation, depending on length of employment.

The status of PHS hospitals is uncertain at this time. There have been periodic attempts by the executive branch of the government to close some of these hospitals. Health officials in both parties have felt that the increasing availability of Medicare, Medicaid, and private health insurance have made these institutions anachronistic. However, members of Congress, particularly from the geographic areas affected, oppose such closings. In September 1973, both houses of Congress passed overwhelmingly a medical services bill to which was attached a proviso that would have forced the administration to keep open these hospitals. The President vetoed the bill, and although the Senate overrode the veto, the House did not. Further successful action to retain the hospitals followed in later legislation, and the hospitals were "saved" again, but the situation still appears unstable.

The eight hospitals involved are in or near major cities of the United States and provide general medical and surgical services as well as a wide range of specialties. The ninth hospital in the system is located at Carville, Louisiana, and provides care and rehabilitation for patients with leprosy and for training and research in that disease.

The Indian Health Service is responsible for the health care of more than 475,000 American Indians, Eskimos, and Aleuts, operating approximately fifty-one hospitals and seventy-seven health centers, most west of the Mississippi River. The clinical nurse in the Indian Service works in the clinics and hospitals. The public health nurse coordinates nursing services between the hospital, clinic, school, and home.

There are a number of other nursing positions in the PHS. The National Institute of Mental Health deals with basic research training activities for specialized manpower, and intensified programs on suicide, crime, and delinquency. The Center for Disease Control conducts national and international programs in research, prevention, and control of infectious diseases. The National Center for Health Services Research Development conducts and supports research and demonstrations related to the availability, organization, and financing of health services. The Maternal and Child Health Service employs nursing specialists in the field in its nationwide programs, providing comprehensive health services for mothers and children.

The Clinical Center under the aegis of the Department of Health and Human Services (DHHS) is a component part of the National Institutes of Health, the principal research arm of the Public Health Service. The National Institutes of Health is composed of a number of institutes—including National Eye Institute; National Cancer Institute; National Institute of Aging; National Institute of Neurological Diseases and Stroke; National Heart and Lung Institute; National Institute of Arthritis, Metabolic and Digestive Diseases; National Institute of Allergy and Infectious Diseases; National Institute of Dental Research; and National Institute of Child Health and Human Development. The hospital of the Clinical Center employs staff nurses to participate with the medical staff in planning for the total care of patients undergoing medical research. They may be assigned to any nursing service for an indefinite period of time or they may choose to rotate from one service to another when vacancies permit. Nurses at the Clinical Center are encouraged to be innovative in the development of new skills and to be active participants in determining their role.

The National Health Service Corps was created in 1970 to provide direct medical care services in urban and rural communities with critical health manpower shortages, but there was some concern about its success and it received considerable political attention. There has been considerable turnover of administrative personnel because of dissatisfaction with funding and governmental policies. Now, a new emphasis on screening in the NHSC is emerging, with legislation giving scholarships to health professions students if they serve in the Corps after graduation.

Although there are other major programs in the PHS, the others do not employ nurses. The Department of Health and Human Services no longer has a national job information center. Local employment information is now available by contacting the nearest federal office building and asking for the Office of Personnel Management.

VETERANS ADMINISTRATION NURSING SERVICE

The Veterans Administration (VA) was established in 1930 as a civilian agency of the federal government. Its purpose is to administer national programs that provide benefits for veterans of this country's armed forces. The VA operates the nation's largest organized health care system, comprised of 172 hospitals, 200 outpatient clinics, eighty-nine nursing home care units, and sixteen domiciliaries. More than one million veterans receive hospital care through the VA system yearly. The VA's Department of Medicine and Surgery employs more than 28,000 professional nurses.

To accomplish its objective of providing high-quality health care, the VA has developed extensive programs in research and education. A majority of VA medical centers are affiliated with medical schools, schools of nursing, and other health-related schools in a network of health care facilities that cover the entire country. Individual hospitals range in size from approximately 100 to 2,000 beds, most of which provide care for patients with medical, surgical, and psychiatric diagnoses. Eighteen hospitals are predominately for the care of patients with psychiatric diagnoses. Many VA health care facilities have outpatient clinics and extended-care facilities, such as nursing home care units.

Veterans Administration medical centers are administered through the Department of Medicine and Surgery headed by a Chief Medical Director. The Nursing Service functions within this Department. The office of the national Director of Nursing Service is located at the Veterans Administration Central Office, Washington, D.C. 20420.

To qualify for an appointment in the VA, a nurse must be a U.S. citizen, a graduate of a state-approved school of professional nursing, currently registered to practice, and meet required physical standards. Graduates from a professional school of nursing may be appointed pending passing state board examinations.

There are several levels of salary grades of VA nurses, ranging upward from junior grade through associate, full, intermediate, senior, chief, assistant director, director, and the executive grade of director, the last reserved for the national leader of the VA Nursing Service.

Specific qualification requirements are related to education, experience, and competencies for appointment or promotion to each grade. However, most nurses do not receive salary for specific positions. The VA salary system recognizes excellence in clinical practice, administration, research, and education. Nurses who prefer to give direct patient care receive salaries commensurate with their qualifications. A Nurse Professional Standards Board reviews performance, recommends promotion, and recommends special salary advancement according to established criteria. A nurse appointed to one VA medical center may transfer to another without loss of salary.

Personnel policies in VA offer low-cost life insurance and group health insurance as well as a liberal retirement plan. Nurses do not accumulate Social Security benefits while employed by the VA.

The VA Nursing Service emphasizes continued learning and advanced education. There is a Nursing Career Development Program to provide opportunities within the system. Nurse researchers are employed in some VA medical centers and in the national office. Clinical nurse specialists work in some VA health care settings. Also, nurse practitioners function in specific units, clinics, or satellite facilities. Applications and inquiries for full- or part-time employment should be directed to the Chief, Nursing Service, at the VA Medical Center at the location of interest.

THE ARMED SERVICES

Despite similarities, there are specific differences among the Army Nurse Corps, Navy Nurse Corps, and Air Force Corps. In recent years there have been a number of changes in qualifications and assignments to meet the changes in society and in the health field. All the armed services have a reserve corps of nurses established by acts of Congress to provide the additional nurses that are needed to care for members of the services and their families in time of war or other national emergency. Nurses may join the reserve without having joined the regular service; the requirements are similar. A certain amount of daily training (which is paid) is required, usually one weekend a month and two consecutive weeks a year, at local medical units related to that particular service. There are opportunities for promotion, continuing education, and fringe benefits

such as low-cost insurance, retirement pay, and PX shopping. More information is available from the reserve recruiter of the particular service. In all the services, nurses have the economic, social, and health care benefits of all officers as well as the opportunity for personal travel. After discharge (or retirement, which is possible in twenty years), veterans' benefits are available.

The Army Nurse Corps

Because it is the oldest of the federal nursing services, the Army Nurse Corps has had considerable influence on the development of nursing and the status of nurses in all of the armed services. When the Army Nurses Corps (ANC) was established as part of the Army Medical Department in 1901, nurses had a status comparable to that of enlisted men. Believing that they needed the authority of officers for disciplinary reasons related to giving nursing care, nurses, principally through the American Nurses' Association, tried unsuccessfully for many years to persuade Congress to give them that recognition. During World War II, the federal government gave nurses serving in all branches of the armed services temporary commissions. But it was not until 1947 that women nurses achieved permanent commissioned status. Men in nursing had to wait until 1955 to be so recognized.

Qualifications for a commission in the Army Nurse Corps are that the person be:

1. A graduate of a baccalaureate school of nursing acceptable to the Department of the Army.
2. Between twenty and thirty-three years of age (unless with prior military service).
3. Currently licensed to practice nursing in the United States, the Commonwealth of Puerto Rico, or the District of Columbia.
4. A citizen of or lawfully admitted to the United States for permanent residence.
5. Able to provide excellent professional, personal, moral, and scholastic references.
6. Able to conform to the physical standards

prescribed for appointment in the U.S. Army.

7. Married or single; both women and men may have dependents of any age.

8. Engaged in practice as a registered nurse on a full-time basis for not less than six months within the one-year period preceding date of application.

An RN just completing a baccalaureate program in nursing comes into the ANC as a second lieutenant. Additional professional experience or education may earn an initial appointment at a higher rank. Ordinarily, the agreed-upon length of service is three years. Generally every newly commissioned officer is in the Army Reserve, in which the individual may continue indefinitely after release from active duty. In the Regular Army Nurse Corps, the nurse may now advance to the rank of brigadier general.

Army nurses may give direct patient care in any clinical specialty as staff nurses, head nurses, or nursing consultants. They may teach as directors or instructors for military courses in various hospitals and the Academy of Health Sciences, or be responsible for nursing education and training within a Department of Nursing. They may become involved in administration in various clinical services or at Army headquarters. They may also function as nursing methods analysts, nurse researchers, nurse counselors, consultants to the surgeon general, or advisor to military nurses of allied nations. Assignments may be in the United States or various parts of the world. There are numerous educational programs, such as the clinical nursing specialty courses. Army Nurse Corps officers may also elect to attend a college or university for advanced degrees with all or part of the costs paid.

Further information may be obtained from the local Army Nurse Corps recruiting station or by writing Army Nurse Opportunities, Box 4444, Mount Vernon, New York 10551.

Navy Nurse Corps

Although the Navy Nurse Corps was officially established by Congress in the twentieth century, Navy nurses were recommended by the first chief of the Bureau of Medicine and Surgery in 1811, and sisters of the Order of the Holy Cross served on the Navy ship *Red Rover* as volunteers in 1862. They were the first female nurses to serve aboard the first U.S. Navy hospital ship. The first Navy nurses (called the Sacred Twenty) and a superintendent reported to Washington for duty in 1908. By 1910 nurses had expanded their activities to include the Far East, Hawaii, and the Caribbean. In World War I, women nurses were assigned to hospitals in England, Ireland, Scotland, and France. Throughout World War II, Navy nurses also brought nursing care to front-line casualties aboard twelve hospital ships and also to air evacuees. They served in foreign lands where American women had never been seen and some were prisoners of war. In 1944, the USS *Highbee* became the first combat ship to be named for a woman, the second superintendent of the Navy Nurse Corps.

Today, many Navy nurses not only care for patients, but also teach patients, corpsmen, and other nurses, and assume administrative positions. They are assigned to clinics, hospitals, regional medical centers, and Hospital Corps schools in the United States and other parts of the world.

Appointments are made in grades of ensign to lieutenant (senior grade), depending upon age, education, and other professional qualifications, but the nurse may advance to the rank of rear admiral. Basic qualifications are that the person be

1. A graduate of an approved nursing school in the United States or Canada.
2. A registered nurse.
3. Twenty to thirty-four and a half years old:
4. Single or married; applicants with dependents will be considered.
5. A citizen of the United States.

6. Physically qualified according to Navy standards.
7. Able to supply excellent professional, personal, moral, and scholastic references.

All Navy nurses are encouraged to continue their education through Navy in-service and continuing education courses, as well as courses leading to academic degrees. Qualified career officers may request assignment to full-time study for a baccalaureate or master's degree.

Further information is available from the local Navy recruiting station or from Nursing Program, Navy Recruiting Command, Naval Department, Washington, D.C.

Air Force Nurse Corps

The Air Force Medical Service became a separate entity from the Army Medical Service in 1949; previous to this, Army nurses and doctors were assigned to duty with the Air Corps. Two specific differences between nursing in the Air Force and other services are that, in addition to providing professional nursing care to military personnel and their families in the United States and foreign countries, Air Force nurses assist in the evacuation of patients by air and are an integal part of the aerospace program through practice in environmental health. When it became obvious during World War II that a better method of patient movement was necessary, the Army Air Force School of Air Evacuation was set up to train carefully selected nurses to care for patients on each evacuation flight. The flight nurse school is now a part of the Aerospace Medical Division at Brooks Air Force Base, Texas, and has graduated approximately 7,000 flight nurses since the Korean conflict. Flight nurses must be medically acceptable for flying. They take a difficult course that includes such subjects as aviation, physiology, psychology, and nursing procedures for in-flight care of patients (usually seriously wounded). Aerospace nurses are now known as Envionmental Health Nurses and are prepared for this function in a one-year course. They are responsible for the entire Air Force aerospace environment, including underground missile sites and stratospheric flights of experimental aircraft. They are part of the medical support for space flights as well as fitting into the everyday working environment in other areas.

Other educational programs available are nursing administration, nurse practitioner, anesthesia, and nurse midwife. A selected number of Air Force nurses study at universities for a graduate or undergraduate degree, during which time they receive full pay and allowances. Generic senior students in NLN-accredited baccalureate nursing programs may apply for selection into the Air Force Nurse Corps. They will be appointed as officers after graduation and passing state board examinations.

Requirements for appointment as an Air Force nurse are that the person be:

1. A graduate of an accredited school of nursing that is acceptable to the surgeon general of the Air Force.
2. A registered professional nurse with current registration.
3. A United States citizen.
4. At least 18 years of age.
5. Physically qualified.

Most appointments are made in the grades of second and first lieutenants, but nurses with added professional experience and education may be appointed at a higher rank. It is now possible to advance to the rank of general.

Additional information may be obtained by contacting a local Air Force recruiter or by writing to United States Air Force Recruiting Service/RSON, Randolph AFB, Texas 78148.

NURSING IN EXTENDED AND LONG-TERM CARE FACILITIES

Under Medicare and Medicaid, nursing homes that qualify for reimbursement are called skilled nursing facilities. The intermediate care facility provides for those who require care beyond room and board but less than that designated as "skilled." These include institutions for victims of cerebral palsy or other neurological conditions and mental retardation. The older term *nursing home,* which might apply to either, is still used by most people. There are some 16,000 nursing homes in the country, about 75 percent under proprietary (for profit) ownership.

Although the average bed capacity is around fifty, the total number of beds is greater than hospital beds. There are more RNs working in nursing homes than there were even five years ago, although the majority of care-givers are practical nurses and aides.

Nurses may have positions in nursing homes similar to those in hospitals, with the additional role of facility administrator being assumed by some nurses. In this case, the nurse must be certified for the position, and although the individual's knowledge of nursing may be extremely helpful in understanding the need for quality care, being a nurse is not a requirement for certification.

The director of nursing, who has the same kinds of responsibilities as any other DN, is sometimes expected to act as the administrator's assistant, whereas some administrators take over some of the director's prerogatives.[43] In small nursing homes, the director might assume both roles. Because of the profit orientation, financial management is extremely important. The administrative nurse should be well-prepared in managerial skills; unfortunately, that is rare.

In most nursing homes the pace is slower and the pressure less. Nurses interested in nursing home care enjoy the opportunity to know the patient better in the relatively long-term stay and to help the patient maintain or attain the best possible health status. This is not the area of practice for someone impatient for quick results. Both rehabilitative and geriatric nursing require a large amount of patience and understanding. In rehabilita-

tion, nurses work closely as a team with related health disciplines—occupational therapy, physical therapy, speech therapy, and others. In geriatric nursing, the nurse works to a great extent with nonprofessional nursing personnel and acts as team leader, teacher, and supervisor. It may well be that there is only one professional nurse in a nursing home per shift, with practical nurses as charge nurses and aides giving much of the day-to-day care.

Because the patients are relatively helpless and often have no family or friends who check on them, the nurse must, in a real sense, be a patient advocate. Physicians make infrequent visits and in some cases, where there are limited or no rehabilitative services, the nurse is the only professional with long-term patient contact.[44]

For this reason, geriatric nurse practitioners (GNPs) are considered a tremendous asset in nursing homes. The GNP is responsible for assessing patients and evaluating their progress, sometimes performing certain diagnostic procedures. She/he usually manages medical problems within a general protocol, but a particularly important function is assessing personal and family relationships, patient and staff relationships, and life situations that may affect the patient's health status. In some nursing homes, the GNP is on twenty-four-hour emergency call and also performs the other usual nurse practitioner functions.[45]

Qualifications and Conditions of Employment. Requirements for employment are similar to those in hospitals for like positions, although often the need for degrees is not emphasized. Conditions of employment and salaries have improved and are now similar to those in hospitals. Because, under Medicare, orientation and subsequent in-service education are mandatory, the nurse has an excellent opportunity to learn about long-term nursing care and the concepts and techniques of geriatric nursing. Because the increase of older people is one of the trends in society, geriatric care is being given greater attention, and workshops, courses, and programs are available in the field. With an aging population, there are also likely to be good job opportunities for some time to come.

PUBLIC HEALTH (COMMUNITY HEALTH) NURSING

Although there is an increasing tendency to refer to public health nursing (PHN) and community health nursing (CHN) interchangeably, there are those who differentiate between the two terms by assigning to CHN a broader scope of practice and a different orientation. Community health nursing is seen as considering the health needs of the *aggregate,* that is, groups of clients or potential clients, who have certain commonalities (expectant mothers, school-age children, the aged, those who have just experienced the death of a child), as opposed to concentrating primarily on the needs of individuals and families. Both may interrelate.[46] The aggregate focus may be less specifically clinical, with consideration given to community needs for services other than health (but affecting health directly or indirectly). However, assessment and diagnosis of community (aggregate) needs can also point the direction for priority services. For instance, in a community in which the older population is increasing and young people are moving away, the types of services needed would be different from those of a suburban housing development. One type of practitioner prepared to assess community needs and assist the community in seeking appropriate help is the community nurse practitioner (CNP), a generally nonclinical role concerned with health care access, fragmentation, health promotion, and disease prevention[47] CNPs, who usually have master's degrees, may be employed in both governmental and non-profit agencies, but there are still too few to determine their impact. Nevertheless, this role obviously fits in with the ANA definition of community health nursing practice.

Community Health Nursing is a synthesis of nursing practice and public health practice applied to promoting and preserving the health of populations. The nature of this practice is general and comprehensive. It is not limited to a particular age or diagnostic group. It is continuing, not episodic. The dominant responsibility is to the population as a whole. Therefore, nursing directed to individuals, families or groups contributes to the health of the total population. Health promotion, health maintenance, health education, coordination and continuity of care are utilized in a holistic approach to the family, group and community. The nurse's actions acknowledge the need for comprehensive health planning, recognize the influences of social and ecological issues, give attention to populations at risk and utilize the dynamic forces which influence change.

In Community Health Nursing Practice the consumer is the client or patient. Consumers include individuals, groups and the community as a whole. For example, the consumer may be a single individual, family (interpreted in the broadest sense), a school population, an industrial population or selected at-risk segments of the population. Professional practitioners of nursing bear primary responsibility and accountability for the nursing care consumers receive.[48]

Translating this concept into specifics, the ANA Division on Community Health Nursing Practice states:

The primary focus of community health nursing is on the prevention of illness and the promotion and maintenance of health. Therefore, community health nursing practice includes the provision of needed therapeutic services, counseling, education, direction, and advocacy activities. The community health nurse who is in constant contact with people in groups who seek and need health care has unique opportunities to identify discrete health problems, as well as potential health problems, and to evaluate current health status. The community health nurse is involved in the planning and coordination of community health programs and services.

The community health nurse, therefore, has responsibility in general and comprehensive areas of health practice for:

a. *Determining health needs of the individual, the family, and the community;*
b. *Assessing health status;*
c. *Implementing health planning;*
d. *Evaluating health practices;*
e. *Providing primary health care.*

The community health nurse needs to be aware of regulations which are developing, as well as new and existing regulations, policies, and laws that directly affect community health nursing practice. [49]

In fulfilling these responsibilities, PHN/CHN nurses practice in many settings. Most are employed by agencies that may carry the title of public health, community health, home health, or visiting nurse. They may be official—governmental and tax-supported (such as a city or county health department); nonofficial or voluntary—agencies supported to a great extent by community funds (such as visiting nurse or home health service); or proprietary—for profit. These agencies range in size and services from small, employing only one or two public health nurses, to very large, employing a sizable staff of professional nurses, other health professionals, practical nurses, and home health aides and homemakers. Some of the latter may be contracted for from an agency (see Chapter 8).

Public health nurses' employment opportunities are not limited, however, to these agencies. They may also be employed by hospitals to conduct home-care programs or to serve as liaison between the hospital and community facilities, or by other institutions and agencies, private and governmental, in need of the kind of services the public health nurse is prepared to provide: schools, outpatient clinics, community health centers, free walk-in clinics for drug addiction and venereal diseases, migrant labor camps, and rural poverty areas.

Public health nurses may also work for various international agencies assisting less developed countries, because the need for public health nursing services in these countries is usually urgent. Because the PHN/CHN field is so broad, it offers almost unlimited employment opportunities for qualified professional nurses. As part of the traditional public health services, every state, every United States territory, and many counties, large towns, and cities have a public health department. (In some states health and welfare units have been merged, but most still have separate health departments.) How effective it is in meeting the needs of the community it serves depends upon its finances, its physical facilities, its staff, and its leadership.

Originally, public health services were concerned with controlling such diseases as typhoid fever, cholera, smallpox, and yellow fever. Programs have expanded rapidly in the last few decades, on local, state, and national levels, to include diagnostic, therapeutic, and rehabilitative services as well as preventive health care and counseling. New areas of concern are mental illness, alcoholism, chronic illness, drug addiction, and the need for primary care. There is also active participation in civil defense.

Public health offers extraordinary opportunities for the imaginative, competent, and resourceful person to originate and develop ideas that may greatly affect the health of the community and, conceivably, of the entire world. Research and education are extremely important phases of public health and are carried on continuously, often under the auspices of, and supported financially by, the Public Health Service.

Professional nurses make up the largest group of professional public health personnel, and their influence is considerable. Workers in the field of public health include physicians, social workers, sanitary engineers, nutritionists, dentists, physical therapists, speech therapists, and others. Members of these groups may work alone or in a team relationship. All public health workers, therefore, need an overview of the entire program to understand their place in the organization and the scope of their own work. An effective public health program requires excellent working relationships with other agencies, both health and nonhealth, because public health activities reach every segment of the community. Although situations differ, nurses in official agencies may make home visits, but their responsibilities are primarily in community health information services and in public health clinics focused on the needs of that agency's population. Traditionally, these have been family planning, maternal-child care, and communicable disease; in a number of communities these agency nurses are also the school nurses and, occasionally, are contracted to do some occupational health nursing. Nurse practitioners are being employed to care for patients in the areas of their expertise, but all nurses observe and evaluate the patients' physical and emotional conditions and are involved in teaching, therapy, counseling and prevention; they make referrals as necessary and act in a liaison capacity with other agencies for needed services.

The visiting nurses, or home health nurses, regardless of their place of employment, also carry out these functions and may, in addition, give physical care and treatments. If the nurse assessment indicates that such care does not require professional nurse services, home health aides/homemakers may be assigned to a patient/family, with nurse supervision and reassessment. Visiting nurses have also set up clinics that they visit periodically in senior citizen centers or apartments, as well as in the SRO (single-room occupancy) hotels commonly used for welfare clients in large cities. There are multiple liaison roles with hospitals, HMOs, clinics, geriatric units, and various residences for the long-term disabled and mentally ill or retarded, primarily to assist in admission and discharge planning, as well as coordinating continuing patient care.

Nurses in managerial positions in PHN/CHN agencies have similar responsibilities as those in hospitals in terms of general managerial skills. A major difference for the top nurse administrator is that that individual is frequently director of the entire agency, with direct responsibility to the agency board of directors (nonofficial agency) or the health officer (governmental agency).

As part of the administrative functions of management and administration of home health care services (planning, developing, and evaluating), certain specific responsibilities of the nurse administrator have been delineated:

- *Uses statistical data to determine the quality and quantity of health services.*
- *Facilitates coordination of services within and outside the agency.*
- *Oversees responsibilities for management, education, and service functions.*
- *Oversees the fiscal affairs of the agency, with responsibility for budget preparation and control; secures financial resources for the agency.*
- *Initiates and participates in local, state, and national health and welfare programs.*
- *Promotes collaboration between the service setting and educational programs preparing service staffs.*
- *Employs, manages, and directs the human resources of the agency.*
- *Provides leadership and vision in developing the long-range plans of the agency in the context of community needs.*
- *Markets agency services.*[50]

Some of the major changes that will affect public health nurses, as seen by some public health administrators are

1. New health delivery systems—such as health maintenance organizations, comprehensive health centers, group practices, satellite primary care centers putting emphasis on preventive care as an incentive to economical operations.
2. New types of health and social manpower emerging in the community, placing a greater responsibility on the public health nurse to coordinate their activities.
3. Expanded responsibilities for service, resulting in public health nurses providing primary care, particularly in areas of physician shortage.
4. Impact of management theory in the health field requiring nurses to be knowledgeable in these concepts and still remain patient advocates.

5. Rising cost of home visits, necessitating great selectivity in patient load and new methods of health teaching.
6. Decentralization of health administration at state and federal level, placing greater decision-making responsibilities at the local level.
7. Impact of profit-making agencies in competition with governmental and voluntary agencies, acting as competitive forces.

Qualifications and Conditions of Employment. Schools of professional nursing have long recognized that nurses who plan to enter the field of public health need special preparation for it. Most diploma and AD schools give students theoretical instruction in public health nursing, conduct orientation visits to community health agencies, provide several hours of experience in prenatal and well-baby clinics, and integrate public health aspects of nursing wherever possible in all clinical areas. One of the problems in giving experience to students in these schools is the lack of clinical facilities (agencies) for practice. What experience is available is usually reserved for baccalaureate programs, because preparation for public health nursing is usually a major educational objective of these programs and students have taken a considerable number of courses in preparation. However, their experiences are also not limited to official and nonofficial agencies, as public health is seen in a broader perspective.

Besides state licensure, and for some agencies, prior nursing experience, one major qualification for public health nursing work is graduation from a baccalaureate nursing program. Many graduates of these schools go on to earn a master's degree and are thus prepared, educationally, for a lifetime career in this field. Because of the shortage of nurses with the prescribed preparation in public health nursing at the present time, however, graduates of diploma and AD programs can and do find positions in this field, working at the beginning level and under supervision. In some areas they work

only in clinics and do not make home visits. Some employers encourage nurses to work toward a baccalaureate degree by providing tuition or scholarship grants.

Pay and advancement at all levels are related to educational and other qualifications. Nurses may be promoted as they assume advanced or expanded role functions or administrative positions.[51] Most agencies make available to all staff written personnel policies and conditions of employment. Many official agencies operate within a civil service system. In the states with strong labor laws permitting collective bargaining for nurses, nurses may organize either through a union or the ANA and bargain for better salaries and working conditions.

In the past, PHN/CHN nurses enjoyed standard daytime hours with most working Monday through Friday. However, with the move toward more care in the community on a twenty-four-hour basis, rather than in institutions, PHN/CHN nurses will be expected to rotate shifts and work weekends, much the same as nurses employed in institutions.

There is another key point that relates to both the nurse as a practitioner and the conditions of employment. Because public health nurses do not generally function in the protected controlling environment of an institution, where there is a degree of implied authority, but rather in the client's setting, where the client determines who will enter his home, and whether he will receive or follow the health teaching and counseling given, these nurses should have the personality characteristics to deal with such situations. Even if the setting is a clinic, there is no force that can make a client come to, or return to, a clinic, or for that matter, follow any regimen given. There have been studies done indicating that the poor, especially the blacks, may reject health services because they feel a prejudicial attitude among the providers of care, whereas at the same time average middle-class white nurses hold, or feel they hold, different values concerning health care.[52,53] Even with the best of intentions, nurses (and other health workers in the community) may not be able to convince their clients that certain preventive measures are necessary. For instance, a measles epidemic in New Jersey in 1974 was attributed to the simple fact that parents had not brought their children to free clinics for the one inoculation needed. Not all nurses can deal with these frustrations or have the skills and personality characteristics that enable them to work and relate effectively with clients not of their own life-style.

Professional nurses who select public health nursing as a career need outstanding ability to adjust to many types of environment with a variety of living conditions, from the well-to-do in a high-rise apartment to the most poverty-stricken in a ghetto or rural area, and to appreciate a wide range of interests, attitudes, educational backgrounds, and cultural differences. They must be able to accept these variations, to understand the differences, to communicate well so as to avoid misunderstandings and misinterpretations, and to be able to give equally good nursing care to all. Public health nurses in any position must use excellent judgment and are expected to use their own initiative. They have the opportunity to work with other disciplines and other social agencies to help provide needed services to the clients, services that may include financial counseling, legal aid, housing problems, family planning, marital counseling, and school difficulties. In some instances, public health nurses are not only case finders, but case coordinators—patient advocates in every sense.

OFFICE NURSING

Office nurses are employed by physicians or dentists to see that their patients receive the nursing they need, usually in the office. Office nurses may give all of this care or assign certain duties to other personnel who work under their direction and supervision. If working for several doctors or dentists in a group practice center, the nurse may need to supervise a staff of several employees.

Nurses may be employed in a one-doctor

general practitioner's office, which requires a nurse with general skills, or they may be employed in a specialist's office, which requires special skills. For instance, a surgeon may employ a nurse who can also act as his scrub nurse in surgery done at the hospital or assist him in office surgery, providing for adequate supplies and equipment and assuring the adherence of aseptic principles. Becoming rapidly more popular is group practice in which physicians of the same or different specialties provide comprehensive medical care for their patients. Usually the several nurses employed are part of a team with other technical and professional personnel service. X-rays, laboratory tests, electrocardiograms, electroencephalograms, physical therapy, and splint and cast application may be done. On the other hand, in some of these offices, and even in certain one-doctor offices, nurses perform some diagnostic procedures.

Giving nursing care, often of a preventive or rehabilitative nature, is the primary function of office nurses, and if given the opportunity, they can contribute a great deal to the health and welfare of patients and their families. Unfortunately, in too many instances the employer expects the nurse to be hostess, secretary, bookkeeper, errand girl, housekeeper, purchasing agent, public relations expert, and laboratory technician as well, tasks that a medical assistant could do. However, although these extraneous nonnursing tasks do not appear to be the best utilization of a professional nurse's time and skills, it should be recognized that some nurses like the variety.

Office nurses responsible for non-nursing duties should learn to do them well. There is literature available on bookkeeping and secretarial procedures to which they can turn for help. Community colleges and adult education programs usually include secretarial and bookkeeping courses in their evening schedules. The nurse can soon master the information and procedures needed and will develop judgment as to which of these duties should have priority in a busy daily schedule.

What the office nurse does in terms of

nursing will depend largely upon the employer's type of practice, philosophy of nurse utilization, and daily schedule of appointments. Tasks may be as routine as giving medications, chaperoning physical examinations, preparing equipment, and seeing that the patients' records are completed and filed at the end of the day. A more complete utilization of nursing skills would include observation, communication, teaching, and coordination with community health agencies. A few nurses even make hospital patient rounds with or without the physician.

As the nurse obtains a health history from the patient or helps him prepare for the doctor's examination, or chats with him informally, there are many opportunities to observe his general physical condition, his mental and emotional health, the signs and symptoms of illness, and attitudes. A nurse can also observe a member of the family who may be with the patient. These observations and impressions can be very helpful to both the doctor and to the nurse.

The experienced office nurse knows how important it is to be sensitive to the patient's personality. Questions and comments must be phrased carefully to elicit the information wanted and, at the same time, to develop the patient's confidence in the nurse, put him at ease, and effect cooperation in all phases of treatment and care. Nurses must know how to communicate with all patients at their own level, neither talking down to them nor confusing and perhaps frightening them with technical terms they cannot comprehend. They must be cognizant of the impact of nonverbal communications and remember to smile now and then no matter how busy or pressured they may be, to look pleasant, and to be both calm and efficient at the same time. (Not that this should be confined to the office nurse; most people respond to a warm, human, nonthreatening attitude.)

The office nurse should be free to do a great deal of teaching and counseling of individual patients and even conduct formal classes for groups of patients at times.

Therefore the ability to teach effectively and evaluate the results is useful. There are pamphlets, charts, posters, and free samples that nurses can use as teaching aids, and, of course, the nurses, like the physician, are expected to keep current in the field, so that any teaching done is based on current data. A teaching program ideally is jointly planned by doctor, nurses, and others involved in health care. Nurses explain, or reinforce explanation of, tests, treatments, and surgical procedures, how to prepare for hospitalization, and what to expect afterward. They teach patients to care for themselves at home and how to give self-medications and simple treatments safely and with a minimum of discomfort and pain; when indicated, they explain how families can take advantage of the health and welfare facilities in the community.

All of the community health agencies are of concern to office nurses. They must know the public health regulations for reporting communicable diseases and how to submit specimens for examination and what to do with laboratory reports. When a patient is going abroad, they must be able to tell him what inoculations he will be required to have. They must be acquainted with the members of the visiting nurse staff and know how to work cooperatively with them in handling patient referrals and promoting community health measures. They must cooperate in all forms of communications with these agencies and others, such as the public schools.

Perhaps one of the most far-reaching effects on office nursing is the development of the nurse practitioner, who is often part of the physician's private practice and assumes much responsibility for patient care. Some office nurses are now being taught by their employer to assume some of these tasks; more are taking continuing education or formal collegiate programs. Office nurses taught on the job are more likely to be (noncredentialed) physician's assistants, and frequently they identify themselves by this title.

Qualifications and Conditions of Practice. All office nurses must be licensed to practice and currently registered in the state in which they work. Although not usually required, education beyond the basic nursing program is desirable. In most cases, nurses have had previous nursing experience.

Salaries and working conditions in this field are, generally speaking, both flexible and variable, representing private arrangements between the individual office nurse and the employer. Office nurses sometimes say they are willing to make some sacrifices in salary because the hours or responsibilities of office nursing fit their tastes or general life situation. This type of nursing often gives the married nurse the morning free for household and family responsibilities, provides her with most, if not all, weekends off, and may not call for a full work week, depending on the doctor's office hours and his expectations of the nurse. There is, however, the possibility of evening hours or overtime if the doctor is delayed by an emergency.

Currently, the conditions of employment appear to be improving, with better salaries, the same as or more than that of the hospital nurse, and a variety of fringe benefits (again depending on the employer). Some of the most common fringe benefits include paid vacation and holidays, paid sick leave, year-end bonus, and free medical care for the nurse and family. Less likely to be paid are medical-surgical or hospitalization insurance and pension or retirement plans. Most office nurses seem to enjoy a friendly and congenial relationship with their employing physician or physicians and usually succeed in working out mutually satisfactory working conditions and remuneration. They appear to stay in the job longer than most nurses, an average of nine years.

Whether the role encompasses traditional or expanded practice, the office nurse is wise to carry personal malpractice insurance, because there is no guarantee that the nurse is covered completely, and certainly not for individual negligence, by the employer's malpractice insurance.

Those considering a career in office nursing will do well to discuss all aspects of their work and employment conditions in detail with their employer. It is important to make sure that they will be free to function primarily as nurses and that the employer understands what the nurse expects the role to be. A job description is highly desirable, and the office nurse who assumes a position without one would do well to formulate one while holding the position.

A written contract setting forth the agreements between the nurse and her employer can also be mutually beneficial.

SCHOOL (STUDENT) HEALTH NURSING

School nursing began in 1900 as a function of disease control, to help cope with such epidemics as diphtheria, influenza, measles, and other communicable diseases. State and federal legislation have a great impact on all aspects of the school nurse position, because funding for almost all schools is somewhat involved with public funding. For instance, Title 1, Elementary and Secondary Education Act of 1965, provided money for school nurses in ghetto and rural poverty areas, and the number of school nurses doubled. On the other hand, some states have cut the number of school nurses, have hired less qualified nurses, or have turned over school nurse functions to public health nurses when budget cuts were felt to be necessary. Nevertheless, the potential is great in terms of actual needs for preventive care, health teaching, and promotion of health.

Some school systems do not clearly delineate the responsibilities of a school nurse, or do not update the job description in line with modern concepts of health care. The nurse accepting such a position must be extremely self-directed and will find the guidelines cited by professional school nurse groups helpful. For instance, the Department of School

Nurses of the NEA states that the primary function of the professional school nurse is to strengthen the educational process of children and youth by assisting them to improve or adapt to their health status. Ideally, a qualified school nurse should be able to

Assess and evaluate health and developmental status of pupil in order to make a nursing diagnosis and to establish priority for action.

Interpret health and developmental status of pupil for parents, school personnel, and for pupil.

Interpret results of medical findings concerning pupil for parents, school personnel, and for pupil.

Counsel pupil, parents and school personnel and plan action for eliminating, minimizing, or accepting health problems that interfere with effective learning by pupil.

Assist persons responsible for pupil's health to find and use appropriate resource material.

Recommend modifications in the educational program to administrator when health or developmental status of pupil indicates need for such action.

Serve as health consultant and resource person in health instruction curriculum planning by providing current scientific information from related fields.

Use direct health services as vehicle for health counseling.

Serve as liaison between parent, school, and community in health matters.

Serve as a member of placement committee for special educational programs.[54]

Again, ideally, this nurse does not wear white uniform and cap, which often symbolizes sickness to the public. She is not a first aid station and should be circulating to the classroom, home, and total community. However, in many job situations the school nurse is still primarily the giver of first aid in illness or emergency; helps in screening programs for diseases of the eyes, ears, and teeth; keeps records; and does some health teaching and case finding. In a large school system the nurse may be supervising practical nurses, aides, volunteers, clerical assist-

ants, vision screening technicians, audiometric technicians, or other personnel, and may even become a supervisor of other nurses. In a small system, a nurse may assume all these responsibilities alone, even to the point of covering several schools in the same system. A physician may be on call or, more likely, may be available at stated times. The nurse–pupil ratio can vary from 1:800 to 1:11,000; most nurses are responsible for 900 to 1,500 pupils.

School nurses become isolated from other nurse colleagues because, among other things, they are expected to become a part of the educational system, even sometimes, to participate in PTA meetings, faculty meetings, and curriculum development (in areas related to health). Some choose to join the National Education Association instead of ANA, and the NEA becomes their economic security bargaining agent as it may be for the teachers.

A fairly recent development is the school nurse practitioner, who functions basically as other nurse practitioners, bringing much more comprehensive care to the pupils in those settings where nurses are permitted to function in this manner. A joint statement by the ANA and the American School Health Association that defines the role of the school nurse practitioner, and the necessary education, describes the added facets of the role. These include serving as a health advocate for the child, helping parents assume greater responsibility for health maintenance of the child; providing health instruction, counseling, and guidance; contributing to the health education of individuals and groups, applying methods designed to increase each person's motivation to take responsibility for his own health care; assessing and arranging management and referrals for children with health problems; securing and evaluating a thorough health and developmental history of the child and recording the findings; performing physical examinations; and the like. The patterns of practice for school nurse practitioners vary according to the needs perceived and limits set by the school boards. In one pattern the nurse might assume responsibility for the total school health program, assisted by an aide to do clerical work and to triage simple conditions. In a second pattern, the nurse may visit a number of schools, assessing and evaluating children and leaving the follow-up to another nurse or aide on location. In another, practice might be limited to doing physical exams, substituting for a physician, or evaluating children with learning difficulties.

Colleges and universities also provide a setting for the nurse interested in student health, although obviously there is considerable adult health involved. Responsibilities vary according to the size of the institution and the types of services offered. College students often pay a health fee which entitles them to specific benefits. Services may include mental health counseling, family planning, and care for minor illnesses or accidents. Nurse practitioners also function in these settings, although there are instances when an affiliation with a teaching hospital or medical school makes student health a learning setting for residents.

Qualifications and Conditions of Employment. Obviously, nurses interested in school nursing must like children and adolescents and be able to relate well to them. Educationally, the nurse should have at least a baccalaureate degree, as recommended by the American School Health Association, ANA, Department of School Nurses, NEA, and the surgeon general's report, as well as specified courses related to the field of school nursing. Master's degrees are encouraged as is continuing education. Individual states or school systems within states may vary from these requirements. Some require no degree; others ask for a few additional specific courses which may or may not relate to the field (in one state these are courses in history of the state and audio-visual aids). In 1972 about 40 per cent had degrees of some kind.[55] The DSN of NEA recommends having a certifi-

cation program in each state, and a number of states require certification for employment as a school nurse. In some cases, the school nurses are expected to have the same educational credentials as teachers and are paid on the same salary scale. School nurse practitioners will often have had a continuing education or degree program as preparation for this role.

Theoretically, nurses would apply to the local school board for a school nurse position, but actually in smaller systems, the nurse may be able to obtain such a position on the basis of personal acquaintance or sheer availability. School nurse positions are often considered particularly desirable for women with families because the time schedule is the same as for teachers, with weekends and summers free. As noted, salaries, particularly in the larger systems, may be equal to that of the teachers, if the qualifications are equal; in smaller communities, the salary may be quite low.

Opportunities for advancement are found primarily in the larger systems, where the nurse may move to a supervisory position. However, there are many satisfactions to be gained and there is the possibility of professional growth in those systems in which nurses are able to assume a full professional role.

NURSING EDUCATION

Teaching is so much a part of the professional nursing student's basic experience that it might seem reasonable to expect a great many young graduates to select teaching as a career. Fortunately, many do, but not nearly enough to fill the positions available to well-prepared teachers in all areas of nursing education. There are not enough nurses at present to meet the need in any field of nursing, but the shortage of qualified teachers is particularly acute. Without enough teachers, the problem of preparing an increased supply of nurses for present and future needs assumes serious proportions.

In January 1978, it was reported that 20,217 full-time and 4,457 part-time nursing faculty members, not including administrators, were employed in RN programs. The number of unfilled budgeted positions was reported as 909. Compared to 1976, there were more part-time and less full-time faculty, and more budgeted positions unfilled. The greatest demand was for faculty in baccalaureate and higher-degree programs, with the least demand in diploma programs.[56] Practical nurse programs also have around 5,000 teaching positions.[57] At any given time the need is probably considerably larger, partially because there are new programs in higher education opening yearly, and also because most nursing education programs, particularly in institutions of higher education, have had financial problems that prohibit budgeting of an adequate number of teaching positions. An even more vital factor is that most programs do not have fully qualified faculty. Master's degrees have been recommended as a minimum for teachers in all nursing programs, and doctorates for deans of collegiate programs and faculty of graduate programs. Because general university standards require a doctorate for almost any level of teaching position, there is now more pressure for nurses to adhere to this standard also.

In 1978, almost 93 percent of baccalaureate and higher-degree nursing faculty had master's or doctoral degrees, as did almost 65 percent of associate degree faculty and about 33 percent of diploma faculty.[58] All rose about 5 to 6 percent from the 1976 figures. Practical nurse faculty have only about 12 percent with graduate education.[59] Faculty with earned doctorates (about 12 percent) function primarily in programs offering baccalaureate or higher degrees.[60] Both NLN criteria and many state board standards for accreditation suggest master's degrees and higher, and it is expected that faculty not holding the appropriate degree be enrolled in a nursing education program that leads to such a degree.

The philosophy, objectives, kinds of students, and conditions of employment vary in different kinds of nursing education programs.[*] Nurses planning to teach should give thought to the kind of program with which they can identify philosophically and in which they can function effectively. The number and types of positions within each program depend upon the size of the student body, the curriculum content, the faculty organization, and the school's philosophy, aims, and budget. There is a place in some schools for a nurse instructor of sciences, but in most schools, students take courses in physical and social sciences taught by nonnurse instructors at their own or another college or university.

Most nurse-teachers are employed to teach nursing in the area of their clinical expertise, but trends toward nursing curriculum "models" may mean the adjustment of the teacher to differing approaches. In associate degree and practical nurse programs, the teacher may be expected to teach a variety of nursing subjects. Other specific differences in setings may also be noted.

There are certain aspects of a faculty position that are the same, regardless of the educational setting. Faculty have certain responsibilities to the total program, usually through committees. Some are development and updating of philosophy, objectives, and conceptual framework, and selecting appropriate courses to meet those objectives; selection, evaluation, and promotion of students; assisting in developing educational and faculty standards, policies, and procedures; participating in promotion and tenure of faculty; developing special projects; planning for the future. In a collegiate setting, the teacher is expected to participate in college committees of the same nature. In relation to the student, a basic role is teaching in the

*See Chapters 12 and 13 for specific details on each program and issues in nursing education.

classroom, laboratory, and clinical setting, individually or in groups, using appropriate and effective techniques with current knowledge and practice in the area of expertise. Advisement and personal and career counseling of students are also important; some teachers are class or student committee advisors and consultants, as well. In the college and university settings, research and publication are a major expectation; generally, the teacher must seek outside funding for research. Almost equally important is service to the profession and the community, as members or officers of organizations, as consultants, or as speakers.

Differences in teaching in the various programs relate to both the setting and level. In universities, particularly medical centers, there is a trend toward joint appointments, with the teacher carrying a patient case load and, occasionally, administrative responsibilities in the clinical setting.[61] Graduate faculty are expected to be scholarly and research-oriented, for, as well as teaching, they will be directing graduate students' research. They are likely to work closely with graduate faculty in other disciplines if courses are interdisciplinary. They may be expert teachers and practitioners in a particular clinical specialty and/or in nursing administration, nursing education, or other graduate-level studies. Working with graduate students on special projects and guiding or supervising their research may mean hours with the student in conference and in committee presentations for the master's thesis or doctoral dissertation, including certain administrative responsibilities. The paper work in most teaching is extensive.

There are students of superior academic and intellectual ability and high motivation in all programs, but certain baccalaureate and almost all graduate programs have a more homogeneous selection, because high admission standards generally screen out those of lesser ability. However, just about all students are much more challenging and demanding than they were ten years ago; they

want participation rights, they ask questions, and they don't accept pat answers.

Faculty in college- or university-based programs have the advantage of being in an academic setting with broad interdisciplinary contacts and campus activities. They may have joint appointments in other departments or schools and other responsibilities there. They also have the benefits and problems of being in such a setting; the policies and regulations are less directly controllable. Students in collegiate programs affiliate or rotate through a number of hospitals, agencies, or facilities. Unless the program is in a medical center, or unless the teacher holds a joint appointment, students and teachers maintain somewhat of a guest status and find it more difficult to affect care. If other students are also present, there is competition for good "teaching" patients.

On the other hand, in diploma programs, basic nursing education is controlled by a hospital. Nursing classes and often clinical practice are given in that particular school and hospital, although students may go to other clinical settings. Because of the geographic proximity and the fact that hospitals often think of the diploma students as "their" students and future employees, there may be a closer relationship between nurses in the clinical area and the faculty. Often the director of nursing has overall responsibility for both nursing service and nursing administration, and there are opportunities for both service and education personnel to plan and work together on joint projects related to the hospital in general. Often there is more national prestige in being affiliated with a university program, although this varies, and other schools with strong community ties are highly respected.

The teaching opportunities in PN programs offer another type of challenge to the nurse educator. The method of teaching and the philosophy of vocational education differ somewhat from those of professional education. The course of study usually is limited to one year. The setting may be in hospitals, public schools, or community colleges, among which both philosophy and environment vary considerably. It is important that the professional nurse teaching in these programs understand and respect the role of practical nurses in giving patient care and be able to teach accordingly.

Qualifications and Conditions of Employment. Besides the educational requirements, teachers in all nursing programs are expected to have a knowledge of nursing in general and continuously updated knowledge and clinical expertise in the subject area in which they expect to teach. They also need knowledge and skill in curriculum development, the teaching-learning process, and teaching methods and techniques. It is equally important for any prospective teacher to establish rapport with students, and be open-minded and secure enough to welcome differences in opinion. Evaluation of teacher effectiveness is an ongoing process in a progressive educational setting and includes self-evaluation and evaluation by students, peers, and administrative heads. The quality of teaching is considered in retention and promotion of faculty.

One classic study on qualities for effective teaching lists knowledge of subject; sympathetic attitude toward, and interest in, students; interest in and enthusiasm for subject; tolerance, broadmindedness, liberality; interesting presentation; personality to put subject across; sense of humor, sense of proportion; ability to stimulate intellectual curiosity; organization; fairness; sincerity, honesty; moral character. Other intangible factors of personality and appearance are also mentioned.[62] One study with nursing students seems to indicate that these qualities are still considered important, particularly in teacher–student relations.[63] That teaching skills, knowledge, and good teacher-student relations are important is seen in another study that describes four major components of primary importance in effective teaching: (1) command of the subject and ability to "put it across," (2) rapport with

class and skill at controlling group participation, (3) one-to-one response between teacher and student, (4) and flair and infectious enthusiasm that awaken interest and stimulate response.[64]

It is also often expected that the teacher be scholarly and make contributions to nursing through participation in professional activities and/or publications. A teacher in an institution of higher education may be appointed at any level from instructor to full professor, depending on qualifications (and the need of that institution for that individual). Tenure and promotion depend on fulfilling stated requirements.[65,66]

Tenure in colleges and universities means basically that the individual has a secure place in that institution, cannot be dismissed except under unusual circumstances, and can be promoted to higher rank (associate or full professor). Usually there is a span of time (seven years or so) by which the person must be tenured or leave, unless put in some special category outside the tenure track. The more prestigious the institution, the higher the standards for appointment, promotion, and tenure.[67,68] If college teaching is to be a nurse's career, plans for doctoral education are a must.

Salaries and fringe benefits vary, and in an institution of higher learning are the same as for an individual in another discipline at the same rank. A full professor at the last salary step may earn as much or more than the administrator of that particular program. Salaries range from less than $20,000 to more than $40,000.

Teaching positions in any educational program usually demand irregular working hours. Except for scheduled classes, the amount of time a teacher will spend at work is unpredictable because there are so many influencing factors, such as class and clinical preparation time, student conferences, student evaluation, participation in school committees and meetings, library study, and participation in student activities.

Teachers are also involved in professional activities, updating their own clinical practice and advancing their education. Depending on where they teach, they may be able to set their own hours as far as presence in the school is concerned (except for scheduled classes) or may be expected to put in a forty-hour or more week on a regular eight-hour daily basis. It is estimated that the average university nurse-teacher spends about fifty-six hours a week on the job. However, faculty are usually more free than other nurses to attend educational and other meetings. Nurses selecting a career in this field will want to analyze the conditions of each employment opportunity to make sure that it offers them as much as possible of what they want most in both material and professional rewards, and an atmosphere in which they can do their best work. For a teacher, often the greatest reward is the intellectual and personal stimulation of an educational environment, including interaction with students and peers.[69]

Administration in Nursing Education

At the head of each educational program in nursing is a professional nurse who is both administrator and teacher. Nursing education administrators need preparation in administration as well as teaching. Again, it is best, and sometimes required, that the director of the program take graduate courses in administration in a college or university.

Courses in nursing education administration are only rarely available in graduate nursing education programs, so those whose goal is educational administration often acquire experience as assistants to a top administrator or in minor administrative positions and apply principles from non-nursing management courses. In some colleges and universities, department chairmen or deans are appointed administratively on recommendation of the faculty for limited terms, after which they return to nonadministrative faculty positions. This approach has advantages and disadvantages. It gives presumably competent faculty members an opportunity in the administrative role, but it may not be considered desirable by the individual whose primary interest is educational administration and who must then relocate in another institution to remain in a top administrative position.

Qualifications for nursing administration positions in education usually include experience in nursing and nursing education and frequently in administration of some kind. This nurse should be able to relate well to others, in the nursing program, in the profession, in the particular setting of the school, and in the community. The need for leadership qualities is frequently cited. A minimum of a master's degree is usual, and the dean, director, or chairman of a collegiate or university program in nursing is expected to have a doctoral degree. It is also not uncommon to expect these candidates to have achieved national prominence in the nursing field, to have published and done research. Frequently, when a top administrative position is open, a search committee, composed according to institutional criteria, looks for, screens, interviews, and recommends an individual after a national search.[70]

The top administrative post of any nursing education program usually requires both long hours of work on the job and active participation in professional activities. If in a college or university, the administrator is expected to be a leader in campus-wide committees and activities. There may be pressure from the faculty, students, administration, and community, all trying to achieve their own ends. Often there are financial problems for the school. There is little time for nurse administrators to keep abreast in their own clinical field, for the demand to keep current on administrative, educational, and general nursing trends is immediate. This is not a position for someone who cannot learn and act quickly and who wilts under pressure. The rewards, however, can be great professionally, in the satisfaction of accomplishments of the nursing program, its faculty, and students, and in the opportunity to be in a leadership position in nursing and in health care.

Salaries, fringe benefits, and, sometimes,

rank and tenure tend to be negotiable and usually depend on a number of factors related to the position, the community, and the qualifications of the nurse.

PRIVATE DUTY NURSING

For many years private duty nursing was second only to hospital nursing in its attraction for professional nurses, but each year has seen a slight decrease in the total number of nurses in this field of practice, particularly younger nurses.

Private duty nurses are independent practitioners in almost complete control of where they will work, when they will work, the type of patients they will care for, and when they will take vacation or days off. They are limited in what they can charge for services only by the prevailing fee in their community, which is not legally binding.

Private duty nurses make their availability for service known through a nurses' registry, an employment agency, local hospitals, and personal contacts with other nurses, doctors, and members of the community. Individual nurses may build up a list of "clients" composed of families and doctors who always try to engage them whenever they need private duty nurses.

A private duty nurse is usually employed (by the patient or family) to nurse one patient. In time of emergency or special need, some agree to take care of two, or perhaps more, patients in the same room or in adjoining rooms. However, the nurses contend that when they care for more than one patient at a time, they cannot give the quality of service they want to give and that their patients are entitled to have; therefore they prefer not to accept these assignments. Some private duty nurses do general duty in hospitals during periods of staff shortage or to relieve general duty nurses on weekends and holidays.

Patients who need a private duty nurse may be either in a hospital or in their own home. Wherever they are, the nurse is responsible for the patient's care while with him or her. When leaving for any length of time—to go to the dining room, for example —the nurse must make the patient as comfortable as possible mentally and physically and must report to the nurses in charge where she/he is going and when she/he will return. If the patient needs constant attention, relief must be arranged for by the nurse. This is also done if the nurse wishes a day or so off after being with a patient continuously for a number of weeks. Patient and family are consulted and prepared for the temporary substitution.

Most patients requesting private duty nurses are quite ill, or at least require a great deal of care physically and/or mentally. More than half the patients cared for are those who have undergone surgery, particularly if they are relatively helpless afterward and have drainage tubes, IVs, catheters, and so on. Such patients may be fearful of being left alone on a busy clinical unit, even though they would receive adequate care. Other patients who often prefer constant attendance are patients with strokes, cancer, and burns. Moreover, there is always a percentage of patients who can afford three nurses around the clock and who simply wish to have someone constantly at hand. Although intensive-care units and recovery rooms have fulfilled some of the needs for constant observation and immediate attention for the critically ill or newly operated, these are short-term units. There are also patients who are not in critical condition but who require an enormous amount of individualized care. Free from the pressures of time and heavy patient care loads that often harass the general duty nurse, private duty nurses have the opportunity to give truly comprehensive professional care to their patients, with limited concern for hospital routines.

Private duty can also be "special duty," as it was once called, because a private duty nurse often specializes in caring for one type of patient, specializing, for example, in obstetric nursing or in nursing patients who have had chest surgery, cardiovascular conditions, or gastrointestinal surgery.

Qualifications and Conditions of Employment. For success in private duty nursing and greatest job satisfaction, the private duty nurse must have a genuine liking for people and must be able to adjust well to a wide variety of personalities, establishing and maintaining warm yet professional relationships with both patients and their families, no matter how long a case may last. This nurse must enjoy giving direct comprehensive nursing care and must communicate this feeling, nonverbally, to the patient. Constant contact with one patient for eight hours a day over a period of weeks can be a strain. It is necessary for any independent practitioner to have the motivation and the ability to understand and practice modern concepts of comprehensive nursing care, with all of its ramifications. Naturally it is necessary to be currently licensed in the state where the nurse practices, with the exception of times when patient and nurse may be traveling and residing temporarily in another state. It is also important to understand the legal implications of the position and use sound judgment to avoid inappropriate ·involvement or activities. Malpractice insurance is advisable.

As self-employed persons or independent contractors, private duty nurses are almost entirely on their own as far as retirement plans, Social Security payments, and payment of taxes are concerned. There is no employer who arranges special benefits, and it is up to the nurses to keep accurate records from day to day and arrange for their own security through wise expenditures, savings, and insurance. They have no sick leave benefits, no paid vacations. They are their own business managers in every sense of the word.

The responsibility to keep updated is likely to be the private duty nurse's individual responsibility. Hospital in-service programs are usually available, as are workshops, institutes, and other programs, but no one makes arrangements for the independently practicing nurse. Such continuing education may be even more important for these nurses than for institutionally employed nurses, because even though theoretically the hospital nursing service is responsible for the overall nursing care of all patients, private duty nurses generally function with little or no supervision. This is obviously more likely if the nursing care is given in the patient's home.

An eight-hour tour of duty is fairly standard throughout the country, but twelve hour shifts are not uncommon. Fees vary considerably from place to place; they may or may not be higher than a staff nurse per diem. Although it is generally agreed that there is sufficient employment available for private duty nurses in most areas, those nurses who limit their practice to the day shift, certain kinds of patients, and limited length of employment may find that they do not have the opportunity to work as much as they would like. Moreover, LPNs are being employed for private duty, particularly in the home, but also in some hospitals. The increased number of well-prepared nurse practitioners who are setting up independent private practice may also bring about changes in the private duty picture.

OCCUPATIONAL HEALTH NURSING

Occupational health nursing was initiated at the Vermont Marble Company in 1895, using the services of Ada Stewart and her sister, Harriet, or, some say, in 1888 in the mining town of Drifton, Pa.

Two department stores were the next industries to provide similar health services for their employees: John Wanamaker Company of New York in 1897; the Frederick Loeser Department Store, Brooklyn, in 1899. Early in the 1900s, more and more industries on both the east and west coasts recognized the economic value of keeping employees healthy and established similar health services. Adding impetus to the trend was the enactment of workmen's compensation laws (beginning in 1911), which place emphasis on the importance of preventing accidents to employees on the job and giving immediate and expert attention to injuries received at work. This development brought industrial nurses into the plants. World Wars I and II were also strong influences in the growth of industrial nursing because they precipitated a great need to conserve manpower.

For many years nurses employed in these positions called themselves industrial nurses. In 1958, however, the industrial nurses within ANA voted to call themselves occupational health nurses because *occupational* embraces banks, hotels, offices, department stores, and so on, whereas *industrial* connotes (in the minds of most persons) manufacturing industries located in plants, factories, foundries, and mills. Other organizations also adopted the newer term, including, most recently, the American Association of Occupational Health Nurses.

A key factor in changes in occupational health nursing was the enactment in 1971 of The Occupational Safety and Health Act.* That created The National Institute for Occupational Safety and Health (NIOSH) to research health problems and recommend safety standards and the Occupational Safety and Health Administration (OSHA) to guarantee a "safe and healthful workplace." A 1972 President's Report on Occupational Safety and Health stated that 100,000 persons die annually of occupational diseases and 390,000 contract disabling illnesses. Since then, OSHA has been inspecting the nation's workplaces for health and safety hazards, but its effectiveness has been blunted by lack of funds and the resistance of employers who have sometimes sued and won to limit the access of OSHA's inspectors. Nevertheless, unions, environmentalists, and other interested citizens have pressed for more action.[71]

Now, OSHA funding for Occupational Health and Safety Centers to prepare professionals in the field includes some funding for nurses. There had been almost no place that OHNs could receive formal, specialized education. New OHN graduate programs usually include nurse practitioner skills and courses on environmental health and safety, although some also emphasize management skills.

The American Association of Occupational Health Nurses states in its philosophy that

> *The occupational health nurse is a vital component of the health care system. Responsibilities are influenced by current patterns of health service, legislation, social and economic factors.*
>
> *The occupational health nurse is accountable to the medical director for all professional and administrative matters. When no medical director is employed the nurse will be directly responsible to a member of management for all administrative matters but will seek guidance on medical problems from the company's designated physician.*
>
> *The primary goal of the nurse working as a member of the occupational health team is promotion and maintenance of the general physical and emotional health of the worker, prevention of disease, and rehabilitation of the sick and injured. The occupational health nurse is concerned with environmental conditions of the work area as well as the physical and mental health requirements of particular jobs. Emphasis is on preventive approaches to health care in which health teaching, counseling and detection are implicit.*[72]

The health department in which an occupational health nurse works may consist of a single room or it may be a large department with several examining and treatment rooms, X-ray and laboratory facilities, and offices for nurses and physicians. Whatever its size, the administrative policies and scope of the program are decided by business management; the health services are under the medical direction of a physician who may work for the company full-time, part-time, or on an on-call basis.

Many occupational health nurses are employed in one-nurse health departments. In these instances, the nurse carries the department's work alone. A major study, still frequently quoted, stated that in 1966, two

---

*Also discussed in Chapters 6 and 19.

thirds of the occupational health nurses worked without direct medical supervision.[73] Whether this nurse functions in a sophisticated manner in the delivery of health care depends on his or her education and experience, and the policies of the employer. As a prepared nurse practitioner or nurse clinician, the nurse may assess the worker's condition through health histories, observation, physical examination, and other selected diagnostic measures; review and interpret findings to differentiate the normal from the abnormal; select appropriate action and referral; counsel; and teach. The occupational health nurse practitioner must also be concerned with the physical and psychosocial phenomena of the workers and their families, their working environment, community, and even recreation. If the nurse is in a more conservative environment and/or without the appropriate background, the activities may be limited to first aid and some emergency treatment, keeping records, assisting with physical examinations, and carrying out certain diagnostic procedures. In many cases, most often when the nurse does not function in an expanded role, standing orders, or directions, prepared and signed by the medical director, give the necessary authority to care for conditions that develop while the employee is on the job. The nurse refers employees with nonoccupational illnesses or injuries to their family doctors. However, a particularly interesting development that broadens the scope of the OHN's practice is a new emphasis of concern on worker health problems that may or may not be directly caused by the job but affect worker performance—alcoholism, emotional problems, stress, drug addiction, and family relations. In many cases, the nurse is involved in counseling and therapy.

In a large health department in an industry that employs one or more full-time physicians, the nurse may also function as a nursing care coordinator to develop, implement, supervise, and evaluate the delivery of health care to employees, working with professional and nonprofessional staff.

In general, occupational health nursing in a health department of any size means much more than meeting the immediate needs of an ill or injured employee. The nurse uses interviewing, observing, and teaching skills, takes health histories, keeps health records, and is responsible for supplies and equipment. The ability to take and recognize abnormalities in electrocardiograms, to do eye screening, audiometer testing, and certain laboratory tests and X-rays is considered useful. In addition, the nurse must be vitally concerned with the safety of the employees and may tour the plant with management and the safety engineer to help them plan a practical safety program.

The nurse may also need to act as interpreter of company health and safety policies and thus learn company policy on personnel matters, sick leave, insurance benefits, pay rates, and the necessary information for myriad records. Health teaching to attain and maintain optimum health, usually done on an individual basis, is generally considered an important aspect of the job. On the other hand, the serious and not infrequent responsibility of giving immediate care to workers with serious injuries, often with no physician present, should not be overlooked. Such situations have major legal implications. Says one author:

> Assessment and legal accountability are key words in dealing with such practical problems as the determination of the severity of the injury, the hazards of transportation versus treatment at the scene of the accident, and the legal implications of swift and accurate thinking to decide whether to act or to withhold action.[74]

As noted earlier, the occupational health nurse, if not a nurse practitioner, needs medical directives that have been prepared or approved by the physician in charge. These are basic to the legal discharge of this nurse's responsibilities as far as the employees and the physician are concerned and to personal legal protection against lawsuits. OHNs should be familiar with the laws governing the practice of nursing and medicine in their state and discuss them with the physician and management to make sure that they all understand the legal scope of nursing functions.

Qualifications and Conditions of Employment. Graduation from a state-approved school of professional nursing and current state registration are basic requirements for the occupational health nurse. Comparatively few employers require a college degree, although many consider it desirable. Both the Surgeon General's report and the ANA recommend a baccalaureate degree, and the ANA also recommends specific courses related to the occupational health nurse's functions. However, approximately 75 per cent of these nurses work in manufacturing industries where it seems that the employers are more interested in experience and self-reliance than education. In 1972, 90 per cent of occupational nurses had no degree.[75] Whether the evolving role of the nurse practitioner, who has more education and can also assume more responsibilities, will change this attitude remains to be seen. Currently, only continuing education related to the job is considered necessary. However, a great percentage of OHNs are nearing retirement age and, as they are replaced with better-prepared nurses, their availability, interest, and the new educational programs will probably make at least baccalaureate education the norm.

Some nursing schools incorporate the concepts of occupational health nursing in the basic curriculum and arrange field trips to observe occupational health services in action. Although such preparation is helpful to the nurse who selects this specialty as a career, it is up to the nurse to apply the principles and to adapt the techniques on the job; to become outstandingly proficient in the skills needed in the practice of occupational health nursing; to become familiar with the physical layout of the business establishment, its operation, and its products or services; to be well acquainted with the community, its resources, and its needs, including the neighborhoods in which most of the employees live; and to establish cordial working relationships with all community health and welfare agencies.

Nurses in a one-nurse occupational health service need to be especially well qualified because they carry almost total responsibility for the program. Nurses without education and experience beyond basic education in nursing will find greater satisfaction working in a multiple-nurse occupational health service where they can learn on the job.

A career OHN will be expected to seek certification by the American Board for Occupational Health Nurses, Roselle Park, N.J., an independent nursing specialty board authorized to certify properly qualified OHNs.

Salaries and fringe benefits vary according to the size of the industry or business and its location. Both tend to be somewhat lower than that of other nurses. Some OHNs belong to a union, but this is discouraged by the AAOHN (and by employers). The usual company benefits include vacations, sick leave, pensions, and insurance. Working hours are those of the workers; thus, in an industry with work shifts around the clock, nurses are usually there also. As a professional person, the nurse may have some of the privileges of management such as temporary absences to attend meetings. Although some industries carry professional liability insurance that supposedly covers the occupational health nurse, it may not apply in all cases of possible litigation. It is advisable, therefore, for these nurses to carry their own individual professional liability insurance.

NURSING IN THE EXPANDED OR EXTENDED ROLE—THE NURSE PRACTITIONER (NP)

In the emergence of any new role, there is considerable controversy in relation to terminology, functions, and education. Not all of this has been resolved concerning the nurse practitioner (NP). There is disagreement as to whether the role is expanded or extended, merely changing, or not new at all. Lillian Wald, pioneer in public health nursing, made house calls, prescribed and dispensed medications and treatments, and counseled her client families as needed. In more recent times, the Frontier Nursing Service of Wendover, Kentucky, which was noted for its "nursing on horseback" midwifery services, has been expanding its practice to overall family services.[76]

It is generally agreed, however, that the new wave of nurse practitioners began with two experiments: a clinic program at the University of Kansas Medical Center, which showed that nurse-run clinics were more effective with chronically ill women than were regular clinics,[77] and the Ford-Silver program at the University of Colorado that became the first PNP program.[78] The term *nurse practitioner,* although coming into common usage for anyone functioning in the expanded role, creates a semantic problem because technically anyone practicing nursing is a nurse practitioner.

Definitions of nurse practitioners also vary, but generally it is conceded that nurse practitioners have acquired additional knowledge and skills, some of which were previously considered medical, either in short-term or degree educational programs, and use fully all aspects of nursing skills, which enable them to provide more extensive health services to the patient/client, often in collaboration with a physician or physicians, but also independently, in consultation with a physician as needed.

Edith Lewis sees as the common denominator:

> First and probably foremost is that the nurse is oriented toward providing care for clients rather than services to institutions . . . she practices independently or interdependently, as the setting dictates; she makes her own decisions, assumes responsibility and accountability for them, and is subject to few if any hierarchal restraints.
>
> For the most part, she maintains a one-to-one relationship with her clients and sees

them as part of the family-community constellation to which they belong. She may or may not possess, or feel the need for physical assessment skills; to the degree that she uses them, she does so to enrich the data base for her nursing judgments. For the nurse practitioner is not practicing medicine; she is practicing nursing.[79]

A useful description of the responsibilities of nurse practitioners in primary health care after completing a formal program is given in the *1977 Federal Rules and Regulations* that govern the educational programs for NPs funded by DHHS through the Nurse Training Act. It lists the ability to:

1. *Assess the health status of individuals and families through health and medical history taking, physical examination, and defining of health and developmental problems;*
2. *Institute and provide continuity of health care to clients (patients), work with the client to insure understanding of and compliance with the therapeutic regimen within established protocols, and recognize when to refer the client to a physician or other health care provider;*
3. *Provide instruction and counseling to individuals, families and groups in the areas of health promotion and maintenance, including involving such persons in planning for their health care; and*
4. *Work in collaboration with other health care providers and agencies to provide, and where appropriate, coordinate services to individuals and families.*

Primary health care means care which may be initiated by the client or provider in a variety of settings and which consists of a broad range of personal health care services including:

1. *Promotion and maintenance of health;*
2. *Prevention of illness and disability;*
3. *Basic care during acute and chronic phases of illness;*
4. *Guidance and counseling of individuals and families; and*
5. *Referral to other health care providers and community resources when appropriate.*

The nurse practitioner practices in a variety of settings such as clinics, health centers, extended care and long-term care facilities, physicians' offices, industries, homes, schools, and acute care settings. A major HEW document on the expanded nursing role delineates extended and expanded functions that are or could be carried out by nurses in primary care, acute care, and long-term care. The major emphasis, in general, has been on services in primary care, defined by that committee as "a person's first contact in any given episode of illness with the health care system that leads to a decision of what must be done to help resolve his problem, and the responsibility for the continuum of care, i.e., maintenance of health, evaluation, and management of symptoms and appropriate referrals.[80]

Within the general framework of the settings and functions cited, nurse practitioners seem to be carving out individualized roles, depending on the needs of a particular community, the legal freedom in that state, and the interests, education, and abilities of the nurse involved.

A HEW-funded, longitudinal study of nurse practitioners, reported in 1977, provides the most current and complete information on NPs' education and practice. One hundred thirty-one certificate-awarding programs and another eighty-four programs granting master's degrees were identified, with a gradual increase of the latter. Most are federally funded, a factor that has stimulated growth. A sample of forty-four institutions offered seventy specialized programs under a variety of designations, including adult nurse practitioner (ANP), community health nurse (CHN), community mental health/psychiatric (CMH-P), community health nurse clinician (CHNC), community nurse specialist (CNS), developmental pediatric nurse practitioner (DPNP), emergency nurse practitioner (ENP), family health practitioner (FHP), family nurse clinician (FNC), family nurse midwife (FNM), family nurse practitioner (FNP), gynecologist/nurse practitioner (GNP), mental health nurse practitioner (MHNP), mental health practitioner (MHP), medical/surgical nurse (MSN), nurse practitioner/midwife (NP/MW), obstetrics/gynecology (OBs/Gyn), pediatric nurse practitioner (PNP), and women's health care (WHC). Certificate programs range from nine to eighteen months; most master's degree programs require two years of study, with the shortest twelve months. Hours of preceptorship with MDs, NPs, or both ranged from 270 to 1440.[81]

The survey of practicing NPs also gives a useful overview.[82] Between 1970 and 1975, 5,656 students had been admitted to NP programs and more than 4,000 graduated. Most were in pediatric, family, and adult NP programs. From a sample of that group it was found that 77.6 percent of the certificate graduates and 53.7 percent of master's graduates were employed, with the highest percentage of employment in the Northeast and lowest in the South. More black than white NPs were employed. Most were working as NPs; the others had joined NP training programs as faculty. There is a great shortage of faculty with appropriate academic credentials plus NP training.

Employment settings varied: more than 63 percent were in ambulatory care settings (private or prepaid group practice, hospital, or community clinics); more than 10 percent were in nonhospital institutions, primarily college and school health programs; 10 percent were in nonhospital community settings (home health or health department agencies and schools of nursing); 7 percent were in hospital practice, and a few were in extended care facilities. Thirty-two percent were located in the inner city and 16.2 percent in rural areas. The majority were employed by physicians, and about 80 percent stated that MDs supervised them.

Probably because of the NPs' expansion into the gray areas between medicine and nursing, especially in the management of disease conditions and the use and interpretation of various diagnostic modes, there has been considerable evaluation of NP performance, acceptance, and cost effectiveness.

Despite justifiable criticism of this research as being largely anecdotal, very specific to certain individuals and frequently done by those involved in their training or employment, almost all the research* shows that NPs have performed at a level comparable to physicians, according to standards of that setting; have provided continuity of care where it had been fragmented; are accepted by consumers; save physician time; and are profitable to some employers, particularly physicians (without comparable financial reward themselves). In some cases, NPs' thoroughness and extensive teaching did not enable them to see as many patients as did MDs, and cost effectiveness was questioned. A few studies have compared NPs with various educational backgrounds, but they have not been definitive. Unfortunately, almost none have evaluated the NP role according to recognized research protocol.

There are several serious problems that interfere with NP practice. The first is the resistance of many physicians who are unfamiliar with and distrustful of nurses in this role, and threatened professionally and economically, particularly when patients other than the poor are involved. Such MDs usually prefer to utilize PAs, if anyone, because PAs are legally under the MDs' supervision and cannot practice independently. Retaliation comes in the form of medical licensing boards harassing NPs and their MD colleagues for, respectively, practicing medicine without a license and aiding and abetting such practice, which can result in loss of license. Although these accusations seldom stand up and are usually not carried through, they sometimes succeed in discouraging NP/MD teams. Some medical boards and associations also lobby against changes in the nurse practice act that would legalize NP practice. Thus, the nurse-physician colleague relationship that is inherent in team

practice is not always present, but more serious is the question of the NPs' right to practice, which will be considered in Chapter 20. A major concern is general lack of reimbursement for services (unless directly under the supervision of the physician). Ironically, HHS funds NP programs through one agency and withholds funding through another (Medicare), except in experimental programs and, to some extent, in approved rural clinics. A few states reimburse (through Medicaid), as do a few private third-party payors. The issue involves nurse autonomy and power, which will be discussed in Chapter 16.

In the following sections, the most common NP roles are discussed in more detail. These roles may vary according to setting, with more or less independence, more or less broadening or narrowing of the role as needed. Sometimes there is a comprehensive role, such as the family nurse practitioner in a health clinic, or the insurance physical examiner. There are many articles and books describing the many NP roles, some of which are listed in the bibliography.

Family Nurse Practitioner

Family nurse practitioners (FNPs) may be functioning alone in clinics in isolated rural areas with only long-distance contact with a physician, in mobile units, in doctors' offices, in urban community health centers, group medical practices, health departments, and hospital outpatient departments, as well as independently. They may be involved in:

1. Management of well children or treatment of their uncomplicated illnesses.
2. Management of uncomplicated maternity patients in the course of pregnancy and the postpartum period.
3. Family planning—counseling and examination.
4. Medical supervision of those patients in a relatively stable phase of their illness, recognizing complications and exacerbations that require physician referral or consultation.

---

*The hundreds of studies reported cannot be listed, but Cohen (bibliography) cites many published in the nursing, medical, and hospital literature.

5. Acute and emergency care as dictated by the situation.

Pediatric Nurse Practitioner

Pediatric nurse practitioners are most likely to function in clinics, doctors' offices, health departments, and group practices. Their activities include (1) management of well children, (2) management of selected common childhood conditions and illnesses, with appropriate referrals when necessary, (3) anticipatory guidance to parents about child rearing and to the child about his needs, (4) health teaching about illnesses, and (5) other counseling.

Adult Nurse Practitioner

The adult nurse practitioner (ANP) role usually includes the care of long-term patients, but may be limited to geriatrics or another specialty. It may also be called medical nurse associate or practitioner. Settings are similar to those of the family nurse practitioner, but are especially out-patient departments, community health centers, and some nursing homes. Responsibilities include:

1. Evaluating history, physical findings, and laboratory data appropriate for patient's illness, making adjustments in drugs, and other therapeutic measures.
2. Aiding patient and family to cope with illness.
3. Utilizing appropriate services to help client solve health-related problems.
4. Taking initiative in providing social, physical, and emotional rehabilitation of the chronically ill when possible.

Obstetric-Gynecologic Nurse Practitioner

Obstetric-gynecologic (OB-Gyn) nurse practitioners may function in similar settings as the other practitioners, but particularly in clinics. They may or may not limit practice to gynecology (depending on the setting and, of course, their education). Among their functions are:

1. Eliciting complete gynecological history and performing breast and pelvic examinations, recognizing abnormalities.
2. Teaching and counseling patients in areas of family planning and general gynecologic health (some insert intra-uterine devices).
3. Detecting venereal disease and counseling patients.
4. Performing cancer screening exams and perhaps other diagnostic tests.

For obstetrics, their functions are:

1. Eliciting complete obstetric history and performing obstetrically oriented examination, recognizing deviations from normal.
2. Performing routine prenatal and post-partum examinations.
3. Counseling patients about normal pregnancy.
4. Checking newborn (in some cases).

In some states the public health nurse in clinics develops and implements a management plan for prenatal care for all "normal" pregnant women, referring those with any abnormality to the physician.

Nurse-Midwife

Although nurse-midwives are sometimes categorized as one of the nurse practitioner roles, the nurse-midwife has been in existence for some time. The first school of nurse-midwifery was started in 1931 in New York City by the Maternity Center Association. According to the American College of Nurse-Midwives:

Nurse-midwifery practice is the independent management of care of essentially normal newborns and women, antepartally, intrapartally, postpartally and/or gynecologically, occurring within a health care system which provides for medical consultation, collaborative management, or referral and is in accord with the Functions, Standards, and Qualifications for Nurse-Midwifery Practice *as defined by the American College of Nurse-Midwives (ACNM).*

A certified nurse-midwife (CNM) is an indi-

vidual educated in the two disciplines of nursing and midwifery, who possesses evidence of certification according to the requirements of the American College of Nurse-Midwives.

Nurse-midwives practice in a variety of settings, where maternity care is given—clinics, doctors' offices, hospitals, and the new birthing centers. Their practice may be interdependent within a health care delivery system, for example, a hospital obstetric service largely staffed by nurse-midwives, where a physician might be a backup as needed. They might also have a formal, written alliance with an obstetrician, or another physician, or a group of physicians who has/have a formal consultative arrangement with an obstetrician-gynecologist. The ACNM states that nurse-midwives practice within the framework of medically approved protocols. The fact that many mothers now seem to prefer a normal/natural birthing process, when there are no potential complications, has brought a resurgence of interest in nurse-midwifery. Ten years ago, few states permitted nurse-midwives to practice, but this new interest has brought about legal changes that permit the nurse-midwife to practice with only a nursing license and ACNM certification or under new nurse-midwifery licensure laws (that also usually require the certification). In the states where nurse-midwives are controlled by the medical practice act, their practice can be arbitrarily limited at the pleasure of that board.

ACNM-approved (accredited) nurse-midwifery programs vary from eight months to two years in length and are usually given by some educational or clinical institution. There are post-RN certificate programs that do not require a baccalaureate degree, but the trend is toward a master's degree. All include theory and practice in prenatal care, management of a patient in labor, normal spontaneous deliveries in the hospital, immediate care of the newborn, care of the postpartum patient, and family planning. After completion of an ACNM-approved program, the nurse-midwife is eligible to take the certi-

fication examination. Licensed registered nurses trained in midwifery in a foreign country may take an approved refresher course or internship and the certifying exam.

Psychiatric-Mental Health Nurse Practitioner

Psychiatric-mental health nurse practitioners function particularly in community mental health centers, including crisis intervention centers, and in interdisciplinary groups, but they frequently carry a private case load in association with physicians, hospitals, or other health care institutions. It is not unusual for them to be called upon to give emergency psychiatric care, and they may specialize in specific areas such as child psychiatry.

The nurse may serve as a therapist in individual or group therapy, participate as a consultant in an interdisciplinary group, and do general mental health and preventive counseling. In many ways the role is similar to that of the clinical specialist in psychiatric nursing, although the latter may tend to function chiefly in subspecialty areas.

Qualifications, Education, and Conditions of Employment. Just what the appropriate educational credentials of a nurse practitioner should be has not really been decided. Probably the eventual decision will be the master's degree, but, just now, NPs prepared in almost any type of structured program will be employed by someone. In some cases, when they are trained on the job, their mobility is limited, without further education. The educational confusion of generic and RN programs teaching assessment skills, certificate, and various degree programs, does nothing for the NP image. One commonality that is gaining acceptance is certification by ANA and/or a specialty organization. Certification for entrance into a specialty provides a certain base line of qualifications, as do legal guidelines, regulations, or the nurse practice act if it is sufficiently specific. Neither is there a clear picture of the conditions of employment, because the situations vary so much. If an employee, the nurse practitioner might expect the same fringe benefits as others on a similar employment level. Salary may or may not be higher than that of another nurse who does not have this additional preparation, as has been discovered by nurses who return to the same place of employment but function in an expanded role. Sometimes it is a matter of individual bargaining. Physicians' assistants who are mostly men (NPs are mostly women) appear to receive higher salaries. However, this is said to be because most PAs work for private MDs and work more than forty-hour weeks.

PRIVATE PRACTICE AND INDEPENDENT PRACTICE

Private practice and independent practice are often used synonymously, but Keller maintains that this misinterprets the nature of activities of private practice and confuses it with practice in the nurse practitioner role. Private practice, she says, "indicates simply that nursing is conducted under the auspices of nurses in solo or group association *and* that the business of that practice belongs to that nurse or those nurses—not to the public, to another profession, or to the government. The responsibilities and delegations of authority are administered within the bounds of said ownership, much as any private duty nurse administers her own practice."[83] However, in a 1973 ANA working paper, the independent practitioner is defined as a "licensed professional nurse who independently contracts with an individual, group, agency, or corporation to provide primary nursing care in a variety of settings," which does not differentiate between NP and non-NP private practice.

This new model of practice is seen as having many advantages; there is one-to-one interaction and continuity of care, maximum participation by nurse and patient, the possibility for consumers to attach more value to

nursing services as distinct from other health services and to recognize that nurses especially can do justice to certain kinds of problems, the chance for the public to exercise more choice in selecting providers of care, and the built-in accountability to the client that is associated with fee-for-service.[84]

A private practice is a business, and setting it up and running it must be a businesslike process or it will not survive. There are basic decisions to be made: what kind of organization should be created (corporation, partnership, for-profit, nonprofit); by whom (nurses and other professionals); to whom; at what fees; what kind and how many employees will be needed; how to get clients (marketing); what about advertising; how to relate to other health professions; where will the services be offered; at what hours; what about telephone counseling and/or home visits (house calls)? Early expenses include lawyers' and accountants' fees, space, furniture, equipment, supplies, telephone, insurance, stationery, postage, flyers or brochures. In 1974, a survey of private practices (called independent practices) reported an initial outlay of between $150 and $15,000 by individuals or groups of nurses starting private practices. Many were undercapitalized to start or were unrealistic about the time it takes to build a practice or the amount of a realistic fee.[85] Repeated obstacles or problems to most were the normal business aspects, employee contracts, salaries, benefits, tax deductions, fee preparation and collection, and the multitude of forms and records that must be kept. When federal or other contracts were involved, still more records were necessary.

What kind of services would nurses offer in private practice? If nurses do not have NP training, the usual services offered are any combination of health teaching and health promotion, home health, professional education (continuing education programs), and consulting. For instance, one nonprofit group started with a free hypertension screening program from which they made no money, but which gave them enough visibility to win a contract to provide health counseling services at a senior citizen center. They also engaged in such diverse activities as acting as preceptors for students in a graduate nursing program and a school of pharmacy and teaching classes in university schools.[86]

Nurse practitioners in private practice may have a backup physician or they may have developed relationships with physicians from whom and to whom referrals are made. Some NPs are in full partnership in a group practice of physicians.[87] These NPs do all the things NPs are legally permitted to do in their state, which may or may not include writing prescriptions. Sometimes these practices are in an urban/suburban area,[88] but frequently they are in rural areas with few physicians available, and the nurse is the only health care provider.[89,90]

Assuming that the nurse does not have legal problems about the scope of practice, a major problem is getting enough patients and reimbursement to earn a living. Many nurses can afford to give only part of their time to the practice because of limited reimbursement and perhaps hold university teaching positions or are subsidized by some organization. Third-party payment is still uncertain and most patients cannot or do not choose to pay an independent practitioner if they can get clinic care which is covered.

Another problem has been individual practice privileges in health care organizations, especially hospitals and nursing homes. What this means basically is the privilege of a nurse not employed by that institution to admit patients and/or write orders for their care or participate in any part of his/her patients' care. The ANA has delineated several levels of appointment privileges and guidelines for appointment. JCAH and AHA have also made statements. For nurses, it is particularly important that the nurse's credentials be reviewed by a *nursing* credentials committee, just as physician's credentials are reviewed by a medical staff committee.

In rural areas where there is no source of health care, the NP may have the same phys-

ical, professional, and psychological problems as physicians—isolation, overwork, and some lack of stimulation. Nevertheless, independent practice provides a degree of professional autonomy that many nurses crave. As one of the first acknowledged independent practitioners stated, ". . . in the twenty-fifth year of my nursing career, I have become professionally free and have removed the impediments to my practice of nursing."[91]

NURSE ANESTHETIST

A certified registered nurse anesthetist (CRNA) is a registered professional nurse who has graduated from an approved school of anesthesia for nurses and has passed the qualifying examination. Lists of approved schools may be obtained from the American Association of Nurse Anesthetists (AANA). The postgraduate course in anesthesia takes about two years, and some programs give courses with credit, which will count toward an advanced college degree. There are also now a few master's degree programs for nurse anesthetists. Most schools of anesthesia charge tuition, but some also pay a monthly stipend.

Anesthetists generally function under the direction of an anesthesiologist (MD), when available, in any setting where anesthesia is given—the operating room, the obstetric department, the inhalation therapy department, the emergency room, or dental offices. Anesthetists provide the patient with preoperative psychological support in many situations, although patient contact in this respect varies according to the setting. In the operating room, oxygen and the appropriate anesthetics, other drugs, and IV solutions are administered while the patient's vital signs and blood loss are carefully monitored. The NA accompanies the patient to the recovery room.[92]

Although salaries equal or exceed other nursing salaries, anesthesia situations are usually considered stressful, the hours may be irregular, and because the service must be covered for twenty-four hours, the anesthetist may be on call in some employment situations. Malpractice (liability) insurance is necessary, sometimes difficult to get, and perhaps fifty times as expensive as that of other nurses. Many men now find this field attractive; the AANA notes that more than 14 percent of the 18,000 plus nurses in this field are men.

NURSE RESEARCHER

For some time nurses have been participating in medical research, often as gatherers of data rather than as researchers. They still do, although some are gaining status as researchers in general health research. Since the 1930s nurses have become more aware of the need for research in nursing, but few were academically prepared to carry it out. At first, most nursing research was directed by social scientists who were concerned with nurses, their attitudes and education. As nurses gained more advanced preparation in the social, physical, and biological sciences, they began to direct and carry out research themselves—first on nursing functions and nursing education, but gradually moving into patient-centered studies of nursing care. A need to develop a knowledge base for nursing and research into nursing practice has also been repeatedly emphasized. Nurses in research may function in a variety of roles, depending on their educational preparation. If the nurse has not had doctoral preparation or research training, working on a research team as research assistant or associate, collecting data or doing a small part of data analysis, may be a start. Fully prepared nurse researchers are in great demand. They may find employment in universities and health institutions or may choose to freelance as consultants. The need is greater than either the supply of qualified nurses or the funds available for research. The majority of nurses with doctoral degrees have taken positions in universities and colleges,

either as professors of nursing or administrators, where they engage in both research and teaching. This is considered a compatible and necessary combination, because they not only increase knowledge of nursing, but train other nurses in research and guide their studies. The need to recruit nursing students early for graduate study and research is important for the development of nursing.

A particularly encouraging trend is the employment of nurse researchers in practice settings, such as medical centers and government. In these positions nurse researchers may have responsibility for studying patients' nursing needs, defining and evaluating patient care effectiveness, setting up testing situations for development of new nursing techniques, equipment, or procedures, acting as advisors or consultants to nurses developing patient research projects, and planning with other disciplines in the improvement of patient care.[93] Nurse researchers may also become research project directors, directors of research institutes, or be full partners in an interdisciplinary research team.

Qualifications and Conditions of Employment. Nurses engaged in research as described here are expected to have research training and ability, and, preferably, a doctoral degree. Personally, they must have the ability to do both creative thinking and to carry through the orderly process of research, which with human beings is seldom static or orderly, and the writing skill to report their findings. Nurses holding university positions earn the same salaries and benefits as other nurse teachers in that setting. Although time may be allotted for research, the funding of this research is often the responsibility of the teacher-researchers, and they must become adept at grantsmanship. There are also nurses hired by universities to head or participate in specific research projects, without teaching responsibilities. These positions are often on a short-term basis and may have been initiated by someone else. Most researchers find that they devote considerable time to their studies, and working hours are often not in a regular forty-hour-a-week framework. This is particularly true if the researcher also has teaching and/or administrative responsibilities.

If employed in a clinical setting, the nurse researcher's salary is probably negotiable, depending on background. Although such positions may be budgeted, there may be very limited budgeting for other personnel, equipment, and so on, needed for specific research projects. Again, funds must be sought from other sources, such as foundations, individuals, or, most frequently, governmental agencies. The availability of these funds has fluctuated, which has been a detriment to nursing research (see Chapter 14).

For nurse researchers, however, the satisfactions are great, both in terms of the personal satisfactions of research and the knowledge that they have made meaningful contributions to the nursing field. With all the opportunities available to nurses with doctoral degrees, it is certain that those engaged in research do so because it is their top preference.

NURSE CONSULTANT

There are professional nurse consultants specializing in all areas of nursing—education, administration, and clinical practice, particularly specialties—who provide assistance to individuals and groups. Because the usual purpose of seeking consultation is to bring about change of some kind, which may be a tension-provoking situation for the consultees, not just specific knowledge, but the ability to understand and communicate in complex human relations situations is especially important. Someone who cannot relate to others in a way appropriate to the situation will not be successful, regardless of expertise. A good consultant must get as clear and accurate a picture of the total situation, attitudes, abilities, and commitment of the people involved, the problems, assets, resources, and other factors that are not al-

ways overtly presented or visible, and have the ability to critique and assist. Because consulting is usually done in a limited time span, the consultees must be stimulated to think productively about what they can and must do to continue the task. There is a difference between giving advice and being a consultant, for the professional role requires the ability to observe, assess, plan, and make accurate judgments and to present them in a way workable for the consultees.[94] Usually consultants are presented with a problem or request to help develop a program or service. The consultant collects data, does a preliminary review, and then an analysis, based on information sent and frequently an on-site visit. The consultee may be given resource materials and a final written report with an analysis of the situation and recommendations for action.

Although many well-prepared nurses in top positions consult apart from their primary jobs (and this kind of prestige is considered desirable by some employers), professional consultants are usually employed in local, state, national, international, private, or governmental agencies and organizations. There are, for instance, consultants with the National League for Nursing, HHS, state health departments, WHO, and private consulting firms, even private businesses, by the nurse and/or a group. In the last case, the facets of business management apply as for nurses in private practice.[95] Fees may be negotiated or set according to specific criteria.

INTERNATIONAL NURSING

The nurse with a taste for adventure and seeing the world may enjoy a position with one of the agencies concerned with nursing in parts of the world outside the United States. Such positions are almost invariably challenging and a little off the beaten track. This nurse has the opportunity of learning to cross cultural barriers and adapt teaching, living, learning, and development as a person appropriately. At the same time, the qualifications are usually high, including special preparation in the area in which the nurse will be working.

World Health Organization

In its early days the World Health Organization asked for nurses to serve chiefly as members of specialized teams concerned with malaria, venereal disease, tuberculosis, and maternal and child health, and such requests are still received from countries. However, the emphasis now is on developing and expanding nursing and midwifery programs, so that more of the available positions are for experienced nurse educators whose duty it is to assist member governments to strengthen health services, develop education and training programs in nursing and midwifery, and plan programs for the control of communicable diseases. Therefore, besides basic qualifications, the candidate must have education and experience appropriate to an assigned post, such as specialization in education, administration, or a clinical specialty. There may also be language requirements. The nurse is paid a basic salary, net of national tax, plus allowances and other benefits. Annual leaves are for six weeks and travel expenses home are paid every two years. Assignments are usually for an initial two years, although short-term consultants are used on occasion. Applications can be obtained from the Chief of Personnel, WHO, Avenue Appia, Geneva, Switzerland, or from the nearest regional WHO office.

The Pan American Health Organization, a regional office of WHO, collaborates with member governments in conducting health improvement programs in the Americas. Many of these programs provide consultation services in nursing service administration, usually as part of a team of physician, engineer, and health educator. Other nursing education positions are advisory for the establishment or strengthening of schools of nursing and for implementation of supplementary training programs in nursing education, public health, midwifery, and preparation of auxiliary personnel. Minimum requirements are a Bachelor of Science degree in nursing, or its equivalent; advanced preparation in public health, education, or administration; substantial and varied experience, including teaching, supervising, or consulting; knowledge of Spanish, Portuguese, and perhaps French (those with all other requirements except language may be considered with the addition of language study). Salary and benefits are generally the same as for other regions covered by WHO. Further information may be obtained at PAHO, 525 23rd St., N.W., Washington, D.C. 20037.

Peace Corps

Since the Peace Corps began in 1961, it has employed both volunteer and staff nurses. Staff nurses serve in many of the sixty Peace Corps countries in the preventive and curative program developed to care for the volunteer. Where once the nurse was primarily a helper to the physician, today Peace Corps nurses (as employees) are responsible for administering and implementing a comprehensive health care program for Peace Corps volunteers living and working in areas of the world where sanitation is inadequate and endemic diseases are common. Their duties include maintaining a preventive health program through inoculation, physical exams, health education, and counseling; providing all primary care for routine illnesses and injuries, utilizing local specialists when possible. (A few Peace Corps physicians may serve as consultants to nurses in three or four adjoining countries.) The nurse maintains an office in the capitol city but travels to rural areas to check on volunteers.

The nurse must be an RN, U.S. citizen, and have appropriate language skills for the country assigned because only a brief exposure to the language is offered, good health, stamina, and, of course, have the appropriate skills to deliver primary care.

Grade and salary are determined according to experience and type of degree held. Housing is provided; there are generous annual leaves and travel to and from the assigned post is paid by the Peace Corps. Each tour of duty is for thirty months and may be extended another thirty months.

As in WHO, Peace Corps volunteer nurses are also primarily engaged in teaching, supervising, or planning positions. However, basic requirements are usually a degree or diploma in nursing, RN registration, and one or two years experience (public health nurses are expected to have a degree). Program training is given. All volunteers serve for two years and receive subsistence allowances that include free transportation, housing, medical care, and forty-eight days paid vacation.

A domestic version of the Peace Corps is VISTA. Volunteers work in those areas in the United States, Puerto Rico, and the Virgin Islands where there are major health problems, such as migrant camps, Indian reservations, inner city or rural areas populated by the poor. Service is usually for one full year after training, with an option to extend service for several months or re-enroll for a second year. ACTION is the federal agency combining the Peace Corps, VISTA, and other voluntary agencies dealing with proverty-related social and economic problems in the United States and developing countries. Further information may be obtained from ACTION, Peace Corps/VISTA, Washington, D.C. 20525.

Project HOPE

The purpose of Project HOPE is to bring the skills and techniques developed by the American health professions to other peoples of the world in their own environment, adapted specifically to their needs and their way of life. HOPE began in 1958, when a prominent Washington, D.C. heart specialist, Dr. William B. Walsh, submitted a plan for the world's first peacetime hospital ship. A reconverted 15,000-ton veteran of two wars consequently became the S.S. HOPE, and Project HOPE was sponsored by the People-to-People Health Foundation, Inc. In 1960 the S.S. HOPE left on her maiden mission to Indonesia and South Vietnam, followed by missions to other countries in various parts of the world; it was retired in 1973. Whereas nurses on the ship's medical staff were highly competent specialists or generalists who worked on a one-to-one basis with host country counterparts in a hospital, the emphasis has shifted. Relatively long-term, land-based programs, always an essential component of Project HOPE, have replaced the ship as the milieu within which HOPE teams carry out their professional activities. Formal educational programs based in hospitals, universities, and other institutions are taking precedence over informal ones in program planning within the host country. As a result, recent recruitment efforts have centered on academically qualified, widely experienced nurses, sensitive to the intricacies of working outside of their own cultural and health care systems. Nurses used to view a position with Project HOPE as a short-term commitment, a once in a lifetime adventure; they are now encouraged to see such service as attractive opportunities for building a career in international health. The philosophy is still to function on a one-to-one basis with all planning, implementing, and evaluating done in collaboration with host country colleagues; HOPE goes only where invited. HOPE is not intended to become a permanent fixture, but continues only as long as a country can benefit from what the project can provide. Although seen as an aid to foreign countries, HOPE also has two projects in the United States, one in Laredo, Texas, and the other on a Navajo Indian reservation in Arizona.

Basic qualifications are listed as:

1. Bachelor's degree in nursing.
2. At least two years professional nursing experience.
3. Formal or informal teaching experience.
4. Ability to establish productive interpersonal relationships in cross-cultural settings.
5. Adaptability to changes in culture, lifestyle, work setting, program plans.

6. Interest and aptitude in learning a foreign language (required in most programs).
7. Interest in problem solving within varying sets of limitations.

Most positions require a two-year commitment, but faculty on sabbatical leave are considered for shorter assignments. Salary depends on the assignment, educational background, and experience of the applicant. Further information can be obtained from Project HOPE, 2233 Wisconsin Avenue, N.W., Washington, D.C. 20007.

OTHER INTERNATIONAL NURSING OPPORTUNITIES

Almost every religious denomination supports some kind of missionary work in foreign countries. Nurses are usually welcomed in such activities because missionary work often includes some form of professional or semiprofessional health care activities. Nurses who select missionary nursing as their life's work must have a strong desire to nurse the sick and underprivileged, often in primitive surroundings; ability to teach religious principles by example, and possibly in religious classes; and knowledge of the language of the people in the regions assigned. They will have many opportunities to teach and sometimes guide citizens and health workers of other lands. Missionary nurses must expect to find their rewards principally in personal satisfaction because positions as missionary nurses usually carry a low salary for long hours of hard work. Nurses can obtain specific information about missionary nursing from their own church. Some mission groups accept volunteers who are not of their own religious faith.

Another major possibility in international nursing is occupational nursing for major industries with overseas branches. On occasion, the governments, universities, hospitals, or industries of foreign countries also seek American nurses with all types of educational preparation. In recent years, Mid-

eastern countries, particularly, have employed recruiters to fill staff and other positions in their hospitals. It is especially important to clarify the role and function, as well as personal living conditions, and to learn about the country, for some American women nurses have found it very difficult to adjust in Moslem countries. Limited opportunities are found with the federal government in countries where federal personnel are stationed, but these positions are first filled by transferring career personnel already in the agency.

In all cases, there are usually advertisements in newspapers or professional journals for these positions. If not, the nurse should make inquiries to the private company concerned or the appropriate federal agency.

OTHER CAREER OPPORTUNITIES

It would probably be impossible, or at least extraordinarily lengthy, to give information about every career possibility available for nurses. A list of specific *positions*, directly related to nursing, not even including specialization or subspecialization, runs into the hundreds when the diverse settings in which nursing is practiced are considered. Overall, these are clinical nursing, administration, education, or research (or a combination of all), but the specific setting brings its own particular challenges. They may require knowledge of another culture and the physical psychosocial needs of these people, such as nursing in an Indian reservation,[96] or a new orientation to practice such as working in an HMO, or in juvenile court,[97] or the prison system,[98] or even camp nursing.[99]

In some cases, specialization or subspecialization, usually requiring additional education and training (because most generic education programs present only a brief exposure), becomes a new career path. There are any number of these, and as each becomes recognized as a distinct subspecialty, involved nurses tend to form a new organization or a subgroup within ANA or some related medical organization to develop standards of practice. For instance, nurses whose major interest is pediatric oncology have, as members of either or both the ANA Division on Maternal and Child Health Practice and Association of Pediatric Oncology Nurses, set standards of practice approved by both groups. There are also more articles in journals and papers given at meetings about nursing in these various areas, so that a practicing specialty nurse can keep abreast of current practice; other nurses may also develop interest in new fields. Specialization and subspecialization are not really new; operating room nurses have been practicing since the beginning of American nursing[100] and coronary care nurses[101] or enterostomal therapists[102] are into their second decade. More recently, there is new emphasis and, consequently, a number of new educational programs in such areas as women's health care,[103,104] family planning,[105] thanatology,[106] and sex education,[107] all of which have an interdisciplinary context that brings additional dimensions to the practice.

When nurses assume positions such as editors of nursing journals, or nursing editors in publishing companies, they draw not only on their nursing background, but must learn about the publishing field and acquire the necessary skills. Editing isn't the same as writing, and the responsibility for putting out a journal or other publication has financial, administrative, legal, philosophical, and policy-making components. In the same vein, nurses employed as lobbyists, labor relations specialists, executive directors or staff of nursing associations, nurse consultants for drug or supply companies, and staff for legislators or governmental committees all use their nursing, but must learn from other disciplines not related to nursing and develop new role concepts. If they choose to maintain a nursing role and orientation as well, nursing is enriched and strengthened; if they abandon all identity with the profession, it may lose valuable input. As health care and nursing expand, some nurses will develop new positions themselves, for which the need and the qualifications cannot now be determined. It seems safe to say, however, that opportunities and challenges in nursing today are practically unlimited.

NURSING SUPPLY AND DEMAND

With all the career opportunities available for nurses, many of them barely emerging, it seems ludicrous to question whether there are too many nurses to fill these positions. However, because so much of nursing education is funded by the federal government, the issue of overproduction seems to arise with each new introduction of the Nurse Training Act. In the 1970s, particularly, attempts by the various Presidents to cut or virtually eliminate funding seemed to escalate. This is not unreasonable in some respects, because the original intent of the NTA (1964) was, in part, to increase the number of nurses (Chapter 19). Since then, the number of nurses has increased tremendously. Does that mean that the shortage has been overcome? By 1974 there were many dire warnings of overproduction of nurses, and it is true that in some geographic areas the job market was relatively tight. (At the same time, foreign nurses were being imported to work in hospitals, with accompanying legal problems.) The federal government engaged the NLN to conduct a study to determine whether new graduates were experiencing difficulty in acquiring positions and contracted with ANA to study the foreign nurse situation. Even before the results were available, there was some evidence that the need for nurses was still not met.

Rather, there was a tendency for some health agencies to "save money" by employing lesser-prepared and, theoretically, less expensive nursing personnel (and fewer of any kind) regardless of need. There was, unquestionably, an unrelenting shortage of nurses prepared at the baccalaureate and higher-degree level, and, overall, a maldistribution of nurses. Poor use of nursing personnel is not new; it is also not resolved. One nurse, not underestimating the employer's problem, also saw a responsibility for nursing.

> Productive change in the system has to start with the values inculcated in nursing education. How do we capture the high motivation, human relatedness, and sense of justice that today's student brings, and channel it to postgraduation employment choices in areas other than affluent ones, for hours other than eight to four, for days other than Monday through Friday? How do we alter the elitism that governs nursing practice? Clearly, any solution to the health manpower problem which fails to explore ways and means of improving distribution and utilization in the broadest sense of these words is doomed to failure.[108]

When the NLN survey was completed, it showed no major changes in the job-seeking experiences of new graduates. Of all new graduates from RN programs, 2.6 percent were not employed but looking for work in 1976, a fraction of a per cent more than in 1972.* However, the figures for PNs had increased from 3 percent to 5.8 percent, a possible indication of the move toward all-RN staffs. A key point made was that the inability of RNs to find work seemed to relate more to personal goals instead of lack of available positions, that is, suitable hours, satisfactory salary, travel distance, desired nursing specialty. As expected, maldistribution of nurses was evident; at the extremes, there was a relatively high shortage in Louisiana and Utah and a low shortage or equilibrium in Vermont and New York.[109] A latter general RN survey from ANA also provided some interesting information, for example, the total numbers of nurses seeking positions was up slightly from 1974 (3 percent versus 2.3 percent), but those nurses having most difficulty finding employment were those who had been in the employ-

ment pool for some time; there were also more nurses seeking part-time than full-time positions.[110] These figures supported other indications that more married women with children, who had been at home, were returning to nursing, at least on a part-time basis. Some of these women were in their fifties and were reactivating licenses that they had allowed to lapse.

The ANA foreign nurse study confirmed problems previously identified: that many foreign nurses recruited to this country had serious difficulties both in language and in practice, and because of these disadvantages were often grossly misused and underpaid. A number of state boards of nursing were already requiring that the state licensing examination be passed before permitting practice, and the failure rate was high. One effect of the ANA report was the formation of the Council of Graduates of Foreign Nursing Schools (CGFNS), which subsequently arranged for foreign nurses to take preliminary qualifying examinations before leaving their country. Regulations by the Immigration and Naturalization Service require that graduates of foreign schools of nursing (except Canada) pass this examination to be eligible for H-1 (occupational preference) visas. This was seen as a protection for both the public and nursing. (See Chapter 20.)

The factors that affect supply and demand in relation to all nursing manpower are currently in a state of flux, as they frequently are. Weighing on one side are the demands of the public—their perceived right to health care and their increased utilization of services. On the other are the overwhelming increase in health care costs and the demands of third-party payors to cut back. In hospitals, the cutbacks have taken a toll on nursing positions, but the shift in funding to HMOs, ambulatory care, and home health care has created a greater demand for nurses in these areas. (Sometimes nurse practitioners are also being employed instead of physicians, either because of a physician shortage or because of the high MD salaries.)

---

*Available 1978 figures showed a drop to 1.9 percent.

Some research has shown that an all-RN staff is less costly and of higher quality than that utilizing LPNs and aides. The latter have been found less cost-effective because of their frequently excessive downtime (including absenteeism and sick time), and their inability, both legally and in terms of knowledge, skill, and judgment, to take independent action, thus requiring RN direction or intervention. Christman advocates (and has implemented) an all-RN staff, who, with the guidance of clinical specialists, meet the therapeutic nursing needs of patients while all-purpose workers, directed by a service supervisor, provide nonclinical comfort services.[111] There is a definite increase in nursing directors who are adopting this hiring pattern, usually within the primary nursing model; there are also some giving preference to baccalaureate graduates. Because all nurse administrators are being pressed to do cost-benefit analyses of nursing services, if the all-RN/primary nursing model data are positive, the demand for RNs may rise; if not, there may again be a tendency to employ the worker whose overt cost is less. At any rate, the serious issue of health care costs will have tremendous impact on utilization of nurses. More than likely, the inevitable passage of some form of comprehensive national health insurance will bring still another measure to the question of supply and demand, involving kinds as well as numbers of nurses needed.

Since 1977 and 1978 figures showed a leveling-off or no-growth status in nursing education, unless there is a sudden return to the profession of the inactive pool of nurses and a major cutback in health services, both of which seem unlikely, there appears *not* to be an oversupply of nurses. However, the entire issue is closely related to the influence and autonomy of nurses. Who decides how many and what kind of nurses are needed where? Who determines what they can or cannot do? Whose advice does the Congress or the administration take when the crucial decisions on nurse education and utilization

are made? The power pendulum has been swinging both to and from nursing. Consider the impact of those outside nursing in influencing these decisions. At a high-level conference on nursing manpower needs and utilization, a variety of prestigious participants, after presenting and critiquing pertinent data, supported increased baccalaureate education and concluded that there was no evidence of any RN oversupply. However, the distinguished economist who had called the conference recommended policy directions in direct opposition to these findings (although admitting that this was only his opinion).[112] Unfortunately, there was some indication that his report, fed into the U.S. Office of Management and Budget, influenced recommendations of major cutbacks in the NTA funding and resulted in President Carter's pocket veto of the NTA.[113] An overwhelming show of nurse power came with the avalanche of organized, well-planned nursing efforts[114] that resulted in newspapers castigating President Carter and the Congress voting to retain most of the 1979 nursing funds that he wished rescinded. However, the battle is not over; manpower planning for nursing personnel continues to be done by non-nurses who look at services delivered from a task orientation, and, too frequently, make recommendations for increases in the lowest level of task-performer, ignoring the need for professional judgment.[115]

Therefore, it is vital for nursing to be involved in and knowledgeable about health manpower planning, particularly in relation to nursing personnel. Several major steps have been taken. The studies undertaken by the Division of Nursing (DHHS) as a result of a mandate in the 1975 Nurse Training Act are expected to have great impact and to be widely utilized. Eight major and rather complex studies undertaken are the WICHE panel of expert consultants; the state model; the national model; an econometric model of the impact of national health insurance; the micro model; supply projections; the ANA sample survey of RNs, and the distribution model.[116]

A unique source of manpower information is HHS' National Health Planning Information Center (NHPIC), which houses, among others, more than 5,000 documents dealing with nursing education and services and nurse manpower planning, resources, and methodologies. This computerized, updated information center contains documents rarely available from other sources, such as theses, federal reports, and local government and association reports. One of the twenty-two depositories in the libraries of large medical centers, nursing schools, and health care organizations is the NLN, which maintains a complete collection of microfiche reproductions of the documents.[117]*

Just how much direct involvement nursing will have in the manpower data game is still undetermined. For various reasons, including the need to centralize all health manpower data, some of these responsibilities have been moved out of the HHS Division of Nursing. Contracts for studies on nurse manpower will go to nursing organizations or groups only if they have the appropriate resources to compete. If they are unable to do so, they begin to be left out of the inner circle of data sources and may also have little input in assuring accuracy. For instance, a simple example is one state survey in which the questionnaire about need for and availability of nurses went to personnel directors of hospitals only (not the director of nursing), and no community agency was included. Yet, the result was used to set manpower policies in that state.

Given the state of the United States economy, federal cutbacks will be an ongoing issue, and nursing must be strong enough and influential enough to hold its own or its potential for serving the public will be severely curtailed.

REFERENCES

1. Aleda Roth et al., *1977 National Sample Survey of Registered Nurses* (Kansas City, MO.: American Nurses' Association, 1979), p. 188.
2. Ibid., pp. 146–158.
3. Ibid., pp. 159–161.
4. American Nurses' Association, *Standards of Nursing Practice* (Kansas City, Mo.: The Association, 1973).
5. Edythe Alexander, *Nursing Administration in the Hospital Health Care System* (St. Louis, Mo.: C. V. Mosby Company, 1978), pp. 230–235.
6. Department of Health, Education, and Welfare, *Toward Quality in Nursing: Report of the Surgeon General's Consultant Group in Nursing* (Washington, D.C. The Department, 1963), p. 19.
7. Gwen Marram et al., *Cost-effectiveness of Primary and Team Nursing* (Wakefield, Ma.: Contemporary Pub., 1976).
8. Ellen Davis and Gladess Crisp, "An Inside Look At Nursing in Outpatient Surgery," *RN*, **42**:38–43 (May 1979).
9. Kathryn Morrow, "Specialize in General Nursing—On An 'Overnight' Unit," *Nursing 79*, **9**:122, 124, 126 (May 1979).
10. Loy Wiley, "Should You Join Rent-A-Nurse for Temporary Service?" *Nursing 76*, **6**:81–88 (Sept. 1976).
11. Dorothy Johnson, Joan Wilcox, and Harriet Moidel, "The Clinical Specialist as a Practitioner," *Am. J. Nurse*, **67**:2298–2303 (Nov. 1967).
12. Rachel Ayers, "Effects and Role Development of the Clinical Nurse Specialist," in *The Clinical Nurse Specialist and Improvement of Nursing Practice*, edited by Geraldine Padilla. Special issue. *Nurs. Digest*, **6**:14–21 (Winter 1979).
13. Helen Donovan, "The Clinical Specialist—Where Does She Fit?" *Supervisor Nurse*, **1**:35 (July 1970).
14. Esther Lucile Brown, *Nursing Reconsidered, a Study of Change* (Philadel-

---

*Use of the data file can be arranged through the Librarian/Records Manager of the NLN Central Files. The center may be utilized by writing to National Health Planning Information Center, Attn.: Nursing Information Center, P.O. Box 1600, Prince Georges Plaza Branch, Hyattsville, Md. 20788, or by calling (301) 927-6410.

phia: J. B. Lippincott Company, 1970), p. 68.

15. American Nurses' Association, *Roles, Responsibilities, and Qualifications for Nurse Administrators* (Kansas City, Mo.: The Association, 1978).

16. Elmira Mary Price, *Learning Needs of Registered Nurses* (New York: Teachers College, Columbia University, 1967), pp. 65–66.

17. Joan Ganong and Warren Ganong, "Are Head Nurses Obsolete?" *J. of Nurs. Admin.,* 5:16–18 (Sept. 1975).

18. Barbara Stevens, "The Problem in Nursing's Middle Management," *J. of Nurs. Admin.,* 2:35–38 (Sept./Oct. 1972).

19. ANA, op. cit., p. 6.

20. American Nurses' Association, *The Position, Role and Qualifications of the Administrator of Nursing Service* (New York: The Association, 1969).

21. American Hospital Association, *Statement on the Position of the Administration of the Department of Nursing Service in Hospitals* (Chicago: The Association, 1971).

22. Ibid., p. 3.

23. Myrtle Aydelotte, *Survey of Hospital Nursing Services* (New York: National League for Nurses, 1968), pp. 4–6.

24. Pam Arnold, "Nurse Administrators Profiled: Big Job, Low Pay," *Am. Nurse,* 7:2 (Apr. 1975).

25. *Roles, Responsibilities and Qualifications for Nurse Administrators,* op. cit., p. 4.

26. Alice Behrens, "The Pleasures and Problems of the Director of Nursing in a Small Hospital," *J. of Nurs. Admin.,* 5:311–334 (Feb. 1975).

27. Juliana Manez, "The Untraditional Nurse Manager: Agent of Change and Changing Agent," *Hospitals,* 52:62–65 (Jan. 1, 1978).

28. *The Position, Role and Qualifications,* op. cit.

29. *Roles, Responsibilities and Qualifications for Nurse Administrators,* op. cit., p. 14.

30. *Toward Quality in Nursing,* op. cit., p. 19.

31. AHA, op. cit.

32. Lucie Young, "Room at the Top—A

33. Place for Nurse Administrators," *J. of Nurs. Admin.,* 11:85 (Nov./Dec. 1972).

33. Agnes Flaherty, "Nursing Service Administrators: Group is Key in Delivery of Health Care," *Am. Nurse,* 7:1, 16 (Apr. 1975).

34. Dorothy del Bueno, "Organizing and Staffing the Inservice Department," *J. of Nurs. Admin.,* 6:12–13 (Dec. 1976).

35. Dorothy del Bueno, "No More Wednesday Matinees," *Nurs. Outlook,* 24:359–361 (June 1976).

36. Katherine Chavigny, "Nurse Epidemiologist in the Hospital," *Am. J. Nurs.,* 75:638–642 (Apr. 1975).

37. Pascal Imperato, et al., "The New York City Nurse-Epidemiology Program," *Bull. N.Y. Acad. Med.,* 53:569–585 (Aug. 1977).

38. Robyn Ravgiala, "A New Role for Nursing: Project Director," *J. Nurs. Admin.,* 9:22–24 (May 1979).

39. Phyllis Schaeffer, "The Utilization Review Coordinator: A Different Kind of Nurse," *Nurs. 76,* 6:95–98 (Feb. 1976).

40. June Orme and Rosemary Lendbeck, "Nurse Participation in Medical Peer Review," *Nurs. Outlook,* 22:27–30 (Jan. 1974).

41. Am. Nurses' Assn., *The Professional Nurse and Health Education* (Kansas City, Mo.: The Association, 1975).

42. Terry Alexander-Rodriguez, "Could Prison Nursing Be the Specialty for You?" *Nurs. 78,* 8:94–97 (Mar. 1978).

43. Ruth Stryker, "What Should the Long-Term Care Director of Nursing Really Do?" *J. of Nurs. Admin.,* 5:79–80 (Sept. 1975).

44. Ruth Stryker, "How Does Nursing Home Administration Differ from Hospital Administration?" *J. of Nurs. Admin.,* 75:16–17 (May 1975).

45. Ginette Pepper, et al., "Geriatric Nurse Practitioner in Nursing Homes," *Am. J. Nurs.,* 76:62–64 (Jan. 1976).

46. Carolyn Williams, "Community Health Nursing—What Is It?" *Nurs. Outlook,* 25:250–254 (Apr. 1977).

47. Clarence Skrovan, et al., "Community Nurse Practitioner—An Emerging Role," *Am. J. Pub. H.,* 64:847–885 (Sept. 1974).

48. Am. Nurses' Assn., *Standards: Com-*

munity Health Nursing Practice (Kansas City, Mo.: The Association, 1973).

49. *Concepts of Community Health Nursing Practice* (Kansas City, Mo.: ANA Division on Community Health Nursing Practice, 1975).

50. Council of Home Health Agencies and Community Health Services, *Characteristics of the Home Health Agency Administrator* (New York: National League for Nursing, 1977).

51. Henrietta Bernal, "Levels of Practice in a Community Health Agency," *Nurs. Outlook,* **26**:364–369 (June 1978).

52. Diana Brinton, "Value Differences Between Nurses and Low-Income Families," *Nurs. Res.,* **21**:46–59 (Jan./Feb. 1972).

53. Jane La Fargare, "Role of Prejudice in Rejection of Health Care," *Nurs. Res.,* 21:53–58 (Jan./Feb. 1972).

54. Department of School Nurses, NEA, *Platform and Policy Statements* (Washington, D.C.: The Association, 1974).

55. Am. Nurses' Assn., *Facts About Nursing, '76–'77* (Kansas City, Mo.: The Association, 1977), p. 13.

56. National League for Nursing, *Nursing Data Book* (New York: The League, 1979), p. 55.

57. National League for Nursing, *Nurse Faculty Census 1976* (New York: The League, 1977).

58. *Nursing Data Book,* op. cit., p. 58.

59. *Nurse Faculty Census,* op. cit.

60. *Nursing Data Book,* op. cit., p. 58.

61. Luther Christman, "The Practitioner Teacher," *Nurse Educator,* **4**:8–11 (Mar./Apr. 1979).

62. John Riley, et al., *The Student Looks at His Teacher* (New Brunswick, N.J.: Rutgers University Press, 1950).

63. Myrlene Kiker, "Characteristics of the Effective Teacher," *Nurs. Outlook,* **21**:721–723 (Nov. 1973).

64. Milton Hildebrand, "The Character and Skills of the Effective Professor," *J. Higher Educ.,* **14**:46–47 (Jan. 1973).

65. Glendola Nash, "Faculty Evaluation," *Nurse Educator,* **2**:9–13 (Nov./Dec. 1977).

66. Shake Ketefian, "A Paradigm for Faculty Evaluation," *Nurs. Outlook,* **25**:718–720 (Nov. 1977).

67. Juanita Murphy, "Tenure: Achieved or Ascribed," *Nurs. Outlook,* **26**:176–179 (Mar. 1978).

68. Joyce Foster, "Tenure: Process and Procedures," *Nurs. Outlook,* **26**:179–181 (Mar. 1978).

69. Shirley Seyfried et al., "Factors Influencing Faculty Choice of Position," *Nurs. Outlook,* **25**:692–696 (Nov. 1977).

70. Karen Nishio, "The Right and the Qualified," *Nurs. Outlook,* **25**:713–717 (Nov. 1977).

71. Nicholas Ashford, *Summary of Crisis in the Workplace: Occupational Disease and Injury (A Report to the Ford Foundation)* (Cambridge, Ma.: M.I.T. Press, 1975).

72. American Association of Occupational Health Nurses, *Guide for Development of Functions and Responsibilities in Occupational Health Nursing* (New York: The Association, 1977), p. 4.

73. M. L. Brown and M. L. Bauer, *Occupational Health Nurse: An Initial Survey* (Washington, D.C.: Department of Health, Education and Welfare, PHS Division of Occupational Health, 1966).

74. Irene A. Murchison, "Role of Law in the Decision-Making Process in Occupational Health Nursing," *Occup. Health Nurs.,* **21**:15 (July 1973).

75. *Facts About Nursing, '76–'77,* op. cit., p. 13.

76. Helen Tirpak, "The Frontier Nursing Service—Fifty Years in the Mountains," *Nurs. Outlook,* **23**:308–310 (May 1975).

77. Charles Lewis and Barbara Resnik, "Nurse Clinics and Progressive Ambulatory Patient Care," *New Engl. J. Med.,* **277**:1236–1241 (Dec. 1967).

78. Loretta Ford and Henry Silver, "The Expanded Role of the Nurse in Child Care," *Nurs. Outlook,* **15**:43–45 (Sept. 1967).

79. "A Role By Any Name," *Nurs. Outlook,* **22**:89 (Feb. 1974).

80. Department of Health, Education and Welfare, *Extending the Scope of Nursing Practice* (Washington, D.C.: The Department, Nov. 1971), pp. 8–12.

81. Vivian Hedrick, "A National Survey: Educating for the Expanded Role," *Nurse Practitioner,* **3**:13–16 (Jan./Feb. 1978).

82. Eugene Levine, "What Do We Know About Nurse Practitioners?" *Am. J. Nurs.,* **77**:1799–1803 (Nov. 1977).

83. Nancy Keller, "The Why's and What's of Private Practice," *J. Nurs. Admin.,* **5**:15 (Mar./Apr. 1975).

84. Ibid.

85. Betty Agree, "Beginning an Independent Nursing Practice," *Am. J. Nurs.,* **74**:636–642 (Apr. 1974).

86. Sarah Archer and Ruth Fleshman, "Doing Our Own Thing: Community Health Nurses in Independent Practice," *J. of Nurs. Admin.,* **8**:44–51 (Nov. 1978).

87. Rosanne Wille, "Sharing Responsibilities and Rewards As A Nurse Associate in a Group Practice," *Nurs. 79,* **9**:120–124 (Apr. 1979).

88. Rothlyn Zahourek, et al., *Creative Health Services—A Model for Group Nursing Practice* (St. Louis, Mo.: C. V. Mosby Company, 1976).

89. John Edwards, et al., "The Cambridge-Council Concept, or Two Nurse Practitioners Make Good," *Am. J. Nurs.,* **72**:460–465 (Mar. 1972).

90. Robert Oseasohn, et al., "Primary Care by a Nurse Practitioner in a Rural Clinic," *Am. J. Nurs.,* **75**:267–271 (Feb. 1975).

91. M. Lucille Kinlein, "Independent Nurse Practitioner," *Nurs. Outlook,* **20**:22–25 (Jan. 1972).

92. Betty Smith, "Should You Become a Nurse Anesthetist?" *Nurs. 77,* **7**:108–111 (Nov. 1977).

93. Susan Steckel, "If You Want to Make a Positive Difference in Nursing, Become a Nurse Researcher," *Nurs. 78,* **8**:78–80 (July 1978).

94. Jo Anna De Meyer, "A Nurse Consultant in Action," *J. Nurs. Admin.,* **2**:42–45 (Mar./Apr. 1972).

95. Catherine Norris, "A Few Notes on Consultation in Nursing," *Nurs. Outlook,* **25**:756–761 (Dec. 1977).

96. Martha Primeaux, "Caring for the American Indian Patient," *Am. J. Nurs.,* **77**:91–94 (Jan. 1977).

97. Mary de Chesnay, "Do You Want to Help Troubled Teen-Agers? Be a Juvenile Court Nurse," *Nurs. 76,* **6**:80–83 (Oct. 1976).

98. Terry Alexander-Rodriguez, "Could Prison Nursing Be the Specialty for You?" *Nurs. 78,* **8**:94–97 (Mar. 1978).

99. Hollis Backman et al., "Camp Nursing: An Opportunity for Independent Practice in a Miniature Community," *MCN,* **1**:88–92 (Mar./Apr. 1976).

100. Margaret Fay, "The Challenge of O.R. Nursing," *Nurs. 77,* **7**:98–100 (Oct. 1977).

101. Frances Storlie, "Do You Want to Specialize in CCU Nursing?" *Nurs. 78,* **8**:71–76 (Jan. 1978).

102. Jacqueline Lamanske, "Want to Specialize? Consider Becoming an Enterostomal Therapist," *Nurs. 77,* **7**:94–96 (Apr. 1977).

103. Jean Colls, "Want to Specialize? Consider Becoming a Women's Health-Care Nurse Practitioner," *Nurs. 77,* **7**:72–74 (Jan. 1977).

104. Donald Ostergard et al., "Training and Functions of a Women's Health-Care Specialist, A Physician's Assistant, A Nurse Practitioner in Obstetrics and Gynecology," *Am. J. Obs. & Gyn.,* **121**:1029–1037 (Apr. 1975).

105. Miriam Manisoff et al., "The Family Planning Nurse Practitioner: Concepts and Results of Training," *Am. J. Pub. Health,* **66**:62–66 (Jan. 1976).

106. Joy Ufema, "Do You Have What It Takes To Be A Nurse Thanatologist?" *Nurs. 77,* **7**:96–99 (May 1977).

107. Beverly Henshaw, "Providing Patient Care As A Sex Educator," *Nurs. 79,* **9**:78–80 (June 1979).

108. Sister Bernadetta Armiger, "Nursing Shortage or Unemployment?" *Nurs. Outlook,* **21**:315 (May 1973).

109. Walter Johnson, "Supply and Current Demand for Nurses in Light of a Survey of Newly Licensed Nurses," in *Nursing Personnel and the Changing Health Care System,* Michael Millman, ed. (Cambridge, Ma.: Ballinger Publishing Co., 1978), pp. 153–187.

110. Aleda Roth et al., *1977 National Sample*

Survey of Registered Nurses (Kansas City, Mo.: American Nurses' Association, 1979).

111. Luther Christman, "On the Horizon: The All-R.N. Nursing Staff," *Nurs. Digest,* 2:27–29 (Oct. 1974).
112. Eli Ginzberg, "Policy Directions" in *Nursing Personnel and the Changing Health Care System,* Michael Millman, ed. (Cambridge, Ma.: Ballinger Publishing Co., 1978), pp. 265–272.
113. Lucie Young Kelly, "End Paper: The Data Game," *Nurs. Outlook,* **26**:728 (Nov. 1978).
114. "Nursing Shortage? Yes!" *Am. J. Nurs.,* **79**:469–480 (Mar. 1979).
115. Timothy Keaveny and Roger Hayden, "Manpower Planning for Nurse Personnel," *Am. J. Pub. Health,* **68**:656–661 (July 1978).
116. "NLN Newsmaker," *NLN News,* **26**:4,8 (Feb. 1978).
117. "New Service Offers Access to Health Planning Data," *NLN News,* **27**:4 (Feb. 1979).

BIBLIOGRAPHY

Aiken, Linda. "Primary Care: The Challenge for Nursing." *Am. J. Nurs.,* **77** (Nov. 1977), 1828–1832. Excellent delineation of reasons that primary care should be encouraged.

ANA Guidelines for Appointment of Nurses for Individual Practice Privileges in Health Care Organizations. Kansas City, Mo.: The Association, 1978.

Anders, Robert. "Matrix Organization: An Alternative for Clinical Specialists." *J. Nurs. Admin.,* **75** (June 1975), 11–14. Particularly interesting description of matrix organization.

Anders, Robert. "Program Consultation by a Clinical Specialist." *J. Nurs. Admin.,* **8** (Nov. 1978), 34. Discusses implementation of a program of consultation for abortion patients by a psychiatric clinical specialist.

Anderson, Margaret, and Mary Jean Denyes. "A Ladder for Clinical Advancement in Nursing Practice: Implementation." *J. Nurs. Admin.,* **5** (Feb. 1975), 16–22. Development of Zimmer's model; includes process, position descriptions, evaluation.

Aradine, Carolyn, and Mary Denyes. "Activities and Pressures of Clinical Nurse Specialists." *Nurs. Res.,* **21** (Sep./Oct. 1972), 411–418. Practicing clinical specialists identify 122 activities and 59 pressures. At first, concentration was in patient care and personal growth; later, community activities, consultation, and education were included.

Armington, Catherine, et al. "Student Evaluation —Threat or Incentive." *Nurs. Outlook,* **20** (Dec. 1972), 789–792. The demand of university nursing students for the right to evaluate teachers resulted in a project to do so. Results indicated that characteristics of a good teacher as cited by these students are similar to those cited in earlier studies, which are also reviewed.

Auld, Margaret, and Grace Ann Ehlke. "What Camp Nurses Need to Know." *Am. J. Nurs.,* **74** (Apr. 1974), 662–663. A survey of camp nurses gives demographic data and the need for additional preparation in terms of both knowledge and performance skills.

Aynes, Edith. *From Nightingale to Eagle: An Army Nurse's History.* Englewood Cliffs, N.J.: Prentice-Hall, Inc., 1973. A controversial, readable book in which the author reflects on past and present problems of nursing chiefly as they relate to nursing education and the Army Nurse Corps.

Backsheider, Joan. "The Clinical Specialist as a Practitioner." *Nurs. Forum,* **10** (Fall 1971), 359–377. A study determining functions of clinical specialists, relationships with staff, and needed education as seen by these clinicians.

Barckley, Virginia. "Cancer Consultant to Nursing Homes." *Am. J. Nurs.,* **70** (Apr. 1970), 804–806. Description of responsibilities of a nurse working for the American Cancer Society who provides consultation, in-service education, and other assistance to nursing home personnel.

Barnett, Sandra and Pati Sellers. "Neonatal Critical Care Nurse Practitioner: A New Role in Neonatalology." *MCN* **4** (Sep./Oct. 1979) 279–280. What this specialist does and the education needed.

Barrett, Jean. "The Nurse Specialist Practitioner: A Study," *Nurs. Outlook,* **20** (Aug. 1972), 524–527. Reports on evolving role and evaluation of clinical specialists who have 24-hour responsibility for patients, give direct care, supervise staff, and maintain a colleague relationship with physicians.

Bates, Barbara. "Doctor and Nurse: Changing Roles and Relationships." *AORN J.,* **15** (Jan.

1972), 53-62. A physician working closely with a nurse practitioner program reviews the literature relevant to these changing roles and relationships and offers a conceptual framework to aid in understanding them. Extensive, valuable bibliography. Similar article in: *N. Engl. J. Med.*, **283** (July 16, 1970), 129-134.

Bellaire, Judith. "School Nurse Practitioner Program." *Am. J. Nurs.*, **71** (Nov. 1971), 2192-2194. Description of program to expand role of school nurse and activities carried out.

Billings, Gloria. "NHSC Carries Health Care to the Community." *Am. J. Nurs.*, **72** (Oct. 1972), 1836-1838. Description of the National Health Service Corps as it brings health services to communities lacking them and helps them set up their own.

Bliss, Ann, and Eva Cohen, Eds. *The New Health Professionals*. Germantown, Md.: Aspen Systems Corp., 1977. Includes papers on both nurse practitioners and physicians' assistants.

Browne, Helen, and Gertrude Isaacs. "The Frontier Nursing Service: The Primary Care Nurse in the Community Hospital." *Am. J. Obstet. & Gynec.*, **124** (Jan. 1976), 14-17. How FNS nurses combine services in the hospital and home. Abridged version in *Nurs. Digest*, **5** (Spring 1977), 71-73.

Browning, Mary, and Edith Lewis, Eds. *The Expanded Role of the Nurse*. New York: American Journal of Nursing Co., 1973. A compilation of articles on concepts, education, role, and settings of nurse practitioners. Includes section on physicians' assistants.

Bullough, Bonnie. "Is the Nurse Practitioner Role a Source of Increased Work Satisfaction?" *Nurs. Res.*, **23** (Jan./Feb. 1974), 14-19. Results of questionnaire given to various groups of nurses showed that pediatric nurse practitioners rated highest, both in intrinsic and overall job satisfaction. However, more RNs without specialized training were satisfied with their choice of career. Underlying causes are explored.

Burkeen, Oleta. "The Nurse and Industrial Hygiene." *Occ. Health Nurs.*, **25** (Apr. 1976), 7-10. Spells out specific industrial hygiene-related nurse functions.

Burkeen, Oleta. "The Role of the Occupational Health Nurse in Performing Health Examinations." *Occup. Health Nurs.*, **21** (May 1972), 22-26. This study showed that a number of occupational health nurses were placed in extended-role positions with little preparation. Recommendations are made in relation to the role of the nurse in these settings.

Burkett, Gary, et al. "A Comparative Study of Physicians' and Nurses' Conceptions of the Role of the Nurse Practitioner." *Am. J. Pub. Health*, **68** (Nov. 1978), 1090-1096. Significant differences shown between MD and NP perceptions of nurse autonomy. Good references.

Burnett, Imodale, and Gary Walsh. "Caring for Single-Room Occupancy Tenants." *Am. J. Nurs.*, **73** (Oct. 1973), 1752-1756. Describes the program of a multiagency, multidisciplinary team caring for individuals in single-room occupancy settings in New York City.

Burosh, Phyllis. "Physicians' Attitudes Toward Nurse-Midwives." *Nurs. Outlook*, **23** (July 1975), 435-456. MDs seem more willing to accept concept of well-trained graduate maternity nurse than nurse-midwife.

Cahill, Imogene. "The Faculty Subculture in the University." *Nurs. Forum*, **12** (Summer 1973), 218-236. A description of a college faculty as a subculture, including images, self-images, value system, relationships, customs, and activities.

Carter, A. B. "Rural Emergency Psychiatric Services." *Am. J. Nurs.*, **73** (May 1973), 868-869. Crisis intervention is provided via phone or field visit at all times by psychiatric emergency personnel.

Castiglia, Patricia, et al. "The Development and Operation of a Professional Nursing Corporation." *MCN* **4** (July/Aug. 1979) 205-208. How four nurses started a child health nursing group practice.

Castle, Mary. "Help Stamp Out Infections: Be An Infection Control Coordinator." *Nurs. 76*, **6** (Sept. 1976), 90-95. Explains role.

Charney, Evan, and Harriet Kitzman. "The Child-Health Nurse (Pediatric Nurse Practitioner) in Private Practice." *N. Engl. J. Med.*, **238** (Dec. 9, 1971), 1353-1358. Evaluation of PNP-MD practice shows team practice gives as good care as pediatrician alone and is accepted by parents and other professionals.

Cipolla, Josephine, and Gilbeart Collings. "Nurse Clinicians in Industry." *Am. J. Nurs.*, **71** (Aug. 1971), 1530-1534. Description of program to prepare nurse clinicians and their function in an individual setting.

Ciske, Karen. "Accountability—The Essence of Primary Nursing." *Am. J. Nurs.*, **79** (May

1979), 890-894. Excellent article stressing basic concepts of primary nursing.

Claiborn, Stephen, and William Walton. "Pediatricians' Acceptance of PNPs." *Am. J. Nurs.*, **79** (Feb. 1979) 300. Survey of Texas pediatricians shows approval by two-thirds, but with limits.

Cohen, Eva, et al. *An Evaluation of Policy-Related Research on New and Expanded Roles of Health Workers.* New Haven, Ct.: Yale University School of Medicine, 1974. Excellent summary of NP/PA research done until that time. Companion volume has extensive annotated bibliography.

Colavecchio, Ruth, et al. "A Clinical Ladder for Nursing Practice." *J. Nurs. Admin.*, **4** (Sept./Oct. 1974), 54-58. Describes behaviorally stated clinical steps of four levels to reward nurse competence, knowledge, and performance.

Collins, Theodora. "Recovery Room Nursing Is a Clinical Specialty." *RN*, **36** (Nov. 1973), 43-50. A description of the nurse's work in the recovery room, qualifications needed, and problems encountered.

Daeffler, Reidun. "Patients' Perception of Care Under Team and Primary Nursing." *J. Nurs. Admin.*, **5** (Mar./Apr. 1975), 20-26. Primary nursing is preferred; weaknesses described and recommendations made.

Danon, Ardis. "Organizing an Abortion Service." *Nurs. Outlook*, **21** (July 1973), 460-464. A nurse writes of the planning and specific organization of an abortion service to provide the patient with psychosocial support as well as physical safety.

Davis, Marcella, Marlene Kramer, and Anselm Strauss, Eds. *Nurses In Practice: A Perspective on Work Environments.* St. Louis, Mo.: C. V. Mosby Company, 1975. Extremely interesting series of vignettes of real nurses practicing in various settings as seen by field researchers.

Denman, Dorothy and George Kavira. "The Essentials of Supervision." *Sup. Nurs*, **5** (Oct. 1974), 46-51. Discusses leadership, authority, aspects of evaluation.

Edwards, Linda, and Eunice Kelly. "A Three-Level School Health Program." *Nurs. Outlook*, **25** (June 1977), 388-391. Local health department offers schools choice of services to meet their needs.

Felton, Geraldene. "Clinical Specialist Preparation for the Nurse Anesthetist." *Nurs. Outlook*,

20 (Sept. 1972), 597-598. Description of a master's program for preparation of the nurse anesthetist.

Fennal, Mildred. "Becoming a CCU Nurse." *Am. J. Nurs.*, **73** (Sept. 1973), 1540-1543. A nurse's description of orientation and adjustment to a coronary care unit.

Ford, Loretta. "A Nurse for All Settings: The Nurse Practitioner." *Nurs. Outlook*, **27** (Aug. 1979), 516-521. NP practice is firmly established says author. Now research is needed to study its present and future impact.

Ford, Loretta. "Opportunities and Obstacles in Occupational Health Nursing." *Occup. Health Nurs.*, **21** (July 1973) 9-14. Nurse educator projects the role of the occupational health nurse as nurse practitioner.

Ford, Loretta, and Henry Silver. "The Expanded Role of the Nurse in Child Care." *Nurs. Outlook*, **15** (Sept. 1967), 43-45. The earliest PNP program directors describe how these nurses make independent judgments in giving comprehensive care to children.

French, Jean. "This I Believe—About Community Nursing in the Future." *Nurs. Outlook*, **19** (Mar. 1971), 173-175. An expert sees future community nurses making more independent judgments, requiring a new direction in education, and becoming involved in research.

Garrison, Roger. "What's Different About Community College Teaching?" *Nurs. Outlook*, **19** (Sept. 1971), 584-586. Concern of one community college educator that these colleges and their faculty are tending to conform instead of being innovative.

Gaspard, Nancy. "Director of Nursing in a Comprehensive Health Center." *Nurs. Outlook*, **19** (Sept. 1971), 590-591. Profile of individuals in this position, including education, experience, problems, responsibilities, and concerns.

Gerhart, M. E. "Competencies of Nursing Directors in Junior Colleges." *J. Nurs. Educ.*, **12** (Apr. 1973), 2-5. This survey indicated that these directors should have knowledge of junior college philosophy, ability to evaluate teachers, knowledge of nursing, and provide continuous enthusiastic support to the nursing program.

Goldsmith, Seth, et al. "Obstetricians' Attitudes Toward Nurse-Midwives." *Am. J. Obstet. & Gynec.*, **111** (Sept. 1, 1971), 111-118. Shows MDs in Maryland generally have negative attitude toward midwives' technical competence.

Also shows differences in attitudes of those who have had prior experiences with nurse-midwives.

Greenidge, Jocelyn, Ann Zimmern, and Mary Kohnke. "Community Nurse Practitioner—A Partnership." *Nurs. Outlook*, **21** (Apr. 1973), 228-231. Three nurses who developed an independent group practice in New York City tell how they set it up, response from the community, and problems.

Harris, Shirlene. "A Model Unit for Baccalaureate RNs." *Hospitals*, **48** (Mar. 1974), 79-84 ff. Describes the development of a decentralized unit that lets recent baccalaureate degree nurses give the bedside care they were taught to give. Results indicate better nursing care and increased job satisfaction.

Herzog, Eric. "The Underutilization of Nurse Practitioners in Ambulatory Care." *Nurse Pract.*, **1** (Sept./Oct. 1976), 26-28. Describes studies showing underutilization, studies explaining why, and approaches to closing the gap.

Hildebrand, Milton. "The Character and Skills of the Effective Professor." *J. Higher Educ.*, **14** (Jan. 1973), 41-50. Reviews a study designed to identify and describe effective teaching. Fifty-five characteristics are noted, discriminating between the best and worst teacher as seen by students.

Holly, Helen. "Jail Matron, R.N." *Am. J. Nurs.*, **72** (Sept. 1972), 1620-1623. Describes the medical and nursing problems in a county jail and the role of a nurse in this setting.

Hutchison, Margaret. "Efficient Occupational Health Service Management." *Occ. Health Nurs.*, **25** (Feb. 1976), 7-9. Good description of role of occupational health nurse.

Igoe, Judith Bellaire. "The School Nurse Practitioner." *Nurs. Outlook*, **23** (June 1975), 381-384. Describes roles of school nurse practitioner.

Isler, Charlotte. "Bright Future for OBG Nursing." *RN*, **37** (Jan. 1974), 31-37. Describes new approaches, facilities, and techniques in OBG nursing; includes advances at specific institutions.

Jelinek, Darlene. "The Longitudinal Study of Nurse Practitioners: Report of Phase II." *Nurse Pract.*, **3** (Jan./Feb. 1978), 17-19. National study of NPs, including demographic data.

Johnson, Nancy. "The Professional-Bureaucratic Conflict." *J. Nurs. Admin.*, **1** (May/June 1971), 31-39. A study of three hospitals reveals the degree and kind of conflict experienced by supervisors and head nurses and suggests the need for reorganization of the nursing departments to enhance their professional functioning.

Jordan, Judith. "The Nurse Practitioner in a Group Practice." *Am. J. Nurs.*, **74** (Aug. 1974), 1447-1449. Nurse describes role working with diabetics and explains why she considers herself an NP, even though without advanced education.

Keith, Pat. "The Preliminary Investigation of the Role of the Public Health Nurse In Evaluation of Services for the Aged." *Am. J. Pub. Health*, **66** (Apr. 1976), 379-380. Lists services both PHNs and elderly rank as most important.

Kiker, Myrlene. "Characteristics of the Effective Teacher." *Nurs. Outlook*, **21** (Nov. 1973), 721-723. Concepts of the effective teacher as seen by undergraduate and graduate students. Includes teaching characteristics, personal attributes, and relationships with students.

Kron, Thora. "Team Nursing—How Viable Is It Today?" *J. Nurs. Admin.*, **1** (Nov./Dec. 1971), 19-22. A new look at team nursing, describing the basic concepts that make it viable. Written by one of the experts on team nursing.

Kubala, Stephanie, and Linda Clever. "Acceptance of the Nurse Practitioner." *Am. J. Nurs.*, **74** (Mar. 1972), 451-452. Study shows that patients do not always accept NPs but that this can be overcome.

Levine, Jules, et al. "The Nurse Practitioner: Role, Physician Utilization, Patient Acceptance." *Nurs. Res.*, **27** (July/August 1978), 245-254. Comprehensive study of NPs from Virginia provides good data.

Lewis, Charles, and Barbara Resnik. "Nurse Clinics and Progressive Ambulatory Patient Care." *New Engl. J. Med.*, **277** (Dec. 1967), 1236-1241. One of the first articles describing expanded role of nurse. Includes evaluation of activities and success of program.

Lewis, Edith, and Mary Browning, Eds. *The Nurse in Community Mental Health*. New York: American Journal of Nursing Co., 1972. A compilation of articles from *Am. J. Nurs.* and *Nurs. Outlook* on the various components of nursing in community mental health.

Little, Marilyn. "Physicians' Attitudes Toward Employment of Nurse Practitioners." *Nurse*

Pract., **3** (July/August 1978), 27-30. California study shows various factors related to MD attitude.

Longest, Virginia. "Expanded Roles for Veterans Administration Nurses." *Am. J. Nurs.*, **73** (Dec. 1973), 2087-2089. Written by the VA director of nursing service, this article describes some of the progressive nursing approaches in the VA.

Lowery, Barbara, et al. "Nursing Students' and Faculty Opinion on Student Evaluation of Teachers." *Nurs. Res.*, **20** (Sept./Oct. 1971), 436-439. Differences in opinions of students and teachers are described, particularly in relationship to objectivity and traits to be rated.

Luneski, Irene. "Temporary Nursing: Is It for You?" *RN*, **36** (Sept. 1973), 47-50. A temporary nurse works for a contracting service, is paid by them, and is placed in a variety of positions on a short-term basis.

Manthey, Marie. "Primary Care Is Alive and Well in the Hospital." *Am. J. Nurs.*, **73** (Jan. 1973), 83-87. Presented are organizational philosophy and framework that enable hospital nurses to practice primary nursing along with reactions to the system.

Masson, VeNeta. "International Nursing: What Is It? Who Does It?" *Am. J. Nurs.*, **79** (July 1979), 1242-1245. Includes what an international nurse is and how it differs from nursing in the United States as to qualifications. Sources of information on employment.

Mauksch, Ingeborg. "Critical Issues of the Nurse Practitioner Movement." *Nurse Pract.*, **3** (Nov./Dec. 1978), 15, 35-36. Interview with a nursing leader brings candid answers, pinpointing key issues.

Meglen, Marie, and Marie Burst. "Nurse-Midwives Make a Difference." *Nurs. Outlook*, **22** (June 1974), 386-389. Description of a midwifery educational program and services in the Mississippi Delta.

Morgan, J. A. "A New Dimension—Nurse Midwifery in Vermont." *J. Nurse-Midwifery*, **18** (Spring 1973), 4-10. A questionnaire on nurse-midwife acceptance by patients showed that the great majority were willing to have the services of the nurse-midwife. Other aspects of adding nurse-midwives to the health team are discussed.

Mundinger, Mary M. "Primary Nurse—Role Evaluation." *Nurs. Outlook*, **21** (Oct. 1973), 642-645. Change of a nursing service to give

responsibility and accountability for total patient care back to the nurses.

Murray, Raymond, and Shirley Ross. "Training the Family Nurse Practitioner." *Hospitals*, **47** (Nov. 1, 1973), 93-98. Preparing the FNP to help relieve the shortage in primary health care is discussed from the employer's point of view, including issues and problems in education and practice.

McGann, Marlene. "The Clinical Specialist: From Hospital to Clinic to Community." *J. Nurs. Admin.*, **5** (Mar./Apr. 1975), 33-37. Describes role as this nurse sees it, with comments added by two nurse administrators. Further comment in July/August issue, p. 6.

McLaren, Phyllis, and Ruth Tappen. "The Community Nurse Goes to Jail." *Nurs. Outlook*, **22** (Jan. 1974), 35-39. Two graduate students provide help for some of the women inmates' health needs and problems. A picture of life in a county jail is also given in relation to environment and attitudes.

McNiff, Martha. "Nursing in a Psychiatric Prison Service." *Am. J. Nurs.*, **73** (Sept. 1973), 1586-1587. Some of the challenges of a nurse in such a setting are discussed. Describes the environment and nurse-patient relationships.

Nelson, Karen. "The Nurse in a Methadone Maintenance Program." *Am. J. Nurs.* **73** (May 1973), 870-874. Description of clinic and nurse's role; importance of counseling and an accepting, friendly attitude are stressed.

"The Nurse Supply: Shortage or Surplus?" *RN*, **37** (June 1974), 34-45. Survey of nurse employment in hospitals done by this journal reveals that the nursing shortage in this area is not severe, and that quality and experience (particularly in specialty areas) are being sought as well as staff for evening and night shifts.

"Operating Room Nursing," Special Issue. *RN*, **36** (Mar. 1973), 33-48. A survey of OR nursing today includes rating of RNs by surgeons, staffing, kinds of responsibilities, and projected future developments.

Orme, June, and Rosemary Lindbeck. "Nurse Participation in Medical Peer Review." *Nurs. Outlook*, **22** (Jan. 1974), 27-30. These nurses check, assess, and coordinate the delivery of medical care services and act as patient advocates in an early PSRO-type situation.

"Overview:New Challenge for With-It Nurses." *RN*, **35** (Jan. 1972), 32-39. Result of *RN* survey reviews type of facilities, personnel, and availability of physicians in intensive-care units.

Palmer, Irene. "The Dreams and Danger of Deanship." *Nurs. Forum*, **10** (Spring 1971), 132-149. A dean discusses the role of nursing deans, the problems of assuming a new position, relationships with faculty, students, and others, and the kind of setting in which deans function.

Pearson, Linda. "The Clinical Specialist as Role Model or Motivator." *Nurs. Forum*, **11** (Winter 1972), 71-77. Discussion of experts' opinions on how clinical specialists may act as role model and bring about change. Author stresses need to be motivator with good interpersonal relationships in order to bring about change.

Pepper, Ginette, et al. "Geriatric Nurse Practitioner in Nursing Homes." *Am. J. Nurs.*, **76** (Jan. 1976), 62-64. Demonstration project shows utilization of GNPs upgraded care.

Perdue, Barbara Lee. "To Be a Good Supervisor." *Nurs. Outlook*, **13** (Sept. 1965), 65-66. Lists and discusses the characteristics and qualifications of an effective supervisor in terms of her roles as an "idea promoter" and a "people developer." Much of the material in this article applies to the process of supervision and is therefore useful to the advanced student or practicing graduate nurse.

Pierik, M. Madaline. "Joint Appointments: Collaboration for Better Patient Care." *Nurs. Outlook*, **21** (Sept. 1973), 576-579. Report of a university setting where nursing education and nursing service share joint appointments and work together for mutual benefit.

Price, Alice. "An Open Letter—Are Nurse Mavericks Any Less Professional?" *Nurs. Outlook*, **18** (Apr. 1970), 38-39. A nurse who works for a pharmaceutical company talks about the role of a nurse away from the mainstream of nursing and what she can bring to nursing.

"Profile of a Training Director," *Nurs. Outlook*, **22** (June 1974), 393. A brief picture of in-service directors based on a survey of 814 directors of education in hospitals and nursing homes.

Rafferty, Rita, and Jean Carver. "Nursing Consultants, Inc.—A Corporation." *Nurs. Outlook*, **21** (Apr. 1973), 232-235. Another approach to independent nursing practice in the community, helping patients, physicians, and institutions through consultation and educational services related to nursing care.

Ramphal, Marjorie. "Clinical and Administrative Judgment." *Am. J. Nurs.*, **72** (Sept. 1972), 1606-1611. Whether the nurse administrator or the practitioner should make key clinical judgments is discussed from the viewpoint of both.

Reinhardt, Adina, and Mildren Quinn, Eds. *Current Practice in Family-Centered Community Nursing*. St. Louis, Mo.: C. V. Mosby Company, 1977. Twenty-four contributors describe different facets of community health nursing. Useful in showing how current problems are met.

Reiter, Frances. "The Nurse-Clinician." *Am. J. Nurs.*, **66** (Feb. 1966), 274-280. Patients, says the writer, are being deprived of professional nursing care. Her views on this subject and on how implementation of the nurse-clinician concept can alleviate this situation are recommended reading. Author is an early originator of the nurse clinician concept.

Riehl, Joan, and Joan McVay. *The Clinical Nurse Specialist: Interpretations*. New York: Appleton-Century-Crofts, 1973. Compilation of articles written by nursing administrators, educators, clinical specialists, and physicians, tracing the historical development of the role, citing educational requirements, functions, and implications for the future.

Rielly, P. A., and Michael Newton. "The Role of the Obstetric, Gynecological, and Neonatal Nurse. Report of Two NAACOG Surveys." *J. Obstet. Gynecol. Nurs.*, **2** (July-August 1973), 17-31. One survey concentrated on forty general or specific tasks in the labor and delivery areas, all of which were done sometimes by nurses in this field. The second covered tasks in the postpartum, gynecologic, neonatal areas, in the hospital, clinic, and doctor's office. Some concern for overlapping responsibilities is expressed.

Roberts, Melville, et al. "Technicians or Nurses in the OR?" *Am. J. Nurs.*, **74** (May 1974), 906-907. Three surgeons describe the role of OR technicians today and examine a trend to eliminate RNs from the OR. They conclude RNs are needed, but nursing must make the effort to remain in control there.

Robinson, Alice. "Intesive Care Today—and Tomorrow: A Summing-Up." *RN*, **35** (Sept. 1972), 56-60. Reviewed are some of the major problems in ICU nursing and proposed solutions; some predictions for the future.

Roueche, Berton, ed. *Together: A Casebook of Joint Practice in Primary Care*. Chicago National Joint Practice Commission, 1977. Compilation of examples of joint MD/nurse (not always NP) practice. Interesting, but tends to underestimate nurses' contributions.

Runnerstrom, Lillian, et al. "The Nurse-Midwife in the Obstetric Health Team." *Nurs. Forum*, **15** (1976), 59-68. Describes role and considers major issues.

Sackett, David, et al. "The Burlington Randomized Trial of the Nurse Practitioner: Health Outcomes of Patients." *Annals of Int. Med.*, **80** (Feb. 1974), 137-142. One of the first NP studies done according to good research protocols. Shows NPs were effective and safe.

Santis, Lydia. "Teaching Others to Teach." *Nurs. Outlook*, **21** (Oct. 1973), 658-663. Description of a cross-cultural program by Project HOPE staff designed to impart basic knowledge about the educational process to nurses in Jamaica. Good principles as well as description of one HOPE program.

Sheahan, Sister Dorothy. "Short Shrift for Hospital Nursing—the Director's Defection." *Am. J. Nurs.*, **73** (Mar. 1973), 485-490. A controversial article that castigates directors of nursing for managing systems rather then leading nursing practice.

Simborg, Donald, et al. "Physicians and Non-Physician Health Practitioners: The Characteristics of Their Practices and Their Relationships." *Am. J. Pub. Health*, **68** (Jan. 1978), 44-48. Study of 1,369 patients in six primary care practices. Skills of MDs and non-MD practitioners were found potentially complementary but non-MD group underutilized.

Spradley, Barbara. *Contemporary Community Nursing*. Boston: Little, Brown and Company, 1975. Purpose is to clarify nature of community nursing. Fifty-two contributors cover such topics as general role of nurse in community health settings, expanded role, cultural dimensions, family communication, assessment, health planning.

Steel, Jean. "Precepts for Practitioners." *Nurs. Outlook*, **26** (Aug. 1978), 498-499. Seasoned nurse practitioner shares experiences with real-life problems.

Steen, Joyce. "Liaison Nurse: Ombudsman for the Chronically Ill." *Am. J. Nurs.*, **73** (Dec. 1973), 2102-2104. A nurse helps to improve the continuity of care of chronically ill through her activities in a new role.

Stevens, Barbara. "The Head Nurse as Manager." *J. Nurs. Admin.*, **4** (Jan./Feb. 1974), 36-40. Problems and guidelines.

Sullivan, Judith, et al. "Overcoming Barriers to the Employment and Utilization of the Nurse Practitioner." *Am. J. Pub. Health*, **68** (Nov. 1978), 1097-1103. Part of NP longitudinal study by HEW. Barriers identified: legal restrictions, limitations of space and facilities, and resistance from other providers.

Vacek, Pamela, and Taka Ashikaga. "Educational Program Evaluation: The University of Vermont Family Nurse Practitioner Program." *Nurs. Res.*, **27** (Jan./Feb. 1978), 36-41. Well-done study compares nurse practitioner and other RN activities.

Wagner, Doris. "Nursing in an HMO." *Am. J. Nurs.*, **74** (Feb. 1974), 236-239. Pictures and text illustrate nursing as done in an HMO and cite satisfactions gained.

Ward, Mary Jane. "Family Nurse Practitioners: Perceived Competencies and Recommendations." *Nurse Res.* **28** (Nov./Dec. 1979), 343-347. Mail questionnaire results show kinds of conditions FNPs handle. Discussion focuses on appropriate education.

Warner, Anne, Ed. *Innovations in Community Health Nursing: Health Care Delivery in Shortage Areas*. St. Louis: C. V. Mosby Company, 1978. Independent nurse practitioners from Alaska to Florida to Maine give marvelous descriptions of what they do.

Wiley, Loy. "Today's Nurse 99-44/100 Per Cent Efficient and She Floats." *Nurs. 78*, **8** (Feb. 1978), 89-92. How to manage assignment as "float" nurse.

Yankauer, Alfred, et al. "The Costs of Training and the Income Generation Potential of Pediatric Nurse Practitioners." *Pediatrics*, **49** (June 1972), 878-887. This study shows that PNPs could generate some $3,000 per year in additional income for a physician employer and that the physician could easily defray the cost of the nurse's new educational program. Costs are described.

Young, Lucie. "Room at the Top—A Place for Nurse Administrators (JCAH Standard I)." *J. Nurs. Admin.*, **2** (Nov./Dec. 1972), 81-85. Description of the qualifications and role of the nurse administrator, with emphasis on the importance of participation in top-level decision making. Recommendations are made for educational preparation.

Zahourek, Rothlyn. "Nurses in a Community Mental Health Center." *Nurs. Outlook*, **19** (Sept. 1971), 592–595. Study of one western community mental health center, including functions, competencies, and satisfactions.

Zimmer, Marie. "Rationale for a Ladder for Clinical Advancement in Nursing Practice." *J. Nurs. Admin.*, **2** (Nov./Dec. 1972), 18-24. The dimensions of a system of recognition for excellence in practice via a promotional ladder.

Zimmern, Anne, Jocelyn Greenidge, and Mary Kohnke. *Independent Nurse Practitioner.* Garden Grove, Ca.: Trainex Press, 1974. Three nurse practitioners who formed an independent practice describe their philosophy, practice, accomplishments, problems.

See also bibliography and references in Chapter 7 which describes settings as well as references in this chapter. Hundreds of articles on nurse practitioners have probably appeared since 1967 in nursing, medical, hospital and public health journals, including information on education and practice, including evaluation research. The February 1974 issue of *Nursing Outlook* is devoted to the education and practice of the NP, and the March 1975 *Nursing Outlook* focuses totally on evaluation of NPs. Also in 1975, the National Joint Practice Commission published an annotated *Selected Bibliography with Abstracts on Joint Practice.* All the articles in the vol. 6, #4 (Winter 1979) issue of *Nursing Digest* are on the clinical nurse specialist and improvement of nursing practice; the Fall 1977 issue (vol. 5, #3) on "The Delicate Art of Nursing Supervision and Leadership". Vol. VII (Winter 1980) of *Nursing Dimensions* and the Vol. 1 (Winter 1977) issue of the *Nursing Administration Quarterly* explore primary nursing and Vol. 3 (Fall 1978) focuses on cost effectiveness for nursing. "Nursepower" *Am. J. Nurs.* (Oct..1979) 1745–1756 is shorter version of Roth (ANA) survey.

Finally, for those who are interested in the variety of careers available to nursing, almost all the nursing journals publish articles on new careers periodically. Most consistent is *Nursing,* which has articles almost monthly. In addition, the October and November 1978 issues of *Nursing 78* present "A Guide to Nursing Specialties."

16

Issues of Autonomy and Influence

Within the overall issues of autonomy and influence lie many other nursing issues and concerns: maintenance of ethical standards and accountability (Chapter 10); direction of nursing education (Chapter 12); growth of nursing research (Chapter 14); utilization of nurse manpower (Chapter 15); and participation in credentialing (Chapter 20). If other disciplines are able to control nursing practice, it will never be able to fulfill its potential. If the voices of other groups override that of nursing, the tremendous contribution the profession can make to improving the delivery of health care will be lost. There is some indication that nursing's perceived lack of autonomy has already been detrimental to its ability to influence public policy. It is therefore essential that nurses understand the meaning of nursing autonomy and their individual and group roles in enhancing what has lately been called nurse power.

NURSING AUTONOMY

Professional *autonomy* has been defined as the right of self-determination and governance without external control. Inherent is the understanding that the freedom and independence thus held also mandates responsibility and accountability. Sociologists have identified autonomy as the most strategic (and cherished) distinction between a profession and an occupation or semiprofession. Identified as components of autonomy are control of the profession's education, legal recognition (licensure), and a code of ethics that persuades the public to grant autonomy. A distinction has been made between "job content" autonomy, the freedom to determine the methods and procedures to be used to deal with a given problem, and "job context" autonomy, the freedom to name and define the boundaries of the problem and the price to be paid for dealing with it.[1] The keys to autonomy as applied to nursing are that no other profession or administrative force can control nursing practice, and that the nurse has latitude in making judgments in patient care within the scope of nursing practice defined by the profession.

There are a number of reasons why nursing does not have full autonomy. Early nursing in America did not assume an autonomous stance. In part, this was because most nurses were women, and female status was low at the time. Nurses, usually female, were constantly admonished to obey the physician, usually male, and to abide by his judgment about the patient's condition. Even though nurses were trained to observe, the next step was to report and wait for further direction. Acting on their own judgment of what to do for the patient lay within a vary narrow area. Added to this was the nurse's position in the male-dominated hierarchy of the hospital (which, as it became larger, became a male-dominated bureaucracy). As Ashley has reported, nurses were expected to be the mother figures, giving freely (in the financial as well as the social sense) of their time and efforts to meet the needs of all members of the hospital family, from patients to physicians. She attributes nurses' lack of progress and accompanying low status to the fact that they are women and maintains that their work has been virtually ignored and trivialized in comparison to that of the physicians. "Nursing's problems, rooted in the tradition of economic exploitation, inadequate education, and long-standing social discrimination, have plagued the profession for the greater part of its history."[2] The fact that there were some early nurses who struggled free and were able to practice independently, primarily in public health settings, is evidence that there was from the beginning health care practice that was uniquely nursing. Unfortunately, the majority of nurses did not seem to resist actively the subordinate role they were given. Many of these deterrents to nursing autonomy still exist.

Concepts of Power and Influence

All of the classic definitions of power include the concepts of influence, control, strength—for instance: "the ability of a person, group, or system to use their concerted strategies, energy or strength to influence the behavior or actions of others."[3] Or, as others have said, the capacity to modify the conduct of others in the manner desired and prevent one's own conduct from being modified in a way one does not want. Power is usually seen as a social relationship, not necessarily the attribute of a person or group; it is given, maintained, or lost within those relationships. Some thirty years ago, in a model that attempted to measure the poten-

tial effects of the influence or power of one person or group (A) over another (B), certain crucial dimensions were identified:

a. The base of power—*economic and other resources, prestige, popularity, numbers.*
b. The means of power—*the specific actions that might be used (promises, threats, providing what the other needs or wants).*
c. The scope of power—*the set of specific actions that A can get B to perform.*
d. The amount of power—*the increase in probability that B will actually take certain specific actions because of A's use of power.*
e. The extension of power—*the set of individuals over whom A has power.*[4]

Power and influence are sometimes equated, because both affect or change the behavior of others; however, when they are separated, it is on the theory that power is the potential that must be tapped and converted to the dynamic thrust of influence. Almost all authorities agree that a person or group must be valued in order to have power or influence. French and Raven have described six sources of such power: reward power and coercive power, which seem self-explanatory; legitimate power (power derived from certain cultural values that are held or from a legitimizing act such as an election); referent power (liking or identifying with another); expert power (based on the knowledge, abilities, and credibility of the person or group); and informational power (arising from the communication activity of the person/group exerting influence).[5]

Considering these concepts, it is clear that nursing has the potential for power with its overwhelming numbers, its special knowledge and skill, its place in public trust, and is, in fact, already beginning to exercise nurse power legislatively, although not as much as it might.[6,7] It would be a pity if nurses wasted their efforts on the limiting power of the powerless, the petty tyranny of the captive nurse with the clock-in, clock-out mentality.[8]

Nursing and Feminism

When the question is asked as to why nurses, with so much potential for influence, do not seem to be able to or want to use it, there is inevitable reference to the fact that nursing is still about 98 percent a woman's profession, and, even with changing legislation and attitudes, women as a whole are still subject to discrimination (See Chapters 6 and 17) and still often victims of female socialization.

For many years, most women nurses looked at nursing as a useful way to earn a living until they were married, one to which they could return if circumstances forced them. Most nurses do marry and most married nurses did drop out to raise families, working only part-time, if at all. Unmarried nurses (like male nurses) were more inclined to stay in nursing but, unlike men, frequently did not plot an orderly path to positions of authority and influence. This is similar to the career patterns of other women. In business, most women have traditionally been in their thirties or forties before they realized that they either wanted to or would be forced to continue working, and by then they were often frozen in dead-end, low-prestige (but productive) jobs. (When they decided to compete for power positions in management, they were up against an "old boy" network that prevented or deterred their progress.) Moreover, they had to overcome their own reluctance to be aggressive and to reject traditional female social goals.[9] Nurses have tended to move into the administrative hierarchy more though default than intent, perhaps gathering credentials on the way, but until the last few decades, relatively few had attained power *outside* nursing, either as recognized expert practitioners within a practice setting, or as representatives of nursing in health policy determination. Why? Do nurses lack a goal-oriented commitment to nursing? Bowman and Culpepper said:

> There must be a conscious decision to use power. It is this conscious decision to assume power which nurses, individually and collec-

tively, have been unable or unwilling to make. Most nurses think they are powerless. Many nurses see themselves as objects of the power of others, and have internalized the attitudes of subordination projected by those in positions of authority and other health professions. This has contributed to the development of a negative self-image within the profession.[10]

However, nurses who did opt for leadership found that they frequently had an additional battle to fight—being women in a woman's profession. In a study of nursing "influentials," that is, leaders in the profession, sexual stereotyping, discrimination of various forms (income, status, education), self-image problems (subservience, low self-esteem and self-confidence, insecurity, passivity, lack of assertiveness), and isolation from the male perspective were listed as disadvantages to being in a woman's profession. Frequently, these leaders were seen by others as deviant from the cultural norms that expect women to seek approval, affection, conciliation, and to be "other directed" and conforming.[11]

Although nurses have not always been supportive of the women's rights movement, there is general agreement that the consciousness raising that helps women see their worth, to love and value themselves, has not only affected individual nurses who were involved, but has made nurses in general more aware of and resistant to discrimination. Moreover, women nurses now entering the field are generally more comfortable with the tenets of feminism and see no need to take an inferior role in a profession they have chosen to make a career. Grissum states that this does not mean that nurses who do not hesitate to question the reasoning behind a doctor's order, or demand more money and better working conditions, who are not intimidated and want more control over their profession and input into overall decision making are necessarily trying to attain omnipotence and dominate men (although some, of course, do). Instead, they demand equality, for which they are still often castigated by women as well as by men.[12] Barriers to such equality that impinge on nursing autonomy still exist, especially as nurses move into new roles.[13] It is particularly unfortunate when women and nurses choose to set up some of these barriers themselves when it comes to other nurses: displaying prejudice against qualified married women with children who seek leadership positions;[14] putting obstacles in the way of those breaking new ground;[15] isolating those who have established joint practice modes and must "prove" themselves not only to nonparticipant physicians but to their own nurse colleagues.[16] There is enough group discrimination against women without such behavior. One shocking, highly visible example is evident in the words of the federal judge who heard the job discrimination case of a group of Denver nurses. Although he acknowledged that nurses working for the city and county of Denver were paid less than male workers with comparable levels of responsibility and education, this judge ruled against them because a favorable ruling would have the potential for "disrupting the entire economic system of the United States of America." He interrupted the testimony of a noted nurse to read from the Declaration of Independence and announced that it didn't say anything about women being created equal. The "put-downs" of women by judge and defense attorney in that trial make incredible reading.[17]

The Dilemma of Nurses in a Bureaucracy

It is generally agreed that one of the major constraints to nursing autonomy and professionalism is the status of most nurses as employees in bureaucratic organizations (especially hospitals) where nursing, unlike medicine, is a department in the institutional hierarchy. The director of nursing (whatever the title) reports to the hospital administrator. Most decision making is at the top hierarchical level, and the goals of the bureaucracy are those that receive first priority. If, in the care of patients, those goals conflict with the nurse's professional goals, the nurse is in

a dilemma that has been called "reality shock" when applied to new graduates and is considered one of the reasons for nurses' restless nomadism, sometimes culminating in flight from the profession. The other alternative has been, too often, acceptance of goals not necessarily in the patient's best interest: getting the work done to suit the hospital's schedule, not nursing to meet the patient's needs—a metamorphosis of nurse professional to nurse bureaucrat. When a nurse is rewarded for this behavioral shift, there is inevitably a slow drift to a survival mentality that precludes creative risk taking. As Nightingale said, "A good nurse does not like to waste herself," and lack of adequate resources and apparent lack of respect by administrators and others for *professional* nursing practice not only creates great job dissatisfaction but may make the nurse's work "slovenly."[18]

Job satisfaction surveys of nurses almost inevitably reflect one major dissatisfaction as their lack of professional autonomy and their perception that they are not respected, or at least not listened to as professionals.* This plaint may not be much different from that of any other employee: nonresponsiveness by management is the basis of many labor disputes. There is no question that some institutional/agency administrators are extremely controlling and some nurse administrators are not strong, all of which has an extremely limiting effect on nurse autonomy. Such a combination of factors has in recent years brought about a number of job actions in which the right of nurses to be involved in patient care decisions was a key issue, and nurses have won.[19] A major breakthrough was probably the 1974 strike of a group of San Francisco nurses, in which a prime issue was their being rotated to intensive care units even if they did not have the expertise to care for those patients. After a bitter struggle, in a union contract negotiated by the state nurses' association, the nurses won a

---

*A number of these surveys, especially those published in *Nursing 78*, are discussed in Chapter 11.

voice in how assignments were made to specialty units, how other staffing arrangements were made, an expansion of the professional performance committees for peer review, and greater opportunity to participate in professional decision making and continuing education.[20] This pattern of demands has been adopted by nurses in other settings.

It is obvious why hospital and other administrators resist such steps; they see it as weakening their management rights and power. That they do not seem to be as negative toward the distinct power held by physicians in the same settings has a lot to do with the community prestige and power of physicians. For instance, it has been noted that physicians are in the same social circles as most hospital trustees and therefore have informal access to them and more acceptance as equals than do hospital administrators who are, in a sense, also employees. But a large part of physician clout is that they are the gatekeepers to the health care delivery system; they are virtually the only health providers who can admit to or discharge from health care facilities. Even in public health and other ambulatory care settings, there is often no reimbursement of services if a physician is not supervising care, at least on paper. Health care agencies depend on patients for income; in most cases, they need physicians to help provide that income, particularly if they are independent, but, to an extent, also if they ar employed by the institution or agency.

Part of the independent stance of physicians is in their collegially oriented organization within the hospital, as described in Chapter 7. Unfortunately, nurses have been slow in adopting either such an organizational pattern for professional decision making or any other that guarantees nurses not only equity in health care endeavors, but parity.

The question has long since been raised as to how to create and use knowledge without undermining an organization, a question particularly pertinent for nursing because it is in organizations that most health care is given.

The answer may lie in *altering* the organization so that nursing knowledge can be created and used effectively. L. L. Wade's neoteric model, adaptable to various organizations and agencies including hospitals and nursing homes, has been used by some in considering conditions that Wade cited as conducive to a high level of personal autonomy.

1. *Decisional autonomy and the absence of general rules. (Unique situations militate against the use by professionals of fixed and general rules in dealing with their clientele.)*
2. *Pragmatically structured system of action and the absence of a rigid hierarchy of authority.*
3. *Moderate professionalization and the absence of hyperprofessionalization. (For example, groups such as the legal profession may resist new techniques and ideas because of an excessive preoccupation with the traditional standards and methods of their profession.)*
4. *Effective personal interactions among the organization's professionals and between professionals and clients.*
5. *Equally distributed material props among the organization's professionals (lest inequality in distribution serve to increase social distance between professionals and introduce status differences in their relationships).*
6. *Some degree of nonconformity among the members of the profession in the organization.*
7. *Belief among the organization's professionals that authority ought to derive from objective and nonsocial sources (i.e., science).*
8. *Role congruity among organizational professionals. (Also, under this heading, is freedom from inhibiting moral obligation to the organization, as well as role strains and incongruent statuses.)*
9. *Evaluation of professional behavior only by fellow professionals. (Evaluation should involve the factors of professional status, salary, hiring, and the application of sanctions against incompetent members. It also applies to the setting of goals and to any formulation of preferred group functions that may be required.)*[21]

That this kind of nurse-initiated action takes a great deal of commitment and struggle has been documented, for to make change to autonomy requires both strong nursing leadership and nurses' willingness to take action and assert appropriate responsibility.[22,23,24] Christman, stressing the accountability to both patients and governing boards that is concomitant to autonomy, has suggested:

> To discharge this responsibility nurses must, in general, use a process similar to that employed by the medical staff. They must: 1) control access to staff and practice privileges; 2) confirm background education and certification; 3) review clinical work through appropriate committees; 4) see that shortfalls (less than adequate care) in practice are determined and remedied; 5) delimit practice privileges; 6) develop quality assurance mechanisms; 7) delineate requirements for continuing education; 8) participate in the educational preparation of nursing students; and 9) engage in research to improve care. Because specialization in nursing is increasing greatly, the departmental responsibility for peer review and quality of care is just as necessary as it is in the medical departments.
>
> Through the committee structure and the directing body, usually an executive committee and an elected chief-of-staff, the autonomous staff will maintain consultative relations: 1) with the board of trustees over qualifications for nursing staff membership and appointments and for standards of care; 2) with administration over logistical, material, and management-related issues; and 3) with the medical staff and the departments of the other health professions, e.g., dietary, social work, physical therapy, occupational therapy, clinical psychology, and with whatever other departments may exist, in order to share power and accountability.[25]

Although nursing autonomy of the type described may possibly need the agreement of the chief administrator in an employment setting, a good nurse administrator can negotiate such arrangements as a requirement for effective and productive nursing practice. This does not mean that a nurse administrator abrogates managerial responsibilities, for

good management can enhance opportunities for nurse autonomy.[26] One model of shared governance that has stood is that at Loeb Center in New York, where nurses have practiced autonomously for many years.[27]

A newer dimension of nurse autonomy is the process by which clinical privileges are granted to nurse practitioners. Currently, the usual pattern is total control by physicians, with or without preliminary screening by nursing administration.[28] If such decisions are to be jointly made, perhaps nursing ought also to have input in the determination of physicians' clinical privileges.[29] The fact that *physicians* can determine which *nurses* have privileges points out the differences in the recognition of autonomy.*

Physician-Nurse Relationships

Physician-nurse relationships are a large, if not major, factor in nurse autonomy. There is necessarily a fine line between overstating or understating the problems, or, as some would have it, between paranoia and servility. Physicians' recognition of nurses as co-professionals and colleagues has been present almost since the beginning of nursing, but a hard core of physicians who see and prefer a nurse-handmaiden role, although less common than even a decade ago, still exists. Some individual physicians and, to some extent, a part of organized medicine seem to have limited, stereotypic images of nurses and resist nurse autonomy—either because they honestly doubt nurses' ability to cope with certain problems (bolstered unfortunately by the behavior of some nurses they work with) or they are threatened by the expansion of nursing roles. One example that showed serious lack of understanding of changes in nursing roles was the report of a committee of a prestigious medical group that concerned itself with the status-seeking behavior of nurses and urged a return to the nurse of yore.[30] More serious is the periodic

---

*See also Porter article in Chapter 21 bibliography for legal aspects.

action of certain medical societies and boards to restrict expanded nursing practice by lobbying against the newer expanded definitions of practice in nurse practice acts, by opposing reimbursement for nursing services unless there is physician supervision or using their power to limit nursing practice in a particular community or health care setting.

The reasons for problems in nurse-physician relationships have been examined repeatedly. One reason given is that physician education tends to impress on the medical student a captain-of-the-ship mentality and a need for both omniscience and omnipotence (Aesculapian authority), whereas often nursing education does not develop nurses as independent and fearless thinkers.[31] This is also seen as one cause of the doctor-nurse game in which the nurse must communicate information and advice to the physician without seeming to do so and the physician acts on it without acknowledging the source, a game Stein calls a transactional neurosis that has an inhibitory effect on open dialog that is both stifling and anti-intellectual.[32] Other reasons include different socioeconomic and educational status of doctors and nurses; the MDs' lack of accurate knowledge about nursing education and practice, and vice versa, which enables them to work side by side without really understanding each other or communicating adequately (prompting some authors to compare their behavior to the parallel play of toddlers); different orientation to practice, including physician disapproval of the nursing emphasis on psychosocial aspects of patient care; the difference in attitudes about their profession as a long-term career commitment; and, of course, the nurses' lack of control over their practice, particularly in hospitals.[33,34,35,36]

With many nurses looking toward expanded practice, the fact that many physicians who have been surveyed do not seem comfortable in having nurses carry out responsibilities that were traditionally medicine has caused considerable misunderstanding.[37] This is particularly so when nurses feel

that they must prove themselves to be accepted in new roles, and that there is a "role-challenge" thrown out by physicians.[38] Again, apparently interrelated is the male-female role, the dominance-deference pattern that has had such strong historical roots that as someone stated, the nurse/woman must ". . . feel like a girl, act like a lady, think like a man and work like a dog."[39] That some nurses demonstrate this deference was illustrated clearly in a study in which various nurses were told over the phone by an unidentified doctor to give an overdose of a so-called research drug. Although all showed by voice and body language that they resisted the order, all but one carried it out.[40]

On the other hand, there are an increasing number of physicians who encourage and promote nurse-physician collegial relationships and see them as inevitable and necessary for good health care.[41] Joint practice, both at the unit level[42] and in various manifestations of physician-nurse-practitioner practice, are evidence of this cooperation, as was the National Joint Practice Committee.*

Glib proposals for cooperation will not solve the problems of conflict, which are detrimental to both professions and to the public. However, sometimes practical suggestions at the grass roots level on how to deal courteously and effectively with each other may be useful for the nurse dealing with physicians on a day-to-day basis.[43] Resolving the overall issue is a part of the challenge that both medicine and nursing must face.

THE ROLE OF NURSING LEADERSHIP

The cry for leadership seems to be universal, but what constitutes *effective leadership* is frequently debated. The term defies simple definition. Leadership has been defined as "a social phenomenon in which a group or aggregation of individuals accepts and acts

---

*See Chapter 27.

upon the ideas of one person,''[44] but in its simplest context, it is the ability to influence others, to lead, guide, and direct.

There are a number of theories and studies about leadership:

- the "great man" theory: leaders are born not made.
- the charismatic theory: there is a personal quality of leadership that arouses a special popular loyalty or enthusiasm and an emotional commitment.
- the situational theory: leadership depends on the situation and a person could be a leader in one situation and a follower in another.
- the contingency theory: the effectiveness of leadership depends on leader-member relations, task structure, and position power.
- the path-goal (expectancy) theory: the leader facilitates accomplishment by minimizing obstacles and rewarding followers for completing their tasks.
- the trait theory: leadership is acquired because the individual inherits or acquires certain traits.

The trait theory has been particularly popular, although there is little agreement on just what the key leadership traits and characteristics are. Among those that a variety of research has seemed to identify are effective interpersonal relationships that include tactfulness; a high level of energy and drive; persistence; assertiveness; aggressiveness; enthusiasm; self-assurance; self-confidence; decisiveness; superior judgment; dependability; integrity; persuasiveness; verbal facility; humor; courage; and friendliness. Superior intelligence was seen as a possible detriment if it interferes with the individual's ability to communicate with the followers; some authorities believe that people desire to be led by someone not too far detached from the group. Data on factors such as age, appearance, sex, and social status are inconsistent; although neither age, appearance, nor sex correlate with ability to lead, most people do not become leaders until middle age, not as many women as men achieve leadership positions, high socioeconomic status may be an advantage, and being a bit above average height and weight can be helpful.[45]

The president of an executive recruiting firm once stated what he considered essential for an effective executive: drive, people sense, communication ability, and calm under pressure, which might be considered a short version of the composite picture developed by a major researcher on leadership:

The leader is characterized by a strong desire for responsibility and task completion, vigor and persistence in the pursuit of goals, venturesomeness and originality in problem solving, drive to exercise initiative in social situations, self-confidence and sense of personal identity, willingness to accept consequences of decision and action, readiness to absorb interpersonal stress, willingness to tolerate frustration and delay, ability to influence other persons' behavior and capacity to structure social interaction systems to the purpose at hand.[46]

Much is written about the price of leadership: the loneliness at the top, for instance, and it has been said that a good leader must get over the need to be loved and must learn to function without the need for approval of others. No leader can please all of his/her constituents all the time. To lead inevitably requires commitment; at times the leader must sacrifice personal desires, interests, time. The rewards, of course, are to see goals that one believes in met and to know that this might not have been without one's leadership.

When the issue of nursing leadership is raised, there is, as in other professions, a demand for more and better. One writer said cynically,

Nursing has an overabundance of silly, odd, inadequate, insecure, sadistic, incompetent, weak "leaders"; now it is time to get our professional house in order with some capable, courageous, intelligent, ethical and sophisticated professional leaders who will have the knowledge and the daring to lead us as a pro-

fession and to meet the challenge of the next century.[47]

Leininger, who is recognized as a leader, maintains that there is a critical shortage of capable, well-prepared nursing leaders. She identified a key factor influencing nursing leadership as conflict between past and present expectations of leadership. She noted that if nurses have been "socialized to the subcultural norms that it is not 'ladylike' to fight, to confront, to negotiate, or to be bold or aggressive, they will experience norm conflicts with present day confrontation-negotiation strategies."[48] Other factors cited were negative attitudes toward authority; image, status, and role of women; size and complexity of organizational structures in which nurses function; new expectations related to interdisciplinary service and education; the diversity of interests and education in nursing; and the positional turnover of nursing leaders. Still, nursing does have recognized and identified competent leaders.

In the last decade, there has been a new interest in learning about contemporary leaders. Safier's oral history gives an exciting insight into the lives and ideas of nurses who attained leadership after and during World War II, a crucial time of change for nursing.[49,50] Vance's doctoral study has probably made available the first profile of contemporary nursing leaders, her so-called "nursing influentials." Among other things, the composite profile of seventy women and one man (sixty-nine white and two black) showed an average age of fifty-five (range thirty-eight to eighty); most coming from lower middle-class (49 percent) and upper middle-class backgrounds (35 percent); 49 percent single and 35 percent married, with 33 percent parents of from one to four children; 27 percent educational administrators; 22 percent educators; more than 11 percent administrators of nursing service, and 11.5 percent retired; 62 percent working in large cities, primarily in the northeast and north central United States; and ninety-five having their master's or doctorate, most from Eastern universities. Nurse influentials worked an average of forty-five to sixty-four hours a week (more than business executives surveyed) and most traveled from ten to sixty days a year. Almost all wrote (professional journals, books) and had appeared on radio or television, and all participated in some sort of political activity, primarily letter writing, testifying, and lobbying. An interesting comparison can be made between the leadership traits described earlier and what these nursing leaders identified as their source of influence. In order of importance, those traits and characteristics cited as highly important by at least half the respondents were communication skills, intellectual ability, willingness to take risks, interpersonal skills, creativity in thinking, ability to mobilize groups, recognized expertise in an area of the profession, charisma, and innovativeness. Having academic credentials, collegial support, and a professional work position of power/prestige were also considered important. Traits listed as most important for future leaders were scholarship, intelligence, courage, humanism, sense of self, vision, communication abilities, commitment, political abilities, competence, adaptability, drive, and integrity.[51]

What are a nursing leader's responsibilities? In the nursing literature, suggestions have been made over the years, many of them related to strengthening nursing and guiding nurses to greater autonomy and speaking for nursing to other disciplines and to the public. But more than a decade ago, a respected nurse offered four major tasks to which nursing leaders must devote themselves, tasks not yet accomplished:

1. *Advancing knowledge through research;*
2. *Making plans for and preparing personnel in sufficient numbers to meet the nursing needs of society;*
3. *Creating social systems in which exemplary nursing care, excellent nursing education, and significant scientific inquiry are demonstrated and can flourish; and*
4. *Identifying and developing nurse leaders who vitalize nursing itself and who utilize their very substantial talents toward iden-*

tifying and promoting worthwhile and cherished values of the larger society of which nursing is a vital part.[52]

NURSES AS CHANGE AGENTS

It is recognized that nurses, the only health professionals in contact with every facet of the health care system, are in key positions to bring about change. However, planned change involves problem-solving and decision-making skills as well as the ability to work well with others. A change agent must be skilled in the theory and practice of planned change. Therefore, a brief introduction to change theory may be helpful.[53] Lewin's theory of change is probably the basis for the adaptations of most other theorists. He identifies three basic stages: *unfreezing*, in which the motivation to create change occurs; *moving*, the actual changing when new responses are developed, based on collected information; and *refreezing*, in which the new changes are integrated and stabilized. A further notion is that in all changes there are *driving forces* that facilitate action and *restraining forces* that impede. Each must be identified—the first so that they can be capitalized on, and the second so that they can be avoided or modified.

Lippit's theory includes seven phases within Lewin's stages, a delineation that is useful in thinking through action:

Unfreezing:

1. Diagnosis of the problem.
2. Assessment of the motivation and capacity for change.
3. Assessment of the change agent's motivation and resources.

Moving:

4. Selecting progressive change objectives.
5. Choosing the appropriate role of the change agent.

Refreezing:

6. Maintenance of the change once it has been started.

7. Termination of a helping relationship.

Welch[54] applies the process of change to a situation a nurse might change, working through these steps in some detail, and Olson[55] uses Lewin's model to go through another situational change a nurse may encounter.

Of interest is the model developed by Reinkemeyer (a nurse), which was used by another nurse in dealing with an alcohol abuse problem in her community.[56] Also based on Lewin's model, its phases are summarized as:

1. *Development of a felt need and desire for the change.*
2. *Development of a change relationship between the agent and the client system.*
3. *Clarification or diagnosis of the client system's problem, need, or objective.*
4. *Examination of alternative routes and tentative goals and intentions of actions.*
5. *Transformation of intentions into actual change behavior.*
6. *Stabilization.*
7. *Termination of the relationship between the change agent and the client system.*[57]

Why do nurses (and others) resist change? There are a number of reasons—some quite understandable: satisfaction with the current situation; a lack of clarity about what the change is; a felt threat from the change agent; a feeling that the process and result of the change has not been thought through; selective perception and retention (hearing and remembering only what one wishes); too much work involved; fear of failure or disorganization; lack of two-way communication; and the change seeming to benefit the change agent, not necessarily the group. It is obvious that some of these objections could be quite valid and, if not solved, would weaken the proposed change. If recognized by the change agent, they can be overcome, if the project is worthwhile and the change agent proficient in human relations. If not all participants are won over, the decision must be made to stop or go ahead, trying to anticipate the negative aspects of what may become covert resistance if the resister is outvoted.

Conflicts of some kind are probably inevitable. It is important that the change agent develop effective methods of dealing with conflict. Action, rather than reaction, is the better course, but it should be recognized that a compromise might quite realistically result. Key steps include keeping the issue in focus, clarifying the problems, encouraging two-way communication, creating dialogue that involves group members in full participation, and always remaining responsive.[58] Just how a nurse handles the resistance may be a matter of individual style and the particular situation. Some nurse change agents function with a ''soft'' approach that can be effective. Smoyak advocates a confrontation model—a direct approach considered useful when there is a clear-cut issue and the situation and individuals concerned are ''healthy'' and not ''sick''.[59]

Being a change agent is part of the leadership role, but it is also a role that can be legitimately and effectively assumed by a nurse not yet at that stage of professional development. Whether working as an insider or outsider, each of which has advantages and disadvantages, knowing the process of change, planning carefully and thoroughly, acting strategically and with an appropriate sense of timing, are essential. Because a change agent is a leader in that instance, the leadership role must be assumed and the individual usually must start out by selling herself or himself first before the idea for change is seen as acceptable for consideration.

Strategies for Action

It should be recognized that nursing has accomplished a great deal in the influence arena. Nurses, as represented by their professional organization and backed by their voting power, have political clout;[60] nursing leaders are being heard in policy-making councils. It is probably a healthy sign that so many nurses are saying, ''But compared to what we can do and should do, it's not enough.'' The major problem within nursing

is the lack of cohesiveness, the lack of agreement on professional goals, the divisiveness of nursing subcultures. The heterogeneity of nurses in background, education, and position, all coping with a rapidly changing society, accounts logically for some of these problems. Nevertheless, if nursing is to have the full autonomy of a profession, there must be unification of purpose and action on major issues. Some specific strategies that may be useful for nursing can be suggested.

Political Action. Politics may be defined as the art or science of influencing policy. There is a legitimate tendency to think of politics in the context of government, but affecting policy and operations at the institutional level is often just as important in the work life of a nurse. The term *in-house law* has been used to describe the power nurses can have if they can determine policies and procedures that affect daily practice, for example, a policy stating that nurses may (or should or must) develop and implement teaching plans for patients or arrange for referrals to the visiting nurse, all of which have been blocked by physicians or administrators in some hospitals.

It is vital that nurses participate actively in the agencies or community groups where decisions are being made, such as local or state planning agencies.[61] The strategy used to gain input may vary a little. A basic principle is applicable: before, during and after gaining entree, nurses must show that they are knowledgeable, that they have something to offer, and that they can put it all together into an action package. There are many places to start, for most community groups are looking for members that work and are willing to hold office (for example, church groups, societies, and PTAs). These activities may be seen as (1) a way of getting experience on boards, using parliamentary procedure to advantage, politicking, gaining some sophistication in participating and guiding decisions, and (2) being visible to other groups and the public. Many community groups interlock and, by being active in some, nurses come into contact with others. It also helps to gain support of women other than nurses. Organized women are becoming more successful in getting representation on policy-making groups. It pays for them to have someone who is ready and able to assume such responsibilities. But participating nurses must be capable; there is nothing worse than having an incompetent as the first nurse on a major board or committee. At this stage of nurses' reach for influence, it could do the profession more damage than having a non-nurse, for it appears that women (and nurses) still have to be better than those already in power to gain initial respect.

Another aspect to consider and use is the potential economic power of nurses. A director who controls a million dollar plus budget wields power in how that money is spent. On the other hand, those nurses who have major responsibility for patient care and have no budgeting control are at an immediate disadvantage. Budgetary control (and administrative control), which may include workers other than nurses, increases nurse administrators' circle of power, but they must act on it. The aura of status enables these nurses to move in power circles where they can cultivate individuals who influence public and private decision making. Community nurses are also particularly good resources, because most make strong community contacts. Today, the participation of the consumer in health care decisions is increasing. An activated consumer who supports nursing has impact on local decision making as well as on state and national legislation. A legislator is more inclined to hear the consumer who presumably is a neutral participant, as opposed to an obvious interest group. But nursing must sell that consumer the profession's point of view and balance consumer needs and nursing goals.

Although it is often through the influence of consumer groups and the community's traditional power figures that nurses get on decision-making committees, boards, and so

on, after that, they're on their own and must be prepared, perceptive, articulate, and under control. In the meetings, at the coffee breaks, the politicking and the formation of coalitions may well determine which way a decision goes. Nurses who haven't learned to play that game had better take lessons: using role play, assertiveness training, group therapy, group process, speech lessons—whatever is necessary.

On the level of governmental politics, nurses can and have influenced not only such issues as national health insurance, quality assurance, patient rights, and care of the long-term patient, but have a vital interest in such issues as reimbursement for nursing services, nurse licensure, and funds for nursing education. The specifics of the legislative process and guidelines for action are described in Chapter 18. However, there is no reason that nurses should not run for office. They are intelligent, frequently well educated, and know a lot about human relations. Although none have yet been elected to national office, those who have won state offices are not only effective, but often offer extraordinary insight into health issues. Some have been responsible for major legislative breakthroughs for nurses. For instance, in Maryland, not only was legislation passed providing reimbursement for the services of nurse-midwives and nurse practitioners, but effective July 1979, the General Assembly passed the first law requiring insurance companies to reimburse for any services "within the lawful scope of practice of a duly licensed health care provider"—all initiated or strongly supported by the nurse legislators. For those nurses who choose to run for office, it is important to learn all the tricks of the trade;[62] amateurs seldom win. The accepted route is by becoming involved first with local politics or working in the campaign of an influential figure. For women, there are advantages and disadvantages. In a recent study of women officeholders in New Jersey, Tambarlane[63] found that some women were given opportunities or encouraged by their parties because they wanted to run one woman against another. However, an interesting finding was noted:

> When women's political work and/or success places strains on existing male dominant power relationships within the family or the party, men, perhaps fearing to lose their privileged positions—subtly or overtly—may withdraw their support.

It was also found that women suffer discrimination by being excluded from certain all-male organizations such as the Jaycees, Kiwanis, Rotary, and Lions, where the groundwork for political and other appointments is often done.

Regardless of the setting, there are some basic guidelines for effective political action. First is to be a lifelong student of the social and technical aspect of professional practice; second, to know the current professional issues and the implications for various alternative actions; third, to be aware of emerging social and political issues and trends that will affect health care and nursing; fourth, to learn others' points of view (potential supporters or opponents) and come to terms with what policy changes are possible, as well as desirable; and fifth, to seek allies who can espouse or at least see the desirability of a particular course of action.[64]

Professional Unity. It has long been a political precept that the most powerful groups are those that are united. Almost always this means that an organization speaks for that group, and that is one of the purposes of a professional organization. Nursing has many organizations representing various interest groups (Chapters 24–28). At times they cooperate, but too often they are at odds or simply act separately. Fortunately, there is more concerted effort being made by most to form political coalitions in relation to important issues for nurses. Of serious concern, however, is what Lewis calls the professionally uncommitted. In an outstanding editorial she states:

> It is scarcely newsworthy to observe that nursing is facing many problems today; that was equally true yesterday and will be tomorrow. But what troubles me today is the magnitude and import of our problems on the one hand, and the relatively small number of nurses taking part in the deliberations and decisions, on the other. Such issues as entry into practice, collective bargaining, and the credentialing recommendations must be resolved by the professional organization; yet the percentage of nurses in this country who are members of it is very small indeed. Sadder yet, some nurses seem almost unaware of the idea of nursing as a profession or of the issues that confront it. Why this alienation, deliberate or unwitting, from the profession of which all nurses are a part?

> Nonmembership in the professional organization, I believe, is only one symptom of a deeper malaise: a pervasive lack of what I will call a professional identity. Many nurses are committed to nursing, as they perceive it within the boundaries of their particular job. Most of them, I'm sure, carry out their individual nursing functions to the best of their abilities, want to do whatever they're doing, better. But they are not committed to nursing as a self-determining, self-regulating profession and an important force in the health care field.[65]

Lewis maintains that it is essential to cultivate a professional identity early in nurses' education and to make the profession and organization more relevant to their daily practice. The fact that nurses in influential positions, including faculty, also seem to lack professional identification deprives young nurses of professional role models. She concludes:

> But unless we take this problem seriously, there is a risk that nursing will cease to speak with a single, forceful voice, but will speak instead in the million and a half voices of individual nurses in this country, or in the fragmented voices of many specialty groups. Under those circumstances, who will listen and who will heed? Not the public, I'm afraid, nor the other health care professions, nor even nurses themselves.

Others have agreed that the need for support of the professional organization, where unity and a resolution of internal problems must occur, is crucial if nursing is to be an autonomous, influential power group.[66,67,68]

Nurse Accountability and Professionalism. Without demonstrating accountability for practice, nursing will never be or be considered an autonomous profession.[69,70] Standard setting, peer review, continued competence, protection of patients' rights* all indicate that nursing is taking on the responsibilities to see that the public is protected. However, more nurses must also recognize that for nurses to be professional, the majority of practitioners must consider it a career and put in the time, effort, and commitment necessary to participate in the key decision making.

Nurse Support Network. Nurses who practice autonomously and who take a stand for patients' rights may get into trouble, especially with physicians and employers. Who will support them? Just as men have a "good old boy network", nurses need a "good new nurse" network[71] that through an informal system of relationships provides advice, information, guidance, contacts, protection, and any other form of support that helps nurses, both men and women. Nurse colleague behavior, demonstrated by showing respect for each other, showing competence, giving feedback, recognizing skills and competencies, and consulting with each other is a vital link in a support network. The term *peer pal* has been used to describe the relationship between peers helping each other, acting as sounding boards, a reciprocal relationship that can provide a powerful boost for success.[72]

Overcoming Sexism and Sexist Stereotyping

It is obvious that sexist attitudes have created problems for women nurses, but men

nurses, too, complain of a reverse discrimination (Chapter 11). There is no more place for sexism, or male or female chauvinism, in nursing than in other aspects of society. Men and women need to support each other as professionals (and as human beings). Stereotypes are useless at best and destructive at worst. There are those who say that the answer is androgeny, the state in which both sexes feel free to choose from a full range of human behavior, not being restricted to the behavior ascribed by socialization.[73]

Nevertheless, given the pervasiveness of female sexual stereotyping, it may well be that women nurses will have to make special efforts to attain overt power and influence.[74] Women and nurses must continue to polish their ability to be assertive, to express their own thoughts or feelings without anxiety and without imposing on the thoughts and feelings of others, and to do so better and more often, especially in the face of opposition. (Assertiveness has been contrasted with aggressiveness, which is not being concerned with others' thoughts and feelings.) Assertiveness helps an individual resist manipulation, to feel more confident and self-assured. Withers says that for women, lack of assertiveness impairs personal and professional relationships and is one reason there is still widespread societal belief that women are incompetent. "Eventually the process becomes circular; women don't feel equal, so they don't act equal, so they aren't treated equally, so they don't feel equal . . . and so on."[75] Assertiveness training[76] has become popular, as have books on the topic,[77,78] but it is, first of all, important for unassertive persons to have confidence that their thoughts and feelings are worthwhile and to *want* to change. Actually, good assertiveness training builds on the effective ways in which an individual has always handled difficult situations, and many women already have the tact and sensitivity that is a useful base for assertiveness. A further step for women nurse leaders is to learn some of the techniques of gaining and holding power at top levels.

---

*Patients' rights are discussed extensively in Chapters 10, 20, and 22; professionalism in Chapter 9 and accountability in Chapter 10.

Nurse Mentors

An active mentor system, historically a formal or informal system between a prestigious, established older person and a younger one, wherein the older guides, counsels, and critiques the younger, teaching him/her survival and advancement in a certain field or profession, is badly needed in nursing. It has been recognized as crucial to the success of many, particularly women.[79] Sometimes, the mentor is equated with a role model, preceptor, or the master in a master-apprentice situation. But it is more than that. Says Williams, "Achieving a mentor relationship with an older person is like falling in love—you can't force it to happen, and it only works if the chemistry is right. You can, however, make yourself receptive to such a relationship by displaying a teachable attitude and an eagerness to learn."[80] In other words, the apprentice has to show that she/he is someone worth investing in, someone who will show a measure of return by success in the field. On the other hand, a role model can be merely that—someone to emulate and admire, even with minimal contact, and some apprenticeships are carried out with almost total impersonality. Preceptors, too, may overtly carry out their responsibilities to their students and yet withhold a vital element of development.

That mentors are important in nursing has been demonstrated in Vance's study[81] in which 83 percent of the leaders reported mentors in their lives, and 93 percent were mentors to others (frequently students).

There are influential nurses in many places. If they are willing to make the commitment of time and effort and caring that makes a true mentor, that influence will expand into more than a nurse's influence and become a nursing influence.[82]

Nurses as Risk Takers and Role Breakers

Grissum, like others, has identified the risk taker and role breaker as essential to changing the nursing image and to acquiring autonomy.[83,84] This involves personal and professional behavior on an individual level, being assertive, taking a stand on an issue, and laying claim to the part of health care that is nursing. It also means making a concerted effort to identify and change those aspects of the nursing image that are incorrect or negative, to help the public understand what nursing is and does.[85] One aspect of this new recognition is the effort made by the ANA to get reimbursement for nurses. Nursing services in institutions are frequently lumped in with the hotel services provided, and the distinct professional services are not winnowed out. Thus, the public often has no idea what nursing care involves. Third-party reimbursement could provide nurses sufficient economic leverage to demand nurse-patient ratios appropriate for rendering of professional services, but nursing must also be able to justify expensive professional nurses in preference to less-prepared personnel. And reimbursement of nurse practitioners would give the public greater choice in access to the health care system (and frequently much better care.)[86]

Another aspect of role breaking is to reinforce the budding colleague relationship between nurses and other health professionals, especially physicians. This should be focused on all aspects of patient care in all places where professional nurses function. Nurse practitioners and clinical specialists may, because of their specialized knowledge and skills, be quickly identified as colleagues. It has already been shown that primary nurses in hospitals and public health nurses who have full responsibility for nursing care of a group of patients are equally able to function effectively in collegial relationships. Joint practice committees on a state and local level should be nurtured. Too often they are token groups that are not effective and have little influence, particularly in changing medical attitudes.

Another responsibility is to change that in nursing which does not contribute to nursing as an autonomous profession. Some nurses look at nursing simply as a job and perhaps they always will, unless there is enough peer pressure to stimulate them toward professionalism. Changes are already occurring. There is some indication that more married nurses are seeing nursing as a career and plan an ongoing commitment;[87] the same is true of many nurses just entering the profession. It is possible that the new or newly awakened professional orientation will be the key to autonomy and influence.

REFERENCES

1. Christy Dachelet and Judith Sullivan, "Autonomy in Practice," *Nurse Practitioner*, **4:**15 (Mar./Apr. 1979).
2. Jo Ann Ashley, *Hospitals, Paternalism, and the Role of the Nurse* (New York: Teachers College Press, 1976), p. 93.
3. Merriam-Webster, *Webster's New Collegiate Dictionary* (Springfield, Ma.: G. & C. Merriam Company, 1975), p. 902.
4. John Harsanyi, "Measurement of Social Power, Opportunity Costs, and the Theory of Two-Person Bargaining Games," in Bell, Roderick, et al., *Political Power* (New York: The Free Press, 1969), p. 226.
5. John French and Bertram Raven, "The Base of Social Power," in Dorwin Cartwright, *Studies in Social Power* (Ann Arbor: Institute of Social Research, University of Michigan, 1959), pp. 150–167.
6. Lucie Young Kelly, "Endpaper: Not Bad, Nursing," *Nurs. Outlook*, **25:**275 (Apr. 1978).
7. Lucie Young Kelly, "Endpaper: Nursing Hegemony," *Nurs. Outlook*, **26:**224 (Mar. 1979).
8. Lucie Young Kelly, "Endpaper: The Power of Powerlessness," *Nurs. Outlook*, **25:**468 (July 1979).
9. Margaret Hennig and Anne Jardim, *The Managerial Woman* (Garden City, N.Y.: Anchor Press/Doubleday, 1977), pp. 108–154.
10. Rosemary Bowman and Rebecca Culpepper, "Power: Rx for Change," *Am. J. Nurs.*, **74:**1054 (June 1974).
11. Connie Vance, "Women Leaders: Modern Day Heroines or Social Deviants?" *Image*, **11:**39–41 (June 1979).
12. Marlene Grissum and Carol Spengler, *Womanpower and Health Care* (Boston:

Little, Brown and Company, 1976), pp. 95–127; 193–213.
13. Bonnie Bullough, "Barriers to the Nurse Practitioner Movement: Problems of Women in a Woman's Field," *Int. J. Health Services*, **5**(2): 225–233 (1975). Also reprinted in *Nurs. Digest*, **6:**58 (Fall 1978).
14. "Outmoded Prejudice," Letters, *Nurs. Outlook*, **26:**344 (June 1978).
15. Donna Wong, "Sounding Board: Private Practice—At a Price," *Nurs. Outlook*, **25:**258–259 (Apr. 1977).
16. Beatrice Thomstad, et al., "Changing the Rules of the Doctor-Nurse Game," *Nurs. Outlook*, **23:**422–427 (July 1975).
17. Bonnie Bullough, "The Struggle for Women's Rights in Denver: A Personal Account," *Nurs. Outlook*, **26:**566–567 (Sept. 1978).
18. Lucie Young Kelly, "Endpaper: In Our Imperfect State," *Nurs. Outlook*, **27:**368 (May 1979).
19. Dorothy Brooten, et al., *Leadership for Change: A Guide for the Frustrated Nurse* (Philadelphia: J. B. Lippincott Company, 1978), pp. 35–41.
20. Ruth Edelstein, "Management in American Nursing," *Int. Nurs. Rev.*, **26**(2):78 (1979).
21. L. L. Wade, "Professionals in Organizations: A Neoteric Model," *Human Org.* (Spring/Summer 1967), as described in Sandra Stone, et al., *Management for Nurses—A Multidisciplinary Approach* (St. Louis, Mo.: C. V. Mosby Company, 1976), pp. 42–46.
22. Meridean Maas, et al., "Nurse Autonomy, Reality Not Rhetoric," *Am. J. Nurs.*, **75:**2201–2208.
23. Anonymous, "Change, Conflict, Continuing Education, Competency," *Sup. Nurse*, **10:**26–34 (Apr. 1979).
24. Juanita Murphy and Mary Schmetz, "The Clinical Nurse Specialist: Implementing the Role in a Hospital Setting," *J. Nurs. Admin.*, **9:**29–31 (Jan. 1979).
25. Luther Christman, "The Autonomous Nursing Staff in the Hospital," *Nurs. Digest*, **6:**72 (Summer 1978).
26. Muriel Poulin, "Nursing Service: Change or Managerial Obsolescence," *J. Nurs. Admin.*, **4:**40–43 (July/August 1974).

27. Genrose J. Alfano, "Healing or Care Taking—Which Will It Be?" *Nurs. Clinics of North America,* **6:**273–280 (June 1971).

28. Paul Bergeson and Nancy Melvin, "Granting Hospital Privileges to Nurse Practitioners," *Hospitals,* **49:**99–101 (Aug. 16, 1975).

29. Nancy Melvin, "Developing Guidelines for Clinical Privileges for Nurse Practitioners," in *Power: Nursing's Challenge for the Future* (Kansas City, Mo.: The American Nurses' Association, 1979), pp. 62–67.

30. Lucie Young Kelly, "Endpaper: The Eternal Fascination of Nursing Education," *Nurs. Outlook,* **26:**403 (June 1978).

31. Beatrice Kalisch, "Of Half-gods and Mortals: Aesculapian Authority," *Nurs. Outlook,* **23:**22–28 (Jan. 1975).

32. Leonard Stein, "The Doctor-Nurse Game," *Arch. Gen. Psychiat.,* **16:**699–703 (June 1967). Reprinted also in *Am. J. Nurs.,* **68:**101–105 (Jan. 1968), and other publications.

33. Beatrice Kalisch and Philip Kalisch, "An Analysis of the Sources of Physician-Nurse Conflict," *J. Nurs. Admin.,* **7:**51–57 (Jan. 1977).

34. Joan Lynaugh and Barbara Bates, "The Two Languages of Nursing and Medicine," *Am. J. Nurs.,* **73:**66–69 (Jan. 1973).

35. Shirley Smoyak, "Problems in Interprofessional Relations," *Bull. N.Y. Acad. Med.,* **77:**51–59 (Jan./Feb. 1977). Reprinted in N. Chaska, *The Nursing Profession: Views Through the Mist* (New York: McGraw-Hill Book Company, 1978).

36. Robert Hoekelman, "Nurse-Physician Relationships," *Am. J. Nurs.,* **75:**1150–1152 (July 1975).

37. Edith Wright, "Family Nurse Clinicians: Physicians' Perspective," *Nurs. Outlook,* **23:**771–773 (Dec. 1975).

38. Jane Record and Merwyn Greenlick, "New Health Professionals and the Physician Role: an Hypothesis from the Kaiser Experience," *Nurs. Digest,* **4:**65–68 (Winter 1976).

39. H. Pratt, "The Doctor's View of the Changing Nurse-Physician Relationship," *J. Med. Educ.,* **40:**767–771 (Aug. 1965).

40. C. K. Hofling, et al., "Experimental Study in Nurse-Physician Relationships," *J. Nerv. Ment. Dis.,* **143:**171–180 (Aug. 1966).

41. Roseanne Krcek and Irving Krcek, "The Necessity for New Colleague Relationships Between Professionals," *Nurs. Digest,* **4:**83–85 (Summer 1976).

42. "At This Hospital, The Captain of the Ship Is Dead," *RN.,* **42:**77–93 (Mar. 1979).

43. Patricia Trinasky, "Nurse-Doctor Dissension Still Thrives," *Sup. Nurse,* **10:**40–43 (Apr. 1979).

44. L. D. Haskew, "Dimensions of Professional Leadership," *J. Natl Ed. Assn.,* **50**(2):30–32 (1961).

45. Helen Yura, et al., *Nursing Leadership: Theory and Process* (New York: Appleton-Century-Crofts, 1976), pp. 17–23.

46. R. M. Stogdill, *Handbook of Leadership —A Survey of Theory and Research* (New York: The Free Press), p. 81.

47. Margaret Colton, "Nursing's Leadership Vacuum," *Sup. Nurs.,* **7:**29 (Oct. 1976).

48. Madeleine Leininger, "The Leadership Crisis in Nursing: A Critical Problem and Challenge," *J. Nurs. Admin.,* **4:**30 (Mar./Apr. 1974).

49. Gwendolyn Safier, "Leaders Among Contemporary U. S. Nurses: An Oral History," in Chaska, op. cit.

50. Gwendolyn Safier, *Contemporary American Leaders in Nursing—An Oral History* (New York: McGraw-Hill Book Company, 1977).

51. Connie Vance, "A Group Profile of Contemporary Influentials in American Nursing," (Unpublished EdD dissertation, Teachers College, Columbia University, 1977).

52. Rozella Schlotfeldt, "Knowledge, Leaders and Progress," *Image,* **2:**2–5 (Feb. 1968).

53. Lynne Welch, "Planned Change in Nursing: The Theory," *Nurs. Clinics of North America,* **14:**307 (June 1979).

54. Ibid., pp. 313–320.

55. Elizabeth Olson, "Strategies and Techniques for the Nurse Change Agent," *Nurs. Clinics of North America,* **14:**323–329 (June 1979).

56. Agnes Reinkemeyer, "Nursing's Need: A Commitment to an Ideology of Change," *Nurs. Forum*, **9**:341–355 (1970).

57. Olson, op. cit., pp. 329–330.

58. Ibid., pp. 334–335.

59. Shirley Smoyak, "The Confrontation Process," *Am. J. Nurs.*, **74**:1632–1635 (Sept. 1974).

60. Julia Thompson, *The ANA in Washington* (Kansas City, Mo.: The ANA, 1972).

61. Melinda McLemore, "Nurses as Health Planners—Our New Legal Status," *Nurs. Digest*, **5**:59–60 (Spring 1977).

62. Thom, Mary, "Running for Office," *MS. Magazine*, **2**:61–68 (Apr. 1974).

63. "A Distaff 'Look' to Politics," *Weekend Dispatch* (New Jersey), Sept. 16, 1978, p. 2.

64. Mary Kelly Mullane, "Nursing Care and the Political Arena," *Nurs. Outlook*, **23**:697–701 (Nov. 1975).

65. Edith Lewis, "The Professionally Uncommitted," Editorial, *Nurs. Outlook*, **27**:323 (May 1979).

66. Beatrice Kalisch, "The Promise of Power," *Nurs. Outlook*, **26**:42–50 (Jan. 1978).

67. Sister Dorothy Sheahan, "Scanning the Seventies," *Nurs. Outlook*, **26**:33–37 (Jan. 1978).

68. Jacqueline Rose Hott, "The Struggles Inside Nursing's Body Politic," *Nurs. Forum*, **15**(4):325–340 (1976).

69. Margaret McClure, "The Long Road to Accountability," *Nurs. Outlook*, **26**:47–50 (Jan. 1978).

70. Lulu Wolf Hassenplug, "Nursing *Can* Move From Here To There," *Nurs. Outlook*, **25**:432–438 (July 1977).

71. Lucie Young Kelly, "Endpaper: The Good New Nurse Network," *Nurs. Outlook*, **26**:70 (Jan. 1978).

72. Geraldine Felton, "On Women, Networks, Patronage and Sponsorship," Editorial, *Image*, **10**:58–59 (Oct. 1978).

73. Patricia Dean, "Toward Androgeny," *Image*, **10**:10–14 (Feb. 1978).

74. Renee Lieb, "Power, Powerlessness and Potential—Nurses' Role Within the Health Care Delivery System," *Image*, **10**:75–82 (Oct. 1978).

75. Jean Withers, "Background: Why Women Are Unassertive," *Nurs. Digest*, **6**:70 (Fall 1978).

76. Holly Hutchings and Louise Colburn, "An Assertiveness Training Program for Nurses," *Nurs. Outlook*, **27**:394–397 (June 1979).

77. Manuel Smith, *When I Say No. I Feel Guilty* (New York: The Dial Press, 1975).

78. *Woman, Assert Your Self: An Instructive Handbook* (New York: Harper & Row, Publishers, 1976).

79. Sheehy, Gail, *Passages: Predictable Crises of Adult Life* (New York: E. P. Dutton & Co., Inc., 1976).

80. Marcelle Williams, *The New Executive Woman* (Radnor, Pa.: Chilton Book Company, 1977).

81. Vance, op. cit.

82. Lucie Young Kelly, "Endpaper: Power Guide—The Mentor Relationship," *Nurs. Outlook*, **26**:339 (May 1978).

83. Marlene Grissum, "How You Can Become a Risk Taker and a Role Breaker," *Nurs. 76*, **6**:89–98 (Nov. 1978).

84. Lucie Young Kelly, "Endpaper: How to Start a Counterculture," *Nurs. Outlook*, **27**:149 (Feb. 1979).

85. Denise Benton, "You Want To Be a What?" *Nurs. Outlook*, **27**:388–393 (June 1979).

86. Carole Jennings, "Nursing's Case for Third Party Reimbursement," *Am. J. Nurs.*, **79**:111–114 (Jan. 1979).

87. Lucie Young Kelly, "Endpaper: Goodbye, Appliance Nurse," *Nurs. Outlook*, **27**:432 (June 1979).

BIBLIOGRAPHY

American Nurses' Association. *Power: Nursing's Challenge for Change* Kansas City, Mo.: The Association, 1979. Major papers presented at 1978 ANA convention on issues such as legal aspects, collective bargaining, education, research, and practice.

Ashley, Jo Ann. *Hospitals, Paternalism, and the Role of the Nurse.* New York: Teachers College Press, 1976. Excellent historical look at how nurses' roles in hospitals mitigated against achieving autonomy. Extensive bibliography.

Pertinent summary of problems of nurses achieving autonomy today.

Ashley, Jo Ann. "Power, Freedom and Professional Practice in Nursing," *Sup. Nurse*, **6** (Jan. 1975), 12–29. A call for nurses to face their exploitation and act.

Ashley, Jo Ann. "This I Believe: About Power in Nursing," *Nurs. Outlook*, **21** (Oct. 1973), 637–647. Another variation of Ashley's thesis about the need for nurses to fight for autonomy.

Bell, Roderick. *Political Power*. New York: The Free Press, 1969. A reader on the theory and research of power.

Bennet, Leland. "This I Believe—That Nurses May Become Extinct," *Nurs. Outlook*, **18** (Jan. 1970), 28–32. Author warns that if nurses do not move with the times and find better ways to give patient-centered care, computers can replace them.

Berkowitz, Norman, and Mary Malone. "Intra-Professional Conflict," *Nurs. Forum*, **7** (Winter 1968), 50–71. Excellent analysis of reasons for problems within nursing.

Bowman, Rosemary. "The Nursing Organization as a Political Pressure Group," *Nurs. Forum*, **12**(1) (1973), 72–81. How ANA can influence legislation.

Bowman, Rosemary, and Rebecca Culpepper. "Power: Rx for Change," *Am. J. Nurs.*, **74** (June 1974), 1054–1056. Authors believe that time for nurse power has come and examine powerlessness, use of power, and the growing power of nurses.

Brooten, Dorothy, et al. *Leadership for Change: A Guide for the Frustrated Nurse*. Philadelphia: J. B. Lippincott Company, 1978. Emphasizes need for change so that nursing can exert leadership in health care. Interesting approach and excellent references.

Bullough, Bonnie and Vern Bullough, eds. *Issues in Nursing*. New York: Springer Publishing Co., Inc., 1966. A selection of readings on issues in education, practice, economics, and patient care. Especially useful because some of the articles are classics dating to nursing's early days, which offer an excellent historical perspective.

Bullough, Bonnie and Vern Bullough, eds. *New Directions for Nurses*. New York: Springer Publishing Co., Inc., 1971. An excellent selection of readings on major nursing issues, including nurse-doctor relationships, the health care system, nursing manpower. Focus is on need for nurses seeking autonomy to become familiar with major issues.

Bullough, Bonnie and Vern Bullough. "Sex Discrimination in Health Care," *Nurs. Outlook*, **23** (Jan. 1975), 40–45. Includes information on disparity in income, physicians' bias toward nurses and women patients. Good references.

Cannings, Kathleen, and William Lazonick. "The Development of the Nursing Labor Force in the United States: A Basic Analysis," *Intl. J. of Health Services*, **5**(2) (1975), 185–216. A comprehensive overview of how nursing became a part of the labor force (from the nineteenth century), including data from some of the major reports. Stresses need for unity if autonomy is to be achieved.

Chaska, Norma, Ed. *The Nursing Profession: Views Through the Mist*. New York: McGraw Hill Book Company, 1978. Pertinent readings, including professionalization, nursing practice, interdisciplinary professional relationships, and the future of nursing.

Claus, Karen, and June Bailey. *Power and Influence in Health Care*. St. Louis, Mo.: C. V. Mosby Company, 1977. Emphasis on leadership and leaders as planners, energizers, initiators, humanizers, and risk takers. Development of Power/Authority/Influence Model. Extensive and good references.

Cleland, Virginia. "Sex Discrimination: Nursing's Most Pervasive Problem," *Am. J. Nurs.*, **71** (Aug. 1971), 1542–1547. Considered a classic that awakened nurses to the fact that they were too often unaware of and indifferent to their lack of autonomy.

Dachelet, Christy. "Nursing's Bid for Increased Status," *Nurs. Forum* **17**(1) (1978) 18–45. Notes factors hampering nursing's bid for status, including nursing's image and attitude of physicians. Extensive bibliography.

Dalrymple, Sara, et al. "Implication of a Study in a Nurse-Physician Relationship," *Nurs. Forum*, **7** (Winter 1968), 21–27. Twenty-one of twenty-two nurses prepared to give an excessive dose of an unknown drug ordered by an unknown telephone caller.

Diamond, Helen. "Patterns of Leadership," *Image*, **11** (June 1979), 42–44. Describes how women are shaped *not* to lead from childhood. Refers to Hennig's study. Good summary of issues.

Diers, Donna. "A Different Kind of Energy: Nurse Power," *Nurs. Outlook*, **26** (Jan. 1978),

51–55. Nurses seen as a potential alternative source of power to avert a health care crisis analogous to the energy crisis.

Diers, Donna. "Lessons on Leadership," *Image* **11** (Oct. 1979), 67–71. Incisive suggestions on leadership presented with humor and humanity.

Edelstein, Ruth. "Equal Rights for Women: Perspectives," *Am. J. Nurs.*, **71** (Feb. 1971), 294–298. Author urges women's lib groups to encourage talented women into nursing. Notes some of the sexist problems in nursing.

Elsberry, Nancy. "Power Relations in Hospital Nursing," *J. Nurs. Admin.*, **2** (Sept./Oct. 1972), 75–77. Describes five types of power applicable to hospital nursing, the factors that limit power, and some methods to counter powerlessness.

Fine, Ruth. "Application of Leadership Theory," *Nurs. Clinics of North America*, **13** (Mar. 1978), 139–153. Overview of leadership theories with specific application to nursing service situations.

Fuller, Sarah. "Humanistic Leadership in a Pragmatic Age," *Nurs. Outlook*, **27** (Dec. 1979), 770–773. If nursing is to remain a humanistic profession, leaders and other nurses should adopt idealogical commitment.

Given, Barbara and Sandra Simmons. "The Interdisciplinary Health Care Team: Fact or Fiction? *Nurs. Forum*, **6**(2) (1977), 165–184. Describes problems as well as elements vital to effective functioning. Good references.

Grissum, Marlene, and Carol Spengler. *Womanpower and Health Care*. Boston: Little, Brown and Company, 1976. Focuses on some of the special problems, issues, and barriers confronting women, especially nurses, with suggestions for action. Excellent references.

Harragan, Betty. *Games Mother Never Taught You*. New York: Warner Books, 1977. Despite unfortunate description of nursing as a "narrow profession that remains the same," this popular book gives practical guidelines for "corporate gamesmanship for women."

Hennig, Margaret, and Anne Jardim. *The Managerial Woman*. Garden City, N.Y.: Anchor Press, 1977. Research of these Harvard graduates. A bestseller, easily read. Traces background of women striving for managerial power and provides useful advice.

Kalisch, Beatrice, and Philip Kalisch. "A Discourse on the Politics of Nursing," *J. Nurs. Admin.*, **6** (Mar./Apr. 1976), 29–34. Educating nurses to the importance of cohesive, strong membership base can thwart continued political neglect that weakens nursing impact. Extensive recommended readings.

Kelly, Lucie Young. "Endpaper: Me-Politics and Nursing," *Nurs. Outlook*, **27** (Apr. 1979), 303. Divisive forces within and without nursing are destructive to the profession.

Kelly, Lucie Young. "Our Nursing Heritage: Have We Renounced It?" *Image*, **8** (Oct. 1976), 43–48. A historical look at where we were and a challenge for the future.

Kelly, Lucie Young. "Endpaper: Who's Got the Dinosaur?" *Nurs. Outlook*, **26** (Sept. 1978), 595. Who will the public choose for primary care—a physician or a nurse?

Kelly, Lucie Young. "Endpaper: The Day Nobody Listened—October, 1979, *Nurs. Outlook*, **27** (Dec. 1979), 809. A description of a destructive use of power.

Kelly, Lucie Young. "Endpaper: Escape By Scapegoat." *Nurs. Outlook*, **27** (Nov. 1979), 752. Putting the blame on others instead of taking individual responsibility.

Kelly, Lucie Young. "Endpaper: Quotidian Nursing," *Nurs. Outlook*, **27** (Oct. 1979), 688. Nursing should appreciate the contributions of the "average nurse" as well as the highly prepared specialists. See also Letter to Editor in response Feb. 1980.

Kelly, Lucie Young. "Endpaper: We Try Harder," *Nurs. Outlook*, **27** (Aug. 1979), 569. Nurses must overcome any feelings of inferiority they have concerning their power and value in health care.

Kritek, Phyllis, and Laurie Glass. "Nursing: A Feminist Perspective," *Nurs. Outlook*, **26** (Mar. 1978), 182–186. Describes a course that enabled students and faculty to learn much about themselves and sexism in society.

Lamb, Karen. "Freedom for Our Sister, Freedom for Ourselves," *Nurs. Forum*, **12**(4) (1973), 328–352. Also reprinted in *Nurs. Digest*, **6** (Oct. 1974), 2–9. Reviews major aspects of discrimination against women and suggests how nursing can help fight the battle.

Lawrence, John. "Confronting Nurses' Political Apathy," *Nurs. Forum*, **15**(4) (1976), 363–371. Underscores need for political action and makes suggestions on what course to take.

Levenstein, Aaron. "What Does a Leader Do?" *Sup. Nurse* **10** (June 1979), 66–67. Management expert presents a checklist of activities and notes the need of loyalty of others to be successful.

Levin, Pamela, and Eric Berne. "Games Nurses Play," *Am. J. Nurs.*, **72** (Mar. 1972), 483–487. A nursing version of transactional analysis.

Lewin, K. "Group Decision and Social Change," In Maccoby, E., ed. *Readings in Social Psychology*, 3rd ed. New York: Holt, Rinehart and Winston, 1958. Describes Lewin's theory of change.

Lewis, Edith, ed. *Changing Patterns of Nursing Practice.* New York: Am. J. Nurs. Co., 1971. Reprint of articles, including some classics, on topics such as need for change and nurse-physician relationships.

Lewis, Frances. "The Nurse as Lackey: A Sociological Perspective," *Sup. Nurse*, **7** (Apr. 1976), 24–27. Nurses are still at the lower end of a stratification system and some nurses perpetuate this by their own behavior.

Machiavelli, Niccolo. *The Prince.* New York: New American Library, 1952. Considered a classic on power, applicable to today and often a requirement for management courses.

McBride, Angela. "A Married Feminist," *Am. J. Nurs.*, **76** (May 1976), 754–757. Excerpts from book of same title. This section focuses on author's job, nursing, and, in part, her attitude about nursing and marriage.

Mullins, Anna and Ruth Barstow. "Care for the Caretakers," *Am. J. Nurs.*, **79** (Aug. 1979), 1425–1427. Describes how to develop a support system for nursing.

Peeples, Edward, and Gloria Francis. "Social-Psychological Obstacles to Effective Health Team Practice," *Nurs. Forum*, **7**(1) (1968), 28–37. Considers such factors as occupational gap, social class orientation, income breach, and other problems of attitudes and beliefs of nurses and doctors.

Powell, Diane. "Nursing and Politics: The Struggles Outside Nursing's Body Politic," *Nurs. Forum*, **15**(4) (1976), 341–362. The beginning of N-CAP and its functioning.

Shapiro, Eileen et al. "Moving Up: Role Models, Mentors, and the Patron System." *Sloan Management Review*, (Spring, 1978), 51–58. Examines concepts of role models and mentors and describes the continuum of a patron system as it can be used to help women toward leadership positions.

Siu, R. G. H. *The Craft of Power.* New York: John Wiley and Sons, Inc., 1979. Described as a practical synthesis of East-West philosophies and psychology, a shrewd blending of the best power strategies of each. Applicable to reality.

Vance, Connie. "A Group Profile of Contemporary Influentials in American Nursing." Unpublished EdD dissertation, Teachers College, Columbia University, 1977. Study of nursing leaders also lists names of the "influentials."

Yura, Helen. "Nursing Leadership Behavior," *Sup. Nurse*, **2** (Feb. 1971), 55 ff. A study of nursing leadership behavior, with behaviors derived from studies of nurses already in leadership positions. Behaviors were rated from least to most important by nursing faculty in universities. The researchers derived from this a definition of nursing leadership to be used as a predictor of leadership role potential in students.

Zimmerman, Beverly. "Changes of the Second Order," *Nurs. Outlook*, **27** (Mar. 1979), 199–201. First order changes within the system do not change it; second order changes directed at the system itself can alter it.

Zungolo, Eileen. "A Study in Alienation: The Nurse Practitioner," *Nurs. Forum*, **7**(1) (1968), 38–49. Term refers to RNs in general, as was common at that time. However, application of principles of alienation is still pertinent.

See also references at end of Chapter 16; references and bibliography of Chapters 6, 10, and 11; entire issue of *Nurs. Digest*, **7**(3) (Fall 1978) on politics of self-esteem, with good annotated bibliography; entire issue of *Nurs. Dimensions*, **7**(1) (Spring 1979) on women's health care; entire issue of *Nurs. Admin. Quarterly*, **2**(3) (Spring 1978) on politics and power; entire issue of *Nurs. Admin. Quarterly*, **3**(2) (Winter 1979) on organization nurses in action, which has implications for leadership and power; publications from the American Academy of Nursing on *Primary Care by Nurses: Sphere of Responsibility and Accountability* (1976). *Primary Care in a Pluralistic Society: Impediments to Health Care Delivery* (1977) and *Nursings Influence on Health Policy for the Eighties.* The new journal *Nursing Leadership* also has many articles on power and autonomy (1978).

LEGAL RIGHTS AND RESPONSIBILITIES

An Introduction to Law

Law has been defined as "the sum total of rules and regulations by which society is governed. It is man-made and regulates social conduct in a formal and binding way. It reflects society's needs, attitudes, and mores."[1] The more complex the society is, the more complicated the legal system that governs it and also the more likely that the law will be in a state of change. Everyone dealing with law knows that there is no final or absolute answer—something that is quite frustrating for those who want to know exactly what they can or cannot do. Yet, there are certain principles that may serve as guidelines and as a basis of understanding American law.

ORIGINS OF MODERN LAW

The first "laws" were set up by the leaders of primitive peoples who found they could not live successfully in groups without rules or codes to govern them. Certain leaders, known as lawgivers, sometimes had prevailing customs and traditions set down as the basic law of the land. One of their early tasks was to distinguish between sensible laws and those that were merely taboos or superstitions.

The most illustrious lawgiver of ancient history was Hammurabi, King of Babylon (2067–2025 B.C.), who developed a detailed code of laws to be used by the courts throughout the empire. Known as the Code of Hammurabi, the text was inscribed on stone columns, the ruins of which are now in the Louvre in Paris.

The laws governing Greece remained unwritten until about 621 B.C. when Draco, an Athenian statesman and lawgiver, codified them. Although the code was a marked advancement toward equal justice under the law for all of the people, it was so stern (demanding the death penalty for nearly all crimes) that the word *Draconian* is still used to describe an unduly cruel person or action. Draco's code was replaced by a milder one prepared under the direction of Solon (c. 638 –558 B.C.) and this was later revised by Plato (c. 428-c. 348 B.C.).

In Rome, Emperor Justinian 1 (A.D. 483– 565) appointed a commission of legal experts to prepare a revision—actually a consolidation—of Rome's inefficient set of laws, which had developed over a period of approximately 1,000 years. This revision, the *Corpus Juris Civilis*, issued in four parts, served as a basis for civil law in most European countries and in England. Later it had considerable influence on the structure of laws in the United States. The third part of the document, the *Digest* (A.D. 533), intended for use by judges and practitioners of the law, contained the law in concrete form and was by far the most important section, influencing jurists and scholars for many years, possibly even to this day.

Another famous code of laws, parts of which are still in effect in France, was prepared under the leadership of Emperor Napoleon of France (1769–1821). The legal system of the state of Louisiana, once a French colony, was originally based on the Napoleon of France (1769–1821). The legal sys-laws on the English system of common law. Quebec, Canada, whose population is largely of French origin, also used the French code as a basis for its laws.

In England, centuries ago, the king reigned supreme, but because of great distances and limited communication facilities, he found it necessary to enlist the help of lords and barons in settling disputes in their geographical areas. He, however, retained the privilege of overriding or vetoing their decisions if he deemed it to the crown's, or kingdom's, advantage to do so.

The lords and barons in turn passed on authority for settling certain disputes to persons of lesser standing, retaining the power of veto over their decisions. To achieve a degree of order and uniformity, the same persons traveled from place to place in the manner of circuit judges to hear arguments pro and con and serve as mediators in settling controversies. It was quite natural for these "judges" to make similar decisions when cases presented similar sets of circumstances.

As so often happens, the administrative official (in this case, the king of England) became concerned lest some of his power be stripped from him, and he took steps to regain and centralize control over the dispensation of justice throughout his land. This he did by assuming responsibility for the appointment of judges to preside over hearings of disputes to be held in designated places

called the king's courts. To help them in their duties and serve as guides for future deliberations, the judges often kept written records of their decisions for their personal use. Later the keeping of such records became mandatory. These records and the principles found therein were the foundation of common law.

With the introduction of written decisions, one of the most important principles known in the law was born, the principle of *stare decisis*, which means to stand as decided or "let the decision stand."

> *When a previous case involving similar facts has been decided in the jurisdiction, the court will be strongly inclined to follow the principles of law laid down in that prior adjudication. Unless precedents are carefully regarded and adhered to, uncertainty would be both perplexing and prejudicial to the public. However, when the precedent is out of date or inapplicable to the case before the court, the principle of stare decisis will not be followed and the court will announce a new rule.*[2]

Courts of law presided over by competent lawyers quickly gained the confidence and respect of the English people. As a result, common law achieved extraordinary power, at times claimed to be even greater than that of the reigning monarch, whose arbitrary despotism remained almost unquestioned until the barons forced King John to sign the Magna Carta in 1215 at Runnymede. The following excerpts from the Magna Carta are applicable to some of the current issues in our society:

> *No freeman shall be taken, or imprisoned, or outlawed, or exiled, or in any way harmed, nor will we go upon or send upon him, save by the lawful judgment of his peers or by the law of the land. [Article 39]*
> *To none will we sell, to none deny or delay, right or justice. [Article 40]*

These clauses were the antecedents of due process of law and the guarantee of trial by jury. The charter also provided for a committee of twenty-five barons to enforce it. This was the beginning in England of a government that provided a system of checks and balances that would keep the monarchy strong but prevent its perversion by a tyrannic or inept king or queen. Though severely tested at times, government in England from then on meant more than the despotic rule of one person; custom and law stood even above the king.

The British parliament, the supreme national legislative body, established in 1295 and actually an outgrowth of the Magna Carta, marked the beginning of self-government in England. It took its name from the French *parlement* (derived from *parler*, "to speak"), which in France was originally used to describe any meeting for discussion or debate. The English form *parliament* was first used to designate a debate, later a formal conference only. The laws enacted by this body were termed statutory law as contrasted with common law. The rules and regulations developed to guide the deliberations of Parliament, and now widely used in other countries, are often called *parliamentary law*. They are not laws, however, and are more correctly termed *parliamentary procedure*.

THE UNITED STATES LEGAL SYSTEM

As the American colonies were founded one by one, the manner in which they would be governed was a vital and primary consideration. The edicts of the governments in the homelands of the settlers were a persuasive force, of course; in addition, the colonists were influenced greatly by their own previous experience and knowledge. From the beginning, self-government became their goal, a goal that seemed more attainable in the English colonies than in those originally settled by the Spanish and French.

One of the early problems was to establish methods of dealing with disputes over property and personal injuries. To handle such disputes, the Pilgrim Fathers adopted a system similar to that of the common law then in effect in England. Judges were appointed and courts established, but because the life and customs were so different here from those in England it often proved impractical and unfair to apply decisions that had been made in the mother country. Furthermore, the problems within the colonies varied so widely that a judge's decision regarding a dispute in one colony was not necessarily applied by another judge to a similar set of circumstances in another. Each colony, therefore, developed its own procedures and laws, both common and statutory, based on its own peculiar needs.

From this evolved the concept of states' rights, which has played such an important role in the history of the United States. For many years any infringement of these rights either from the federal government or from other states was vigorously opposed, although in recent years there is less resistance to the initiation of federal programs that assume or share responsibilities that for years were carried by the individual states alone.

It is not unusual, of course, for several states to adopt in their separate legislatures an identical law, such as that governing the age at which a person may vote if he meets other qualifications. The fact remains, however, that a state that enacts its own laws can retain, revise, or repeal them without interference from other states or the federal government. Relinquishment of this right is a serious matter in a democracy, because doing so sets a precedent that may be difficult to overcome. On the other hand, variance in state laws also gives rise to a great deal of confusion, misunderstanding, and red tape. How much simpler it would be, for example, if the laws governing the licensure of nurses and the practice of nursing were uniform throughout the country—providing they were adequate laws, of course.

Road signs for many legal problems are not as easily seen as the speed limits posted along an interstate highway. One may quite innocently get into legal difficulty in one state while doing something that would not be against the law in another. The accused usually has no recourse, however, because ignorance of the law is not a defense in court.

The founders of the United States did not depend on common law alone to govern the colonies; neither did they give unlimited power to the governors and councils appointed by the governments of their homelands. To establish and maintain a degree of control, each of the original thirteen colonies early in its history established legislative bodies elected by the voters. The first was the House of Burgesses, which met in Jamestown, Virginia, in 1619 and which was attended by two burgesses (citizens) from each of twenty-seven plantations.

Such localized government was considered adequate as well as advisable until 1774, when the colonies felt the need to unite to voice their collective grievances against England's colonial policies. In that year, the First Continental Congress, attended by representatives of all colonies except Georgia, met in Philadelphia from September 5 to October 26. The Congress did more than express grievances; it also created an association to impose extensive boycotts against British trade, thus firmly establishing the tradition of pooling strengths and resources in time of national stress and emergency.

By the next year, war had begun and the Second Continental Congress, meeting in session from May 10, 1775, until December 12, 1776, created a Continental army under the direction of George Washington to oppose the British. With the Declaration of Independence, formalized on July 4, 1776, the colonies were launched on a course of liberty from which they—and the states that were later formed—never retreated, although discussions, disagreements, financial difficulties, jealousies, and friction hampered progress time after time.

The Continental Congress continued to meet annually for varying periods of time in several different cities. With limited funds and little experience in affairs of state, the representatives retained the will and courage to continue to advance toward full independence. In 1778, the Congress submitted the Articles of Confederation to the legislatures of the states for ratification; this was accomplished in 1781. The states considered themselves practically as separate countries, however, delegating to the central government only those powers which they could not handle individually, such as the authority to wage war, establish a uniform currency, and make treaties with other nations. They made no provision for an executive head of the central government.

The Articles of Confederation proved to be too weak to hold the colonies together, giving rise to fears that foreign powers might reconquer part or all of the country. Under the leadership of farsighted patriots such as George Washington and Alexander Hamilton, a movement toward nationalization was given impetus and, as a result, in 1787 a Constitutional Convention met in Philadelphia to draw up the Constitution of the United States, the idea for which had originated in English and earlier colonial history. Ratification of the Constitution by a majority of the thirteen colonies established the permanent structure of the Congress of the United States, which held its first meeting in New York, March 4, 1789. Its first meeting in our present capital, Washington, D.C., was held in 1800. The Constitution also designated that a president, elected by the people, should be at the head of the government.

Since then, the volume and complexity of problems facing the legislature have increased tremendously. Departments and councils by the score have been set up to assist in the work of making laws. But at the hub of the work, guiding the action, is always the Constitution of the United States—the law of the land—which, although amended twenty-six times (to 1979), could scarcely be improved upon were it rewritten from the start today. Its basic principles are as pertinent now as they were in 1789.

Constitutional Amendments

Shortly after the adoption of the Constitution, it became apparent that the government's police power needed to be limited by spelling out the rights of the states and the individual citizen. Congress, therefore, submitted to the states twelve amendments to the Constitution intended to clarify these rights, ten of which were ratified by the states in 1791, thus establishing the Bill of Rights, on which social and political developments in the last few decades have placed renewed emphasis. It may be well, therefore, to review these amendments here to help form a basis for later discussion of the legal rights and responsibilities of citizens including nurses.

The *First Amendment* guarantees United States citizens freedom of religion, speech, press, and the right "peaceably to assemble and to petition the Government for a redress of grievances." This amendment is often the center of controversy in disputes related to the freedom guaranteed herein.

The *Second Amendment* gives the people (governmental bodies) the right to keep and bear arms, because a well-regulated militia is necessary to the security of a free state. The *Third* refers to the quartering of soldiers in a private home in time of peace or war.

The last seven amendments included in the Bill of Rights have direct or indirect bearing on crimes, trials, and other legal matters in which nurses might become involved. They, therefore, are reproduced here, in full.

Article IV [Fourth Amendment] Protection Against Search

The right of the people to be secure in their persons, houses, papers, and effects, against unreasonable searches and seizures, shall not be violated, and no warrants shall issue, but upon probable cause, supported by oath or affirmation, and particularly describing the place to be searched, and the persons or things to be seized.

Article V [Fifth Amendment] Due Process of Law Assured

No person shall be held to answer for a capital, or otherwise infamous crime, unless on a presentment or indictment of a grand jury, except in cases arising in the land or naval forces, or in the militia, when in actual service in time of war or public danger; nor shall any person be subject for the same offense to be twice put in jeopardy of life or limb; nor shall be compelled in any criminal case to be witness against himself, nor be deprived of life, liberty, or property without due process of law; nor shall private property be taken for public use, without just compensation.

Article VI [Sixth Amendment] Rights of Accused in Criminal Cases

In all criminal prosecutions, the accused shall enjoy the rights to a speedy and public trial, by an impartial jury of the state and district wherein the crime shall have been committed, which district shall have been previously ascertained by law, and to be informed of the nature and cause of the accusation; to be confronted with the witnesses against him; to have compulsory process for obtaining witnesses in his favor, and to have the assistance of counsel for his defense.

Article VII [Seventh Amendment] Jury Trial in Civil Cases

In suits at common law, where the value in controversy shall exceed twenty dollars, the right of trial by jury shall be preserved, and no fact tried by jury shall be otherwise reexamined in any court of the United States, than according to the rules of the common law.

Article VIII [Eighth Amendment] Excessive Punishments Forbidden

Excessive bail shall not be required, nor excessive fines imposed, nor cruel and unusual punishments inflicted.

Article IX [Ninth Amendment] Unenumerated Rights of the People

The enumeration in the Constitution, of certain rights, shall not be construed to deny or disparage others retained by the people.

Article X [Tenth Amendment] The Rights of States

The powers not delegated to the United States by the Constitution, nor prohibited by it to the states, are reserved to the states respectively, or to the people.

Later Amendments. The *Eleventh Amend-*

ment (1798) is concerned with judicial powers; the *Twelfth* (1804), with the method of electing a president and vice-president; the *Thirteenth* (1865) abolished slavery. The *Fourteenth Amendment*, added in 1868 during the reconstruction period following the Civil War, states, in part:

> *No state shall make or enforce any law which shall abridge the privileges or immunities of citizens of the United States; nor shall any state deprive any person of life, liberty, or property, without due process of law; nor deny to any person within its jurisdiction the equal protection of the laws.*

The *Fifteenth Amendment*, ratified in 1870, reads:

> 1. *The right of the citizens of the United States to vote shall not be denied or abridged by the United States or by any State on account of race, color, or previous condition of servitude.*
> 2. *The Congress shall have power to enforce this article by appropriate legislation.*

The *Sixteenth Amendment* (1913) authorized Congress to "lay and collect taxes on income"; the *Seventeenth* (1913) refers to the election of United States senators; the *Eighteenth*, adopted in 1920 and repealed in 1933, prohibited the manufacture, sale, or transportation of intoxicating liquors for beverage purposes within the United States and all territories subject to its jurisdiction.

The *Nineteenth Amendment*, known as the Women's Suffrage Amendment, went into effect August 26, 1920. It reads as follows:

> 1. *The right of citizens of the United States to vote shall not be denied or abridged by the United States or by any state on account of sex.*
> 2. *Congress shall have power to enforce this article by appropriate legislation.*

The *Twentieth Amendment* (1933) specifies the dates on which the terms of the president, vice-president, senators, and representatives shall assume office.

The *Twenty-first Amendment* (1933) repealed the *Eighteenth Amendment;* the *Twenty-second* (1951) limited the presidential terms of office to two; the *Twenty-third* (1961) gave citizens of the District of Columbia the right to vote for presidential and vice-presidential candidates.

The *Twenty-fourth Amendment* (1964) states:

> *The right of citizens of the United States to vote in any primary or other election for President or Vice President, for electors for President or Vice President, or for Senator or Representative in Congress shall not be denied or abridged by the United States or any State by reason of failure to pay any poll tax or other tax.*

The *Twenty-fifth Amendment* (1965) deals with the disability of a president or a vacancy in the office of vice-president and stipulates how the offices shall be filled in the event of an emergency.

The *Twenty-sixth Amendment* (1971) reduced the voting age to eighteen.

There is the possibility that the Twenty-seventh Amendment will bar legal discrimination against women based on sex. The bill, passed by Congress (1971-1972) and sent to the states for ratification, reads, "Equality of rights under the law shall not be denied or abridged by the United States or any State on account of sex." To be adopted, two thirds of the states (thirty-eight) must ratify the amendment by a specific time. When it was apparent that this goal would not be reached by the legal deadline of March 22, 1979, (three were still needed by mid-1978), both the House and Senate voted to extend the deadline to June 30, 1982. At the same time, a proposal to allow states that had already ratified the amendment to rescind their decisions was defeated, but the final decision on whether rescinding is possible remains open. Most of the states in which the equal rights amendment (ERA) was defeated by 1978 were in the South (Florida, Georgia, Alabama, Mississippi, Louisiana, North Carolina, South Carolina, Virginia, Oklahoma, Arkansas), but the legislators of Nevada, Utah, Arizona, Missouri, and Illinois also voted not to ratify.

Some sixteen states, at that time, had

passed their own laws to prohibit discrimination on the basis of sex, but the degree of confusion can be demonstrated by the fact that some states that approved the constitutional amendment defeated a similar one in their own state.

The Constitution and its amendments are some of the provisions made by the federal government to ensure the rights of individuals to protection under the law and to fair and just practices in the application of laws at any political level. Guards against usurpation of the privileges and authority of individuals, as well as state and local jurisdictions, also are provided. Beyond this, it is up to the states, counties, townships, and municipalities to develop laws and legal procedures to protect their citizens. It is the individual's responsibility to be well informed about the laws governing his/her geographical area and especially those that are applicable to his/her status and vocation. This will help avoid legal infractions and provide some protection against miscarriage of justice should an individual become involved in litigation.

LEGAL STRUCTURE OF THE UNITED STATES

Under the United States government, the law is carried out at a number of levels. The Constitution is the highest law of the land. Whatever the Constitution (federal law) does not spell out, the states retain for themselves (Tenth Constitutional amendment). Because they can create political subdivisions, units of local government, counties, cities, towns, townships, boroughs, and villages, all have certain legal powers within their geographic boundaries. On all levels, but most obviously on the federal and state levels, there is a separation of power: legislative, executive, and judicial. The first makes the laws, the second carries them out, and the third reviews them, a system which the founders of the United States believed would create a balance of power.

There are three basic sources of law: statutory law, executive or regulatory law, and judicial law.

Statutory law refers to statutes that are acts of legislative bodies declaring, commanding, or prohibiting something.* Statutes are always written, are firmly established, and can only be altered by amendment or repeal. The Nurse Training Act is one example of a federal law. A state law requiring professional nurses to be licensed before they can legally practice nursing is another example.

Executive or regulatory law refers to the rules, regulations, and decisions of administrative bodies. For example, the HEW Division of Nursing developed the regulations that determined the requirements for the nurse practitioner programs (part of the NTA finding); the State Board of Nursing spells out the requirements for a nursing school; a State Health Code may adopt a patients' bill of rights as a requirement for all hospitals in the state. All have the effect of law.

Judicial law, also called decisional, case, or common law, as distinguished from law created by the enactment of legislatures, comprises a body of legal principles and rules of action that derive their authority from usage and custom or from judgments and decrees of courts based on these usages and customs. Courts are agencies established by the government to decide disputes. (The term *court* is also sometimes used to refer to the person or persons hearing a case.) There is usually only one judge for a trial (with or without a jury); two or more to hear the appeals (with no jury). The kind of court in which a case is brought depends upon the offense or complaint.

There are also various classifications of law.

Criminal or penal law deals with action harmful to the public and the individual and designates punishment for offenders. Three gradations of criminal acts are recognized by

---

*The legislative process is described in Chapter 18.

the law: (1) *offenses*, such as traffic violations or disorderly conduct; (2) *misdemeanors*, such as small thefts, perjury, conspiracies, and assaults without the use of weapons; and (3) *felonies*, which include major robberies, assault with a dangerous weapon, arson, rape, and murder.

Civil law states the rights of persons and stipulates methods for maintaining or regaining them. The word *civil* means "citizen"; civil laws, therefore, pertain to the individual citizen. The system of civil law is derived, in greatly modified form, from the law of Rome established by the Emperor Justinian. Many acts of negligence, libel and slander, and commercial disputes are examples of cases that are subject to the application of civil law. It is distinct from criminal law.

There are many subdivisions of civil law. One of these of particular interest to nurses is **contract law.** Laws of contract govern all legal actions related to the making, keeping, or breaking of legal contracts of any type—for example, employment contracts, marriage contracts, and contracts for the sale of property. Contract law also deals with fraudulent contracts. No fraudulent contract against an innocent person is binding unless he wants to make it so.

Laws are additionally classified by subject matter, such as labor laws, maritime laws, mercantile laws, tax laws, motor vehicle laws, and others. Two other major categories of law are martial and military law.

Martial law means the suspension of civil law in time of emergency and the enforcement of military law on the civilian population.

Military law is a branch of national (or state) law which governs the conduct of national (or state) military organizations in peace or war. The rules or laws are enacted by the legislative body and administered in court-martial—a court consisting of military officers where personnel are tried for breaches of military law or discipline. Nurses enrolled in the armed forces as commissioned officers are subject to military law, which applies to all branches of the military services.

Enforcement of Laws

Besides generally adhering to the principle of *stare decisis*, courts also abide by another basic legal principle—that the court must have jurisdiction over the person or thing involved, that is, that the proceeding commences in a court located where the defendant lives or is served a subpoena or where the property in dispute is located. An exception occurs when, because of extraordinary publicity or emotionalism about a situation, the defendant claims that she/he cannot get a fair trial in that place and requests a change of venue—to be tried in some other jurisdiction.

The Constitution of the United States provides for the enforcement of federal laws by establishing a system of courts (sometimes called Constitutional Courts because they hear cases about matters mentioned in the Constitution), headed by the Supreme Court, the only one specifically mentioned in the Constitution. Other federal courts—courts of appeal, district courts, and others—have been established in all states and territories either on a permanent or temporary basis. Staffed by judges, lawyers, and other personnel employed by the federal government, they try all cases arising under the Constitution and laws of the United States except those over which the Supreme Court has original jurisdiction. For example, cases involving violations of federal income tax laws and the passing of counterfeit money are tried in federal courts. These courts have no jurisdiction over state and local courts.

Most citizens are not involved in legal action handled by a federal court. Misdemeanors are usually dealt with on a local level, often by a justice-of-the-peace court, common in rural areas and small towns, or, in urban areas, a magistrates court, sometimes called a municipal or police court. A district court, often called a county court, may hear cases in one county or in several. Matters related to estates and wills often are handled at the county level in surrogate courts (sometimes called probate courts) under the direction of surrogate, or probate, judges.

At the state level, no two states have court

systems that are identical. They may differ in the names of the courts, their methods of selecting and removing judges, the number of jurors needed to convict the defendant in criminal cases, and in other ways. They do not differ widely, however, on fundamental principles or in their conduct of judicial affairs.

State courts have jurisdiction over all cases arising under common law and statutory laws in their respective states, except in Louisiana, which still operates partially under the Code of Napoleon, which makes other provisions. All states have a high court for the trial of cases, usually called a supreme court.

To meet changing times in general and advances in the legal profession particularly, reform of the courts at all levels is almost constantly under consideration by the state legislatures. It is a slow process, however, because it involves a change in the law and possibly the enactment of a new one; in some states a constitutional amendment is necessary.

Juries

A **petit jury** is a group of persons, usually twelve, sworn to listen to the evidence of a trial and pronounce a verdict. The right to trial by jury is guaranteed by the Constitution of the United States and by the constitutions of the individual states.

A juror must have the qualifications specified by the statute that applies in a particular situation and be free from any bias because of personal relationships or interests. A person cannot serve as juror on a criminal case if she/he has formed an opinion beforehand on the guilt or innocence of the accused.

Jurors are selected impartially. Jury duty is one of the privileges of a citizen in a democratic society, and many persons find it challenging, educational, and enjoyable. It may also be boring. Some jurors never participate in a trial because they are not the type of person wanted by one or the other of the lawyers, who have a number of peremptory challenges, which require no explanation.

Prospective jurors may spend their entire time of service in a jury room. There is a **definite technique to jury selection, intended** to be most favorable to a lawyer's client. In malpractice or accident cases, nurses are usually not selected to serve; they know too much and may be unsympathetic, say some lawyers.[3]

A woman is often excused from jury duty if she has home and family responsibilities that would suffer because of her absence, or if she is pregnant. In some states, however, nurses, or women in general, have not been called or were quickly excused. Because this violates the woman's right to serve if she so chooses and is able, women's rights groups have fought those restrictive laws. In 1975 the Supreme Court ruled that it is constitutionally unacceptable for states to deny women equal opportunity to serve on juries. The decision was based on the Sixth Amendment guarantee of a jury trial from a cross-sectional representation of the community. Women comprise about 53 percent of the population; therefore, systematically excluding them would deny those rights.

A man must have a very good reason to be excused, although those with pressing duties, such as doctors, lawyers, members of a fire or police department and the armed forces, are usually exempt. Various reasons for requesting release from a call to jury duty are accepted in all states.

A juror receives a modest daily fee. Many employers keep an employee on full salary while he is on jury duty, usually for two weeks or a month, although he is expected to report for work when not actually in court.

A **grand jury** is a group of persons, usually numbering from twelve to twenty-three, whose principal function is to examine the accusations against someone charged with crime and determine whether or not she/he should be indicted; that is, brought to trial before a petit jury. The grand jury system is based on the English system dating from the thirteenth century and is guaranteed to citizens by the Constitution.

Members of the grand jury are selected

even more carefully than members of a petit jury; they are called for a month of duty at more or less regular intervals and are paid more for their services.

LEGAL STATUS OF YOUNG PEOPLE

United States citizens of any age are endowed with the rights of freedom of religion, speech, press, petition, and others as set forth in the Bill of Rights. Furthermore most people agree that all are entitled morally (at least until they forfeit the privilege through their own actions) to respect, tolerance, and understanding from their fellow man. Children born into citizenship in the United States have certain civil rights and responsibilities, some of which are in effect all of their lives; others they relinquish when they become adults and take on new ones.

In the last few years that point of legal adulthood or majority has been in a state of flux, but even more so has been the question of the rights of young people in the nebulous state between minority and the age of majority. Legislation has begun to deal with the rights of children in relation to privacy, informed consent, and many health-related matters. Some of the major legal decisions concerning health care and youth are discussed in Chapter 22, but a few basic facts on the legal status of young people should provide useful background.

Infant, minor, child, or *juvenile* are terms, usually used interchangeably, for someone who has not yet attained majority. The *age of majority* is the age designated by state law at which a citizen of the United States becomes legally adult and is entitled, therefore, to assume full civil rights and responsibilities. This term, sometimes abbreviated to majority, is synonymous with *full* or *legal age.* Each state adopts its own law setting the age of majority. In most states, this had been twenty-one; however, since the passage of the Twenty-sixth Amendment, most states have changed to eighteen, the voting age. On attaining legal age, individuals are permitted

by statutory state law to perform certain acts with or without the consent of parents or guardian. Nevertheless, even within a particular state, the law varies with respect to the activities or purposes involved. The state has the right to set the age of qualification for such activities as voting, serving on a jury, marrying without parental consent, buying, possessing, and drinking alcoholic beverages, making a contract, drawing a will, inheriting money, working for wages, obtaining a license to drive a motor vehicle, attending school, receiving juvenile court treatment for illegal or criminal conduct, using the court to sue another person or one's parents, and receiving medical care without parental consent.

In 1975, the United States Supreme Court forbade setting separate ages of majority for males and females, but some state laws have retained sexual differentiation in setting majority status. Moreover, young people under the age of majority are not only denied certain rights enjoyed by adults, but are denied others by their parents as well, although they also have certain protections.

Emancipation describes the condition whereby children are released from some or all of the disabilities of childhood and receive the rights and duties of adulthood before the age of majority. Emancipation may be total, partial, or complete. Theoretically, only the court or a specific state law can determine emancipation except under certain classic circumstances such as the young person's marriage or membership in the armed services. Parents can petition the court for a declaration of emancipation, which releases them from their legal obligation to the child —the duty to support, maintain, protect, and educate. They give up the custody and control of their child and the right to receive services and earnings. When parents abandon their parental duties, it implies consent, even when formal action is not taken. On the other hand, when young people leave home, and/or earn an independent living, and are otherwise free from the authority and control of parents, this may be grounds for emancipation. Usually young people cannot petition for emancipation without parental consent, but the reality is that unless there is a serious problem, an individual in those circumstances is considered emancipated for all general purposes.

In cases involving consent for medical treatment, the term *mature minor* may be used, indicating that the child is sufficiently intelligent to understand the nature and consequences of treatment.

Right of Sustenance and Shelter

Besides the constitutional rights cited earlier, minors have additional legal rights. From the moment of birth until legal age, children are entitled by state law to such food, shelter, medical care, and clothing (legally termed necessities) as the parents can reasonably afford.*

Wherever minors may be—in school, recreation camp, hospital—they always have the right to food, clothing, and shelter as provided by their parents, either directly or through written or unwritten contract with the agency or individual under whose care any children have been placed temporarily. Failure to provide for a child in this way (including medical care) is termed *child neglect.*

In case of extreme parental neglect or abandonment, the state is obligated to intervene and either see that the parents resume their responsibility for the child's care or take him/her from them, temporarily or permanently, and place him/her in the custody of a guardian, foster family, or institution. The state also must assume financial responsibility for the child until or unless other means of support is available.

Although many young people are earning money—sometimes enough to live on—before they are eighteen or twenty-one, they theoretically are entitled by law to continue receiving sustenance and shelter as provided by their parents or a legally appointed guardian. Also theoretically, the parents are enti-

tled to the minor's earnings. It is unlikely, however, that a court would require a parent to support a wage-earning child under circumstances of hardship without requiring the child to contribute at least part of his/her earnings. Neither is it likely to require the child to turn over a full paycheck to the parent.

When a person reaches legal age, parents no longer are liable for child support; neither are they permitted to confiscate his/her earnings. If the child is mentally or physically incapable of assuming the responsibilities of adulthood, however, the law will usually require the parents or legal guardian to continue to provide the necessities.

Right of Protection

The law requires parents to protect their children from danger and harmful exposures of all kinds. Failure to do so constitutes *negligence.* A parent who in a fit of rage or as a means of inflicting punishment seriously injures a child, is guilty of *assault,* which is unlawful beating or other physical violence inflicted upon a person without his consent.

Child abuse is reportable in every state. Hospitals, all health professionals (including nurses), and sometimes schoolteachers are *requested* to report reasonable suspicion of child abuse. Failure to do so is punishable as a misdemeanor; those reporting in good faith are rendered free from civil liability for having made the report. The minor's right of protection extends to her/his school where, in most states, the law stipulates what punishment a teacher can employ to maintain discipline in a classroom or school. Private schools are not always subject to the same legal restrictions as public schools in this respect.

The law requires the administrative officers of schools, hospitals, places of amusement, all public buildings and vehicles, transportation systems, health and beauty salons, and others to observe specific rules of safety for the protection of all citizens, minors and adults alike. Such establishments must have and enforce regulations intended especially

---

*State laws are changing from the traditional focus on "father" to include the mother or the term *parent.*

to protect the young child or else risk getting into legal difficulties of various degrees of seriousness. Furthermore, they must employ persons capable of providing the services they offer safely and competently.

Right to an Education

Children are legally entitled to an education until they complete elementary school, without cost, except indirectly in the form of taxes, transportation charges, and the like. This right makes it mandatory for parents or legal guardians to see that they attend school regularly. Children cannot legally be deprived of their rights even if they are needed at home, without special permission from school authorities.

Rights of Marriage and Parenthood

Every state has its own statutory laws governing the right of a couple to marry with or without the consent of their parents, guardian, or a superior court, and with or without reputable witnesses. The majority of states permit a couple to marry without the consent of their parents or anyone else at age eighteen. The ages at which a couple can marry with the consent of their parents or other responsible person are also stipulated by state laws. They are usually lower than the ages required for marriage without consent.

Although changing, many marriage laws are also very specific about other legal requirements such as mental ability, freedom from syphilitic infection, and family relationships.

Minors who marry declare their independence by so doing and, therefore, assume the same legal responsibilities as adults who marry. The husband becomes head of the household and, under the law, must support his wife and any children they may have. The parents of the very young husband or wife often continue to help them financially, but the law does not make it obligatory. Neither are parents responsible for debts the minors incur for education or any other purpose after their marriage.

A number of states recognize common law marriages as legal. A couple is married at common law by declaring themselves man and wife and thereafter living together as such. (An increasing number of court decisions concerning persons living together, whether homosexual or heterosexual, juvenile or adult, are expected to set new precedents in the legal status and rights of each.) There are also new rulings emerging on the rights of single parents or unmarried parents. For instance, in 1979 the teen-age father of a child born out of wedlock was able to prevent adoption of the child and was given custody himself. Minors in general have the right of custody over their children, but whether or not the mother can consent to adoption of her child without parental consent varies from state to state. Illegitimate children, those born when their parents are not married, have most of the legal rights of legitimate children, particularly within the last few years when courts and legislation have overturned old statutes discriminating against these individuals.

Right to Give Consent

Under the law, consent means that a person gives permission in writing or orally for the performance of a certain act. In many cases, minors have not been able to consent to health care,* but many changes are occurring.

A minor can consent, of course, to such ordinary procedures as having his/her hair cut, but performers of any service tend to use caution because it is easier and less expensive to keep out of trouble with parents than to prove one's point after the damage is done.

Female minors are protected against sex crimes to a certain extent by penal laws that state at what age a girl can legally consent to sexual intercourse. The age varies in different states—from ten to eighteen. A man who violates the law is guilty of rape and subject to the punishment prescribed by law. The

---

*Consent to medical treatment is discussed in Chapter 22.

law is frequently inadequate in its handling of sex offenses against both young boys and girls.

Right to Make Contracts, Wills, Inherit Property, and Sue

Most states do not consider a contract binding if one of the parties is a minor. This does not mean that the contract cannot be carried out but that the child may disaffirm it. Therefore, many adults do not enter into contracts with minors unless there is a parental signature; the parent, as an adult, cannot repudiate legal contractual obligations. Contracts that cannot be voided by minors are those for "necessaries" (food, clothing, shelter, and medical care), marriage, enlistment in the armed forces, and, in some states, educational loans and automobile and motorcycle insurance.

A contractual agreement to work, written or unwritten, can be legal, subject to the laws of the state that delineate the kinds of jobs that children can hold and at what age and under what circumstances (hours, hazards, and so on). Most states require work permits, which, in turn, require parental consent and proof of age. Acquisition of a social security card is also necessary. Generally, salaries and fringe benefits should be the same for adult and child, male or female. Exceptions may be in the areas of baby-sitting, housework, and agricultural work.

In most states, the law does not recognize a will made by a minor as a legal document. Exceptions are sometimes made, however, particularly if a minor is married. A minor may inherit money or property, but usually does not have control over it until a specific age or the age of majority, on the assumption that the minor cannot manage an estate. Therefore, the court or an adult designated in the will acts as a guardian of the minor. The guardian or trustee has the legal responsibility of safeguarding the estate. Sometimes the disbursement of money inherited by an infant is subject to the discretion of an Orphans Court, which might release money

to pay for the minor's education or medical expenses or for other purposes.

There appears to be no hard-and-fast rule that states at exactly what age a person may witness a will or other legal document or serve as a witness in legal action, or as a legal witness at marriages and other ceremonies. The courts have permitted testimony of children as young as seven years old. It is not so much a question of age as of intelligence and understanding. Some children have more ability and demonstrate better judgment than persons of considerably older age.

A witness must be mentally capable of knowing what he is doing. This obviously excludes the mentally deficient witness and the child who is too young to realize the import of his/her acts.

A minor can sue or be sued to enforce any civil right or obligation. Before any action against the child can be taken, however, if there is no parent or legal guardian, a court of law must be asked to appoint a guardian to institute the action on behalf of the minor or to act for him/her. This person is generally referred to as a guardian *ad litem*, that is, the capacity as guardian ceases when the action or claim is settled.

If the child is suing, an adult—a lawyer, parent, guardian or "next friend"—must bring the suit for him/her. In a few states a child may bring suit against parents or other family members for negligent or injurious harm; other states have an "intrafamily tort immunity" law. Even in the latter circumstances, a child can often sue for damage to personal property or *willful* personal injury.

Other legal action against juveniles in relation to arrest, detention, trial, and punishment has been in a constant state of change in recent years, both in terms of protecting the minor and protecting the public from the minor.

THE LEGAL RIGHTS OF WOMEN[5]

There was a time when adult women were considerably restricted by the law, simply because they were females.* Married women were even more limited than single women, because husbands were entitled to the wife's worldly goods and usually represented them in the execution of all legal procedures. Even if the woman was not married, she was usually under the control of a male family member. The history of women's struggle for equal rights precedes the Constitution, at which time Abigail Adams warned her husband that if the new legal codes did not give attention to women, they would foment a rebellion; two hundred years later, women were still at a legal disadvantage.

The women's suffrage amendment drafted by Susan B. Anthony was introduced into the Senate in 1875, but ratification was not certified until 1920. Efforts toward an equal rights amendment have been under way for more than fifty years.

Between 1920 and 1963, little legislation useful in securing women equal rights was passed, but, probably because of the civil rights, black power and women's rights movements that gained strength in the 1960s, new energies seemed to be released. Dumas cites and describes forty-three pieces of legislation related to women's rights or of special interest to women that were enacted into law between 1963 and 1978.[6] Among these were:

P.L. 88-38 (1963)—*Equal Pay Act;* P.L. 88-352—*Title VII of Civil Rights Act of 1964;* P.L. 92-157—*Comprehensive Health and Manpower Training Act of 1971;* P.L. 92-261 —*Equal Employment Opportunity Act of 1972;* P.L. 92-318—*The Higher Education Amendments of 1972;* P.L. 92-496—*Civil Rights Commission Act of 1972;* P.L. 93-203 (1973)—*Comprehensive Manpower Act;* P.L. 93-259—*Fair Labor Standards Act Amendments of 1974;* P.L. 93-380—*The Education Amendments of 1974;* P.L. 94-106—*Department of Defense Appropriation Authoriza-*

tion Act of 1976; P.L. 94-482—*Education Amendments of 1976;* P.L. 94-566—*Unemployment Compensation Amendments of 1976;* P.L. 95-79—*Department of Defense Appropriation Authorization;* P.L. 95-99— *National Science Foundation Authorization Act, 1978;* P.L. 95-207 (1977)—*Career Education Incentive Act.*

All of the laws cited by Dumas specifically prohibit sex discrimination in employment, military service, or education. However, with legal protection, women are not necessarily granted equal work opportunities and equal pay for equal work, even in state and federal agencies. Within the first five years of the Equal Pay Act, hundreds of corporations were found in violation of the law and owed 46,000 women some $15 million in back pay. There were at the same time more than 7,800 complaints of sex discrimination filed under the 1964 Civil Rights Act.[7] Discrimination that is most difficult to combat is in the area of job promotion, appointment to key positions, or in gaining tenure in academia.

Women have encountered discrimination both subtle and blatant in establishing their own credit, purchasing property, organizing a business, and receiving fair insurance or pension credits. Women have at least some recourse to the law through the enactment of

P.L. 93-237 (1974)—*Small Business Act;* P.L. 93-383—*Housing and Community Development Act of 1974;* P.L. 93-495 (1974)— *Equal Credit Opportunity Act;* P.L. 94-63— *Public Health Service Act Amendments and Special Health Revenue Sharing Act of 1975;* P.L. 94-455—*Tax Reform Act of 1976;* P.L. 95-216—*Social Security Amendments of 1977.*

Many, if not most, insurance companies and retirement plans have not yet agreed to give women the same retirement benefits as men. They may also discriminate in the availability and amount of disability insurance on the "grounds that women are more inclined to fake illness." Moreover, married

---

*See Chapters 3, 4, 6, and 16 for additional information on sexism.

women frequently have no control over common property and are still a target of housing and credit bias.

Other women's rights issues that have resulted in legislation include rape prevention and control, family planning such as: *Public Health Service Act Amendments and Special Health Revenue Sharing Act*—P.L. 94-63 (1975) and *Health Planning and Health Services Research and Statistics Extension Act* —P.L. 95-83 (1977); assistance in child care for working mothers: P.L. 94-401 (1976) *Child Day Care and Social Service Amendment* and P.L. 95-171 (1977) *Social Security Amendment*. A new concern is for "displaced homemakers," widowed or divorced spouses who have lost their source of income. A bill was first introduced in 1977 that would provide counseling, training, and referral centers, but no action was taken. The problem of sexual harassment of women by their employers or professors has also had some visibility, but with limited positive legal response.[8]

Supreme Court and state high court rulings have handed down mixed decisions concerning women's issues. Pregnant women have been both upheld and rejected on the question of time and/or pay for pregnancy leave (remedied in part by legislation). Courts have ruled for and against alimony for *either* husband or wife, and custody of children by either. Although the Supreme Court supported a woman's right to have an abortion, it also agreed that abortions need not be paid for by public funds, thus encouraging legislation that severely limited the ability of poor women to have legal abortions. There have been a number of other rulings in which supporters of women's rights believe that Supreme Court decisions were made only on an individual case basis not considering sound overall legal principles.[9]

Women have become more militant about seeking legal relief from discrimination on the job or elsewhere. Cross suggests some ways to proceed:[10]

1. *File charges with the federal agency that has jurisdiction, following the specific protocol for action. For instance, in filing with the Equal Employment Opportunity Commission (EEOC), there are certain steps that have to be followed and time periods elapsed. If the EEOC (as an example) cannot get the company to end the discriminatory behavior, it gives the woman "notice of right to sue" and she must then get a lawyer and sue. The EEOC itself also sues in some instances. (Unfortunately, with the backlog of cases for many of these agencies, a two- to three-year time span may elapse before any action is taken.)*

2. *File a class action suit, getting help from your own lawyer or the American Civil Liberties Union. The process and validity of class action suits is now in question, so this too might be lengthy.*

Cross also provides information about action to be taken in specific cases and how to attain legal assistance.

The fact that action on women's rights has been so fragmented, frequently contradictory, and not always implemented is a major reason that passage of the ERA is considered so important. The great degree of misunderstanding about what it will or won't do has been widespread, particularly in relation to support and protection of women. (It is important to remember that the ERA prohibits discrimination against either sex.) Some of the projections of what ratification of ERA would mean in relation to some controversial issues are:

1. Decisions about the support obligation of each spouse and about alimony after divorce would be based on individual circumstances and resources, instead of on sex. It is unclear what would happen in the distribution and control of marital property.

2. Women would be permitted to volunteer for military service, or be drafted, if necessary, with appropriate exemption. They would be assigned to duty compatible with their physical and other qualifications and service needs.

3. In a school, enrollment in certain kinds of courses could not be limited to a particu-

lar sex; only legitimate, activity-related **physical qualifications could be used to set restrictions.**

4. Labor laws that provide real protection for women would probably remain and be extended to men also, but those barring women from certain occupations would be invalidated.
5. The constitutional right to privacy is expected to permit continued segregation of public toilets and sleeping quarters in dormitories, prisons, and so on.
6. A woman would not be required to take her husband's name, but could if she wished.
7. Homosexual marriages would not automatically be permitted or prevented; this is generally a state decision.
8. Private or business relationships between men and women would not be affected in any legal sense.
9. In some cases, private institutions would not be affected, but probably they would be eventually.

Because some of these changes are already occurring as a result of the action of individual states, courts, or a lack of objection, there are attorneys and others who say that ratification of the ERA is not necessary and that the trend toward equality between women and men is so strong that lack of a constitutional amendment will not stop it. Nevertheless, because trends do not take care of the problems of here and now and equal rights decisions and laws are so inconsistent, grossly unjust treatments for thousands have resulted. **The fight for passage of the ERA will undoubtedly continue.**[11]

REFERENCES

1. Mary Hemelt and Mary Ellen Mackert, *Dynamics of Law in Nursing and Health Care* (Reston, Va.: Reston Publishing Co., 1978), p. 3.
2. Helen Creighton, *Law Every Nurse Should Know*, 3rd ed. (Philadelphia: W. B. Saunders Company, 1975), p. 7.
3. Robert Cartwright, "Jury Selection," *Trial*, **13**:26–31 (Dec. 1977).
4. Much of the material in this section has been taken from Alan Sussman, *The Rights of Young People: An American Civil Liberties Union Handbook* (New York: Discus Books, 1977), pp. 15–18.
5. Some of the material in this section has been taken from Susan Cross, *The Rights of Women: An ACLU Handbook* (New York: Discus Books, 1973).
6. Rhetaugh Dumas, "Women and Power: Historical Perspective," in *Nursing's Influence in Health Policy for the Eighties* (Kansas City, Mo.: American Academy of Nursing, 1979), pp. 68–73.
7. "The Women—They Want Action," *Dun's*, (June 1970).
8. Karen Lindsey, "Sexual Harassment on the Job and How to Stop It," *Ms.* **5**:47-51, 74–79, (Sept. 1977).
9. Lesley Oelsner, "Recent Supreme Court Rulings Have Set Back Women's Rights," *New York Times*, (July 8, 1977), p. A8.
10. Cross, op. cit., pp. 68–79.
11. Toby Golick, "The Equal Rights Amendment: Do Women Need It?" *Amer. J. Nurs.*, **71**:284–287 (Feb. 1971).

BIBLIOGRAPHY

Listed here are a number of books on health and/or nursing law that are valuable not only as resources for this chapter but for the succeeding chapters. The styles and format vary, but the basic information on law is the same. Later editions and the tremendous number of new books on nursing law are more current and therefore more accurate, but some of those published at earlier dates are included because of the clarity of information on basic principles of law. References cited in Chapter 17 are also useful. To keep current on legal decisions and legislation concerning women's rights and children's rights, or any changes in basic principles of law, one may read major newspapers, news and business magazines, women's magazines, some health professional journals, and law journals.

Creighton, Helen. *Law Every Nurse Should Know.* 3rd ed. Philadelphia: W. B. Saunders Company, 1975. The author, a registered nurse and member of the bar, presents the basic facts of law in a concise, nontechnical style.

Hayt, Emanuel, Lillian Hayt and August Groeschel. *Law of Hospital, Physician and Patient.* Berwyn, Ill.: Physicians' Record Company, 1972. Detailed book with focus on the hospital and emphasis on protecting the hospital.

Hemelt, Mary, and Mary Ellen Mackert. *Dynamics of Law in Nursing And Health Care.* Reston, Va.: Reston Publishing Co., 1978. Intended as a resource to all workers in the health field, it gives in simplified language an overview of medical-legal problems and explains how the practitioner can protect himself from being sued or being found liable.

Murchison, Irene, Thomas Nichols, and Rachel Hanson. *Legal Accountability in the Nursing Process.* St. Louis: C. V. Mosby Company, 1978. Focus is on incorporating the law into the nursing process to support independent nursing action. A series of hypothetical situations is used to focus on a variety of legal concepts particularly relevant to nursing.

Murchison, Irene, and Thomas Nichols. *Legal Foundations of Nursing Practice.* New York: Macmillan Publishing Co., Inc., 1970. An outstanding text on legal aspects of nursing with an approach that encourages critical thinking. Selection of legal case summaries given to illustrate various issues.

Problems in Hospital Law. 2nd ed. Rochelle, Md.: Aspen Systems Corp., 1974. Intended as a desk reference for all personnel who exercise some administrative responsibilities in a hospital and written by a legal staff. Also has good section on introduction to law.

Rothman, Daniel, and Nancy Rothman. *The Professional Nurse and the Law.* Boston: Little, Brown and Company, 1977. A readable text tracing the broad outlines of those areas of law of particular concern to nurses. Generally good overview.

Springer, Eric, ed. *Nursing and the Law.* Pittsburgh: Aspen Systems Corp., 1970. A relatively concise and realistic approach to the subject. Focuses particularly on changes that occur in practice before new legislation is created and attempts to help nurses deal with this conflict.

Willig, Sidney. *Nurse's Guide to the Law.* New York: McGraw-Hill Book Company, 1970. Author displays understanding of nursing today in terms of independent functions. Includes glossary and other useful data in appendix.

Wing, Kenneth. *The Law and the Public Health.* St. Louis: C. V. Mosby Company, 1976. Intended as an overview of public health law for students and practitioners in public health fields. Includes basic principles of constitutional law, the United States legal system, power of state governments, Medicare, Medicaid, and malpractice.

See also the Public Affairs pamphlets of the nonprofit Public Affairs Committee, which can be obtained from them at 381 Park Avenue South, New York 10016, by yearly subscription or at a few cents a copy. Examples: No. 469, *Women's Rights—Unfinished Business*; No. 489, *The Bill of Rights Today*; No. 492, *Securing the Legal Rights of Retarded Persons.* Mancini in her useful legal column differentiates laws, regulations, and policies in *Am. J. Nurs.*, **78**:681 (Apr. 1978).

The Legislative Process

IMPORTANCE OF ACTION

The successful functioning of a democracy depends on the willingness of its citizens to participate in their government. Perhaps the most important activity involved in a successful democracy is exercising the right to vote, with understanding of the issues concerned and the potential impact of election of the candidates. Further involvement might include participating actively in campaigns, participating in organizations that promote or oppose certain legislative issues; contacting legislators about issues; giving testimony at hearings; and even helping to originate and encourage the passage of specific legislation.

Nurses, particularly, need to take on these responsibilities of citizenship, not only on general principles, but because so much of their professional lives are, and will continue to be, affected by legislation. The Nursing Practice Act of each state controls nursing education and practice and can be eliminated, amended, or totally rewritten in the legislative process. Any law involving health care, general education, or almost any other social issue might well have an impact on nursing. For example, at the end of one session of the California legislature there had

been 149 bills of interest to nurses in some way. Included were bills for changes in the Practice Act of professional nurses, vocational nurses, physicians, physical therapists, podiatrists; pharmacists, dentists, and chiropractors; licensing of certain paramedical workers; practice of other paramedical workers; treatment of drug addiction; use of certain drugs; funds for nursing education; funds for scholarships; funds for health facilities; abortion; birth control; health profession planning grants; malpractice; venereal disease; and matters related to consumer protection. On the national level, existing or pending legislation such as Medicare, Social Security, health projects, health care planning, Nurse Training Act, development of health maintenance organizations, national health insurance, health research, mental health grants, public health services, and labor relations all have an impact on nursing practice.

Although there has been a tendency for nurses to underestimate their strength in influencing legislation, there has also been an increasing recognition that they must become involved or suddenly find that someone else is making the legislative decisions on health care in which nurses should have a major part. An interesting development is that a number of nurses have successfully run for office. Many students, tuned in to political know-how and recognizing the power of the new youth vote, are taking a part in legislation at all levels. (However, studies to determine the effect of the eighteen-year-old vote have shown that powerful though the youth vote can be and has been in certain geographic areas, many of the young are as lax in voting as their elders.) Nursing students, in their heterogeneous groups of the young and the not so young, with their variety of backgrounds, have become increasingly active, and their impact has been felt. In one state they were a powerful influence in the passage of child-abuse legislation. They have been effective in testimony given on federal funding for nursing education. As a group, nurses have become more sophisticated in the legislative process, but they have not yet reached their full potential of influence as individuals, as members of a profession that numbers over a million, and as members of other power groups. In part this results from a lack of knowledge of the process itself, the ways in which they can make their power felt, and the *best time* to take action. To help remedy this situation, this chapter presents a pragmatic view of the legislative process.

BECOMING KNOWLEDGEABLE IN THE LEGISLATIVE PROCESS

There are a number of ways in which nurses can become more knowledgeable in the legislative arena. To begin with, the American Nurses' Association and its state and local constituent groups take an active part in legislation. Because the ANA represents a profession, it may take part in developing a bill, testifying, and lobbying in behalf of its members, and has the responsibility to do so. (For example, the ANA is responsible for nurses coming under the Social Security law; state organizations initiated the Nurse Practice Acts.) The major legislative activi-

ties of the nursing organizations are discussed in the chapters on these organizations. Pertinent at this point is the means by which members are kept informed about legislation. All major nursing journals, particularly the *American Journal of Nursing and Nursing Outlook*, report key legislative movements on the national level, and, if particularly significant, those on the state level. *Capital Commentary*, written by the ANA Washington staff, who are also the ANA lobbyists, is included in the *American Nurse*, and special legislative alerts are sent to state and district offices, legislative committee members, directors of nursing service, heads of nursing education programs and selected others. States or districts are permitted to reproduce this information which is particularly important if membership action is required. They may also produce legislative newsletters or have legislative sections that describe legislation activities on national, state, or local levels in their journals or other means of communicating with members. Directors of nursing or heads of nursing education programs often post these legislative newsletters so that all nursing personnel have access to them. (And if not, they can certainly be requested to do so.) Some institutions have special legislative groups who keep abreast of pertinent legislation and see that other nurses are informed. Students may be involved in these groups or their own. The Student Nurses' Association with its various communications is also a means of gaining current information about legislation important to nursing. NLN's newsletters and *Public Affairs Report* are excellent.

The kind of legislative information available in the newspapers depends on their editorial policies. Feature articles, news stories, and editorials on particular legislation are usually found, but these may not include legislation necessarily of special interest to nurses. Some newspapers list the major bills in the state legislature and/or in the Congress, report action taken, and current status. They may also report the vote of the legislators of that particular region on major bills. This enables readers not only to follow the action of a particular bill, but also to see how their own legislators vote in general. The League of Women Voters and other political action groups often publish some sort of legislative roundup for varying subscription prices. Legislators may also send newsletters to voters.

There are several ways for individuals to find out the names of their legislators. Calling the local municipal building or the county clerk's office will usually elicit this information, as well as the numbers of the legislative districts in which one lives. (It is politically expedient for local legislators to know those on a state or national level, because, at the least, local areas may benefit or suffer from such legislation.) However, some patience may be required because experience has shown that a prompt and complete answer is seldom forthcoming at the first extension to which one is connected.

A local or state League of Women Voters branch will usually give this information, and for a minimum fee will often send pamphlets or more detailed and useful information, such as the committes on which the legislators serve. Similar detailed information should be available from the district and state Nurses's Association. It is quite possible that other organizations to which a nurse belongs may also have such information because other groups are also oriented to legislative action. It is always possible to call the local newspaper, asking for the political editor or reporter, but the request for information may be greeted with more or less enthusiasm, depending on the newspaper. Another possible source is local political clubs. It might even be educational to see whether family, friends, or neighbors know the names of their legislators. Although most pertinent health legislation is usually at a state or national level, it is also useful to become acquainted with local legislators, because of their potential contacts and influence.

Because a voter is more influential than a nonvoter, registration and voting are impor-

tant. Local registration boards can give all necessary information, including the place and time of registration and the polling places.

THE LEGISLATIVE SETTING

It is not possible to influence legislation unless there is a clear understanding of how a bill becomes a law and the setting in which this happens. Presumably, legislators, whether state or national, are elected on platforms of their own and/or their party's which set their goals, and on certain promises for action that they make to their constituents. Fulfillment of these goals and promises, of course, means successful passage of appropriate legislation, but also voting on other, perhaps unforeseen, legislation to the general satisfaction of the "folks back home." *It is important to remember that most legislators want to be re-elected at the same or a higher level, and many of their actions reflect this desire.* It is equally important to know that it is not unusual to have hundreds or even thousands of bills introduced in a State Assembly (or House) and Senate. On the national level, some 25,000 bills may be introduced in the two-year course of a congressional session. Although not all of these are voted on finally, and not all are of interest to nurses, a legislator must have pertinent information on at least those that are likely to be of importance to his* areas of interest and his constituents. For this, legislators have staffs of varying size, depending on seniority and other factors. In 1978, the staff total for both Houses was over 13,000 and rising. Some perform secretarial and other similar duties, but others act as aides, assistants, and/or researchers. These are individuals who gather, sort out, and sum up background material on key bills and brief the

---

*In order to avoid constant reiteration of the his/her phrase, the masculine pronoun is used in this chapter when referring to legislators; most legislators in the Congress are men.

legislator on specific issues and on his constituents' feedback. The legislator generally uses this information to decide how he will vote. The men and women who are administrative assistants (AAs) share the power of the legislators, if not the glory.[1] Committee staff do the preparatory work that comes before committees and subcommittees, drafting bills, writing amendments to bills, arranging and preparing for public hearings, consulting with people in the areas about which the committee is concerned, providing information, and frequently writing speeches for the chairman.

Because these assistants get information from numerous sources, representatives of organizations, individuals, and lobbyists find it wise to become acquainted with them, maintain good relations, and provide accurate, pertinent information about the issues with which that particular legislator must deal. When representatives of nursing have not done so, they have found that the information about nursing that a legislator gets may be inaccurate, incomplete, out of date, or simply skewed in the direction another informant favors. A reported instance of the danger of maintaining poor relations with legislative staff was the difficulty that the National Institute of Education, a presidentially appointed agency for research in education, had getting the appropriations they wanted from the Congress in 1973. It was clearly pointed out that the institute staff's indifference to the congressional staff and their negligence in keeping them informed of the institute's plans and activities caused a negative reaction in the appropriations committees.[2]

A measure of the influence a legislator has is his placement on committees, where most of the preliminary action on bills occurs. Appointments are influenced or made by party leaders in the House or Senate. It is customary that the chairmanships of committees, extremely powerful positions, are awarded to members of the majority party, usually senior members of the House or Senate. Some committees are more prestigious than others and are eagerly sought after. Although there

are cases in which the chairman of some of these committees, particularly on a national level, has remained for years, the makeup of a committee may change with each new session. The legislator's performance on his assigned committees may be a means of gaining attention and prestige with his colleagues and his constituents, particularly if major issues arise and there is attendant news media coverage. It is, however, not unknown for him to lose a favorable position because of clashes with his party heads. It is vital to know on which committee one's legislators sit, because the action of committees affects the future of a bill.

Another useful person to know is the party "whip," both at the state and national levels. They are selected by their party/delegation and have the job of "whipping in" the vote, seeing that all party members are present for a particular vote, and/or persuading the recalcitrant to vote a certain way. In times of stress, the whips can offer all kinds of political favors. If they fail, the party leaders take over. The function of the whip goes back to 1769, when the British parliamentarian Edmund Burke, in a historic debate in the House of Commons, used the term to describe the ministers who had sent for their friends as "whipping them in"—derived from the term *whipper-in*, the man who keeps the hounds from leaving the pack.

LOBBYING

Lobbying means that nonmembers of an official body attempt to influence, by legitimate means, members of the body to vote for or against proposed legislation. Lobbyists are paid representatives of interest groups, many of which, such as business, labor, medicine, and hospital administration, wield considerable power in a capitol. Much of the influence of the power groups is traceable to their campaign contributions, which has caused some public and legislative concern and repeatedly results in state and national legislation regulating these contributions. In 1974, interest groups gave candidates $8.5 million. In 1975, the AFL-CIO Committee on Political Education gave almost a half million dollars. The AMA is considered the largest individual contributor to congressional races, having donated $1.79 million in congressional campaigns in 1976. "While substantial contributions may not actually 'buy' votes," stated Common Cause, "they do ensure easy access to public officials and create an unhealthy atmosphere of familiarity."[3]

There are also other ways of assisting candidates, using union dues (or company funds) and resources to provide computers, telephone banks, printing, mailing, sound equipment, and the salaries of union or company people assigned to specific campaigns.[4] The legality of these practices is being questioned, as is much of the technique of lobbying.

Common Cause, a consumer lobbying group that seeks to limit this kind of influence, reports that other than campaign contributions, $1 billion is spent in congressional lobbying efforts, only a small part of which is disclosed.

Professional lobbyists must be registered, and there are regulations concerning the type of organizations that may employ lobbyists. There are numerous ways in which lobbyists attempt to influence legislators, and much is on a direct-contact basis, sometimes in the semisocial settings of a lunch, dinner, cocktails, golf, or other such activity. Lobbyists provide information to the legislators and their staff (not necessarily objectively) and introduce resource people to them. Lobbyists are knowledgeable in the ways of legislation and are often familiar with legislators' personalities and idiosyncrasies. They are invaluable in keeping their interest group informed about any pertinent legislation and the problems involved, and in aiding the group in effective action.

A skilled lobbyist can have great influence on lawmakers and many times this is all to the good. When it is done properly and is controlled, lobbying is a desirable and ac-

cepted way of bringing important information and sound arguments to the attention of legislators, frequently by giving testimony before them. Unfortunately, it has also been used to present biased information to seek to influence opinions and decisions in a group's favor. It may lead to bribery, which has already created state and national scandals and caused great public concern. Legal measures have been taken to curb dishonest lobbying, rarely with complete success. The Congressional Reform Act of 1946 requires lobbyists to register and file statements of expenses made to influence legislation, and there are now laws that regulate the giving of campaign funds to candidates. Individual states vary in their laws regulating lobbying and campaign contributions.

This organized approach to lobbying, effective though it is, should not overshadow the efforts of the individual who, in effect, lobbies, when she/he contacts the appropriate legislator about an issue. Lobbying at this level is a constitutional right to petition the government. Groups such as nurses, who do not necessarily have millions of dollars to spend, have proven to be very effective in lobbying by coordinating the efforts of individuals toward unified action on an issue important to nursing. Therefore, how well and how much the individual citizen lobbies can be crucial in political action. The citizen who does not know how the state or federal government functions, how legislators and others are elected, and for how long, now has available many free or inexpensive brochures. Some that are particularly useful to nurses are listed in the bibliography at the end of this chapter.

HOW A BILL BECOMES A LAW*

Anyone can initiate a bill. Legislation is basically a citizen's demand for action because of discontentment with an existing situation or because of an emerging need. It

---

*See diagram.

may well be that a bill is not a result of the voice of the majority of people, but it may be what the legislators or governmental officials think is wanted by the majority with whom they are concerned. A vocal group is more likely to get action than one that is silent. A citizen who takes his complaints to a legislator is more likely to get a response than one who just complains. And the larger and more politically active the complainer group, the better the chance of being heard. There have been instances of legislation based on the concerns of one individual, but most commonly ideas for a bill are suggested by groups, which may or may not be organized. Some common originators of bills are organizations representing various interest groups, a governmental administrator, agency, or department, a delegation of citizens in a legislator's district, a legislative committee, or the legislator himself. A prolific source of legislation is the executive communication—a letter from the President, a member of his Cabinet, or the head of an independent agency transmitting a draft of a proposed bill to the Speaker of the House and the President of the Senate. This communication is then referred to the standing committee having jurisdiction over that particular subject matter. The chairman of that committee usually introduces the bill promptly, either in the form received or with changes he considers necessary or desirable.

In general, the enactment of a law follows the same procedure in all states and the federal government. The differences are slight and do not have an effect on the citizen's participation in the legislative process. To keep the matter as simple as possible, introduction of a bill in the House of Representatives will be used as an illustration. Only the major steps are given, but the details which can be quite complex are both useful and interesting.[5]

A bill may be sponsored or introduced by one or more legislators. The legislator whose name appears first on the bill is often known as the author and has the responsibility for the procedural handling of the bill. Although it may happen that a legislator is requested to sponsor a bill simply because he is from an interested citizen's district, sophisticates in legislation choose more carefully. The more senior, more prestigious a legislator is, the better the chance for a bill's enactment. Bipartisan sponsorship is desirable, but on occasion a key member of the majority party alone can be just as effective. To have one or more sponsors who are members of the committees to which the bill will be sent is also a highly positive factor. Junior members of Congress often seek senior cosponsors to enhance the opportunity for their bills to succeed.

Before a bill can be introduced, it must be couched in legal language. Although an organization may have its own knowledgeable attorney to do this, the bill is always put in its final form by a government legislative counsel; drafting of statutes is an art requiring considerable skill and experience.

After introduction in the House (which is commonly called "putting the bill in the hopper"), the bill is assigned a number by the Speaker.* Numbers are given consecutively as bills are introduced in each session; if the bill is reintroduced in the next session, it is unlikely to have the same number. The number is preceded by an HR in the House (an A or AB for Assembly in some states), or an S in the Senate. When the bill is "read" in the House by its number only, that is known as the first reading. (In a Senate the sponsor introduces the bill more fully.) The Speaker then refers the bill to an appropriate committee or subcommittee (health, education, judiciary, and so on), and the bill is released for printing. Usually the printed bill includes which House it is, the legislative session, bill number, by whom introduced, date, reference committee, and amendment to particular law (if pertinent). Consecutive numbers precede each line of the bill for easy reference. Definitions of key words may be given.

---

*The Speaker of the House is a member selected by the House membership to preside. He is usually of the majority party.

The Legislative Process

HOW A BILL BECOMES A LAW AT THE FEDERAL LEVEL

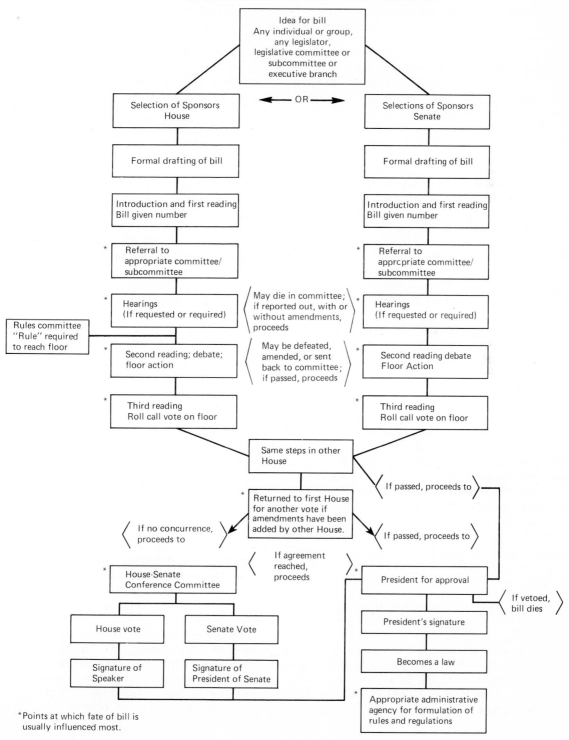

*Points at which fate of bill is usually influenced most.

Amendments to an existing law may be shown by having deleted words or phrases crossed out or put in parentheses and having new words or phrases put in italics or underlined. Bills may be obtained from the bill's sponsor or from one's own senator or representative. However, it is preferable to obtain them personally or by mail, from House Document Room, U.S. Capitol H226, Washington, D.C. 20515. (For Senate bills: Senate Document Room, U.S. Capitol 5321, Washington, D.C. 20510. States also have document or bill rooms.) The bill title and number should be given, if possible, or at least the subject of the bill and approximate date of introduction. Free copies are limited to one of each bill requested, and a self-addressed mailing label should be included.

A great deal of a legislator's time is spent in committee. Some committees may go on simultaneously with the House session, and when the bell rings to indicate a roll call, members quickly go to vote, presumably having made their decisions previously. The committee to which the bill is referred is the first place where its fate can be influenced. If the bill is never put on the committee agenda or is not approved, it will generally proceed no further. The chairman has the power to keep the bill off the agenda or conversely to introduce it early or at a favorable time.

Open or public hearings may be held, at which any interested person may present testimony. The date and time of public hearings are published. The committee then considers the bill—sometimes in executive (closed) session, if it is so agreed by open roll-call vote—and either kills it or approves it (reports it out) with or without amendments, or drafts a new bill. This activity is called "mark-up."

Committee action is determined by a voice vote or roll call but no record is kept of individual votes. (For this reason, there is some pressure toward having open committee meetings and voting.) For favorable action, the majority of the total committee must vote affirmatively. To get the desired vote, interested persons begin their legislative ac-

tion at the committee level. Letters, phone calls, telegrams, and personal contact are used in reaching the chairman and other committee members. This is usually most effective if done by the legislator's own constituents, by whom he is understandably more influenced. Here, also, written testimony and/or oral statements can be given. The techniques for such action, which are highly important, will be given at a later point.

In Congress, the Director of the Congressional Budget Office submits a financial estimate of the cost of the measure enacted. This is included in the Committee Report written by a member of the committee. If the bill is recommended for passage, it is listed on the calender and is sent to the Rules Committee (House only). In the House, the Rules Committee, with more majority than minority members, is most powerful; it can block the bill or clear it for debate. Presumably, the purpose is to provide some degree of selectivity in the consideration of measures by the House. The Rules Committee may also limit debate on the bill at the second reading. If a bill is blocked (no rule obtained), the discharge petition signed by a certain percentage of the House members can clear it, but this seldom succeeds.

A bill that survives all committee action is then scheduled for action "on the floor," meaning the total membership of the House. When the bill and number are read, that becomes the second reading. Amendments may be proposed at this stage and are approved or rejected by the majority. Lobbyists and interested citizens may view the proceedings from the gallery but cannot express their views. (These views should have been expressed through contact with their legislators by now.) The sponsor usually "manages" the bill (sees it through).

Debate is cut off by moving the previous question. If carried, the Speaker asks, "Shall the bill be engrossed and read a third time?" If approved, first the amendments and then the bill are voted on; but if there are the required number of objections, action may be postponed. If a group whose bill of interest seems to be in danger of defeat (or the reverse, if the aim is defeat) can influence at least the minimum number of Congressmen to object, they can buy time to try some other approach to achieve their goals. Delay may also be desired if the amendments appended in committee or in the House are undesirable to concerned individuals. Locking on amendments to a bill that seems sure to pass is a technique for putting through some action that might not succeed on its own and that may be only remotely or not at all connected to the content of the original bill. (For instance, in 1973, President Nixon signed a bill on military spending, which he wanted, to which was attached an amendment for the continuation of federal hospitals that he strongly opposed.) On the other hand, amendments that are totally unacceptable to the bill's sponsors may be added as a mechanism to force withdrawal or defeat of the bill. In general, amendments are introduced to strengthen, broaden, or curtail the intent of the original bill or law. If passed, they may change its character considerably. When debate is closed, the vote is taken by roll call and recorded. Passage requires a majority vote of the total House or a two-thirds vote for certain types of legislation. (Some legislators who, for some reason, do not wish to commit themselves to a vote find it convenient to be absent at the roll call.) If a House member expects to be unavoidably absent, he may arrange to have his vote recorded by being ''paired'', with another absent member who would be voting on the opposite side of the question.

If the bill is passed, it goes to the Senate for a complete repetition of the process it went through in the House and with the same opportunities to influence its passage. A bill introduced in the Senate follows the same general route with certain procedural differences.

A major difference is that bills that are not objected to are taken up in their order and debated. Filibustering is also a unique Senatorial process—a motion to consider a bill that has been objected to is debatable, and Senators opposed to it may speak to it as long as they please, thus preventing or defeating action by long delays. The President of the Senate is the Vice-President of the United States. At times, the same or a similar bill is introduced in both houses on certain important issues. The introduction of bills for nursing funding is an example. If these bills are not the same when passed by each house, or if another single bill has been amended by the second house after passing the first and the first does not concur on the amendments, the bill is sent to a conference committee consisting of an equal number of members of each house. The conference committee tries to work out a compromise that will be accepted by both houses. Sometimes, the two houses are not able to arrive at a compromise and the bill dies, but usually an agreement is reached.

After passing both houses and being signed by each presider, the bill goes to the President, who may obtain opinions from federal agencies, the Cabinet, and other sources. If he signs it or fails to take action within ten days, the bill becomes law. The President may choose the latter route if he does not approve of the bill but for political reasons, such as a big margin of votes, cannot afford to veto it. He may also veto the bill and return it to the house of origin with his objections. A two-thirds affirmative vote in both houses for repassage is necessary to override the veto. Because voting on a veto is often along party lines, overriding a veto in both houses is difficult. If the Congress adjourns before the ten days in which the President should sign the bill, it does not become law. This is known as a pocket veto.

Another type of legislation is a resolution. Joint resolutions originating in either house, are, for all practical purposes, treated as a bill, but have the whereas-resolved format. They are identified as *HJ Res.* or *SJ Res.* with a number. Concurrent resolutions usually relate to matters affecting both houses. They are not legislative but are used to express facts, principles, opinions, and purposes of the two houses. They do not require the President's signature if passed. These are identified as *H. Com. Res. or S. Com. Res.* with a number. Simple resolutions concern the operation of one house alone and are considered only by the body in which they are introduced. They are designated as *H. Res.* or *S. Res.* with a number. State legislatures use similar procedures.

All bills that become law are assigned numbers, not the same as their original number, are printed, and attached to the proper volume of statutes.

One of the criticisms of the legislative process is that action is slow at the beginning of a session and relatively few bills are introduced, debated, and voted on. Often, many bills are introduced near the end of a session and receive inadequate attention. A tremendous number of bills are frequently acted on in the last weeks of a session (often passed) with some question as to whether they have been studied carefully. A technique used by some state legislatures is "stopping the clock"; the clock is figuratively stopped before midnight of the last day of the session (which has been predetermined), and all-night legislative action goes on until the necessary bills, often budgetary in nature, are acted on.

With so many checks and balances provided by "due process of law" in this democratic government, often accompanied by extreme political pressure from within the government and the influence of lobbyists, one can readily understand why it is so difficult and time-consuming to translate an idea for legislation into statutory law, urgent through the need may seem to those who originated and promoted it.

Moreover, action on a law does not end with its passage. Laws are usually general, for too much specificity makes them obsolete too rapidly and requires another trip through the legislative process to add amendments. Therefore, rules and regulations are developed by the governmental agency or department within whose purview the law falls. For instance, amendments to the Nurs-

ing Practice Act are the responsibility of the department under which the state board of nurse examiners falls, and this group will develop the regulations. On the national level, health legislation is sent to the Department of Health and Human Services. Advisory committees of citizens are usually appointed as spelled out by the law or the department. There is public notice of hearings for the proposed rules so that interested individuals may respond. These are published in the *Federal Register.* (States have counterparts.) Regulations are as important as the law itself, because they have the force of law and spell out the specifics of how it is to be carried out. It is possible to influence legislation at this point also and to strengthen or weaken the intent of the law. For example, rules and regulations that delineate the curriculum for a nursing education program may be flexible, rigid, or extremely loose, and a nursing school must adhere to them to become and remain approved. The opportunity to contribute to the development of regulations is available to interested organizations, which may make recommendations for individual appointments on advisory committees or offer informal participation and cooperation. They may also testify at the hearings on regulations. Regulations have been changed after hearings because of major protests by interested groups or the presentation of well-thought-out alternative regulations.

On the national level a law that has had appropriations made for its enactment can be weakened by a cutback or withdrawal (rescission) by the President or a governmental agency, of the funds appropriated by Congress. In 1973, President Nixon refused to release funds appropriated for the Nurse Training Act and other health and social legislation. Nursing schools that had committed themselves to certain projects and to increased enrollment on the basis of these funds were put in a difficult situation. Congress responded to this action by various legislative maneuvers and later passed legislation that would permit Congress to overturn or change the amount of the cutbacks designated by the President. The kind of impoundment power that Nixon had was no longer permitted.

For nursing, precedent-breaking action was initiated by the National League for Nursing, which in June 1973, filed a suit in the federal courts against the HEW secretary and federal budget director concerning impoundment of the $21.7 million budgeted by Congress for grants for schools of nursing. It was filed on behalf of 793 schools of nursing. A temporary restraining order froze the funds and prevented their reversion to the United States Treasury at the close of the fiscal year on June 30. In November, a federal judge ordered the release of the funds, and eventually they were released.

NURSES AND POLITICAL ACTION

Nurses and students of nursing have a large stake in legislation. Acting as individuals or part of a group, they can make an impact on public policy. However, learning how to be effective in communication with legislators is essential. Legislators want to hear from their constituents, but because they are extremely busy, carefully planned and organized contacts are most effective.

Personal Contact

It is sensible for nurses to become acquainted with their legislators before a legislative crisis occurs. This gives them the advantage of having made personal contact and shown general interest, and gives the legislator or staff member the advantage of a reference point. In small communities, legislators often know many of their constituents on a first-name basis through frequent contacts. This personal relationship may be more difficult to achieve in large areas, but the effort to meet and talk with legislators is never wasted.

Having identified and located the legislator, the nurse may call for an appointment or check when the legislator is available in his local office (or in his capital office if this is convenient for both). Before the visit, it is helpful to know

1. The geography of his legislative district and district number.
2. His present or past leadership in civic, cultural, or other community affairs.
3. How he voted on major controversial issues recently under consideration.
4. How he has voted in the past on major bills of concern to nurses.
5. The subject areas of his special interest such as health, consumer affairs, and so on.
6. His political party affiliation.
7. His previous occupation or profession with which he may still have some involvement.
8. What bills of major importance he has authored or coauthored.

This information may be available from the state nurses' association, political action groups (of which a partial list is included in this chapter), or literature about him from his own office.

No one can say how such a visit should be conducted—it is obviously a matter of personal style—but generally it is wise to be dressed appropriately, to be friendly, to keep the visit short, to identify oneself as a nurse and, depending on the nurse's own level of expertise, to offer to be a resource. It is always thoughtful to comment on any of his bills or votes of which the nurse approves. If the first visit coincides with pending health legislation, it is suitable to ask whether he has taken a stand and perhaps add a few pertinent comments. Not more than three major issues should probably be discussed, and it is useful to recommend specific solutions to problems if at all possible. A *brief* written account of the key points and/or documentation of facts can be left, along with an offer to provide additional information if he wants it. Legislators respond best if what is discussed is within the context of what his other constituents might want. In other words, is it good for the public and not just for nursing?

It is important to be prompt for the visit,

but the constituent must be ready to accept the fact that the legislator may be late or not able to keep the appointment. The administrative assistant who substitutes will probably be knowledgeable and attentive, and the time will not be wasted. If distance and time make visiting difficult, a telephone call is a good approach. The same general guidelines can be followed, and here also speaking to the legislator's administrative assistant serves almost as good a purpose as speaking to the legislator.

Although personal visits and calls are considered useful in trying to influence a legislator, especially if an initial introductory visit has already been made, letter writing is also effective. Legislators are particularly sensitive to communications from their constituents. They give far less attention to correspondence from outside their state or district and are often annoyed by it. If a local address is not known, addressing the letter to the state or federal House or Senate is satis-factory. However, addresses should be on hand before the need arises.

After the proper salutation, the writer should identify herself as a nurse and a constituent and state the reason for the letter. A good letter persuades not by emotionalism, vague opinion, threats, or hostility, but by reason, good sense, and facts. The letter should be brief, to the point, specific, and without trivia. In developing arguments to support a position, it is best, when possible, to cite specific local situations that will be affected by the legislation of concern. It is vital that the information about the bill be complete and accurate and the reasons for a particular stand honest and reasonable. A simple objection without reason may have some influence on the legislator, if he tends to count letters, but has little value in educating him on the issues. The writer should include in the letter the bill number, author or authors, or at least its popular title, its status (if in committee, is this legislator on the com-

How to Address Public Officials

Official	Address	Official	Address
President	The President of the United States The White House Washington, D.C.: 20500 Dear Mr. President:	Assemblyman	The Hon. Mary Doe * The State House Trenton, N.J. 08625 Dear Ms. Doe:
Governor	The Hon. John Doe Executive Chamber Albany, N.Y. 12224 Dear Governor Doe:	Mayor	The Hon. John Doe City Hall New York, N.Y. 10007 Dear Mayor Doe:
U.S. Senator	Senator John Doe *Senate Office Building Washington, D.C. 20510 Dear Senator Doe:	City Councilman	The Hon. John Doe City Council New York, N.Y. 10007 Dear Mr. Doe:
Congressman	The Hon. John Doe *House Office Building Washington, D.C. 20515 Dear Mr. Doe: or Dear Congressman:	Judge	The Hon. Mary Doe (Address of Court) Dear Judge Doe:
State Senator	The Hon. John Doe *Senate Chambers Albany, N.Y. 12224 Dear Senator:	Other officials	(not included above) The Hon. John Doe Dear Mr. Doe:

*Local office, or if none, home address may be used. *Note:* Addresses at state capitals vary.

mittee?), the general purpose or interest of the bill, the specific recommendation to the legislator regarding the bill, how this stand is justified in terms of public interest, not just the profession, and what other organizations or groups have a parallel stand.

Berating or threatening the congressman, pretending to wield vast political influence, making promises, or demanding a commitment before the facts are all detrimental. Writing too often or too lengthily on nothing much is just as bad. For professional nurses, incorrect grammar or spelling reinforce a negative image and are inexcusable.

A letter requesting support on an issue is obviously more effective if letters are also written by other nurses and especially by non-nurses in the community. Nurses who can persuade family, friends, neighbors, or groups to support their viewpoints may supply guidelines for writing, if desired, but a form letter should *never* be written. Mimeographed letters and petitions could end up in the legislator's waste-basket.

Some information can best be communicated to a legislator by telephone, telegram, and night letter, particularly if speed is important as when a vote is pending. Night letters are generous in the number of words allowed and inexpensive, and a fifteen-word public interest telegram can be sent to any Congressman, President, or Vice-President for about a dollar.

Nurses using these methods should find that they have an increasing amount of influence with their legislators. Over a period of time the legislator will come to recognize these nurses as persons of integrity and reliability who are accurate and confident about their facts and who are interested in the legislators' positions, attitudes, and problems. Nurses who generally agree with their legislator's approach will find that it is also politically astute to contribute to his re-election campaign and/or offer their services in the campaign. These might include house-to-house canvassing to check voter registration or to register voters, transportation to the polls, making telephone calls to stimulate registration and voting, acting as registration clerk and watcher, poll clerk and watcher, block leader, or precinct captain, raising funds, preparing mailing pieces, planning publicity, writing and distributing news releases, making speeches, manning telephones and information booths, planning campaign events, or having "coffees" to meet the candidate. Groups or organizations can become more extensively involved if they are able to do so legally and financially. Most nurses who have participated in political action have found it stimulating and educational.

Testifying at Hearings

Committee hearings are intended to get the opinions of citizens on particular bills or issues. Student nurses and nurses can be effective speakers for health care, but, if poorly prepared, can cause just as negative an impact. Criticisms made by legislators about nurse testimony include unfamiliarity with the bill and its revisions; a tendency to "talk down" to legislators and use professional jargon; losing equanimity when questioning becomes abrupt or abrasive; an appearance of having more concern for their own well-being than that of the patient or public.

Attending public hearings of the committee to which health issues are referred is both an educational experience and a good preliminary before testifying oneself. It gives the opportunity to become more familiar with the atmosphere and setting of hearings as well as the attitudes and personalities of the committee members and to become acquainted with them individually. Although hearing rooms vary in appearance, and small states often have much simpler arrangements, generally the committee members are seated behind a raised table on which are microphones, nameplates, and copies of pertinent materials. Committee staff members and perhaps a stenotypist are seated below and to one side. A table with microphones is placed directly below for those testifying. It may be disconcerting for someone testifying to find only the chairman present at a hearing or, on the other hand, to find a full committee and hundreds in the audience. A nurse or organization may or may not be specifically invited to give testimony. Either way, it is a courtesy to notify the committee in writing of intent to appear or to request placement on the agenda and to provide a copy of the testimony if possible. Prior presentation of testimony does not exclude the possibility of adding appropriate remarks verbally or in answer to committee questions.

It is detrimental to request the opportunity to present testimony on bills of marginal interest or if a written statement inserted in the record would serve as well. Testimony should be prepared well in advance, or as much so as possible, because hearings may be called on short notice and sloppy testimony is worse than none. The ground rules applicable to the hearing (time limitations, length of testimony, number of copies to be submitted, deadline for submitting advance copies) should be requested from the committee staff and be followed.

Legislators, lobbyists, and others interested in legislative action have suggested some guidelines for giving testimony before legislative bodies:

1. If the testimony is in writing and has been given to the committee, they may prefer that the information be briefly recapitulated rather than read completely. It is vital that the person testifying be secure in her/his knowledge of the facts, totally honest, and comfortable in speaking to a group. It is useful to have additional data available to help in answering questions accurately. It is disastrous to present false information or a dishonest interpretation. If at all possible, the individual should know the data on which her/his testimony is based and not simply read a statement prepared by someone else.

2. Nurses should identify themselves and indicate whether they are testifying personally or for a group or an organization.

3. Although nurses have the right to disagree with their professional organizations, totally independent action confuses the issues for legislators. It is better to work within the organization, ironing out differences. A collective voice usually carries more weight than isolated testimony.

4. It should be understood that everyone appearing before a committee represents a special interest group; legislators weigh conflicting views to make their own decision.

5. Testifiers should be prepared to adjust their schedule so that they can participate as the committee schedule permits. Hearings may start late, be cut short, run late into the night, be recessed and reconvened later, or otherwise changed.

6. In testifying, the nurse should be brief, about ten to fifteen minutes, discuss only the specific bill or issue concerned, refrain from irrelevant comments, and speak plainly and without professional jargon.

7. When being questioned, it helps to be able to think under pressure, remain cool, not become angry, and have a sense of humor. (Some legislators use committee hearings as stages; some may not be friendly to the nurse's cause; others have predetermined ideas and prefer to keep them.) The nurse should never try to bluff; if she/he does not know the answer, it is best to say so and perhaps volunteer to provide the answer to the committee before the vote.

8. As in any other situation, appearance is important and the nurse should be appropriately dressed; a uniform is not appropriate except in unusual circumstances.

9. Nurses should be aware that appearing at a hearing is often all that is necessary. Testifying may not be the best action for various reasons and should not be forced. The appearance of a large number of nurses and students at a hearing indicates that it is of major concern to

them. Behavior should be courteous. This is also no time for intraprofessional quarreling.

10. Nurses should not be shocked or disillusioned if the vote goes against them at the hearing. Votes may have been promised to colleagues at this initial stage, even before the hearing, but may be reversed on the floor. If the bill is filed, a new version may be introduced, with changes made to minimize the opposition.

Politics is often a matter of compromise. Adherents of a bill must be prepared to yield on some issues as necessary, meanwhile holding firm on the most vital issues and allowing opponents to compromise on these points. Most of all, it is essential that nurses continue to be involved in political action, becoming ever more knowledgeable, sophisticated, and effective.

Other Means of Influencing Legislation

There are times when individual nurses are selected to participate in legislative and governmental advisory committees on the local, state, and national level. Most often such a nurse comes to the attention of the appointing individual through professional achievements, political or professional activities, or recommendation by organizations. Organizations such as the ANA and NLN keep alert for the inception of pertinent committees and exert pressure to have nurses included. More and more nurses and students are being appointed to such multidisciplinary and advisory groups. The contributions of thoughtful and informed nurses to committee deliberations, actions, and recommendations can change the course of health care.

Efforts are also being made by interested nurses to educate and involve all nurses in legislation through state political action groups and N-CAP, described in Chapter 25.

These organizations and constituencies of ANA, as well as other organized groups, often make an impact on legislation because they have systems for keeping members in-

formed and active. Legislative teach-ins are held and have been well attended. There are receptions for and meetings with legislators; newsletters and telephone networks set up to alert members to necessary action; and sometimes particular nurses are assigned to particular legislators, whose legislative activities they follow and report on. Nurses have shown that they can be a positive force in legislation, and have found, in addition, personal and professional satisfaction in participation in what Woodrow Wilson called the dance of legislation: "Once begin the dance of legislation, and you must struggle through its mazes as best you can to the breathless end—if any end there be."

REFERENCE SOURCES FOR POLITICAL ACTION AND/OR LEGISLATION

Organizations

Americans for
Democratic Action
1424—16th Street, N.W.
Washington, D.C. 20036

American Nurses'
Association and
N-CAP (Nurses' Coalition for
    Action in Politics)
Government Relations Department
American Nurses' Association
1030—15th Street, N.W.
Suite 516
Washington, D.C. 20005

Common Cause
2030 M Street, N.W.
Washington, D.C. 20036

League of
Women Voters
1730 M Street, N.W.
Washington, D.C. 20036

National Health Council, Inc.
Government Relations
1740 Broadway
New York, N.Y. 10019

National League for Nursing
Public Information Division
10 Columbus Circle
New York, N.Y. 10019

National Organization for Women
53 West Jackson
Chicago, Ill. 60604

Women's Political Caucus
1302 18th Street, N.W.
Room 603
Washington, D.C. 20036

Inexpensive or Free Sources of Written Information (Prices Subject to Change)

Public Affairs Handbook; Sperry and Hutchinson Co., Consumer Services; P.O. Box 935, Fort Worth, Texas 76101. Ten cents.

Action Course in Practical Politics (2600), U.S. Chamber of Commerce; Washington, D.C. 20006. Free.

Primer for Patriotism, Voter's Manual, Nat'l Association of Manufacturers, 277 Park Ave.; New York, N.Y. 10017. Free.

National League for Nursing; Government Relations Pamphlets, Twenty-five Cents Each

Guidelines for Meeting with Legislators

Guidelines for Presenting Testimony on Legislation

Guidelines for Writing to Your Congressman

INFORMATION ABOUT CONGRESSIONAL ACTIVITY

For vacation, adjournments and recess, or scheduling of bills for floor debate or vote, phone the Senate or House majority whips' offices or the Senate or House Democratic or Republican Cloakroom (recorded message). For committee hearings and schedule, see *Congressional Record* for next day; last issue of week lists the following week's schedule; United Press International or Associated Press Datebook; *Washington Post,* "Today's Activities in the Senate and House." To check if the president has signed a particular bill passed by the Congress, White House Records Office (give bill number) or Archives.

For rules covering current debate, House or Senate parliamentarian.

REFERENCES

1. Linda Charlton, "Administrative Assistants: The Powers Behind Congressmen Share in All But the Glory," *New York Times,* Apr. 8, 1975, p. 27.
2. "Institute of Education Gets a Lesson on How Not to Win More Money from Congress," *New York Times,* Oct. 22, 1973, p. 64.
3. "Common Cause: Money Talks on Health Issues," *The Nation's Health,* **8:**5 (Dec. 1978).
4. "Labor Power in Elections," *New York Times,* Jan. 18, 1976, p. 1.
5. The legislative process is given in full detail in Charles Zinn, *How Our Laws Are Made* (Washington, D.C.: U.S. Government Printing Office, 1978).

BIBLIOGRAPHY

Bowman, Rosemary. "The Nursing Organization as a Political Pressure Group," *Nurs. Forum,* **12** (Winter 1973), 73–81. Author reviews reason for influencing government and legislation, factors affecting success, and techniques.

Cnudde, Charles, and Donald McCrane. "The Linkage Between Constituency Attitudes and Congressional Voting Behavior: A Causal Model." In Bell, Roderick, et al. *Political Power.* New York: The Free Press, 1969, pp. 202–208. A sophisticated analysis of how legislators respond to constituency pressure shows that they usually vote as they perceive their constituents want. This book also has other essays on political power in the Congress.

Congress and Health: An Introduction to the Legislative Process and its Key Participants. New York: National Health Council, 1979. First published in 1976, and periodically updated, it contains valuable information on the legislative process, sources of information, jurisdiction, and purpose of actions of committees and key legislators.

Donley, Sister Rosemary. "An Inside View of the Washington Health Scene," *Am. J. Nurs* **79** (Nov. 1979) 1946–1949. Nurse who was a Robert Wood Johnson health policy fellow gives amusing and useful description of legislative machinations in a "small southern town."

Nathanson, Iric. "Getting a Bill Through Congress". *Am. J. Nurs.* **75** (July 1975), 1179–1181. A brief explanation of the legislative process.

Nursing and the Political Process. Indianapolis: Sigma Theta Tau, 1978. A monograph with useful information including extensive bibliography.

People, Power, Politics for Health Care. New York: National League for Nursing, 1976. Report of conference, with good papers on the Nurse Training Act and other major federal legislation, and the politics of legislation.

Redman, Eric. *The Dance of Legislation.* New York: Simon & Schuster, Inc., 1973. A fascinating, exuberant account, tracing a piece of health legislation from drafting to final passage, written by a legislative aide to a U.S. Senator. Includes all the maneuvers, plots, claims, triumphs, despairs, and dedication involved.

Shapley, L.S., and Martin Shubik. "A Method for Evaluating the Distribution of Power in a Committee System." In Bell, Roderick, et al. *Political Power.* New York: The Free Press, 1969, pp. 209–213. Analysis of distribution of committee power and factors influencing decisions.

Smith, Judith, ed. *Political Brokers, People, Organizations, Money, Power.* New York: Liveright National Journal, 1972. Discusses political action groups such as those of AMA, AFL-CIO, and others.

Stanhope, Marcia. *Politics: The Nurse and the Health Care Consumer.* New York: NLN (1979). A paper by one of the NLN summer fellows, exploring relationships and cooperation of nurses and consumers.

Stratton, Robert. "Strategy for Influencing Pro-Life Legislation." *Hosp. Prog.,* **55** (Feb. 1974), 60–61. Guidance is given for specific ways in which hospital administrators can identify and influence proposed legislation and/or regulations in relation to abortions.

The Emergence of Nursing as a Political Force. New York: NLN, 1979. Report of the second health policy seminar, with excellent papers on lobbying, financing health care, and how to work with committees.

"The Swarming Lobbyists." *Time,* Aug. 7, 1978, pp. 14–18. The cover story about the "billion dollar game of who can influence whom."

Wildonsky, Aaron. *The Politics of the Budgetary Process.* Boston: Little, Brown and Company, 1974. Describes how a budget is developed.

Wood, Lucille. "Continuing Education: The Nurse and the Legislative Process." *J. Contin. Educ. Nurs.,* **4** (Mar./Apr. 1973), 19–23. A nurse gives suggestions for participation in the legislative process, including guidelines for giving testimony at a hearing.

Zinn, Charles. *How Our Laws Are Made.* Washington, D.C.: U.S. Government Printing Office, 1978. Definitive description of legislative process includes information on committees and voting process in considerable detail.

See also References at the end of Chapter 19; references and bibliography of Chapters 6, 16, 17, 25, and 26. Many publications of ANA, N-CAP, and NLN relate to legislation and politics, as do those of most other large health associations and the National Health Council. Useful government publications include *Congressional Record* (verbatim transcript of the proceedings of the Senate and House, twenty-five cents per single copy from *Congressional Record* Office, H-112, Capitol, Washington, D.C. 20515, and annual subscription $45 from Superintendent of Documents, Government Printing Office, Washington, D.C. 20401); *Digest of Public General Bills,* also from Superintendent of Documents; *Committee Prints and Hearing Records,* available about two months after the close of hearing, is free but requires self-addressed label sent to Publications Clerk of the committee from which the document is issued; and a *Catalogue of Washington Health Newsletters,* developed by some congressional staffs, available from the Health Policy Center, The Graduate School, Georgetown University, Washington, D.C. 20057. Major newspapers and news magazines always carry political-legislative news, with or without editorials.

Federal Legislation Affecting Nursing

Both federal and state laws have major impact on nursing practice and education. At the state level, nurses need to know about their own nursing practice acts and should be acquainted with the licensure laws of other health practitioners. These are discussed in Chapter 20. Other state legislation affecting the health and welfare of nurses may be equally important, and nurses should keep abreast of both proposed and enacted legislation.

In this chapter, the focus will be on federal legislation that affects the practice of nursing and the rights of nurses; occasionally, state laws that are almost universal or closely related to federal laws will be included. Obviously, all health legislation fits into that category, but those laws that seem to have particular significance will be highlighted here.

SOCIAL INSURANCE

Social insurance differs from personal, or private, insurance in that it is compulsory and, for the most part, operated under governmental auspices. The local, state, or federal government raises funds by taxation to pay the benefits of social insurance. This type of insurance is common in many European countries, but because of the traditional American belief that the individual should be as self-sufficient as possible, the United States was slow to establish a system of social insurance.

Workmen's Compensation

The first such insurance to be held constitutional was the *Workmen's Compensation Act* enacted by the state of Washington in 1911. Today all states require employers in industry to carry workmen's compensation, but in some states, nonprofit organizations, including hospitals, are exempted. However, most nurses are covered by one or another of this type of insurance. Federally, employees are usually covered by the *Federal Employees' Compensation Act* enacted in 1952.

Workmen's compensation insurance, the cost of which is carried entirely by the employer, pays to employees who are injured on the job a proportion of their regular salaries for the time they are unable to work because of their injuries. If they are permanently disabled, they are entitled to additional compensation.

Workmen's compensation insurance laws do away with the requirement of proof that the employee was negligent or that the employee was free from contributory negligence. They also prevent court action for injuries and provide instead an administrative procedure for securing awards of compensation.[1]

Many states have extended the coverage provided by workmen's compensation laws to include occupational diseases; other states have enacted separate occupational disease acts, some of which cover all types of occupational disease; others specify which ones are covered. The major breakthrough on the federal level was the enactment of the *Occupational Safety and Health Act of 1970* (also discussed in Chapters 6 and 15), which established administrative machinery for the development and enforcement of standards of occupational health and safety.[2] There are still no standards for the health care industry, which means, according to the law, that state safety rules remain in effect. These vary from state to state and even among specific communities. Of course, in case of negligence, the employer is liable to employee suits. This is important to the nurse who may acquire a communicable disease, a staphylococcal infection, or other illness on the job, for which she/he might be entitled to benefits under the state law.

State laws governing workmen's compensation are not all alike, but most cover the majority of employees. They do not cover those employees who were intoxicated at the time of their accidents or those who willfully injured themselves. Every employee and every employer should know the terms of the workmen's compensation law in a given state.

Social Security

Beginning in the early 1930s, the tradition in this country that every person was almost entirely responsible for his/her own health and welfare began to be challenged by many forces, particularly the federal government. As time went on, social welfare legislation to help the masses and sometimes specialized groups was enacted more and more often with less and less resistance by the legislators and their constituents who had elected them.

As the social movement grew, the federal government became aware of needs of the people that they either had not seen or had not considered their business in the past. Many believed that the individual states should shoulder this responsibility and objected to the usurping of states' rights by the federal government. As the composition of the Congress changed with each new election, attitudes toward government involvement in social welfare also changed, to the extent that under President Dwight D. Eisenhower a Department of Health, Education, and Welfare was created by Act of Congress in April 1953. The then existing United States Public Health Service became part of the new department. From that time on, health care facilities and personnel received increasing attention in the White House and on Capitol Hill.

The *Social Security Act*, passed in 1935 and amended several times since, is administered by the Department of Health and Human Services (HHS), of which the Social Security Administration is a part. The lawmakers who produced the original act based it on the conviction that a program of economic security must "have as its primary aim the assurance of an adequate income to each human being in childhood, youth, middle age, or old age—in sickness or in health" and that it must "provide safeguards against all of the hazards leading to destitution and dependency."

The attainment of that goal requires, above all else, the broad economic objective of productive employment for those who are able and want to work. Second, and in proper perspective, is the goal to prevent dependency, which requires, on an ever-broadening scale, highly organized and efficient administrative procedures, and adequate financing.

The Social Security Act and its later amendments provide many benefits: federal Old-Age, Survivors', and Disability Insurance; unemployment compensation; federal grants-in-aid to states to promote special health and welfare services for children; matching funds to help finance state-administered relief programs for dependent children and needy persons who are aged, blind, or permanently disabled. Since 1965, the Medicare program (Title 18) has financed a large share of the hospital, nursing home, and home health care costs (and, on an optional basis contingent on the payment of a small monthly premium, the medical care costs) of persons over sixty-five who are eligible for social security benefits. Title 19, Medicaid, passed at the same time, was a hasty compromise on the part of the Congress and can probably be best described as a cooperative federal-state medical assistance program for the poor. By 1965, the Social Security Act provided four welfare programs administered by the state: Aid to the Totally Disabled (ATD) and the Blind (AB), Old Age Security (OAS), Aid to Families with Dependent Children (AFDC), and Medicaid; as well as the social security program for the retired and disabled wage earner and Medicare. The Social Security Amendment of 1972 federalized ATD, AB, and OAS, and these programs became known as the Supplemental Security Income program (SSI). The level of these federal payments to recipients is uniform throughout the states and higher than that paid by some states previously. Total assistance received by the SSI recipient must be no lower than before SSI; states may also add to the benefits voluntarily.

To a great extent, social security was originally and still is slanted toward the male wage earner, with the assumption made that most couples would remain married, that the husband would be the main breadwinner, and the wife would stay at home.

Old-Age and Survivors' Insurance. The average citizen who talks about his social security benefits is usually referring to the federal Old-Age and Survivors' Insurance program. It provides him with a monthly payment from the government after he reaches retirement age; an income for his widow (if she is over sixty-two years of age) and for his dependent children (if they are under eighteen) if he dies; and a small lump-sum payment to help cover his funeral expenses.

The amount of these benefits is based on the individual's average earnings and length of employment during his working life. Retirement age is, officially, sixty-two for both men and women. If she/he prefers, however, an individual may wait until sixty-five to start drawing benefits; if so, monthly checks will be larger than if begun at sixty-two. If a person continues to work for a salary after retirement age, the amount of annual earnings affects the social security benefits.

If both a husband and wife work, each is eligible for retirement benefits in his or her own right. The working wife, on retirement, is entitled to her own retirement benefit and also to a wife's benefit, based on her husband's earnings, on a prorated basis. She would not receive the *full amount* of both her own retirement benefit and her wife's benefit, but if the husband dies, the wife receives the larger of the two benefits, or her own plus part of her husband's to make the highest possible benefit.

Because of the male-female differentiations and inequities in the Social Security Act, these benefits are changed periodically through amendments or by Supreme Court decisions. For instance, child care benefits can no longer be denied to the widower of a deceased female wage earner, and widowers now have the same survivor's pension rights as widows.

Major areas of inequity that still exist include no pension for divorced women if not married for ten years or if the husband is not retired at the time of divorce; no individual pension for women who work at home only; and less coverage for a two-earner family than for a one-earner (the wife usually gets no extra benefits for working). Of further concern is the limited amount a person can earn without losing social security insurance benefits between the ages of sixty-two and seventy, a serious problem in inflationary times.

The report of the Social Security Advisory Council, a group of prominent private citizens established by the law, has periodically made several suggestions (with no guarantee of acceptance), among them that all social security credits and benefits be shared equally by husbands and wives and that every retired person have minimal social security benefits at age sixty-five plus whatever benefits may be earned as workers.

Some employers and some states not participating in social security, notably the federal government, have plans of their own and therefore feel that they are giving their employees adequate protection without social security coverage.

Disability Insurance. If an insured worker of any age, male or female, becomes totally disabled, she/he can begin receiving benefits after a six-month waiting period. To be eligible for these benefits, she/he must (1) have been covered by social security for a specified number of years (five to ten); (2) have a physical or mental disability of indefinite duration; and (3) be so badly disabled that she/he cannot work at gainful employment.

Again, women are at a disadvantage because benefits are not given to anyone who has dropped out of the work force for five years unless she/he has worked five years after that. This does not take into consideration that many women drop out of full-time work for child care.

Unemployment Insurance. Another major provision of the Social Security Act of 1935 is a system of unemployment insurance to protect the worker who is unemployed through no fault of his/her own. Although it seems unlikely that many professional nurses will need this kind of financial assistance because jobs are generally available for qualified nurses, it is possible that a nurse may, for various reasons, need this protection. Situations involving discharge of a nurse are not always clear-cut. For example,

one nurse, discharged from her position in one hospital because of her legitimate activities in behalf of her state nurses' association's economic security program, found other hospitals reluctant to employ her. Having demonstrated to her local employment service office that she was unemployed "through no fault of her own" (her association activities were entirely ethical), she claimed and received unemployment insurance until she found a more openminded employer.

Unemployment insurance is administered by the state governments. Federal law specifies a maximum and minimum benefit, and the states must remain within these limits. Each state has its own law governing the amount of weekly benefits allowed the unemployed person and the number of weeks for which it will be continued. This is realistic because the cost of living and employment conditions vary so widely in different sections of the country.

To collect unemployment insurance, a person must have been out of work for at least a week; be able to work and willing to take a job in his line of work at the prevailing rate; must not have left his previous job without good cause or have been asked to resign because of misconduct. In some states, marriage, pregnancy, and further education do not qualify one to claim unemployment insurance, and a mother cannot collect unemployment benefits for a certain period after childbirth.

Some states do not qualify certain classes of workers for unemployment insurance. These may include farm and domestic workers, members of the employer's family, workers in nonprofit organizations, students, medical interns, and others.

Employers of fewer than four employees were not included until 1972, when states were also required to extend to each of their subdivisions the option of participating. In 1969, only 12 per cent of management and 19 per cent of government nurses had unemployment insurance coverage, but federal legislation required that by January 1972, this coverage be extended to all nurses except those employed by local government.

Medicare-Medicaid

Medicare-Medicaid is a form of national health insurance proposed in one way or another since 1915. Health insurance provisions were deleted from the 1935 Social Security Act by President Roosevelt because he believed this would be necessary to ensure passage of the bill. When enacted into law in 1965, the Medicare title provided hospitalization for social security recipients, as well as allowing purchase of insurance for physicians' services at a nominal monthly fee. The Medicaid title expanded the Kerr–Mills law, which provided payments to states for health care of the "medically needy" aged, to include persons in programs for aid to dependent children, the blind, and the permanently disabled. This law was extremely controversial with some citizens and legislators not completely committed to the idea and the American Medical Association rigorously and uncompromisingly opposed to it. The American Nurses' Association, however, supported it. Passed in 1965, Medicare went into effect on July 1, 1966.

Benefits and Coverage. There are two parts to Medicare and in both the benefits are limited to those who are sixty-five years of age or older and some under sixty-five who are disabled. Upon its initiation, Medicare benefits were available to any citizen of the United States within this age group who had lived in this country more than five years and regardless of whether or not he was covered by social security. However, at that time it was stated that after 1968 individuals would have to have social security coverage to qualify for Medicare.

Part 1 of Medicare (HI) is designed to pay the major share of the costs for the individual over sixty-five who needs care in a hospital, health maintenance organization, extended care facility (a nursing home, for instance), or care at home. The coverage is not total: the patient pays a small deductible to begin with for his hospital care, and the government pays the rest for a given period. Hospital stays longer than that period are financed partly by the patient, partly by the government. There are also limitations on the circumstances under which costs of care in an extended care facility will be paid for, and on the number of days coverage. Outpatient hospital diagnostic services are paid for, again after a deductible, and with certain other stipulations. Payment is also made for visits by staff of a home health agency—a visiting nurse association, for instance—to care for a patient at home, if "skilled" nursing services are required. Part 1 is financed by social security taxes.

Part 2 of Medicare is an optional supplemental medical insurance program (SMI), available to the person over sixty-five upon payment of a small monthly premium matched by the government. This plan pays 80 per cent of the individual's costs for physician's services (in the hospital, home, or office), diagnostic tests and X-rays, therapeutic equipment such as braces and artificial limbs, and additional home health visits over and above those provided by Part 1 of Medicare. The patient must pay the first x number of dollars of these expenses in each calendar year; after that, the 80 per cent coverage goes into effect. Individuals have the same right to choose their own physicians that they always had.

SMI is financed through premiums paid by those enrolled or by someone (the state) paying in their behalf, plus general revenues.

Care covered in all cases must be "necessary and reasonable." Custodial care that could be provided by people without training is not included. Also not covered are certain services the elderly often need: drugs, routine eye and dental care, preventive care, or long-term care.

The Medicare program is the responsibility of the Social Security Administration, which enters into contracts with Blue Cross–Blue Shield, commercial carriers, and group practice prepayment plans to serve as administrative agents.* This arrangement is considered by some as not only adding another layer of bureaucracy, but also increasing costs.

In 1966, Medicare covered all "aged" persons (over sixty-five). Beginning in 1968, at least three calendar quarters in covered (social security) employment was needed; by 1975, the individual had to have the required number of quarters for retired worker benefits. This automatically excluded from HI those not covered by social security, although the 1972 amendments allowed the noneligible to enroll in the program by voluntarily paying a monthly premium that was rather high. Any aged person can enroll in SMI. At the end of the first ten years of Medicare, of all the the aged enrolled in HI, about 98 per cent were also enrolled in SMI.[3]

The Medicaid program had two major objectives: ensuring that covered persons received adequate medical care, and reducing the financial burden of medical expenditures for those with severely limited financial resources. Before Medicaid, most poor people had little or no health insurance and often went without needed care or had to depend on charity. Medicaid was intended to cover all people eligible for welfare (ATD, AB, OAS, and AFDC) plus at the option of the state, other poor people not eligible for welfare, such as the aged, blind, disabled, or dependent children whose incomes were slightly more than the welfare level. As the program became more and more expensive, legislative amendments altered and cut back eligibility requirements. The categories are complex and, unfortunately, many who need Medicaid's health care fall into the cracks. The law does not define the amount and duration of the service for which it requires the state to pay, and, as the program becomes more burdensome, many states have cut

drastically the amount of services.[4] An instance of this might be the denial of payment for abortion except under limited circumstances, although in this case there are also other related emotional factors. The Hyde Amendment (attached as a rider to the appropriation bill since 1977), which outlawed most federal fundings for abortions, and its counterparts in some thirty-nine states that prevented use of state funds cut payment for abortion by public monies by 99 per cent, as estimated by the Alan Guttmacher Institute in 1979. Some 34,000 women annually were probably denied legal abortions. However a ruling by a federal judge early in 1980 declaring that abortion aid limits for the poor was unlawful had the potential for change. The potential evaporated when, some months later, the Supreme Court upheld the constitutionality of the Congressional ban on Federal financing for abortions.

Nevertheless, the long history of lower utilization of health services by the poor changed with Medicaid. By 1974, there was evidence that the poor saw physicians 13 per cent more than did persons with high incomes; and children of poor families increased their use of physician services whereas those of high-income families reduced theirs. Also improved was the care of pregnant women. However, whether the quality of the care is the same is moot.[5] Moreover, there is some question whether services still reach those who need them. This is especially true of some of the special programs related to Medicaid such as the Early and Periodic Screening, Diagnosis, and Treatment Program (EPSDT) that served only about two million of an eligible twelve million children. The more broad-based Child Health Assessment Program (CHAP) was suggested by President Carter in 1977 to replace it, but it was lost in the 95th Congress (1978).

Financing of Social Security

All federal benefits under the Social Security Act are financed by special taxes paid by employees, employers, and self-employed

---

*The term *intermediaries* is used for those handling claims from hospitals, home health agencies, and skilled nursing facilities; *carriers* is used for those handling claims from doctors and other suppliers of services covered.

persons (certain groups are excluded). The tax is calculated on a percentage of the worker's income on which the employee pays on half, the employer the other half. The self-employed person, earning more than a minimal, set amount, pays the entire tax, but at a lower percentage of income rate than the employed person whose employer pays half the tax. Deductions on a paycheck stud appear under *FICA*.

In recent years, there has been some concern about the fiscal stability of social security. FICA payments by the working person are increasing dramatically to support the older and disabled, as people live longer and receive increased (and necessary) benefits. Eliminating inequities will increase the cost even more. Whether or not social security can continue to be funded in the same way is being questioned.

Major Social Security Amendments Affecting Health Care

In the years following enactment, much criticism was directed toward Medicare-Medicaid because of the cost of the program. Increased costs were in part caused by the compromises forced by opposition to the bill, which established private insurance companies as fiscal intermediaries and allowed physicians and health care providers to set their own fees. Cost abuses received considerable publicity, and the frequent subsequent amendments were aimed at reducing cost. A number of amendments since 1966 have been geared, to a great extent, to controlling the soaring costs of the program. There are now rigid regulations about the length of institutional stay that will be reimbursed, the level of care requirements for skilled nursing home services, payment for specific services, and coverage of particular groups. The second major concern, quality of care, also resulted in legislative amendments, for despite the fact that any institutions participating in Medicare had to be certified by DHEW and those participating in Medicaid abide by standards set by each

state, the quality of care was not consistently good.

These amendments affected not only the consumer, but the providers. Probably the various Medicare-Medicaid amendments have had as much, if not more, impact on health care than any other federal law. One of the most important was the Professional Standards Review Organization (PSRO) amendment in 1972, which mandated the establishment of PSROs within all states to improve the quality of health care and make it more cost-effective. The intent was to involve local practicing physicians in the ongoing reviews and evaluation of health care service rendered under Medicare, Medicaid, and the Maternal and Child programs. PSROs, voluntary, nonprofit, and government-supported, are currently primarily the responsibility of and under the control of physicians. The National Council on PSRO is composed of physicians. Although statewide councils and their supportive local units consist of both physicians and nonphysicians, nurses are often, perhaps usually, not included. The purpose of the state council is to develop appropriate criteria and standards, using the National Council's guidelines for review of the services rendered to clients. Each PSRO is responsible for defining its own data set that makes up the uniform hospital discharge data (UHDDS). The National Council is under the direction of an assistant secretary of DHHS, assisted by the Bureau of Quality Assurance (BQA). PSROs must report to BQA. Although there seemed to be some improvement of care, the costs of PSROs was so great that by 1979 zero funding was suggested by the Office of Management and Budget. Nevertheless, funding was provided with expansion of PSROs to review hospital ancillary services, outpatient departments, and long-term care. Inclusion of other health professionals seems inevitable. In 1974 HEW awarded a contract to ANA to develop criteria for measuring effective nursing care and to recommend ways in which nursing can participate in PSROs. Legislation was introduced in 1978 and 1979, mandating inclusion of nurses in the state advisory group and the national councils, but was not passed.

Also in these crucial 1972 amendments (PL 92–603) were provisions that would:

Encourage the increased use of health maintenance organizations.

Establish cost-sharing mechanisms whereby medically indigent patients are required to pay a portion of the cost of services that were formerly free.

Provide new coverage for disabled persons and patients needing long-term kidney treatment.

Modify the rules for the use of extended care facilities.

Set penalties for those states failing to provide screening examinations for children and family planning services for mothers who receive aid to families with dependent children.

Encourage the use of a wider variety of health care personnel, including nurse practitioners.

Section 222 was particularly important for nursing, because it authorized experimentation and demonstration projects to determine under what circumstances payment would be appropriate for independent services by PAs and NPs. Since then, there have been periodic legislative attempts to have nurses, especially nurse practitioners, reimbursed for services. For instance, in 1979, reimbursement for nurse-midwives was included in the proposed CHAP bill. A "sleeper" was the clause that provided payment for the care of people with permanent kidney failure, including kidney transplants. It set up chains of dialysis maintenance centers (for which nurses seem to have acquired primary responsibility) and the cost has become astronomical. The HMO clause resulted in the mushrooming of HMOs and, to some extent, increased utilization of NPs in these settings. Many of these beginnings under Medicare-Medicaid resulted in separate follow-up legislation.

Since its initiation, amendments to the Medicare-Medicaid portion of the Social Security Act have changed it considerably and, undoubtedly, such changes will continue. New bills tend toward expansion of services and control of fraud and abuse. The possibility of the enactment of a national health insurance plan may change it completely. However, it would seem that the major significance of the law will remain the same—that the aged, covered by social security, will no longer be threatened with possible dissipation of lifetime savings to meet the costs of long-term or catastrophic illness.

Health Service and Planning Legislation

One of the early health services laws that provided funds (on a matching grant basis) for constructing and expanding health care facilities was the *Hospital Survey and Construction Act of 1946*, popularly known as the *Hill-Burton Act*. It was highly successful, providing funds for more than 30 percent of the hospital beds in this country in its first twenty years, and funding was renewed several times.

Part of the original intent of Hill-Burton was planning. States received money for developing a planning program, supposedly based on need. As might be expected, however, politics was a more important factor than any rational basis for planning. This resulted in a substantial oversupply of hospital beds and contributed to inflation of health care costs as it became imperative to keep those beds filled.

Another carrot-and-stick approach to planning, as Wing calls it,[6] was the Regional Medical Program (RMP), originally labeled the Heart Disease, Cancer, and Stroke Amendments of 1965, although never limited to those diseases. RMP did not involve direct financial aid to health facilities, but was intended to finance the coordination of research efforts and to finance the distribution of information from research institutions to the whole health care system. More than one billion dollars was spent in the first ten years of the program to both local RMPs and the projects they sponsored. Projects included research, training, data exchange, direct patient care on a demonstration basis, or the construction of equipment and facilities related to these activities. (Nurses were involved in RMPs on a secondary level but benefited from the many educational programs.) RMP was federal funding for "needed" change in health care delivery; it was planning money for private providers to change the system. Partly because of medical politics, it failed its purpose; there is little evidence that the money was well spent.

The first real federal attempt to institute a national system of health planning was through the *Comprehensive Health Planning and Public Health Services Amendments of 1966*, known as Partnership for Health. This legislation set up five new programs related to health planning. Two are most pertinent. One provided funds to state governments to maintain a state health planning agency and a consumer-dominated advisory council and to establish a state plan for health planning activities (CHP "A" agency). The second provided funds to locally based, nonprofit private or publicly owned agencies designated by the state CHP agency as the approved areawide planning agency (CHP "B" agency). Although a nationwide network of planning agencies was established under CHP, both money and authority were limited. The only comprehensive authority was to "review and comment" on requests for federal funding. "Most CHP agencies (were) so ineffective, understaffed, and administratively inept that this review and comment process was little more than added paperwork for the funding applicants,"[7] especially since the federal agencies paid little attention to the comments. CHP also failed.

The latest and most comprehensive of these planning laws is the *National Health Planning and Resources Development Act of 1974*, designed to set up a new system of state and local health planning agencies and

to integrate into those agencies a program for the support of certain kinds of health facility construction. It has been described by some as a mere reorganization and revitalization of the CHP, RMP, and Hill-Burton programs after their statutory authorization drew to a close. The objectives of the act include (1) increasing access to health services; (2) maintaining continuity of care; (3) restoring increases in health care costs; (4) preventing unnecessary duplication of services; and (5) assuring effective utilization of manpower resources. Each state is required to establish a state health planning and development agency (SHPDA) and a state health coordinating council (SHCC) that serves as advisor to the agency. SPHDA prepares state health plans for budget review. (A national council develops guidelines for state councils). The SHPDA is delegated to conduct state health planning and functions related to both the state and health systems agencies (HSAs). The HSAs in various geographic areas of the state have the responsibility to collect and analyze data concerning the health care status of the residents in their designated health service area, the state of the area's health care delivery system, and its utilization, among other things. Each HSA must develop a health systems plan (HSP) and an overall implementation plan (AIP). Most are private, not-for-profit organizations with governing boards of ten to thirty persons, the majority of whom must be consumers.[8] Nurses serve on a number of these boards. Their power lies in their ability to review and approve or disapprove use of certain federal funds in their areas. PL 93–641 is an immensely complex, many-faceted law. HSAs have already been accused of "playing politics." Communication and coordination among HSAs, state, and national agencies are not adequate, and there have been multiple objections to the health planning guidelines that were four years in the process and did not go into effect until 1978.

In 1979, the Health Planning and Resources Development Amendments of 1979 were signed into law, with some weakening of the planning agencies' authority to rein in spending and unneeded facility building. Agreement in the amendments had been delayed for three years because of the various conflicts about the effectiveness of the law. Too much provider influence was one accusation. Another related to the "certificate of need" power of the HSAs, without which existing health facilities cannot buy certain expensive equipment, and none can be developed in the first place without a certificate. One non-controversial facet of the original planning law was the creation of the National Health Planning Information Center, administered by the Bureau of Health Planning and Resources Development of the HRA in DHHS. The Center acquires, analyzes, synthesizes, and disseminates information on a wide variety of topics relevant to health planning and resources development. (See Chapter 29.)

Various other laws providing health care programs and services of interest to nurses include the following:

The Community Mental Health Center Act of 1963 was a three-year program authorizing $150 million for the construction of community mental health centers. The Act also provided for increased federal aid to state and local communities in conducting research to lessen the incidence of mental retardation through inproved maternal and child health programs at the state and local levels. In 1965, an amendment to the Act provided funds for staffing the centers as well as for providing physical facilities.

The Maternal and Child Health Law (1963) gave matching grants to help the states provide better care, particularly for mothers and children in low-income families.

The *Older Americans Act of 1965*, amended again in 1975 to substantially increase appropriations for senior citizens' social, health, and nutrition services and funded through 1978, was the first major law besides social security to concentrate on the needs of the elderly.

The Health Maintenance Organization Act of 1973 authorized the spending of $375 mil-

lion during the next five years to help set up and evaluate HMOs in communities throughout the country. The concept is an arrangement in which subscribers pay a predetermined flat fee monthly or yearly that entitles them to basic health care services as needed. Emphasis is on preventive care and health teaching. This was extended and amended in 1976, relieving some of the rigid requirements imposed in 1973. All funding was to end by September 1980 but in 1979 the federal government announced a ten year plan to encourage the growth of HMOs. Discrimination for or against HMOs concerning certificates of need was an issue in the amendments to PL 93–641; the final result was exemption of HMOs from having to get certificates of need.

The Indian Health Care Improvement Act (PL 94–437) of 1976, designed to improve federal health programs for Indians, includes provisions to recruit and prepare more Indians for the health professions and to authorize continuing education allowances to encourage health professionals to join or continue in the Indian Health Service.

The Alcoholic Abuse and Alcoholism Prevention Treatment and Rehabilitation Act of 1970 provides and increases service in this area of health care. Extended in 1976, the *National Health Service Corps Program* (PL 91–623) of 1971 provided for health services in underserved areas. (The story of its enactment is told in Eric Redman's *Dance of Legislation*.)

The Emergency Medical Services Act of 1973 authorized $185 million over three years to states, counties, and other nonprofit agencies to plan, expand, and modernize emergency medical services. After its expiration, the law was extended.

The Disease Control and Health Promotion Act (PL 94–316), 1976, to provide authority for health information, education, and promotion programs and to extend disease prevention control programs is a long-awaited health education law, but the health education aspects were meagerly funded.

It is sometimes confusing to follow the

changes in these and other programs, or even their continuation. Some are amended or continued in a straightforward way as amendments to a given law. If extension of funding is defeated or vetoed, a program may be carried by a continuing resolution until a new bill can be introduced. Sometimes, a substitute bill providing a variation of the same services is passed. Other times, funding is picked up in an omnibus bill such as the amendments to the Public Health Services Act. For instance, in 1978 the health services bill extended through fiscal 1981 federal support for community health centers, migrant health centers, venereal disease programs, genetic disease and hemophilia programs, and home health services; one year of assistance to hypertension programs, immunization, lead-based paint poison control, and grants to states for comprehensive public health services; as well as two new programs for primary care centers with care provided by a primary care group (including nonphysician providers), and a program for teen-age pregnancy prevention and health care.

If a particular program is extended by one of these omnibus bills, it retains its name. This type of political maneuvering is one reason that legislative information provided by the professional nursing and other health organizations is so useful, although it must be read with the understanding that each organization or group presents such information colored by its own interests.

EDUCATION IN THE HEALTH FIELD

It was not until the *Health Amendments Act* of 1956 was passed after fourteen years of effort by devoted and dedicated citizens that *people* in the health professions received substantial financial assistance. This Act, now a section of the Public Health Service Law, provided funds (called traineeships) to prepare nurses for administration, teaching, and supervision, and nurses and physicians for public health work. The traineeship pro-

gram was successful—more than 67,000 nurses took advantage of funds for long-term full-time study and/or short-term courses from 1956 to 1971—and the fact that it came up for periodic renewal before Congress helped to emphasize the importance of advanced preparation within the nursing profession.

As the population of the country and the world increased rapidly and as the federal government urged the enactment of legislation to provide care for the aged under social security, health facilities and personnel became matters of urgency to Washington. More and more funds were channeled into health and education projects. At the same time, nurses were becoming more vocal, their organizations stronger, more self-assured, and more convincing when their representatives met with legislators and appeared before legislative committees. As a result of these and other factors, several new laws were enacted in the early 1960s that supported nursing and the individual nurse.

Most significant among these was the *Nurse Training Act* of 1964 (Title VIII of the Public Health Service Act). The purpose of this law, based on the report of the Surgeon General's Consultant Group on Nursing (Chapter 5) was to increase the number of nurses through financial assistance to diploma, associate degree, and baccalaureate degree nursing schools, students, and graduates taking advanced courses, and thus to help assure more and better schools of nursing, more carefully selected students, a high standard of teaching, and better health care for the people. Signed into law by President Lyndon B. Johnson on September 4, 1964, the law, which provided $287.6 million for a five-year program, was supported by both the American Nurses' Association and the National League for Nursing. In passing through the legislative process, the bill was altered considerably, but it still emerged a strong law, acceptable to most nursing leaders and nursing organizations. Subsequently, aid to students and schools of nursing was continued for two years under Title II (Nurse Training) of the Health Manpower Act of 1968.

The enactment of the *Nurse Training Act of 1971* expanded and extended federal aid to nursing education until June 30, 1974: the maximum federal share of costs for nursing school construction was increased; funds could be used to construct interim educational facilities and authority was granted for guarantees and interest subsidies on nonfederal loans for the building of nonprofit private nursing schools. In addition, funds were allotted for financial-distress grants, to help schools of nursing achieve quality nursing education or meet accreditation standards, and start-up grants, to plan, develop, and establish nursing schools. New capitation provision grants were made to encourage nursing schools to expand their enrollment. (At the same time, this law added to the standing prohibition against race discrimination, a prohibition against sex discrimination.) Variable amounts were granted to schools according to the number of full-time students they enrolled and graduated. Additional support was given for schools preparing nurse practitioners such as family nurse practitioners, nurse-midwives, and pediatric nurse practitioners.[9] However, to receive these grants, the schools were required to develop and/or maintain three special projects related to recruitment and retention of minorities, interdisciplinary education, preparation of nurse practitioners, innovations in curriculum and other specified areas. It was possible to include projects that were already supported by a special project grant from the division, also available under the Nurse Training Act, but continued commitment was required even if these funds were cut or eliminated. Although far short of the 1972 authorizations, the allocation still increased federal support for nurse training significantly. Then in 1973, the Nixon administration refused to release a large amount of the appropriated funds, withholding completely those allotted for capitation. Although a suit

against HEW by the National League for Nursing resulted in a favorable judgment for release of the capitation funds by the end of the year, limitations on traineeship funds prevented large numbers of students from beginning or continuing in baccalaureate and graduate programs.

Overall, it was estimated that the Department of Health, Education, and Welfare withheld (impounded) a total of $1.1 billion in health funds in fiscal year 1973. Other health groups also initiated suits for release of these funds, with usually favorable action. The struggle for adequate health funding in 1974 resulted in repeated vetoes by the president and a failure of the Congress to override the vetoes. In a final bill of 1973, approved congressional appropriations for nurse training were still approximately three times more than requested by the president, and a veto was expected. In his budgetary plan, the president had eliminated *any* funding for capitation, financial distress, traineeships, construction grants, and educational grants and contracts; and alloted considerably less than had the Congress in all other areas. After months of prodding by the Congress and national organizations, the president signed the 1974 HEW appropriations bill, in part because it contained an agreement that the administration could withhold up to $400 million of the total appropriation where the Congress had voted larger amounts for specific programs than the presidential budget.

This negative administrative attitude was particularly unfortunate because the funds granted as of 1964 had been well utilized. Some of the accomplishments included starting of forty new nursing education programs, salvaging and/or increasing 26,000 places for first-year students; providing remedial services for disadvantaged students in twenty-four programs; supporting a number of innovative open-curriculum programs; providing nurses with training for primary care responsibilities; aiding recruitment of minorities, including men; providing traineeships for

67,000 nurses in teaching, supervision, administration, and clinical specialties.[10] In addition, federal nursing funds over the years have supported nursing research and preparation of nurses in research, a great need in the development of the profession.[11] An elimination or cut in federal funds also endangered growth in this area.

The Nurse Training Act and three other health training acts were to expire June 30, 1974, but for various reasons, including consideration of a study on health manpower education costs, no legislation was introduced by mid-year. By that time, the funding had run out and the NTA and the other education acts were supported by a continuing resolution. As a matter of interest, the *Congressional Budget and Improvement Act,* which would allow the Congress more control over the budgetary process and force it into long-term planning, had just been signed into law. This law also prevented the president from impounding unremitted funds, although rescission, cutting back on allotted program funds, was legal. Rescission had to be approved by the Congress within a specified time period. In the last minutes of the 93rd Congress, the NTA of 1974 was passed. It was vetoed by President Ford on January 3, a pocket veto because the Congress had adjourned.

In the 1975 session, a new bill was introduced, passed, and again vetoed, but the veto was overriden by large margins of both Houses—the first successful over-ride of that session. Grass roots support by nurses was given much of the credit by both Rogers and Kennedy. In all, $106.5 million were appropriated for the NTA for fiscal 1976, including capitation, traineeships, and special projects. Again, the president vetoed and again there was an over-ride.[12] The Nurse Training Act of 1975 became Title IX, PL 94.63.

In 1978, the Congress, ignoring President Carter's claim that there was no longer a shortage of nurses, passed a two-year extension of nurse training programs. Without such authority, the program would have run out at the end of 1978. President Carter pocket-vetoed the NTA, claiming that the measure was inflationary. He later attempted massive rescission of NTA funds, but through the extensive lobbying of nurses and their supporters, the Congress refused to go along with Carter and nursing did better than any other health profession. Meanwhile, when the Congress reconvened in January 1979, a new NTA was introduced, later passed, and finally signed by President Carter. Funding was at $103 million, almost $3 million over 1979 spending levels. Included was funding for capitation, nurse practitioner, nurse anesthetist, and advanced nurse training programs, traineeships, student loans, special projects and construction. A special stipulation was that HEW contract out a two-year study of the supply, demand, and education of nurses. In 1980, it was time for introduction of a new Nurse Training Act, and considerable attention was focused on the need to improve the clinical practice of students.

grams had been supported by such early laws as the *Health Professions Education Assistance Act of 1963,* which provided matching grants over a three-year period for the construction of new teaching facilities for health personnel, including collegiate schools of nursing. Later, PL 94–484, *The Health Professions Educational Assistance Act of 1976* made the first important changes in federal support for medical education since 1971 when Congress had instituted basic federal aid to medical schools because of the growing physician shortage. PL 94–484 authorized a total of $2.3 billion for fiscal 1978–80 for basic federal aid to health profession schools, student assistance and scholarships, and other health manpower training projects. Although designed to assist medical, osteopathic, and dental schools, the act contained provisions for other health professionals, including nursing. *The National Health Service Corps* program (NHSC) and the *Area Health Education Center* program (AHECs) both encouraged utilization of nurse practitioners. The Corps program also provides scholarships for nurses who agree to work in under-served areas. Other workers in health care may be federally funded and such funding tends to increase their numbers tremendously. Among these are practical nurses, aides, emergency medical technicians, and physicians' assistants.

The Manpower Development and Training Act of 1962 was designed to prepare unskilled and poorly educated workers for jobs that require some degree of technological skill and to reduce unemployment by training quickly at government expense large numbers of these unskilled persons to fill available jobs. MDTA covered such health workers as practical nurses, orderlies, nurses' aides, psychiatric aides, and surgical technicians. Many hospitals, educational programs, and other groups took advantage of this law, and large numbers of these ancillary workers were trained. Because of the variety of programs and a tendency to produce subspecialty categories of workers this not only tended to increase fragmentation of care, but also resulted in many dead-end jobs.

In 1963 *the Vocational Education Act* provided funds to help provide training facilities for practical nurses, and in 1965 this was broadened to include enrollees in associate degree programs (for practical nurse training). Continued federal funding of practical nurse programs has been responsible, to a large degree, for the major increase of both programs and students enrolled. A leveling-off appeared to be occurring in the 1970s, however.

The Health Manpower Act of 1972 provided the stimulus for substantial development of PA programs. *The Emergency Medical Services Act of 1973*, mentioned earlier, also funded training programs for EMTs.

CIVIL RIGHTS, EMPLOYMENT, AND LABOR RELATIONS

Beginning in the 1960s, there were a number of laws passed to prohibit discrimination based on sex as well as race, color, religion, and national origin. Many of these are particularly meaningful to women and are cited in Chapter 17. Some of the most important are the following:

The Equal Pay Act of 1963 was intended primarily to end wage inequities based on sex and thus to assure women the same financial return as men receive for the same work. This did not apply to hospital employees, because it applied only to workers in industries covered by the Fair Labor Standards Act, and hospitals were not among these.

The Civil Rights Act of 1964, called by some the most far-reaching social legislation since Reconstruction, intended to create a rule of law under which the United States could deal with its race problems peaceably through orderly, legal process in federal courts. Title VII of the Civil Rights Act (Equal Employment Opportunity Law) has affected the job status of nurses because it includes a section forbidding discrimination against women in job hiring and job promotion among private employers of more than twenty-five persons. Executive order No. 11246 as amended extended the law to include federal contractors and subcontractors. Hospitals and colleges are subject to this order because of their acceptance of federal grants of various kinds.

One year later, the *1965 Voting Rights Act.*, with direct bearing on the Civil Rights Act, was passed, requiring that the procedure for registering persons to vote within a given county must be the same for everyone. Intended to ensure the right to vote promised in the Fifteenth Amendment, this law attempted to eliminate the practice of disqualifying potential voters on the basis of discriminatory literacy tests. This legislation represented an alteration in federal-state power, for the separate states had had the authority for nearly two centuries to set, for the most part, the standards for voting eligibility within their own borders.

The *Educational Amendments* of 1972 had three provisions of economic importance to women: (1) equal treatment between men and women in federally funded educational programs (especially admissions to programs); (2) minimum wage and overtime pay benefits to employees of nursery school, private kindergartens, and other preschool enterprises; (3) extension of the federal Equal Pay Act of 1963 to executives, administrators, and professional employees. The same pay was guaranteed to men and women doing substantially equal work, requiring substantially equal skill, effort, and responsibility under similar working conditions in the same establishment.

The Employee Retirement Income Security Act, 1974 (ERISA) established minimum federal standards for private pension plans to protect workers already covered by pension plans. The rigidity of the enacted programs and the confusion and overlap caused by dual enforcement by both the Department of Labor and Department of the Treasury caused many problems, and a delineation of functions was offered in later legislation.

The Age in Employment Discrimination Act Amendments of 1975 was intended to eliminate "unreasonable discrimination on the basis of age." Among other things, it banned certain kinds of mandatory retirement. The *Fair Labor Standards Act Amendments* of 1974 (originally 1938) increased the minimum wage and extended coverage to seven million workers, including state, county, and municipal employees.

Among other civil rights that have been given new protection are the rights of patients, children, the mentally ill, prisoners, the elderly, and, most recently, the handicapped.* Action on protecting these rights have come through a variety of legal means at state and national levels. Protection has increasingly been specified through regulations of various laws such as the amendments and subsequent regulations of the Social Security Act. Another is the *Rehabilitation Act of 1973.* Section 504 reads, ". . . no otherwise qualified handi-

capped individual in the United States shall, solely by reason of his handicap, be excluded from the participation in, be denied the benefit of, or be subjected to discrimination under any program or activity receiving federal financial assistance." The definition for *handicapped* includes drug addicts and alcoholics as well as those having overt physical impairment such as blindness, deafness, or paralysis of some kind. Because most health facilities and health professional educational programs have some federal support, this law applies both to admission into a nursing school, for instance, or employment in a hospital. Some cases have already reached the Supreme Court. In 1979, a PN with serious impairment of hearing sought admission to an AD nursing program. The Court upheld denial of admission because "nothing in the language or history (of the law) reflects an intention to limit the freedom of an educational institution to require reasonable physical qualifications for admission to a clinical training program."[13]

The right to privacy also affects nurses. One of the most important federal laws in this area is the *Freedom of Information Act* (FOIA) of 1966 and the *Privacy Act* of 1974. The purpose of the FOIA is to give the public access to files maintained by the executive branch of government. Recognizing that there were valid reasons for withholding certain records, the law exempted broad categories of records from compulsory public inspection, including medical records. To further clarify the situation, the FOI Act of 1974 was passed to amend the 1966 law. It had been necessary to set some time and expense limits for federal agencies because, in their frequent reluctance to give up information, they tended to use bureaucratic red tape to delay transmission of the requested records and imposed high fees to photocopy them. The next question that arose was whether a person shouldn't have the right to see all information about himself/herself in government files and know how much is kept secret from other people. The result was passage of the Privacy Act. Its purpose was to

---

*These rights are discussed in Chapter 22.

provide certain safeguards for an individual against an invasion of personal privacy by requesting the federal government, with some exceptions, to:

1. Permit an individual to determine what records pertaining to him are collected, maintained, used, or disseminated by such agencies.
2. Permit an individual to prevent records pertaining to him and obtained by such agencies for a particular purpose from being used or made available for another purpose without his consent.
3. Permit an individual to gain access to information pertaining to him in federal agency records, to have a copy made of all or any portion thereof, and to correct or amend such records.
4. Collect, maintain, use, or disseminate any record of identifiable personal information in a manner that assures that such action is for a necessary and lawful purpose, that the information is current and accurate for its intended use, and that adequate safeguards are provided to prevent misuse of such information.
5. Permit exemptions from the requirements with respect to records provided in this Act only in those cases where there is an important public policy need for such exemption as has been determined by specific statutory authority.
6. Be subject to civil suit for any damages which occur as a result of willful or intentional action which violates any individual's rights under the Act.

Such access includes the hospital record of patients in federal hospitals and, possibly, under Medicare/Medicaid. Another part of the law was aimed at protecting the confidentiality of patients' records.*

Another step in this direction of access to one's own records was enactment of the

---

*Some states have also enacted FOI Acts relating not only to records, but to meetings which must be open to the public (sometimes called sunshine laws).

Family Educational Rights and Privacy Act of 1974, also known as the Buckley Amendment. The basic intent of this law was to provide students, their parents and guardians with easier access and control over the information contained in academic records. Educational records are defined broadly and include files, documents, and other materials containing information about the student and maintained by a school. Students must be allowed to inspect these records within forty-five days of their request. They need not be allowed access to confidential letters of reference preceding January 1975, records about students made by teachers and administrators for their own use and not shown to others, certain campus police records, certain parental financial records, and certain psychiatric treatment records (if not available to anyone else). Students may challenge the content, secure the correction of inaccurate information, and insert a written explanation regarding the content of their records. The law also lists who has access to the records (teachers, educational administrators, organizations such as testing services, state and other officials to whom certain information must be reported according to the law). Otherwise, the records cannot be released without the student's consent. The law applies to nursing education programs as well as others.

The rights of research subjects have also been incorporated in diverse federal legislation, especially in the last decade. PL 93-348, the *National Research Act* of 1974 not only provided some funds for nursing research, but also set controls on research, including the establishment of a committee to identify requirements for informed consent for children, prisoners, the mentally disabled, and those not covered by the HEW regulations, and required an institutional committee to review a research project to protect the patient's rights. The 1974 Privacy Act required a clear, informed consent for those participating in research. The 1971 *Food and Drug Act* also gave some protection in regulating use of experimental drugs, including notification to the patient that a drug is experimental. *The Drug Regulation Reform Act* of 1978 took further steps in protecting the patient receiving research drugs. Other drug and narcotics laws* also affect nursing.

In recent years, drug manufacturers have been developing many highly potent drugs in their attempt to supply an increasingly numerous and aware public with medicine to prevent and cure their ailments. Many of these drugs produce side effects ranging from a slight rash or a mild gastrointestinal upset to much more serious consequences, sometimes even death. When one drug—thalidomide—was proved in 1962 to cause major deformities in babies born of mothers who took the drug, Congress was motivated to enact legislation to control more rigidly the production and distribution of new pharmaceuticals and thus protect the public against dangerous drugs.

The main provision of the law passed by Congress in 1962, called the Drug Amendments of 1962 (to the Food, Drug, and Cosmetic Act of 1938), provides that manufacturers of drugs who seek Food and Drug Administration (FDA) approval must prove through extensive preliminary clinical testing, often a long, slow process, that the drug is safe to use and that it will have the intended therapeutic effect; misleading or false labeling and advertising by drug manufacturers is forbidden; and drug manufacturers, processors, and packagers must register with the FDA each year, be inspected by FDA at least once every two years, and be open to inspection at any time.

The Comprehensive Drug Abuse Prevention and Control Act of 1970 (Controlled Substance Act) replaced virtually all other federal laws dealing with narcotics, depressants, stimulants, and hallucinagens. It controls how drugs must be handled by providers, including hospitals. The *Drug Regulation Reform Act* of 1978 took further steps in protecting the patient; at the same

*The Harrison Narcotics Act is discussed in Chapter 21.

time the FDA also set requirements about sharing product information on drugs with consumers.

Also within the broad categories of rights are those laws related to labor relations. The first was the *National Labor Relations Act* (NLRA), one of several laws enacted to pull the country out of the Great Depression. The thesis, according to Werther,[14] was that labor unions could prevent employers from lowering wages, resulting in higher incomes and more spending. To achieve the growth of unions, employers had to be limited; for instance, they could no longer legally fire employees who tried to unionize. The National Labor Relations Board (NLRB), created by the law, was empowered to investigate and initiate administrative proceedings against those employers who violated the law. (If these administrative actions did not curtail the illegal acts, court action followed. Only employer violations were listed.)

In 1947, the NLRA was substantially amended, and the amended law, entitled the *Labor Management Relations Act (or Taft-Hartley Act)*, listed prohibitions for unions. Section 14(b), for instance, contained the so-called "right-to-work" clause, which authorizes states to enact more stringent union security provisions than those contained in the federal laws. More than twenty states have enacted such laws. Usually they prohibit union security clauses in contracts that make membership or nonmembership in a labor union a requirement for obtaining or retaining employment. Such laws prohibit closed shop, union shop, and, sometimes, agency shop, whereby employees who do not join a union must pay a fixed sum monthly as a condition of employment to help defray expenses.

In 1959, a third major modification was made. One of the purposes of the law, the *Labor-Management Reporting and Disclosure Act* or *Landrum-Griffin Act*, was to curb documented abuses such as corrupt financial and election procedures. For this reason, it is sometimes called the union members' Bill of Rights. The result is a series of rights and responsibilities of members of a union or a professional organization, such as ANA, that engages in collective bargaining. Required are reporting and disclosure of certain financial transactions and administrative practices and the use of democratic election procedures. That is, every member in good standing must be able to nominate candidates and run for election and must be allowed to vote and support candidates; there must be secret ballot elections; union funds must not be used to assist the candidacy of an individual seeking union office; candidates must have access to the membership list; records of the election must be preserved for one year; and elections must be conducted according to by-laws procedures.[15]

Highly significant for nurses is the 1974 law that again amended the Taft-Hartley Act. PL 93-360, the *Nonprofit Health Care Amendments*. This law made nonprofit health care facilities that had through considerable lobbying been excluded in the 1947 law subject to national labor laws. These employees were now free to join or not join a union without employer retribution, a right previously denied to them unless they worked in a state that had its own law allowing them to unionize. It also created special notification procedures that must precede any strike action. Included in the definition of health care facility were hospitals, HMOs, health clinics, nursing homes, ECFs, or "other institutions devoted to the care of sick, infirm, or aged persons." Whether doctors' offices could be included was left to be settled by the NLRB.[16] Employers of all kinds, however, must abide by the various civil rights and other protective laws noted earlier. The *Civil Service Reform Act* of 1978 also had an influence in the labor relations activities of nursing because its definition of *supervisor*, discussed in Chapter 25, opened the door for nurse supervisors to be included in collective bargaining units. It also wrote into law collective bargaining, previously only sanctioned by executive order.

Another right that should be reported is the revision of the *Copyright Law*, amended in 1976 to supersede the 1909 law. The categories of work covered include writings, works of art, music, and pantomimes. The owner is given exclusive right to reproduce the copyrighted work. The new law has some significance in this time of photocopying from journals and books; there are certain limits and need for permission to copy anything beyond certain minimums. Libraries can provide the appropriate information. Some books and journals specify their copying permission requirements.

National health insurance has been debated in Congress for more than a decade. The plans offered are diverse and still changing. As expected, a crucial question is that of cost.[17] Opposing viewpoints are along the lines of comprehensive versus catastrophic plans, with some inclination to a phasing in of any plan by first concentrating on certain groups (infants and children, mothers, or the elderly). NHI tends to be a political football because of the public's "right to health" stance and the problem of funding (total governmental funding or private insurance plans).[18,19]

These differences can be seen in the varying opinions of physicians[20] and those who look toward national health service. A differentiation must be made between national health *service* and national health *insurance*. NHS would make all health workers government employees and all care would be provided in government hospitals and health centers (as in many European countries). Financing is mainly by general revenues, but some insurance funds are used. In NHI plans such as Canada's[21] the crucial feature is that all health providers, including institutions, are independent entrepreneurs who contract with the government to provide services.[22] Both the ANA[23] and the NLN[24] favor a comprehensive NHI plan that includes inpatient and outpatient care, twenty-four-hour emergency care, home care, clinic services, rehabilitative care, and preventive and supportive care.

Follow-up of federal legislation requires

close attention. It is not just the law itself that affects the public, but the proliferating federal regulations. Legislators have charged that regulations have been used to specifically circumvent the intent of the law; at the least, regulations often shape the legislation they are intended to carry out. Among President Carter's goals was clarification of the language of regulation (plain English, please) and allowance of sufficient time for comment by consumers. Otherwise, the process can become the exclusive prerogative of the federal agencies. Of equal importance are the agencies created by the various laws, such as the Federal Drug Administration and Federal Trade Commission. The FTC, for instance, goes back to 1914 when the Federal Trade Commission Act was passed. It has extensive power—it can represent itself in court, enforce its own orders and conduct its own litigation in civil courts, and seems to have relative freedom from the executive branch of government. Its forays into the health field with rulings on professional advertising, licensure and other aspects of health care delivery never thought of in 1914, may point a direction for other administrative agencies.[25] On the other hand, the subjects of the FTC rulings have banded together to lobby for limitation of FTC powers. The struggle will not be immediately resolved.

REFERENCES

1. Helen Creighton, *Law Every Nurse Should Know* (Philadelphia: W. B. Saunders Company, 1975), pp. 60–61.
2. William Curran, "Major Reform in the Oldest of Health Insurance Programs: Workmen's Compensation and Industrial Health and Safety," *N. Eng. J. Med.,* **288:**35–36 (Jan. 4, 1973).
3. Marian Gornick, "Ten Years of Medicare: Impact on the Covered Population," DHEW Publication No. 55A, **76:**1170 (1976).
4. Kenneth Wing, *The Law and the Public Health* (St. Louis: C. V. Mosby Company, 1976), pp. 70–90.
5. Karen Davis, "Achievements and Problems of Medicaid," *Public Health Reports,* **97:**309–316.
6. Wing, op. cit., pp. 132–134.
7. Ibid., p. 135.
8. Edyth Alexander, *Nursing Administration in the Hospital Health Care System* (St. Louis: C. V. Mosby Company, 1978), pp. 49–51.
9. Jessie M. Scott, "Federal Support for Nursing Education 1964–1972," *Am. J. Nurs.,* **72:**1855–1861 (Oct. 1972).
10. Ibid.
11. Susan Gortner, "Research in Nursing; the Federal Interest and Grant Program," *Am. J. Nurs.,* **73:**1052–1055 (June 1973).
12. Lucie Young Kelly, "The Nurse Training Act—How Legislation is Formulated, Adopted, and Implemented," in *People. Power. Politics for Health Care* (New York: NLN, 1976), pp. 37–48. (This article encludes considerable detail on how the 1975 NTA become law.)
13. "Supreme Court Rules Against Handicapped," *Am. Nurs.,* **11:**6 (June 20, 1979).
14. William Werther and Carol Ann Lockhart, *Labor Relations in the Health Professions* (Boston: Little, Brown and Company, 1976), pp. 6–8.
15. Ibid., pp. 22–27.
16. Yvonne Bryant, "Labor Relations in Health Care Institutions: An Analysis of Public Law 93–360," *J. Nurs. Admin.,* **8:**28–39 (Mar. 1978).
17. "Paying for Medical Care," in Victor Fuchs' *Who Shall Live?* (New York: Basic Books, Inc., 1974), pp. 127–146.
18. Theodore Marmor, "NHI in Crisis: Politics, Predictions, Proposals," *Hosp. Prog.,* **59:**68–72 (Jan. 1978).
19. Jeffrey Prussin, "National Health Insurance: A Political Issue at the Crossroads," *Nurse Educator,* **3:**23–27 (Nov.-Dec. 1978).
20. John Colombotos, et al., "Physicians View National Health Insurance: A National Survey," *Medical Care,* **13:**369–396 (May 1975).
21. Gordon Hatcher, "Canadian Approaches to Health Policy Decisions," *Am. J. Pub. Health,* **68:**881–889 (Sept. 1978).

22. Milton Terris, et al., "The Case for a National Health Service," *Am. J. Pub. Health*, **67**:1183–1185 (Dec. 1977).

23. American Nurses' Association, *Position Statement on National Health Insurance* (Kansas City, Mo.: The Association, 1979).

24. National League for Nursing, *Position Statement on National Health Insurance* (New York: The League, 1979).

25. Joseph Avellone and Francis Moore, "The Federal Trade Commission Enters a New Arena: Health Services," *N. Eng. J. Med.*, **291**:478–483 (Aug. 31, 1978).

BIBLIOGRAPHY

Amundson, Norman. "The Rules of the Game are Changing." *J. Nurs. Admin.*, **1** (May-June 1971), 45–49. A description of the changes in federal and state laws in relation to collective bargaining in health care institutions and their effects on nursing.

Atkisson, Arthur, and Richard Grimes. "Health Planning in the United States: An Old Idea With a New Significance." *J. Health Politics. Policy and Law.* **1** (Fall 1976). 295–318. Examines major failures of P.L. 93–641.

Blum, John et al. *PSROs and the Law.* Germantown, Md.: Aspen Systems Inc. 1977. A comprehensive review of the legislation.

Bullough, Bonnie. "The Medicare-Medicaid Amendments." *Am. J. Nurs.*, **73** (Nov. 1973), 1926–1929. An excellent exploration of the 1972 amendments and their impact on the public as well as on nurses.

"Challenges to Nursing in Medicare." *Am. J. Nurs.*, **65** (Nov. 1965), 68–75. Seven experts in nursing examine the meaning of Medicare in terms of opportunities for nursing and the improvement of patient care. Implications for nursing education and service, as well as community action, are explored. Historical interest.

Fischer, Gary. "Rehab Act Calls for New Approach to Interviewing Job Applicants." *Hospitals*, **52** (May 16, 1978), 81–83. Shows how compliance with section 504 will require revision of hospital hiring practices.

Frankenhoff, Charles. "The Planning Environment of Health Systems Agencies: A Strategy for Intervention." *Inquiry*, **14** (Sept. 1977), 217–227. Geared to the health administrator, article discusses the implementation of P.L. 93–641.

Kasner, Marilyn. "Analysis of Select Federal Health Legislation in Relation to Nursing." *Journal, NYSNA*, **7** (June 1976), 29–37. Author concludes that nurses have been ignored or minimally considered.

Legislative History of Professional Standards Review Organization. Wash. D.C.: USDHEW (US Government Printing Office 720–337/8073) 1978. Legislation through Oct. 1977 including amendments and committee reports on the laws related to PSRO.

McKibbin, Richard. "Public Policy for Health Manpower: Nursing Student Loans." *J. Health Politics, Policy and Law*, **2** (Fall, 1977), 349–361. Tries to determine the extent to which nursing student loan program has accomplished its primary objectives of increasing the nurse supply and decreasing the maldistribution of nurses.

Kleiman, Mark. "What's In It For Us? A Consumer Analysis of the 1979 Health Planning Act Amendments," *Health Law Proj. Lib. Bull.* **4** (Oct. 1979) 328–336. Interesting analysis pointing out strength and weaknesses as they affect the consumer.

Mosesman, Barry. "Team Approach to Comprehensive Health Planning." *Nurs. Dig.*, **1** (Aug. 1973), 50–55. Gives good background of CHP agencies and performance.

Regulatory Agencies—The Effect on Health Care Institutions. (New York: Natl. League for Nursing) 1974. Papers presented at meeting. Describes kinds of regulations and agencies involved as well as role of nurses in compliance.

Welch, Claude. "Professional Standards Review Organizations—Problems and Prospects." *N. Engl. J. Med.*, **289** (Aug. 9, 1973), 291–295. Cites importance of PSROs as a method of improving medical care. Specifically describes some of the problems involved.

West, Jonathan, and Michael Stevens. "Comparative Analysis of Community Health Planning: Transition from CHPs to HSAs." *J. Health, Politics, Policy and Law*, **1** (Summer, 1976), 173–195. Reviews organizational and operational characteristics of the relatively successful local CHPs and delineates problems that HSAs will probably have also.

Zimmerman, Anne. "Taft-Hartley Amended: Implications for Nursing." *Am. J. Nurs.*, **75** (Feb. 1975), 284–288. Former president of ANA and activist in collective bargaining discusses amendments as related to ANA particularly.

See also references in Chapter 19; references and bibliography in Chapters 6, 16, 17, 22, and 25; all issues of *American Nurse* and the NLN *Public Affairs Report;* and *Public Health Reports,* **91** (July-August 1976), 299–342. The latter presents an extensive perspective on Medicare-Medicaid ten years after enactment. Nursing, hospital ad-ministration, health law, and health policy journals all have news reports and, frequently, articles and editorials on federal legislation affecting health care delivery. *A.J.N* periodically has columns on nurse's finances that are affected by the law, such as pensions and ERISA (Oct. 1978) and Workmen's Compensation (Nov. 1978).

20

Licensure and Health Manpower Credentialing

Despite a variety of patchwork reforms, the health care system remains the target of serious criticism. Major focus has been directed toward the undeniable fragmentation of services, accelerating costs, and poor utilization and maldistribution of health manpower. Therefore, credentialing of health manpower, as one of the factors that probably contributes to these problems, has been given special attention by legislative, governmental, and consumer groups for some years. This pointed scrutiny has subsequently aroused new, or at least renewed, interest on the part of the health occupations and professions.

Licensing of individuals is probably one of the most authoritative mechanisms of credentialing, because it is a function of the police power of the state. Its primary purpose is to protect the public; therefore, the state, through its licensure laws, sets standards and qualifications for the licensed practitioner and holds the power to punish those who violate the law. At the same time, licensure, as it stands currently, has definite advantages for the licensee: status, protection of title (RN, LPN, MD), and certain economic gains. Other methods of credentialing for individuals or institutions have also evolved. Whether official, quasiofficial, or voluntary,

most purport to provide a certain assurance of quality or safety to the public as well as benefits for the credentialed. And therein lies the dilemma. As one expert in the credentialing field noted:

It is true that any professional society or group, no matter how socially oriented, will tend to develop barriers to protect itself . . . Among the contemporary protective mechanisms for the health professions are accreditation, certification, licensure, and registration. All four of these mechanisms medicine has employed with excellent results, if not always for the benefit of society, at least for the benefit of most members of the profession. And now many of the numerous other health professions wish to adopt, if they have not already done so, the same steps which medicine had fashioned to meet the needs of society and its own protection. (emphasis mine)[1]

This phenomenon has not escaped the notice of the consumer or the government. Because the health professions, as a whole, did not seem to show any rapid progress in remedying the more questionable aspects of credentialing, particularly licensure, a series of blue-ribbon panels, high-level committees, and prestigious task forces at state and national levels were formed. For instance, since 1968, DHEW committees have produced at least six major publications on credentialing of health manpower personnel.[2,3,4,5,6,7] Furthermore, in 1970-71 the Carnegie Commission on Higher Education looked at both higher education and some aspects of health professional education.[8,9] In 1972, the Commonwealth Fund supported an extensive study of accreditation (Study of Accreditation of Selected Health Education Programs, or SASHEP).[10] All of these groups presented firm recommendations for strengthening, changing, or eliminating various forms of credentialing, but it was the 1971 HEW (PHS) report that first gave official recognition to the concept of institutional licensure.

This report made clear not only that health manpower credentialing was no longer immune from public criticism and that it must be fused with the public interest, but also that the federal government had every intention of seeing that action was taken by using its authority in very specific ways. Preceding the recommendations was an invitation—and a warning:

> This department has a definite role in the process of credentialing progress—a role for catalytic action and support. While the Federal Government cannot solve these problems by itself, it is also apparent that meaningful solutions may not be forthcoming, on a timely basis, without a greater Federal interest. The needs in this field offer great opportunity for significant public-private cooperation.[11]

Of the recommendations—support of a moratorium on licensure of new health personnel and expansion of current acts to extend broader delegational authority, the use of national examinations and development of meaningful equivalency and proficiency examinations, strengthening of licensing boards to help maintain quality health services, including requiring assurance of the practitioner's continued competence—the most immediately controversial was probably the last:

> The concept of extending institutional licensure—to include the regulation of health personnel beyond the traditional facility licensure—has important potential as a supplement or alternative to existing forms of individual licensure. Demonstration projects should be initiated as soon as possible.[12]

The 1971 PHS report also gave definitions for the major credentialing processes[13] that have, since then, been used almost universally:

Accreditation*: The process by which an agency or organization evaluates and recognizes an institution or program of study as meeting certain predetermined criteria or standards.

Licensure: The process by which an agency of government grants permission to persons to engage in a given profession or occupation by certifying that those licensed have attained the minimal degree of competency necessary to ensure that the public health, safety, and welfare will be reasonably well protected.

Certification or Registration: The process by which a nongovernmental agency or association grants recognition to an individual who has met certain predetermined qualifications specified by that agency or association. Such qualifications may include: (a) graduation from an accredited or approved program; (b) acceptable performance on a qualifying examination or series of examinations; and/or (c) completion of a given amount of work experience.

Another acceptable definition of registration given in the working papers of the nurse credentialing study is: the process by which individuals are assessed and given status on a registry attesting to the individual's ability and current competency. Its purpose is to keep a continuous record of the past and current achievements of an individual.

_____

*Accreditation is discussed in Chapters 12 and 26.

PROBLEMS OF INDIVIDUAL LICENSURE

As noted earlier, licensure is a police power of the state; that is, it is through the state legislative process that the decision is made as to what group is licensed, with what limits, and it is the responsibility of a specific part of the state government to see that that law is carried out, including punishment for its violation. Although licensure laws differ somewhat in format from state to state, the elements contained in each are similar. For instance, in the health professions laws, there are sections on definition of the profession that delineates the scope of practice; requirements for licensure, such as education, age, character; exemptions from licensure; grounds for revocation of license; creation of a licensing board (for example, state board of nursing), including member qualifications and responsibilities; and penalties for practicing without a license.

Licensure laws are either mandatory (compulsory) or permissive (voluntary). If mandatory, the law forbids anyone to practice that profession or occupation without a license on pain of fine or imprisonment. If permissive, the law allows anyone to practice as long as she/he does not claim to hold the title of the practitioner (such as registered nurse).

Licensing of the health occupations was advocated in the early nineteenth century, but it was not until the early 1900s that a significant number of such licensing laws were enacted. They were generally initiated by the associations of practitioners who were interested in raising standards and establishing codes for ethical behavior. Because voluntary compliance was not always forthcoming, the associations sought passage of regulatory legislation. To some critics, this movement is also seen as a means of giving members of an occupation or profession as much status and compensation as the community would give, as well as a means for self-control of that profession.

It is true that as the health occupations proliferate, each group begins to organize and seek licensure. Because many of these occupations are subgroups of the major health professions, licensure could create problems in further fragmentation and increased cost in health care.

In all of the proposals for changes in health manpower credentialing, criticism of individual licensure is implicit or explicit. Particularly in the last ten years, the evils were cited, but there was little recognition of actions taken to remedy the faults. Evolving changes (often slow in evolving) were dismissed as too little and too late. Edward Forgotson, a physician-lawyer who directed a study of licensure for the National Advisory Commission on Health Manpower, enumerated some of the key criticisms of individual licensing.

1. *Most licensure laws for the health professions do not mandate continuing education or other requirements to prevent educational obsolescence. Therefore, the minimal standards of safety, theoretically guaranteed by granting the initial license, may no longer be met by some (perhaps many) practitioners.*
2. *Educational innovations in the health professions may be stifled by the rigidity of statutorily specified courses and curricular requirements. Changing these requirements to make them responsive to the rapid informational and technological explosion is a difficult and time-consuming process, and the result is the possibility that existing minimal standards may lag behind the practice realities.*
3. *Definitions of the area of practice are generally not specific, so that allocation of tasks is often determined by legal decisions or interpretations by lay people. On the other hand, some limitations of practice—ones that are not congruent with changing health care needs—are delineated.*
4. *Most licensing boards are composed of members of that particular profession (or, in some cases, the professional superior of that group), without representation by*

competent lay members or allied health professions. This is seen as allowing these professionals to control the kind and number of individuals who may enter their field, with the possibility of shutting out other health workers climbing the occupational ladder, and also limiting the number of practitioners for economic reasons. Moreover, the members of a one-profession board may lack overall knowledge of total expertise in the health care field, so that the scope of functions which could be delegated to other workers is not clearly determined. This creates the possibility that others capable of performing a particular activity may be prevented from doing so by another profession's licensing law.[14]

In addition to these generally reiterated criticisms, the 1971 HEW report also pointed to the lack of geographic mobility for some health professionals, who may be licensed in one state but barred from another unless a new license is obtained.[15] Only nursing, with its State Board Test Pool Examinations that are used in every state, allows for licensure by endorsement (that is, assuming that other criteria for licensure are met, a nurse need not take another examination when relocating to another state). Even then, nursing does not completely escape the mobility criticism, because, in the last few years, various nursing state boards have adopted rather idiosyncratic internal criteria. And, of course, not all health occupations are licensed; of the more than thirty-two,* only thirteen are licensed in every state: chiropractors, dental hygienists, dentists, nursing home administrators, optometrists, pharmacists, physical therapists, physicians (MD and DO), podiatrists, professional and practical nurses, and veterinarians.[16]

Nevertheless, it seems that almost all of the established or fledgling health occupations, more than 250 at last count, look toward licensing as a primary means of credentialing. The licensure problems of one health

occupation obviously are not necessarily the same as those of all the others. Yet, because the majority of all kinds of health workers function in institutional settings, the various weaknesses of all health occupations' licensing laws, the inconsistencies and varying standards of those seeking licensure, and the sheer numbers involved appear to be the bases for whatever enthusiasm exists for alternatives to licensure, such as institutional licensure.

Institutional Licensure

Institutional licensure is a process by which a state government regulates health institutions; it has existed for more than thirty years. Usually, requirements for establishing and operating a health facility have been concerned primarily with such matters as administration, accounting requirements, equipment specifications, structural integrity, sanitation, and fire safety. In some cases, there are also minimal standards of square footage per bed and minimal nursing staff requirements. The issue in the new institutional licensure dispute is whether personnel credentialing or licensing should be a part of the institution's responsibility under the general aegis of the state licensing authority.

There are a number of interpretations of just what institutional licensing means and how it would be implemented. Lawrence Miike, a physician-lawyer, considers it "instructive to view institutional licensure not as a developed concept, but, more appropriately, as a convenient descriptive term applied to the concept of a unified health delivery system."[17] He adds that the *Hershey model* has become synonymous with institutional licensure to many people and has led to some confusion.

Nathan Hershey, professor of health law at the University of Pittsburgh, has criticized individual licensure for years. In a number of papers, he advocated, instead, that institutionally based health workers be regulated by that institution within bounds established by state institutional licensing bodies:

---

*Health occupations seem to be designated differently in various publications, even within HHS.

Because the provision of services is becoming more and more institution-based, individual licensing of practitioners might be legitimately replaced by investing health services institutions and agencies with the responsibility for regulating the provision of services, within bounds established by the state institutional licensing bodies.

The state licensing agency could establish, with the advice of experts in the health care field, job descriptions for various hospital positions, and establish qualifications in terms of education and experience for individuals who would hold these posts. Administrators certainly recognize the fact that although a professional nurse is licensed, her license does not automatically indicate which positions within the hospital she is qualified to fill. Individuals, because of their personal attainments, are selected to fill specific posts. Educational qualifications, based on both formal and inservice programs, along with prior job experience, determine if and how personnel should be employed.[18]

Hershey further suggested the development of a job description classification similar to that used in civil service. Personnel categories could be stated in terms of levels and grades along with descriptive job titles. Under such a system, the individual's education and work experience would be taken into consideration by the employing institution for the individual's placement in a grade; basic qualifications for the position, expressed in terms of education and experience, would be set by the state's hospital licensing agency.

Thus, a professional nurse returning to work after ten or fifteen years, Hershey indicates, might be placed in a nurse aide or practical nurse position, moving on to a higher grade when she "regained her skills and became familiar with professional and technological advances through inservice programs."[19] Hershey was, then and later, rather evasive as to the place of the physician in this new credentialing picture, implying that the current practice of hospital staff review was really a pioneer effort along the same lines and might as well continue to

function. However, he did list as sites all institutions and agencies providing health services, nursing homes, physician offices, clinics, and the all-inclusive "et cetera."

In the next three years after Hershey's article (and prior to the HEW report), institutional licensure as an alternative, or, in some cases, an adjunct to individual licensure, was a point of some discussion by assorted groups, especially the American Hospital Association and its affiliates. (This interest is not immediately visible in the nursing literature, however.) A survey of papers, articles, and position statements issued in that period, some of which are cited in the 1971 credentialing study,[20] indicates some variations on the theme. These include institutional licensing for personnel directly involved in the operation of an institution (administrators), added to expanded and broad licensing categories of groups of health professionals, certification of technical groups, and licensure of health teams.[21]

Nurses are often reassured that institutional licensure would not include or affect them or their practice. But it is difficult to see how institutional licensure would *not* affect them when, at the least, others would decide upon the duties of nursing personnel whom nurses would supervise. It is also unrealistic for nurses to expect to be exempted when many of the tasks once considered in the realm of professional nursing have now been assigned to those with less preparation, when expedient. Or, on the other hand, tasks that have been part of another group's responsibility suddenly become nursing's, when it serves the purposes of the institution.

One advantage cited for institutional licensure is that job descriptions and classifications, combined with inservice training or other experiences and education, would allow health practitioners to move from one classification to another. But is this new? This plan has already been adopted by some of the more progressive hospitals. More to the point is to determine whether all agencies would be willing to initiate the expensive and extensive educational, evaluative, and supervisory programs necessary to fulfill the basic tenets of institutional licensure. Hospital administrators, especially, have been complaining about the expense of orientation and inservice education programs, cutting back on them as much as possible (sometimes more than is acceptable by the Joint Commission on Accreditation of Hospitals). This raises the specter of a return to the corrupted apprentice system of early hospital nursing in the United States. Probably a hospital's own personnel would be used as teacher-preceptors. Who then would do their job? How would they be compensated? How long would a "student" be expected to function in his/her current position with the current salary while he/she "practices" the new role? And with what kind of supervision? What kind of testing program for each level? Testing by whom? With what kind of standards? Such sliding positions might well cut manpower costs, but might they not also indenture workers instead of freeing them to new mobility? Problems of criteria for standards are obvious. If fifty states cannot now agree on criteria for individual licensure, why would institutional licensure be any different? Considering the 7,000 plus profit and nonprofit hospitals with bed capacity ranging from the tens to the thousands, in rural areas and urban, with administrators and other key personnel prepared in widely varied ways, and the even larger number of extended care facilities, clinics, and home care agencies equally dissimilar, a state of confusion, diversity, and parochialism becomes an overwhelming probability. Instead of facilitating interstate mobility, institutional licensure would more likely limit even interinstitutional mobility. A worker could qualify for X position in institution A, with absolutely no guarantee that this would be acceptable to institution B. Moreover, the disadvantages to those health professions that have fought to attain, maintain, and raise standards might be disastrous to patient welfare. Nurses, particularly, who are just beginning to fulfill their potential for total health care, account-

able to the patient and not to an administrative hierarchy or a physician for their professional acts, may find themselves relegated to increasingly technical tasks, substituting for a more expensive physician and being substituted for by the less prepared. (Not a nurse practitioner, but a physician's assistant; not giving primary nursing, but resurrecting nursing by direction.) Will this save the patient money, or cost him optimum health?

Whether or not it is argued that many of these practices exist today—de facto institutional licensure—as one proponent asserted, it hardly seems progressive to legalize what is already considered an unsatisfactory situation. And let there be no mistake, under this proposed system an institution would have the power to determine the specific tasks and functions of each job and indicate the skill and proficiency levels required, regardless of the employee's licensure, certification, or education. Control would be almost complete, because guidelines to be developed by the state institutional licensing agency are intended to be general.

But, then, would not the state guidelines protect the consumer, if not the employee? Presumably, the state licensing agency would be empowered to review the institution's utilization and supervision of health personnel to determine whether employees are performing functions for which they are qualified, but how realistic or feasible could such an evaluation possibly be? No one believes that an army of experts knowledgeable in all the subcategories of health care could be recruited, employed, and dispersed to check the hundreds of thousands employed in the multiple subcategories of workers in the thousands of care-giving facilities in any state. Therefore, one more paper tiger would be created—inspection by paper work. To determine the effectiveness of such surveillance, it is only necessary to look at the nursing home scandals and the admitted deficiencies of various municipal, state, and proprietary hospitals, to name a few. In all of these situations, the institution reviewed was given an official blessing; in truth, the conditions varied from unsafe to life-threatening. Generally, approval was given on the basis of the written self-report, with or without a visit by harassed, overworked surveyors. (What's more, when surveyors did recommend closings of the institutions, they were frequently overruled or ignored, if it was politically expedient.) Would institutional licensure suddenly, miraculously avoid these pitfalls?

A final question remains concerning those health professionals who provide care outside the walls of a health institution. Is the possibility of independent practice eliminated? Or will multiple systems of certification—individual and institutional licensure—add to the confusion?

Given the inconsistencies of institutional licensure, the economic advantages to certain employers, and the perceived threat to established professions, a polarity of reactions was to be expected. Continuing to voice general approval were the hospital and hospital administrator groups, but organized nursing arose to rally an opposing constituency. The first major action was a strong resolution approved by the ANA House of Delegates, followed by a statement by the NLN asserting unalterable opposition to the institutional licensure concept. Soon, most of the major RN and PN organizations, as well as the AMA, stated like opposition.

Meanwhile, the federal government funded two institutional licensure projects, one in Pennsylvania and one in Illinois. The first never seemed to get off the ground; the Illinois project was completed, but the recommendations of the final report concluded that although technically the concept could probably be carried out, "Implementation of the institutional licensure concept should not be undertaken at this time unless a significant commitment to this concept, far greater than exists now, occurs. This commitment would have to be on the part of those in government health agencies."[22]

The strong protests plus the report seemed to cool HEW's enthusiasm for this particular means of solving the credentialing problems.

In 1977's *Credentialing Health Manpower*, the only reference to institutional licensure was that on the basis of "studies of the feasibility of a national certification system and institutional licensure as alternatives to the traditional model of occupational licensure in health . . . the Public Health Service (PHS) has concluded that the certification alternative should be further developed, whereas the institutional licensure approach—because of the intense controversy that it generated—should not receive further consideration at this time."[23]

Does this eliminate the threat of institutional licensure? Not really, for it seems now that the concept is reappearing, if it ever disappeared, without its label.[24] In some states, overt attempts to legislate institutional licensure (which had been kept in committee or killed primarily through the efforts of organized nursing) keep emerging. Attempts to consolidate or eliminate the licensure boards of the various health occupations, seen by some nurses as an indirect approach to institutional licensure because they tend to attenuate nursing's control over its practice, have had varied success. In a number of states, boards have been consolidated under committees of lay people (or at least a majority of consumers), which make the decisions about licensing, with the individual boards acting in an advisory capacity. The many new sunset laws that require governmental agencies to assess themselves periodically and make a case for their continued existence or be eliminated also include nursing boards. Unhappy though all health professionals might be about these actions, the point is that the public, as represented by the state and national legislators, still does not see that credentialing (especially licensing) is doing what it should: serve the public. Should not the public have some controls then? Shouldn't a board be able to prove that it is performing a needed public service?

Other Approaches

When the 1971 credentialing report suggested that there be a two-year moratorium

CREDENTIALING HEALTH MANPOWER
DHEW 1977 Recommendations

RECOMMENDATION I: A NATIONAL VOLUNTARY SYSTEM FOR ALLIED HEALTH CERTIFICATION

A broadly representative national (non-Federal) certification commission should be established to perform the following functions for allied health occupations:

1. Develop and continually evaluate criteria and policies for the purpose of recognizing certification organizations and monitoring their adherence to these criteria.
2. Participate in the development of national standards as proposed in Recommendation II.
3. Provide consultation and technical assistance to certification organizations.

RECOMMENDATION II: NATIONAL STANDARDS

National standards for the credentialing of selected health occupations should be developed and continually evaluated. Professional organizations, other elements in the private sector, and State governments should play a significant role in this process. The standards thus developed should be utilized for the various purposes for which standards are required, including professional certification, licensure, private sector and civil service employment, and third party reimbursement.

RECOMMENDATION III: CRITERIA FOR FUTURE STATE LICENSURE DECISIONS

States should entertain proposals to license additional categories of health personnel with caution and deliberation. Before enacting any legislation that would license additional categories of health manpower, States should consider the following factors:

1. In what way will the unregulated practice clearly endanger the health, safety and welfare of the public, and is the potential for harm easily recognizable and not remote or dependent on tenuous argument?
2. How will the public benefit by an assurance of initial and continuing professional competence?
3. Can the public be effectively protected by means other than licensure?
4. Why is licensure the most appropriate form of regulation?
5. How will the newly licensed category impact upon the statutory and administrative authority and scopes of practice of previously licensed categories in the State?

RECOMMENDATION IV: IMPROVED LICENSURE PROCEDURES

States should take new steps to strengthen the accountability and effectiveness of licensure boards that will allow them to play an active role in assuring high-quality health services. These include:

1. Allocate increased funding, staffing, legal assistance and other resources.
2. Assign high priority to disciplinary procedures and responsibilities.
3. Adopt relevant national examinations and standards.
4. Expand membership on boards to include effective representation of consumers and other functionally-related professionals.
5. Establish appropriate linkages with the various health licensing boards and between such boards and other governmental health agencies responsible for the planning, development and monitoring of health manpower and services.
6. Develop a data capacity that is relevant to the formulation of health manpower policy.

RECOMMENDATION V: COMPETENCY MEASUREMENT

Certification organizations, licensure boards, and professional associations should take steps to recognize and promote the widespread adoption of effective competency measures to determine the qualifications of health personnel. Special attention should be given to the further development of proficiency and equivalency measures for appropriate categories of health manpower.

RECOMMENDATION VI: CONTINUED COMPETENCE

Certification organizations, licensure boards and professional associations should adopt requirements and procedures that will assure the continued competence of health personnel. Additional studies of the best mechanisms to assure continued competence should be supported on a high-priority basis by professional organizations, the proposed national certification commission, State agencies, and the Federal Government.

on licensing new categories of health personnel, with "statutorily defined scopes of functions", there seemed to be a reasonable response. AMA, AHA, ANA, and others had already suggested such action, and many state legislatures were becoming concerned as each emerging health occupation sought recognition through licensure. Still, the recommendation for an additional two years' moratorium in the 1973 report was only a stopgap. What were the alternatives?

It is essential that every health professional become familiar with the final 1977 HEW recommendations because they point the direction for future action. The ultimate weapon is the government's power to give or withhold funding. For instance, if requirements that health personnel must be certified or licensed under national standards and must give evidence of continued competence were written into regulations for Medicare-Medicaid reimbursement, few employees or practitioners could afford to ignore the matter. Because concern for the public is shared by state government, some of the recommendations on licensure are already being adopted.

Certification, among the first suggestions of the credentialing reports, had already been adopted by some health professionals, such as sanitarians, nurse-midwives, and anesthetists. There were several criticisms: the practitioner frequently had to graduate from a program accredited by the same group that did the certifying (which gave rather complete control to that group), and because of the lack of legal enforcement power, there was no guarantee that the certified person maintained continuing competence any more than the licensed.

The first problem was resolved to a large extent by the FTC rulings that such arrangements were illegal restraint of trade. Professions then gradually separated these functions into independent entities. As a follow-up to the 1971 credentialing report, a project to determine the feasibility of a national certification system, aimed particularly at allied health personnel, was explored with federal funding. The results seemed to be positive, and the PHS concluded that this concept, a voluntary national certification system, should be developed further.

By 1978, a Certification Council had organized. The general purpose was to certify the certifiers—an overall group that would include the organizations that certified allied health professionals, but also set certain uniform standards and guidelines. At the same time, certification of nurses* was also undergoing reorganization and expansion, as was certification for PAs.** In almost all cases, the practitioner had to show evidence of continued competence for recertification. Although in itself certification has no *legal* clout, the increasing tendency for states to require certification as a component of the right to practice, either under licensure or other statutes, and sometimes to reimburse services has made certification a necessity for some.

Improving the licensure process also became a national mandate. Although the speed of the action taken varied from state to state, steps taken almost universally at one level or another included adding consumers and sometimes other functionally related health professionals to each board, more attention being given to disciplinary procedures, and gradual development of proficiency and equivalency examinations.

In nursing, certain positive steps were and are being taken. The ANA and NLN took action on the issues of open curriculum, mandatory continuing education for relicensure, and certification. Most state associations have initiated revision of their nursing practice acts, broadening the scope of practice, adding consumers to their boards, and sometimes requiring evidence of current competence through various means, including continuing education. Nurses in the field have continued to strive toward improving techniques of peer evaluation, implementing

---

* See Chapter 25.
** See Chapter 8.

standards of practice, and encouraging voluntary continuing education. State boards have given increased attention to removing and/or rehabilitating incompetent nurses. Educators are working seriously on equivalency and proficiency examinations and other methods of providing flexibility and upward mobility for nursing candidates. Finally, a major study of credentialing, sponsored by the ANA,[25] made some daring proposals in 1979, suggesting the establishment of a national nursing credentialing center, possibly a federation of organizations with "legitimate interests" in nursing and credentialing, "as the means of achieving a unified, coordinated, comprehensive credentialing system for nursing."

Other professions have also given increased attention to these same matters, some admittedly for the first time.[26] The criticisms of current credentialing processes involve all. Therefore, none of the concerns belongs exclusively to any one health discipline. It is entirely possible that they cannot be resolved by any one health discipline.

LICENSURE, THE LEGAL BASIS OF NURSING PRACTICE

Enactment of nurse licensure laws was one of the primary purposes of ANA at its inception. The first permissive nursing practice law in this country was enacted in North Carolina on March 3, 1903. Weak though it was as compared with present-day laws, it represented a great achievement for nursing leaders who had been working toward this goal for a decade. Within a month New Jersey passed a state nursing practice act, followed closely by New York and Virginia. In 1904, Maryland was the only state to pass such an act, but in each succeeding year from 1905 until 1917, legislation was effected to govern the practice of nursing, although it was not always just what nurses desired. By 1917, forty-five states and the District of Columbia had nursing practice acts; by 1923 the last of the forty-eight states in existence

adopted such an act. In 1952 all states and territories had such laws. Hawaii's first nursing practice act was passed in 1917 and Alaska's in 1941.

In every instance the original state law was permissive. The first mandatory nursing practice act was enacted in New York in 1938, but it was not put into effect until 1947.

One of the real dangers in permissive licensing is that correspondence and other schools with poor curricula and inadequate clinical experience produce workers who can legally "nurse" although they are potentially dangerous practitioners. Such programs also tend to defraud unsuspecting students who do not know that they will not be eligible for licensure, because a school must maintain minimum standards set by the state board before graduates may sit for licensing examinations. As of 1980 there were no states with permissive licensure laws for professional nurses; a few states had permissive licensure for practical nurses. A 1980 review and report of the state boards indicated that only the District of Columbia lacked a mandatory RN law, although others were loose in their interpretation of mandatory.

Objections to making licensure laws mandatory come from many sources. Some feel that mandatory laws are used to keep out individuals who might be capable but lack the formal education and other requirements for licensure. It is true that some laws are rigid in these requirements, but more and more states are beginning to consider the use of equivalency and proficiency examinations and other means of demonstrating knowledge and skills.

Another voiced concern is that those already practicing in the field will be abruptly removed and deprived of their livelihood. This is, however, untrue because mandatory laws are forced, for political and constitutional reasons, to include a grandfather clause. A grandfather or waiver clause is a standard feature when a licensure law is enacted or a present law is repealed and a new law enacted. The grandfather clause allows persons to continue to practice the profession/occupation when new qualifications are enacted into law. Although the concept goes back to post-Civil War days, it is also related to the Fifth and Fourteenth amendments of the Constitution. The U.S. Supreme Court has repeatedly ruled that the license to practice a profession/occupation is a property right and that the Fourteenth Amendment extends the due process requirement to state laws. Even though this property right is honored, the individual licensee must continue to be a safe practitioner, for that is the purpose of licensure. Many nurses currently licensed were protected by the grandfather clause when a new law was passed or new requirements made, although most probably never realized it. For instance, when the Missouri Nursing Practic Act was repealed in 1976, the new law had a grandfather clause, and all nurses holding a valid license continued to be licensed. When the various states began to require psychiatric nursing as a condition of licensure, those who had not had those courses in their educational programs did not forfeit licensure. When the grandfather clause is enacted in relation to mandatory licensure, those who can produce evidence, frequently including an affidavit of a physician or RN, that they practiced as, say, a PN, if applying for LPN status, must be granted a license. Some PNs who went through this process had had no formal schooling at all, and, therefore, despite the waiver license, they may have had difficulty in finding employment or found their interstate mobility limited. Because of these problems and often because they became aware of their own inadequacies, many took courses to fill the gaps in their knowledge and chose to take the state board examinations later.

CONTENT OF NURSING PRACTICE ACTS

Unfortunately, many nurses know no more about the law that regulates their practice than that it requires their taking state board examinations in order to become licensed. More details about the procedure for obtaining a license will be given later; however, it is vital that nurses understand the components of their licensure law and how these affect their practice.

Because each state law differs to a degree in its content, nurses should have available a copy of the law of the state in which they practice and the regulations that spell out how the law is carried out. These may be obtained from the state board or whichever agency in the state government has copies of laws for distribution. The language in all laws often seems stilted because they are written in legal terms. However, a little effort or discussion with someone familiar with the law will soon enable the nurse to become almost as familiar with legal jargon as with nursing jargon.

Such understanding will become increasingly important, for the majority of states anticipate some change in their nursing practice act in the near future or have already passed amendments. Changes made or contemplated are generally in relation to the definition of nursing practice, the makeup of the nursing board, and ensuring competency (mandatory continuing education). Nurses in the states with pending or newly passed legislation must know what these changes are and how their practice will be affected.

Most nursing practice acts have basically the same major components, although not necessarily in the same order: definition of nursing, requirements for licensure, exemption from licensure, grounds for revocation of license, provision for reciprocity for persons licensed in other states, creation of a board of nurse examiners, responsibilities of the board, penalties for practicing without a license. All states do not, unfortunately, have the same requirements in these categories. Pertinent examples will be given as the components of the nursing practice law are presented, as well as suggestions made by the ANA Ad Hoc Committee on Legal Aspects of Nursing Practice, Congress for Nursing Practice, in 1979. Only the RN licensure law or component of the Nursing Practice Act will be considered at this time. However, the ANA committee recommended that because nursing is one occupational field it should be controlled by one law and one state board. (Definitions and requirements would, of course, still be separate.)

Definition and Scope of Practice

The definition of nursing in the licensure law determines not only the legal responsibilities, but also the scope of practice of nurses. It will be immediately noted that although the definition of nursing in all nursing practice acts is stated in terms of functions that can be carried out by a licensed nurse, it is quite broad. This is generally frustrating to nurses who turn to the definition to determine if they are practicing legally because it does not spell out specific procedures or activities (such as starting intravenous injections or giving inoculations). Often such activities are not even spelled out in the regulations of the laws. Usually a broad definition is preferable because of the problems of including specific activities in a law. Changes in health care and nursing practice often move more rapidly than a law can be changed, and the amending process can be long and complex. If particular activities were named, the nurse would be limited to just those listed. Not only would the list be overwhelmingly long, but it is conceivable that any new technique easily and, perhaps necessarily, performed by a nurse would require an amendment to the law. However, it is interesting to note that one of the newest definitions (California) does specify certain procedures, but always includes a "not limited to" phrase.

A practicing nurse soon finds that the nursing functions taught in an educational program may differ from those expected by an employer. The differences may be small and caused by differences in the various settings of nursing care. Nursing in a medical center may require knowing more sophisticated techniques or assuming more comprehensive responsibilities in nursing care. Sometimes, whether in a large or small agency, there are procedures performed that the nurse has not learned. If the nurse has not practiced for some time, this is even more likely. In other cases, the responsibilities expected in the nursing role are not in nursing care but in clerical and administrative tasks. Although this may not be desirable, it is not illegal. What concerns the nurse is whether the patient-oriented care expected in the employment situation is legal or in the domain of another health profession. Many of the activities in health care overlap. A common example might be the giving of drugs, which could be done by physician, registered nurse, licensed practical nurse, and various technicians in other hospital departments if related to a diagnostic procedure or treatment. Yet dispensing a drug from the hospital pharmacy, so commonly done by hospital supervisors at night when no pharmacist is on duty, is in most states a violation of the pharmacy licensing law.

Obviously, one of the greatest concerns for nurses is the possible violation of the Medical Practice Act. Nursing has gradually been performing more and more of the technical procedures that once belonged exclusively to medicine, but often these are delegated willingly by physicians. Whether nurses are always properly prepared to understand and perform them well is seldom questioned. However, as some nurses assume more comprehensive overall responsibilities in care, cure, and coordination of patient care, questions have been raised by both nurses and physicians. Some are resistant to such changes; others are supportive but concerned about the legality of such acts.*

In a 1970 position statement on nursing, the American Medical Association stated support of the expanding role of the nurse in

---

*In some states, NPs have been cited as practicing medicine without a license, which endangers their own license as well or subjects them to a fine if guilty. Most have been attempts at harassment by MDs and have failed.

providing patient care. In this paper as in the HEW report on *Extending the Scope of Nursing Practice*, there is a statement that the identical act or procedure "may be the practice of medicine when carried out by a physician and the practice of nursing when carried out by the nurse."[27,28] The AMA statement appears to allude particularly to technical procedures, but the HEW report looks at the situation more broadly.

> *There is an every-widening area of independent nursing practice entailing nursing judgment, procedures, and techniques. This is due to natural evolution, commencing with the nurse's assumption of certain activities carried out under medical direction, and the subsequent relaxation or removal of that direction.*
>
> *Concomitant with increasingly complex nursing practice is the continual realignment of the functions of the professional nurse and physician. The boundaries of responsibility for nurses are not shifting more rapidly simply because of increased demands for health services. The functions of nurses are changing primarily because nurses have demonstrated their competence to perform a greater variety of functions and have been willing to discontinue performing less important functions that were once performed only by nurses.*[29]

The same report states that there are no legal barriers to extending the scope of practice because the statutory laws governing nursing practice (the licensing laws) are broad enough to permit such extension, providing that the nurse has the proper skills and necessary knowledge of the underlying service. It *does* acknowledge that at times common law, essentially judge-made law, has made interpretations of nursing practice not specifically defined by statute through legal decisions and that the profession must then look at these decisions to determine the need to change the statutory law.[30] After reviewing some of the problems concerned with specific acts in changing nursing practice, the report concluded that as nursing changes, both nursing and the law must evaluate these changes and make the necessary

adaptations to meet society's changing needs.[31]

To understand how the scope of practice is determined by the definition in the licensure law, the first step is to look at some of the nursing practice acts and then to consider how specific practice decisions are made.*

Until 1974 the nursing practice acts of most states had as their definition of nursing one similar to a model suggested by the American Nurses' Association in 1955. (See Chapter 9.) In the 1970s, with expanded functions being assumed by nursing, state nursing associations increasingly became concerned about the adequacy of this definition. Therefore the first states to change their laws concentrated on broadening the definition to encompass these roles.[32]

Professional nursing literature had been distinguishing between the independent acts that a nurse must undertake and the dependent acts that must be carried out under the supervision or "orders" of the physician, such as medications and treatments.† The problem in the 1955 definition, in terms of the needs of the 1970s was that although the first sentence did not *prohibit* the nurse from carrying out medical acts or making diagnoses the last sentence effectively prohibited a broad interpretation by the courts.

As nurses in their "expanded role" seemed to be moving into the gray areas between medicine and nursing, it was evident that, if a state had a licensure law with a dependent clause, nurses might be seen as practicing medicine. The 1971 and 1973 credentialing reports suggested extending dele-

---

*Nurse-midwives and nurse anesthetists may be included within a nurse practice act, a medical practice act, separately, or totally ignored legislatively. If mentioned, usually certification is a prerequisite for legal practice.

† A new concern in the late 1970s was the ruling by some judges and attorneys general that nurses must also follow the orders of PAs who act as the MD's representative. Other rulings have required that these orders be signed within twenty-four hours; still others have stated that nurses need not carry out such orders.

gation of authority in all fields, but nursing was concerned that such delegation might mean including nurses specifically in the exception clause of medical practice acts, thus permitting the practice, but placing control totally in the hands of physicians. Perhaps as a compromise or in the hope that medicine and nursing could work together as they should in providing new health care options to the public, ANA counsel suggested that a new clause be added to the ANA model definition:

> *A professional nurse may also perform such additional acts, under emergency or other special conditions, which may include special training, as are recognized by the medical and nursing professions as proper to be performed by a professional nurse under such conditions, even though such acts might otherwise be considered diagnosis and prescription.*[33]

Later, after various states had amended their laws with this phrase or changed it altogether, with varying success, an ANA ad hoc committee revised the definition entirely in 1976 and again in 1979. Both definitions are presented in Chapter 9.

Given the problems of changing licensure laws and the fact that each state has its own political milieu favoring or opposing expanded practice, just how extensive the adoption of the ANA model will be remains questionable. Up to now, state legislatures have chosen three general means of dealing with expanded nursing practice in the legal definition of the licensure law.[34] The first category could be called the nonamended statutes. These states either have made no changes and allow for a liberal interpretation of the definition by the state board or have made minor changes. In some, the word *medical* has been inserted to describe prohibited acts. Thus, presumably certain acts of diagnosis and treatment would be identified as nursing. Other states have retained portions of the traditional definition but omitted or substituted certain other phrases. Although all these states maintain that their acts allow expanded practice, interpretation

is the key, so a change in attitude or political/medical pressures could bring a rapid about-face. The second trend, and by far the largest, is the administrative statute. These permit nurses to perform expanded duties, as authorized by the professional licensing boards: nursing alone, nursing and medicine, or medicine alone. Regulations are an integral part of that mechanism. The first of these states was Idaho; New Hampshire enacted a slightly different version shortly thereafter. Both are similar to the ANA interim suggestion.

> Idaho: *[1955 model definition with following addition:] The foregoing shall not be deemed to include acts of medical diagnosis or prescription of medical therapeutic or corrective measures,* except *as may be authorized by rules and regulations jointly promulgated by the Idaho State Board of Medicine and the Idaho Board of Nursing which shall be implemented by the Idaho Board of Nursing.*

> New Hampshire: *[1955 model definition with following addition:] The foregoing shall not be deemed to include acts of diagnosis or prescription of therapeutic or corrective measures, unless such acts under emergency or other special conditions, which may include special training, are recognized by the medical and nursing professions as proper to be performed by a professional nurse under such conditions, even though such acts might otherwise be considered diagnosis and prescription.*

Various reasons (with positive ad negative connotations) are given for this approach: regulations can spell out specific criteria and protect the public from incompetents and promote use of nurse practitioners by increasing competence and awareness; nursing can limit the role to nurses and exclude others; physicians can extend some control over the degree of nurse expansion; nurses and physicians can respond rapidly to changing needs and patterns of practice, because regulations do not go through the legislative process; state professional boards, familiar with both fields as well as the idiosyncrasies of regulation formulation can act rapidly and effectively. All have some legitimacy. Some states, such as Idaho, found that at first co-operation between the two boards went well, regulations were formulated rapidly, and nurse practitioners were able to practice freely at a time when they were badly needed. Then, physicians decided to pull back, and legal obstacles were put in the way of such practice. (The law required *joint* agreement). In some states, regulations could not be agreed upon, even by nurses alone, or there was considerable internal group pressure, and legal practice stayed in limbo. On the other hand, Oregon, using this approach, provides both recognition of and authority for nurse practitioners by its rules, which include standards for necessary education and training, permissible practice, and procedures for continuing education. The board of nursing is given considerable flexibility in implementing this' statutory directive. For instance, NPs may expand their practice to physical diagnosis and treatment of "common episodic and chronic problems" and may utilize these powers "in collaboration" with physicians, removing the strict supervision concept. The opposite is true in Virginia where all such activities can be performed only under the direction of a physician.

In a minority are the states choosing the "authorization" alternative, developing their own new definition, intended to permit expanded practice. The first of them was New York, and several states copied that definition almost verbatim. California developed its own definition. The two make an interesting comparison.

New York: *The practice of the profession of nursing as a registered professional nurse is defined as dignosing and treating human responses to actual or potential health problems through such services as casefinding, health teaching, health counseling, and provision of care supportive to or restorative of life and well-being, and executing medical regimens as prescribed by a licensed or otherwise legally authorized physician or dentist. A nursing regimen shall be consistent with*

and shall not vary any existing medical regimen.

California: *The practice of nursing within the meaning of this chapter means those functions helping people cope with difficulties in daily living which are associated with their actual or potential health or illness problems or the treatment thereof which require a substantial amount of scientific knowledge or technical skill, and includes all of the following:*

(a) Direct and indirect patient care services that insure the safety, comfort, personal hygiene, and protection of patients; and the performance of disease prevention and restorative measures.

(b) Direct and indirect patient care services, including, but not limited to, the administration of medications and therapeutic agents necessary to implement a treatment, disease prevention, or rehabilitative regimen prescribed by a physician, dentist, or podiatrist.

(c) The performance, according to standardized procedures, of basic health care, testing, and prevention procedures, including, but not limited to, skin tests, immunization techniques, and the withdrawal of human blood from veins and arteries.

(d) Observation of signs and symptoms of illness, reactions to treatment, general behavior, or general physical condition, and (1) determination of whether such signs, symptoms, reactions, behavior, or general appearance exhibit abnormal characteristics; and (2) implementation, based on observed abnormalities, of appropriate reporting, or referral, or standardized procedures, or changes in treatment regimen in accordance with standardized procedures, or the initiation of emergency procedures.

"Standardized procedures," as used in this section, means either of the following:

(1) Policies and protocols developed by a health facility licensed pursuant to Chapter 2 (commencing with Section 1250) of Division 2 of the Health and Safety Code through collaboration among administrators and health professionals including physicians and nurses;

(2) Policies and protocols developed through collaboration among administrators and health professionals, including physi-

cians and nurses, by an organized health care system which is not a health facility licensed pursuant to Chapter 2 (commencing with Section 1250) of Division 2 of the Health and Safety Code. Such policies and protocols shall be subject to any guidelines for standardized procedures which the Board of Medical Examiners and the Board of Nursing Education and Nurse Registration may jointly promulgate; and if promulgated shall be administered by the Board of Nursing Education and Nurse Registration.

The nurses in the states adopting the New York model (including New York) have had serious problems in achieving acceptance of the overall definitions as adequate to protect the public; that is, it included no educational training requirements or delineation of practice. Organized medicine in those states is insisting that medical diagnosing and treating is off-limits. There are also attorneys and others who see the definition of diagnosis and treating as worded in the New York statute as self-limiting:

1. *"Diagnosing" in the context of nursing practice means identification of and discrimination between physical and psychosocial signs and symptoms essential to effective execution and management of the nursing regimen. Such diagnostic privilege is distinct from a medical diagnosis.*
2. *"Treating" means selection and performance of those therapeutic measures essential to the effective execution and management of the nursing regimen, and execution of any prescribed medical regimen.*
3. *"Human Responses" means those signs, symptoms and processes which denote the individual's interaction with an actual or potential health problem.*

Frequently, limitations are due to the compromises necessary to get the law passed, for instance excluding medical diagnosis in the definition. Although there are those who say that everything NPs do is nursing because *they* are nurses, the argument has not yet been accepted legally.

The California law is seen to have its own limitations in the use of "protocol" and "policies," but some legal interpretations maintain that they are equally important and allow adequate initiative.[35]

Several other legislative approaches have also been adopted.[36] Pennsylvania regulations allow nurses to perform medical acts under the supervision of the physician but define the limits of supervision. A few states allow the nurse deciding to function in the expanded role to submit a proposal and credentials to the state board, which can then authorize these specifically. (This could be a problem if there were many proposals). Another handful of states have designated in the law or in regulations an advanced nurse practitioner (New Hampshire) or a "certified registered nurse" (Washington), requiring either certification or other examinations determined by the board; these could be national tests.

Which of these legislative approaches is best can probably not be decided definitively. Some states have switched from one approach to another; others have concentrated on the rules and regulations. Still of concern are the words *diagnosing, prescribing,* and *treating,* which have heretofore been reserved as the physician's prerogative. The question of whether or not a nurse can, or indeed, already does, diagnose remains a point of controversy. It has been noted that:

> *The ability for critical thinking and to make decisions, either deliberately or with great speed, has ever been a part of the standard of conduct of the practitioner of professional nursing. This function shifts in complexity with scientific advancement in health care, for to do critical thinking and take appropriate action the nurse must be able to draw from the biological and physical sciences that are continually feeding new knowledge into the field of medical science. The function has long been recognized as an indisputable part of nursing practice, but selection of the proper word to describe the function is a controversial issue.[37]*

Although for years the observational function of the nurse included only observing, recording, and reporting the results, research shows the modern function to be more complex. It is conceived to include "observation—recognition of signs and symptoms presented by the patient, inference—making the judgment about the state of the patient and/or nursing needs of the patient, and decision making—determining the action to be taken that will be of optimal benefit to the patient."[38] One definition of *diagnosis* as "the utilization of intelligence to interpret known facts, and acting upon the decision reached from this interpretation"[39] appears to bring into context these more modern functions.

In differentiating between medical and nursing diagnosis, one study sees medical diagnosis as determining the cause of disease and seeking to eradicate it through specifics, and nursing diagnosis as making a determination of a symptom and its alleviation.[40] There are those who say that simply prefacing the word *diagnosis* by *medical* will allow nurses to make *nursing* diagnoses.

Because the nurse's actions based on professional inferences do involve the risk of error, there can be serious consequences for the patient, for which the nurse must take responsibility. There is certainly no question that some of these inferences and subsequent actions are being made almost instantly in today's nursing practice, for example, a coronary-care nurse's action (treatment) to recognize and terminate a potentially fatal heart arrhythmia. It is ironic and anachronistic that many nursing practice acts specifically forbid diagnosing, whereas at the same time some court decisions have held nurses negligent because they have *not* made a diagnosis.[41]

Again, this reiterates the overlap of responsibilities in medicine and nursing (and other health disciplines, as well). The only state that has given legal recognition to it is the California law where the statement of legislative intent says:

[to] recognize the existence of overlapping functions between physicians and registered nurses and to permit additional sharing of

functions within organized health care systems which provide for collaboration between physicians and registered nurses.

It can be seen why in California NPs and PAs are prescribing drugs as part of a four-year test project to evaluate possible changes in laws to expand roles of some health workers.

One further point must be made regarding definitions. Given the variety of licensure laws, how can nurses determine if they are practicing legally on a day-to-day basis, whether they are going beyond their legal scope of practice, or neglecting a legal requirement. The law itself is the first source of information; almost all have some specifics. For instance, teaching and/or counseling are identified in more than 75 percent. Other processes of legalizing specific practices all have advantages and disadvantages as has been seen in the discussion of regulations. A summary may prove useful.

Process: The attorney general of a state may make a ruling concerning a particular activity of the nurse.

Problem: A new attorney general may make a new ruling at any time. Even if the original ruling stands, it may actually be obsolete with the passing of time and changing health care.

Process: The attorney of a health agency or an individual may give an opinion on the legality of an activity.

Problem: A legal opinion, although based on careful study of the law, remains only an opinion and a judge could differ from it. It is not a protection if legal action should result from performing a particular activity.

Process: A judge may make a ruling.

Problem: Such rulings are always based on an event in the past, and on a specific act done at a specific time and place and under specific circumstances, which may never again be duplicated. The quality of the decision also depends on the competence of the judge and the accuracy of advice by experts. Another judge in another situation may make a different ruling, even though circumstances may be very similar.

Process: The doctrines of common practice or custom and usage may be invoked. This means basically that the act is performed in that particular community or at that current time and is acceptable as within the responsibility of the nurse by the individuals' employer and/or physicians in the area. It usually assumes appropriate training for that function.

Problem: Although this has been considered acceptable in some courts, it has been denied in others. It is possible that a nurse may be prosecuted for practicing medicine without a license, a criminal violation of the Medical Practice Act, but such a situation is not common, particularly if the activities are performed in a hospital—unless the nurse makes an error.

Practically speaking, statutes cannot be changed informally by mass violation, although they may be changed through the legislative process eventually, because of evidence that a nurse has been taught to perform such a function and is capable of carrying it out safely.

Process: The ANA and State Nurses' Associations have on occasion made statements regarding nursing functions.

Problem: Although all professional organizations see one of their roles as that of determining the functions of their practitioners, this has no legal impact, if that profession is also regulated by law. The organization can, of course, take a stand on this issue and can initiate legislation along these lines.

Process: The American Medical Association and other organizations, including nursing groups other than the ANA, have made statements regarding the function of nurses.

Problem: The AMA may consider its statements appropriate if the function is one that is or has been generally regarded as medical in scope. However, this profession cannot make a unilateral decision, be-

cause nursing is separately licensed and not under medical control. It may be dangerous for both an individual physician and a nurse to function within such a statement, because its lack of legality makes the nurse liable for practicing medicine and the physician for aiding and abetting. This has already occurred with physician's assistants.[42] Nor do other organizations have the legal right to determine functions of nurses.

Process: The National Joint Practice Commission, initiated by the National Commission for the Study of Nursing and Nursing Education (see Chapter 27), has made joint statements relating to emerging nursing practice, because this was one of its responsibilities.

Problem: Although prestigious and nationally oriented, the commission statements face the same problems as the state joint statements—they are not really legal.

Process: Some states are amending their medical practice acts to include a delegation statute. This, in effect, permits a person under certain circumstances to perform medical activities *under the direct supervision and control of a licensed physician.* Often this amendment is meant to allow for the legal practice of the physician's assistant, but at least two states, Oklahoma and Connecticut, have specifically included registered and practical nurses. A number of health law experts as well as HEW have recommended such actions as one answer to the dilemma of licensing the multiple health occupation groups.[43]

Problem: Although such an amendment will legalize certain activities of the nurse that are considered in the gray areas between medicine and nursing, it also puts the nurse under the direct supervision of the physician, as more of a physician's assistant than a professional nurse. This cannot, as currently understood, endanger the nurse's own licensure, but does limit the expanded nursing role because the questioned activities are still seen as medical activities, which require physician supervision.

Process: Joint statements of practice (or function) have been issued by professional organizations within states concerning a specific function of the nurse, for example, intravenous therapy, inoculations, closed-chest cardiac resuscitation, cardiac defibrillation, drawing blood. These statements are usually jointly agreed upon by the nurses' association, medical association, and hospital association, and occasionally other professional groups. They are not intended to tell nurses how to practice nursing, but set criteria that attorneys believe would make it possible for them to defend a nurse if legal defense were necessary in relation to the emerging, questioned areas of nursing practice.

When joint agreement is reached after a meeting of representatives and attorneys of the concerned associations, the statement is published and distributed by each group and often by the state medical licensing board and nursing licensing board.[44] The statements usually include specific criteria for performance of the acts concerned and always include the need for appropriate education and training. Frequently there is a preliminary statement advocating the formation, in each health care institution, of a committee of medicine, nursing, and administration to state responsibilities of doctors and nurses, and set criteria for determining the role and responsibility of each, considering newer developments in health care and education.

Problem: Because these organizations do not have legal status in relation to changing the law (although they can initiate such changes), these statements are in a way only formalizing the custom and usage doctrine. The chances of prosecution of the nurse by the medical licensure board are slight, for usually the board has been involved in the issuance of the statement. However, these statements do not have the effect of law unless the groups are given the legal authority to make them.

Theoretically, a case could still be made against the nurse, particularly if a civil malpractice suit is involved. To remedy this situation, several actions were taken to legalize the statements. Pennsylvania had them put in legal form with agreement of the association and boards concerned and filed by the nursing board as regulations under the Nursing Practice Act. In California, a resolution of the state legislature gave the joint statements recognition as a "responsible, effective method of recognizing and responding to the development of needs and methods of providing new patient care." The resolution called for the use of these statements "in cases of conflicting or absent statutory definition to validate generally accepted practice or patterns of care" and aiding appropriate groups "in anticipating new needs, and making responsible innovations in practice patterns."[45] A number of states have developed and used joint statements, with or without legal sanction.

It is not always easy for nurses to determine immediately which or how many of these alternatives are operative in the state where they practice. Except for those practices that may be limited to a particular hospital or agency, the State Board of Nursing can usually provide information as to whether a certain activity is permitted or specifically prohibited. When this information is not available, it is essential to remember that whatever nurses do they must be competent in their performance, which implies education, training, and currency.

Creighton, writing about the enlarged scope of nursing practice, predicted:

> . . . the professional nurse will become more of an independent practitioner directly involved in decision making. Legally she will be responsible for her decisions. The more independent she becomes as a practitioner, the greater her unshared legal responsibility.[46]

Creation of a Board of Nursing Examiners

The name of the state administrative agency varies from state to state as does the number of members. Traditionally this board has been made up entirely of nurses, who may or may not be designated as to area of practice. In most states, members are appointed by the governor from a list of names submitted by the state nurses' association. In recent years there has been some public outcry against such total control by professionals, with the result that gradually the addition of non-nurses, either public members or other health professionals, has been legally required. Although some nurses have considered this a danger to the profession, it can be to the advantage of nursing to have the input and support of the public and others on the health team, for these public members can be educated to understand and appreciate the problems of the profession. The danger exists when political pressure seeks to force the creation of a board with a majority of non-nurses, so that nursing practice and education can be totally controlled by others. Some forty states had consumers or other professionals as members in 1977. The ANA guidelines support consumer participation. Board size ranges from five to thirteen appointed members, who make policy. Employed staff carry out the day-to-day activities.

Responsibilities of the Board of Nurse Examiners

The major responsibility of a board is to see that the nursing practice act is carried out. This involves establishing rules and regulations to implement the broad terms in the law itself. Usual responsibilities include approval of programs of nursing and development of criteria for approval (minimum standards) such as facilities, curriculum, faculty, and so on; evaluating the personal and educational qualifications of applicants for licensure; determining by examination applicants' competence to practice nursing; issuing licenses to qualified applicants and disciplining those who violate the law or are found to be unfit to practice nursing.

Nursing boards may also collect certain data and cooperate in various ways with other nursing boards or the boards of other disciplines. If under an overall board, certain administrative responsibilities will be carried out on a central level. If a "sunset" law is in effect, the data and justification for existence is a joint staff-board responsibility.

National Council of State Boards of Nursing

Although not written into the laws, all nursing boards participate in the National Council of State Boards of Nursing, an independent organization since it separated from the ANA in 1978. The NCSBN consists of four "Areas" with separate officers, which meet primarily to share information. A representative of each is a member of the board of directors. The major objectives of NCSBN are as follows:

1. Develop, establish policy and procedure, and regulate the use of the licensing examinations for nursing to be available for use by states and territories.
2. Identify and promote desirable and reasonable uniformity in standards and expected outcomes in nursing education and nursing practice.
3. Identify and assist in efforts to promote continued competence of practitioners of nursing.
4. Collect, analyze, and disseminate data and statistics relating to nurse licensure.
5. Provide means and promote effective communication with related organizations, groups, and individuals.

Policy is set by action of a delegate assembly. Their responsibilities include the following:

1. Establish the criteria for selection of the testing service to be utilized by the Council unless the Council provides such services itself.
2. Adopt test plans to be used for the development of licensing examinations in nursing.

3. Adopt criteria and procedures for maintaining the security of the licensing examination within jurisdictions.
4. Establish dates for the administration of licensing examinations in nursing.

NCSBN headquarters is at 303 E. Ohio Street, Suite 2010, Chicago, Ill. 60611.

Requirements for Licensure as a Nurse

Licensure is based on fulfilling certain requirements.[47] The following points are usually included.

1. The applicant must have completed an educational program in a state-approved school of nursing and received a diploma or degree from that program; usually the school must send the student's transcript. Some states ask for evidence of high school education. There is increasing legislative pressure that the applicant not be required to have completed the program, particularly if the uncompleted courses are in a non-nursing area such as liberal arts. This is now true in California. In at least California and West Virginia an amendment permits military corpsmen to take the examination, providing that there have been certain components in their military courses. Some former corpsmen have passed the state board examinations and become licensed in California, but find it difficult to become licensed in other states or to find employment in agencies that require graduation from an approved school. Still, other states have bills pending with the same amendment.
2. The applicant must pass the State Board Test Pool Examination for Professional Nurses. These examinations are the same for all jurisdictions in the United States and are an effective means of facilitating the interstate licensing process for nurses. Each state has the right to determine the passing score, but almost all agree to a passing score of 350 out of some 800 points of the standardized examinations. At one time many states had various cut-off (passing) points, which

created problems in state-to-state mobility.
3. Some states require evidence of good physical and mental health.
4. As of 1977, nine states still had a minimum age for receiving licensure.
5. As of 1977, seven states still required citizenship or a legal declaration of intent. However, this has been declared unconstitutional.
6. Most states maintain a statement that the applicant must be of good moral character, as determined by the licensing board.
7. No experience is required.
8. A fee must be paid for admission to the examination. This varies considerably among states.
9. Many states allow the nurse a period of time in which to become licensed, usually from graduation to the time in which the licensure examination is given. The nurse may work during this time as a graduate nurse, not as an RN.

Provisions for Endorsement of Persons Licensed in Other States*

Nurses have more mobility than any other licensed health professional because of the use of a national standardized examination. However, usually the individual must still fulfill the other requirements for licensure in the state in which he or she seeks licensure. The nurse's nursing school record is usually evaluated to determine whether the program is generally equivalent to this state's program requirements of the same time period. If not, the nurse may be required to take the courses lacking and the pertinent state board examination.

If all requirements are satisfactorily fulfilled, the nurse is granted a license without retaking the state board examination. A fee is also required for endorsement. Endorsement is not the same as reciprocity; the latter means acceptance of a licensee by one state only if the other state does likewise.

---

*See p. 437 for specifics.

Renewal of Licensure

Until the early 1970s, nursing licenses were renewed simply by sending in the renewal fee when notified, usually every two years. For nurses licensed in more than one state, as long as the license was not revoked in any state, the process was the same. Usually the form asked for information about employment and highest degree (and still does), but there was no attempt made to determine if the nurse was competent. At about that time (also the time of the credentialing reports) there was increased concern about the current competency of practicing health professionals, and an estimate was made that perhaps five per cent of all health professionals, were not competent for one reason or another. Moreover, there was some question as to whether the professions made any real effort to either rehabilitate these people or to revoke their licenses. The credentialing reports emphasized the need for continuing education as a requirement for relicensure. One outcome was the enactment of a mandatory continuing education clause in a number of licensure laws; that is, a practitioner's license would not be renewed unless she/he showed evidence of continuing education. A number of health disciplines have such legislation. By 1977, a variety of states (not all) made mandatory continuing education a requirement for relicensure (or a legal practice requirement) for audiologists, chiropractors, dental hygienists, dentists, emergency medical personnel, nursing home administrators, nurses (RN and PN), opticians, optometrists, physicians (MD and DO), pharmacists, physicians' assistants, podiatrists, psychologists, social workers, speech pathologists, and veterinarians. Not all are well enforced. Some states also have permissive legislation for possible later implementation. In addition, some national associations and state medical societies require continuing education for renewal of certification.[48]

In nursing, the California licensure law was amended in 1971 to require evidence of continuing education by RNs and LVNs for relicensure, beginning in 1975, and it was again amended in 1972 to postpone compliance until 1977. It finally went into effect in 1978. There was some feeling that the postponements resulted from the immense complexity and expense of instituting a mandatory system for California's many thousands of nurses, and by 1979, there was some talk of rescinding the requirement.

In 1972 New Mexico also supported mandatory continuing education, in this instance by amending the Nurse Practice Act's regulations, which had the same effect as passage of a law. Actually, according to HEW, any state could use regulations to require continuing education without changing the law because all practice acts give the licensing boards the authority to determine standards of competence and these are usually delineated in the regulations.[49] Nevertheless, in the 1970s a number of state nurses' associations introduced legislation either requiring continuing education or specifically directing the state board to study or plan such a requirement. Realistically, this action may have been attributable, as much to the fear of externally introduced legislation that might remove control of the measure from nursing as to the conviction that this was a necessary amendment.

By 1979, California, Colorado, Florida, Iowa, Kansas, Kentucky, Massachusetts, Michigan, Minnesota, Nebraska, and New Mexico had laws requiring continuing education for all nurses. States that required a certain category of nurses to engage in continuing education activities were Alaska, (inactive nurse seeking renewal); Delaware (applicant inactive for five years); Louisiana (required if board desires, for inactive to active status and for nurse anesthetist); New Hampshire (for the advanced registered nurse practitioner); Oregon (may require if board desires for those with inactive, lapsed or revoked licenses and nurse practitioners); Utah (for those wishing to return to practice if licenses were inactive for five years). Some of these states will recognize only continuing education offerings approved by their boards or given by an agency, group, or institution that has been given a provider (or approval) number.[50] This may create problems for those licensed in more than one state, or living in a state other than where licensed. In the latter situation, some states permit the nurse to maintain his/her license on an inactive status, which can be reactivated when evidence of continuing education is shown. Forms of continuing education accepted by states include various formal academic studies in institutions of higher learning converted to CEU credit; college extension courses and studies; grand rounds in the health care setting; home study programs; inservice education; institutes; lectures; seminars; workshops; audiovisual learning systems, including educational television, audiovisual cassettes, tapes, and records with self-study packets; challenge examinations for a course or program; self-learning systems such as community service, controlled independent study, delivery of a paper, preparation and participation in a panel; preparation and publication of articles, monographs, books, and so on; and special research. The required number of hours of continuing education, or CEUs, varies considerably among states.

No law requires formal education directed toward advanced degrees. In fact, although additional formal education is acceptable, the emphasis is on continuous, *updated competence in practice.* The fears and anger of many nurses have been misdirected because they assumed that advanced degrees would be required. Obviously, there are innumerable ways in which an individual can maintain competence and increase knowledge and skills. How to measure achievement for the large numbers concerned is the real problem.

Objections to mandatory continuing education focus on the difficulty of assessing true learning; the question of whether learning can be forced (attendance does not mean retention or change in behavior); the danger in breeding mediocrity; the lack of research in effectiveness of continuing education in relation to performance; limitation of re-

sources, particularly in rural areas; the cost to nurses; the cost to government; the usual rigidity of governmental regulations; the problems in record keeping; and the lack of accreditation or evaluation procedures for many continuing education programs.[51]

On the other hand, many nursing leaders have advocated the mandatory route. Early on, the National League for Nursing stated, "In the belief that a continuing education requirement as a requisite for renewal of licensure of nurses will promote the delivery of optimum nursing care, the NLN Board of Directors supports the *gradual and carefully planned* implementation of such a requirement."[52] The ANA later agreed.*

The reasons for a mandatory approach are clear, but rather depressing; there appears to be considerable evidence that RNs do *not* continue in professional learning, particularly if they are not employed. Even if they are employed, there appears to be a prevalent notion in nursing that working in itself equals learning and subsequent competence. Unfortunately, this is not necessarily true. Yet their nursing license gives these nurses the right to practice. The hope that nurses would take advantage of the educational opportunities offered by their professional organization is dimmed when one realizes that less than a third belong to ANA.

The entire issue is far from resolved, although the threat of mandatory laws have increased interest in continuing education. It is also possible that another trend, peer evaluation, and other kinds of performance evaluation may provide a more effective answer to continued competence. Nurses, of course, must assume greater responsibility for nursing evaluation before it too is legislated, as the Medicare Professional Services Review Organization (PSRO). An implied threat (or suggestion?) has already been made.[53] Peer evaluation, like continuing education, is a professional responsibility; to abdicate this responsibility is professional suicide.

---

*See Chapter 25.

Exemptions from Licensure

Generally exempted are basic students in a nursing program; anyone employed previously in a domestic capacity, not as a nurse, and administering family remedies; anyone furnishing nursing assistance in an emergency; anyone licensed in another state and caring for a patient temporarily in the state involved; anyone employed by the U.S. government as a nurse (Veterans Administration, public health, or armed services); any legally qualified nurse recruited by the Red Cross during a disaster; anyone caring for the sick if done in connection with the practice of religious tenets of any church. In all these cases, the person cannot claim to be a registered nurse of the state concerned. Against strong nursing protests, some states have also incorporated in the exemptions nursing services of attendants in state institutions, if supervised by nurses or doctors as well as other kinds of nursing assistants under various circumstances. This, of course, weakens the mandatory aspect of the law.

Grounds for Revocation of Licensure

The board has the right to revoke or suspend any nurse's license or otherwise discipline the licensee. The reasons most commonly found in practice acts for revoking a license are acts that might directly endanger the public, such as practicing while ability is impaired by alcohol, drugs, physical or mental disability; being habitually drunk or a habitual user of certain drugs; practicing with incompetence or negligence beyond the scope of practice. Other reasons are obtaining a license fraudulently, being convicted of a felony or crime involving moral turpitude, practicing while the license is suspended, aiding and abetting a nonlicensed person to perform activities requiring a license; and committing unprofessional conduct or immoral acts as defined by the board. Recently, the refusal to provide service to a person because of race, color, creed, or national origin may also have been added. Although this seems to protect the public, data show that relatively few nurses have had licenses revoked or suspended. The reason is believed, in part, to be the reluctance of other nurses to report and consequently testify to these acts by their colleagues before either the nursing board or a court of law. Nursing associations and state boards are now emphasizing the responsibility of professional nurses to report incompetent practice.

When a report is filed with the state board, charging a nurse with violation of any of the grounds of disciplinary action, in most cases it is first investigated. If the charge is found to be valid, a hearing is set and subpoenas issued (by the board, attorney general, or a hearing officer). The accused has the right to appear personally or be represented by counsel, who may cross-examine witnesses. If the license is revoked or suspended, it may be reissued at the discretion of the board. (Sometimes the individual is only censured or reprimanded.)

The most common reason that nurses lose their licenses is the same as that of physicians—drug use, abuse, or theft. It is rather shocking that not all states specify incompetence as a reason for professional discipline and only a tiny fraction of a percentage of nurses lose their licenses for this reason. In some states, incompetence is subsumed under unprofessional conduct "as defined by the board." In 1977 and 1978, the New York State Board of Regents, which controls all health professional licensing boards, published a set of rules related to unprofessional conduct. Some particularly pertinent to nurses included abandoning, neglecting, harassing, abusing, or intimidating a patient; failing to maintain accurate patient records; claiming professional superiority or special professional abilities and skills unless so certified by an agency recognized by the Board of Regents; failing to exercise appropriate supervision over persons authorized to practice only under supervision of a licensed professional; claiming to use a secret method of treatment; failing to make available to a patient, at the patient's request, copies of records and reports; failing to wear an identifying badge, indicating the practitioner's name and professional status while practicing in a place where health care is given.

Not all states have such specific rules, but a 1979 court action may make this step more likely. In Idaho, in 1977, Jolene Tuma, an instructor in an associate degree program, went with a student to the bedside of a terminally ill woman to start chemotherapy, after the patient's "informed" consent. When the patient asked Ms. Tuma about alternate treatment for cancer, she was told about several. The son, upset because the mother stopped the chemotherapy, told the physician, who brought charges against Ms. Tuma. Subsequently, she was not only fired, but her license was suspended for six months by the Idaho board of nursing for unprofessional conduct, because her actions "disrupted the physician-patient relationship."[54] The case aroused a national nursing furor.[55] Ms. Tuma took her case through the courts, and on April 17, 1979, the Idaho Supreme Court handed down a decision that Ms. Tuma could not be found guilty of unprofessional conduct because the Idaho Nurse Practice Act neither defines unprofessional conduct nor sets guidelines for providing warnings. The judge also questioned the ability of the hearing officer, who lacked the "personal knowledge and experience" of nursing to determine if Ms. Tuma's behavior was unprofessional.[56] Unfortunately, the court did not address itself to Ms. Tuma's actions, which leaves the nurse's right to inform the patient in some question—at least in Idaho.

Another issue is what a nurse should do about reporting incompetence or unprofessional conduct on the part of physicians or other health professionals. Because the nurses' code of ethics requires that she/he safeguard the patient, incompetent or unprofessional practitioners should be reported. One survey indicated that a large percentage of nurses would take some sort of action, usually speaking with the doctor, head nurse, or supervisor, if the patient were endangered by medical action. Few would report the physician to a peer review or licensing board.[57] Some nurses who have reported a physician have either been dismissed from their jobs or harassed. All but six states (Massachusetts, New Hampshire, North Carolina, Oklahoma, South Dakota, and Vermont) have laws giving immunity from civil action to any person who reports to a peer review board, but this does not preclude being sued, even though legally the accused must be cleared. In New York, a statute was enacted in 1977, requiring physicians to report other physicians' misconduct on penalty of being cited for unprofessional conduct themselves; nurses and others are encouraged to report such misconduct also.[58] (Some have interpreted the law as *requiring* such reporting by all licensed professionals.) Similar statutes are also on the books in Arizona, Alabama, Connecticut, Idaho, Iowa, Maine, Montana, Ohio, Oregion, and Virginia.

Penalties for Practicing Without a License

Penalties for practicing without a license are only included in the mandatory laws. Penalties vary a great deal from a minimum fine to a large fine and/or imprisonment. Usually legal action is taken. This is being strengthened to deter illegal practice.

Other Components

In recent years, it has become increasingly popular to add a "good samaritan" clause to medical and nursing laws, although these are not always a part of the licensure law. This clause protects the professional from being liable for damages for alleged injuries or death after rendering first aid or emergency treatment in an emergency situation away from proper medical equipment, unless there is proven gross negligence.[59] Although such laws exist in all fifty states, there is some feeling that they are really counterproductive.[60]

Another recent addition has been the requirement that equivalency and proficiency exams be used to determine the qualification of those wishing to enter RN schools. Again,

California is the frontrunner in this legislation.

Licensing laws for practical nurses have a similar format. It is wise for a nurse who is expected to supervise practical nurses to also become familiar with laws concerning them.

PROCEDURE FOR OBTAINING A LICENSE

Almost all new graduates of a nursing program apply for RN licensure, because in all states it is otherwise impossible to practice. Even where licensure is permissive, it is wise to become licensed, for licensure is the legal indication that an individual has at least the minimum knowledge and skills for safe and effective practice. Without this it may become increasingly difficult to find a nursing position and impossible if one relocates to another state with mandatory licensure. Although there is nothing to prohibit a graduate from postponing licensure, it is generally more difficult psychologically and because of lack of practice to take the state board examinations much later.

As a rule, the graduate's school makes available all the data and even the application forms necessary for beginning the licensure procedure. Should a graduate wish to become licensed in another state, because of planned relocation, an application should be requested from that nursing board. Correct titles and addresses of the nursing boards of all states are found in the directory issues of the *American Journal of Nursing*. This board will then advise the graduate of the proper procedure, the cost, and the data needed. For this initial licensing, the nurse must take the state board examinations in the state where licensure is sought.

After receiving the completed necessary data fee, and application, the appropriate state board notifies the graduate of the time and place of the examination. These are given at least once, but usually twice a year; examinations are now given simultaneously throughout the nation. The State Board Test Pool Examinations were first developed in 1944 through the cooperative efforts of state boards of nursing, the American Nurses' Association, and the National League of Nursing Education. The examinations continue to be developed and administered by the state boards of nursing in cooperation with the Council of State Boards of Nursing and the National League for Nursing Department of Test Development.

For some years, the examination for licensure as a registered nurse consisted of one or more test in the following areas: medical nursing, surgical nursing, obstetric nursing, nursing of children, and psychiatric nursing. Each was an integrated test and included questions in areas such as the physical and social sciences, nutrition and diet therapy, and pharmacology as they relate to the particular clinical nursing subject. Each test for RN licensure includes 60 to 120 multiple-choice questions.* Two days are allowed for writing the examination for licensure as a registered nurse. The tests are the same for all nurses seeking an RN, whether graduating from a diploma, associate degree, or baccalaureate program. This has been the subject of considerable criticism, because the stated goals of all three programs are different. However, proponents of a single licensing exam state that the purpose is to determine safe and effective practice, at a minimal level, and that this criterion applies to all levels of nurses.

Great precautions are taken to preserve the security of the tests. Teachers in schools of nursing do not know the specific questions on the State Board Test Pool Examinations, but they are familiar with the types of questions with which the applicant will be confronted, and this type of test is often used in

---

*In 1979 NCSBN voted to adopt a new test plan, effective July, 1982. The structure of the new test plan was expected to combine "nursing behaviors, nursing systems to meet client health requirements, and levels of cognitive ability." Results of the integrated examination were to be reported as a single score.

the classroom. Although books of review and special review classes or courses are available to assist the nurse to study for the examinations, the best preparation is, of course, a sound educational background. Currently, there are no "practical" examinations, testing proficiency in real patient care situations or laboratories.

Nurses who pass the licensing examination receive a certificate bearing a registration number which remains the same as long as they are registered in that state. The certificate (or registration card) also will carry the expiration date—usually one, two, or three years hence—an important date to keep in mind, for failure to renew promptly may mean that the nurse must pay a special fee to be reinstated.

It is advisable to keep one's registration in effect, whether actively engaged in nursing or not. The expense is nominal, and more and more nurses who "retire" temporarily to have families return to nursing. These nurses do have the responsibility (and sometimes the legal requirement) to keep their nursing knowledge updated through continuing education.

One director of a State Board of Nursing has made this excellent point concerning the responsibilities of the licensed nurse:

> Many nurses seem to have the impression it is their right to be granted a license and to retain it, once issued, regardless of their abilities or actions. With the license, however, goes a responsibility for keeping abreast of the advancements in medical science and the changes in nursing practice. As the years go by, progress will be made and standards of competency will also change. As a professional practitioner the nurse is expected to keep pace with change. In 1975, the nurse cannot be expected to be considered a safe practitioner if her level of performance is of the 1959 vintage.[61]

To become licensed or registered by endorsement, applicants must already be registered in one state, territory, or foreign country. They must make application to the state board of nursing in the new state and present credentials, as requested, to substantiate that they have completed preparation equal to that required. A temporary permit is usually issued to allow the nurse to work until the new license is issued.

Nurses who wish to be reregistered after allowing their licenses to lapse should contact their state board for directions. A registered nurse wishing to practice nursing in another country also needs to investigate its legal requirements for practice. Members of the armed forces or the Peace Corps, or those under the auspices of an organization such as WHO or a religious denomination will be advised by the sponsoring group. Registration in one state is usually sufficient.

Nurses from other countries are expected to meet the same qualifications for licensure as graduates of schools of nursing in the United States. The procedure for obtaining a license is the same as for graduates of schools here; however, nurses from other countries are now expected to take the CGFNS Qualifying Examination, which screens and examines foreign nursing school graduates while they are still in their own countries to determine their eligibility for professional practice in the United States. (See Chapter 27.) The one-day examination covers proficiency in both nursing practice and English comprehension; both exams are given in English. If the applicant passes, she/he is given a CGFNS certificate which is presented to the US embassy or consulate when applying for a visa and to the SBNE in the state where the nurse wishes to practice.

The nurse still must take the state board examination and otherwise fulfill the licensing requirements for that state. Specific information about requirements for licensure must be obtained directly from the board of nursing in the state in which the foreign nurse wishes to be licensed.

Nursing's Responsibility

Only the Washington state nursing practice act states specifically that the nurse is accountable to the public, the consumers. However, as a professional privileged by the public to be licensed, the responsibility lies beyond personal accountability. There is a serious need to help resolve the health manpower credentialing mess.

The moratorium on licensing new health personnel is over, according to the calendar, but the problems that instigated the moratorium are not over; they continue unabated. Even if individual licensure is improved, what of the unlicensed worker? Will certification provide the answer or simply duplicate the problems of licensure with no legal recourse? Has the geometric increase of numbers of health care workers improved patient care? Is there another answer? Resolution of the problems posed could well result in helping to resolve some of the other problems of health care delivery. And, if some one must take the lead in initiating cooperative action, it may well be nursing.

REFERENCES

1. Study of Accreditation of Selected Health Education Programs. *Part 1: Staff Working Papers: Accreditation of Health Educational Programs* (Washington, D.C.: National Committee on Accrediting, 1972), p. A–6.
2. U.S. Department of Health, Education, and Welfare. *Report of the National Advisory Commission on Health Manpower.* Volume 1. (Washington, D.C.: U.S. Government Printing Office, 1967).
3. ———. *Report, Volume 2.* (Washington, D.C.: U.S. Government Printing Office, 1968).
4. U.S. Department of Labor. *Occupational Licensing and the Supply of Nonprofessional Manpower,* by Karen Green. Manpower Research Monograph No. 11 (Washington, D.C.: U.S. Government Printing Office, 1969).
5. U.S. Department of Health, Education, and Welfare. *Report on Licensure and Related Health Personnel Credentialing.* (DHEW Publ. No. (HSM) 72–11), 1971.
6. ———. *Developments in Health Manpower Licensure.* (DHEW Publ. No. (HRA) 74–3000), 1973.
7. ———. *Credentialing Health Manpower.* (DHEW Publ. No. (OS) 77-50057), 1977.

8. Carnegie Commission on Higher Education. *Higher Education and the Nation's Health: Policies for Medical and Dental Education. Special Report and Recommendations* (New York; McGraw-Hill Book Company, 1970).
9. ———. *Less Time, More Options: Education Beyond the High School, Special Report and Recommendations* (New York: McGraw-Hill Book Company, 1971).
10. *Study of Accreditation of Selected Health Education Programs. Commission Report* (Washington, D.C.: National Committee on Accrediting, 1972).
11. *Licensure and Related Health Personnel Credentialing,* op. cit., p. 71.
12. Ibid., p. 77.
13. Ibid., p. 7.
14. Edward Forgotson, *Licensure, Accreditation and Certification as Assurance of High Quality Health Care* (Paper Presented at National Health Forum meeting, Los Angeles, March 1968).
15. *Licensing and Related Health Personnel Credentialing,* op. cit., p. 43.
16. United States Department of Health, Education and Welfare: *State Regulation of Health Manpower* (DHEW Pub. No. (HRA) 77–49, 1977, pp. 5–6.
17. Laurence Miike, *Institutional Licensure: An Experimental Model, Not a Solution* (Paper presented at New Jersey League for Nursing Symposium on Institutional Licensure: What it Means To You, Mimeographed, Feb. 27, 1973).
18. Nathan Hershey, "Alternative to Mandatory Licensure of Health Professionals," *Hosp. Prog.,* **50:**73 (Mar. 1969).
19. Ibid., p. 74.
20. DHEW, 1971, op. cit., pp. 65-70.
21. Lucie Y. Kelly, "Institutional Licensure," *Nurs. Outlook,* **21:**566–572 (Sept. 1973).
22. Randolph Tucker and B. Wetterau, *Credentialing Health Personnel by Licensed Hospitals: The Report of a Study of Institutional Licensure* (Chicago: Rush-Presbyterian-St. Luke's Medical Center, 1975), p. 63.
23. *Credentialing Health Manpower,* p. 6.
24. Lucie Y. Kelly, "End Paper: Danger: Creeping Instatutional Licensure," *Nurs. Outlook,* **27:**624 (Sept. 1979).

25. *The Study of Credentialing in Nursing: A New Approach*, Vol. 1, The Report of the Committee (Milwaukee, Wisconsin, 1979). Vol. 2 has excellent background papers. See also Chapter 5 for more details on this study.
26. *Credentialing of Health Manpower-Conference Report* (New York: National Health Council, 1978).
27. AMA Committee on Nursing, *Medicine and Nursing in the 1970s, a Position Statement* (Chicago: American Medical Association, June 1970), p. 2.
28. Department of Health, Education, and Welfare, *Extending the Scope of Nursing Practice* (Washington, D.C.: The Department, Nov. 1971), p. 12.
29. Ibid., p. 12.
30. Ibid., p. 13.
31. Ibid., p. 14.
32. Lucie Young Kelly. "Nursing Practice Acts," *Am. J. Nurs.* **74:**1310 (July 1974).
33. Ibid., pp. 1314–1315.
34. Darlene Trandel-Korenchuk and Keith Trandel-Korenchuk, "How State Laws Recognize Advanced Nursing Practice," *Nurs. Outlook* **66:**713–719 (Nov. 1978).
35. Ibid., pp. 715–716.
36. Ibid., pp. 718–719.
37. Irene Murchison and Thomas Nichols, *Legal Foundations of Nursing Practice* (New York: Macmillan Publishing Co., Inc., 1970), p. 89.
38. Ibid., p. 90.
39. Ibid., p. 92.
40. Ibid., p. 90.
41. Ibid., pp. 90-99.
42. *Whittaker v. Superior Ct. of Shasta Co.*, 438. P. 2d 358 (Calif. 1968).
43. *Report on Licensure and Related Health Personnel Credentialing*, op. cit., p. 74.
44. *All About Joint Statements* (San Francisco: California Nurses' Association, 1967).
45. "California Legislature Recognizes Joint Statements on Practice," *Am. J. Nurs.* **73:**788 (May 1973).
46. Helen Creighton, "Changes in the Legal Aspects of Nursing," *Hospital Progress*, **52:**89 (Sept. 1971).
47. *State Regulation of Health Manpower*, op. cit., pp. 97–98.
48. *State Regulation of Health Manpower*, op. cit., pp. 9–10.
49. *Developments in Health Manpower*, op. cit., p. 44.
50. ANA *Mandatory Continuing Education: The Legislative State of the Art* (Kansas City, Mo.: The Association, 1979), pp. 1–5.
51. *Report on Licensure and Related Health Personnel Credentaling*, op. cit., pp. 57-63.
52. National League for Nursing, *NLN's Role in Continuing Education in Nursing* (New York: The Association, 1974.)
53. *Credentealing Health Manpower*, op. cit., pp. 16-17.
54. "Professional Misconduct?" Letters. *Nurs. Outlook* **25:**546 (Sept. 1977). See also editorial, p. 561.
55. Follow-up letters in Dec. 1977 issue, pp. 738–743; Jan. 1975 issue, pp. 8–9; Feb. 1978, p. 78; Mar. 1978 issue, pp. 142–143.
56. "Jolene Tuma Wins: Court Rules Practice Act Did Not Define Unprofessional Conduct," *Nurs. Outlook* **27:** 376 (June 1979).
57. Linda Stanley, "Dangerous Doctors: What To Do When the MD Is Wrong," *RN* **42:**22–27, 29–30 (Mar. 1979).
58. "Going Beyond the Hospital," *RN* **42:**28 (Mar. 1979).
59. Miles Zarenski, "Good Samaritan Statutes: Do They Protect the Emergency Care Provider?" *Medicolegal News*, **7:**5-7, 14 (Spring 1979).
60. George Annas, "Negligent Samaritans Are No Good," *Medicolegal News*, **7:** 4 (Spring 1979).
61. Adele Stahl, "Prelude to Licensure," *Am. J. Nurs.* **59:**1259–1260 (Sept. 1959).

BIBLIOGRAPHY

Accountability of the Nurse. Kansas City, Mo.: American Nurses' Association, 1973. Speeches presented at 48th ANA convention by various legal experts concerning legal barriers, if any, to nurse accountability, particularly in relation to nursing practice acts.

Agree, Betty. "The Threat of Institutional Licensure." *Am. J. Nurs.*, **73** (Oct. 1973), 1758–1763. Emphasizes the two projects funded by DHEW.

Anderson, Betty Jane. "Orderly Transfer of Procedural Responsibilities from Medical to Nursing Practice." *Nurs. Clin. North Am.*, **5** (June

1971), 311–319. Some legal aspects of nursing in relation to the "gray" areas of practice are discussed.

Bullough, Bonnie. "Nurse Practice Acts: How They Affect Your Expanding Role." *Nurs. 77,* **7** (Feb. 1977), 73–81. Overview of law regulating practice at that time. Taken from first edition of the following book.

Bullough, Bonnie. *The Law and the Expanding Nursing Role.* 2nd ed. New York: Appleton-Century-Crofts, 1980. Articles by variety of experts on licensure. Includes update on institutional licensure by Kelly. First edition also worth reading.

Bullough, Bonnie. "The Law and the Expanding Nursing Role." *Am. J. Pub. Health,* **66** (Mar. 1976), 249–254. Another version of nursing licensure update. Includes list of states with amended laws (as of 1975).

Cohen, Harris. "Professional Licensure, Organizational Behavior, and the Public Interest." *The Milbank Memorial Fund Quarterly,* **51** (Winter 1973), 73–88. Analyzes the close nexus between professional organizations and state licensure. Discusses proposals for change, particularly in board makeup.

"Credentialing in Nursing: A New Approach." *Am. J. Nurs.* **79** (Apr. 1979), 674–683. Report and recommendation of nursing credentialing study.

Creighton, Helen. "Who Is the Professional Nurse?" *Sup. Nurs,* **7** (July 1978), 14–18. Attempts to identify differences between professional and "other" nurse in legal context. Also gives example of nurse cited for unprofessional conduct.

De Tornyay, Rheba. "State Board Member." *Am. J. Nurs.,* **69** (Mar. 1969), 570–572. Still useful discussion of role of state board member.

Dickey, Frank. "Accreditation—What About the Public?" *Nurs. Outlook,* **19** (Oct. 1971), 668–669. The executive director of the National Commission on Accrediting cites the need for accountability to the public, with the need to consider the relevance of accrediting criteria to the quality of the product of the educational programs.

Forni, Patricia. "Trends in Licensure and Certification," *J. Nurs. Admin.,* **3** (Sept.-Oct. 1973), 17–23. Current issues surrounding licensure practices, professional obsolescence, and institutional licensure are discussed. Reference is made to the 1971 HEW Report on Licensure.

Fox, John, and Steven Zatkin. "Innovations in

Family and Community Health Practice and the Law." *Fam.-Comm. Health,* **1** (Apr. 1978), 19–30. Reviews manpower credentialing reports but concentrates on PAs and NPs. Extensive bibliography.

Hall, Virginia. *Statutory Regulation of the Scope of Nursing Practice.* Chicago: Nat'l. Joint Practice Commission 1975. First thorough step by step comparison and analysis.

Hershey, Nathan. "A Court's View of Mandatory Licensure." *Am. J. Nurs.,* **66** (Nov. 1966), 2461–2462. Defines mandatory licensure and illustrates its implications for nurses by use of case material.

Hershey, Nathan. "Expanded Roles for Professional Nurses." *J. Nurs. Admin.,* **3** (Nov.-Dec. 1973), 30–33. New legislation offers two expanded role concepts for the nurse: independence to practice nursing fully and provision of medical services. Author advocates increase in latter. Also in *Nurs. Dig.* (Jan. 1974), pp. 18–19.

Hershey, Nathan. "An Alternative to Mandatory Licensure of Health Professionals." *Hosp. Prog.,* **50** (Mar. 1969), 71–74. The "classic" article in which this noted health law expert describes his concept of, and support for, institutional licensure.

Hershey, Nathan. "Nursing Practice Acts." *J. Nurs. Admin.* **4** (July-August 1974), 36–39. Suggests nurse participation in institutional licensure projects. Criticizes mandatory licensure.

Hershey, Nathan. "The State's Right to Police Health." *Am. J. Nurs.,* **67** (Mar. 1967), 557–558. Examines the police power of the state in providing for the needs of the public, specifically in the areas of health and welfare. Discusses public health legislation, mandatory licensure of health personnel, and constitutional limitations upon a state's police power.

Isler, Charlotte. "Six Mistakes That Could Land You in Jail," *RN.* **42** (Feb. 1979), 64–71. Ways in which a nurse can lose her license and suffer additional penalties.

Kelly, Lucie. "Credentialing of Health Care Personnel." *Nurs. Outlook,* **25** (Sept. 1977), 567–569. Clear delineation of problems in credentialing with discussion of alternatives.

Kelly, Lucie Young. "Nursing Practice Acts," *Am. J. Nurs.,* **74** (July 1974), 1310–1319. A review of the status of nursing practice acts in relation to the components that comprise all practice acts. Includes the criticisms of licensure laws, trends and problems.

Kelly, Lucie Young. "Institutional Licensure,"

Nurs. Outlook, **21** (Sept. 1973), 566–572. A comprehensive overview of concepts of institutional licensure, including the proponents' rationales and problems and dangers involved for public and nurses. Extensive bibliography.

Kinkela, Gabrielle, and Robert Kinkela. "Licensure: What's It All About?" *J. Nurs. Admin.*, **4** (Mar.-Apr. 1974), 18–19. Review of licensure from a different angle—court rulings and how state exercises its police power.

Lipman, Michel. "Your Rights Before a State Disciplinary Board." *RN*, **36** (Dec. 1973), 44–49. Discusses power of boards, grounds for action, right of appeal, preparation of nurse for action.

McGriff, Erline. "A Case for Mandatory Continuing Education in Nursing." *Nurs. Outlook*, **20** (Nov. 1972), 712–713. Author describes types of continuing education available and points out why the mandatory approach is necessary.

Peterson, Paul, and Joan Guy. "Should Institutional Licensure Replace Individual Licensure?" *Am. J. Nurs.*, **74** (Mar. 1974), 444–447. The chairman of the first pilot project and the executive secretary of a nurse's association take opposing views as to the value of institutional licensure.

Regan, Andrew. "License Suspended! A Nursing Board Bares Its Teeth." *RN*. **42** (Oct. 1979), 65–66. Real examples of why nurses have their licenses suspended.

Shimberg, Benjamin, et al. *Occupational Licensing: Practices and Policies.* Washington, D.C.: Public Affairs Press, 1972. A study of licensing often referred to in other publications on licensure. Has a section on health occupations, including practical nursing.

Stevens, Barbara. "Mandatory Continuing Education for Professional Nurse Relicensure—What Are the Issues?" *J. Nurs. Admin.*, **3** (Sept.-Oct. 1973), 25–28. The objectives for legislating mandatory continuing education, the problems anticipated, and other issues are discussed.

"Sunset Laws Affect RN Boards and Acts." *Am. J. Nurs.* **79** (July 1979), 1182, 1196, 1202. Review of sunset laws and experience of Florida specifically.

"The Study of Credentialing in Nursing: A New Approach." *Nurs. Outlook* **27** (Apr. 1979), 263–271. Report and recommendations of the study. Entire report should be read as well (citation in Chapter 5).

See also references at end of Chapter 20 (HEW credentialing reports are especially important and contain many good additional references as do many of the articles cited); references and bibliography of Chapters 6, 13, and 16. Follow-ups on credentialing reports should be read as they appear. News items on changes in licensure and appropriate articles appear in almost all nursing journals. Nov.-Dec. issues of *Nurse Practitioner* has several articles on credentialing, particularly as related to nurse practitioners.

21

Nursing Practice and the Law

United States citizens who enter schools of nursing of any type take with them all of the citizen's legal rights and responsibilities. As nursing students, however, they gradually take on duties and responsibilities that may involve them in litigation, directly or indirectly, trivial or serious, that would not concern them as citizens only. Upon graduation and licensure they may be held liable for actions that apply only to registered nurses, as well as for other acts of a more general nature. With gains in nursing experience and knowledge, responsibilities will increase still further, because a court of law takes these facts into consideration.

There are numerous ways in which nurses become involved with the law in their practice. The impact of statutory law has been discussed previously. In this chapter, other legal aspects will be considered, primarily within the common law of torts, that is, an intentional or unintentional civil wrong.* This is the kind of law that relates to the daily practice of most nurses. As an overview of some of these legal principles is given, it is essential to know that there is no such thing as *the law*.

---

*See Chapter 17 for a review of common civil law and the judicial process.

There is no fixed system of rules that can be mechanically applied to reach results that are fair and just for everyone. Rather, law must be interpreted in relation to specific situations. It is sensitive and moves with social change; it reflects recognition and understanding of advances in social and scientific thought. [1]

BASIC LEGAL CONCEPTS AND TERMS

As any profession, law has its own terminology. Short definitions and illustrations of key words and phrases used in tort law follow.

Borrowed servant—an employee temporarily under the control of someone other than the employer (a hospital OR scrub nurse placed under the direction of a surgeon).

Breach of duty—under law of torts, not behaving in a reasonable manner; in the legal sense, causing injury to someone.

Captain of the ship doctrine—similar to borrowed servant concept that physicians are responsible for all those presumably under their supervision. Courts have ruled both for and against this doctrine, but the trend is to hold the individual responsible for that individual's own acts (example, incorrect sponge count done by nurses) although this does not preclude the hospital's being sued under the doctrine of *respondeat superior.*

Charitable immunity—originating in English common law, holding that a hospital would not be held for negligence to a patient receiving care on a charitable basis. In 1969, the Massachusetts Supreme Court abolished prospectively the immunity of charitable institutions. In other states it varies, but the trend is toward recognizing the liability of charitable institutions. For government hospitals, the old *doctrine of sovereign immunity* granted them freedom from liability ("the government can't be sued" concept). However, the Federal Tort Claims Act (1946) partially waived sovereign immunity of the federal government and a U.S. Supreme Court ruling in 1950 made the government liable for harm inflicted by its employees. Immunity of state and municipal hospitals varies, but the trend is toward liability. Immunity does not include the individual's liability.[3,4]

Damages or monetary damages—redress sought by plaintiff for injury or loss. *Nominal damages* (usually $1) are token damages when the plaintiff has proven his case but actual injury or loss could not be proven. *Compensatory damages* are the *actual damages*, with amounts awarded for proven loss. These include *general damages* (pain, suffering, loss of limb) and *special damages* which must be proven (wage loss, medical expenses). *Punitive* or *exemplary damages* may be awarded when the defendant has acted with "wanton, reckless disregard." The *deep pocket* concept means that the person theoretically most able to pay damages is named in a suit.

Defendant—person accused in a court trial.

Employee—someone who works for a person, institution, or company for pay.

Employer—one who selects, pays, can dismiss the employee, and controls his/her conduct during working hours.

Expert Witness—Someone with special training, knowledge, skill, or experience who is permitted to offer his/her opinion in court. The expert witness gives "expert testimony."

Foreseeability—holds individual liable for all consequences of any negligent act which could or should have been foreseen under the circumstances (example, a suicidal patient is left unattended by an open window and jumps).

Indemnification—if the employer is blameless in a negligence case but must pay the plaintiff under *respondeat superior*, the employer may recover the amount of damage paid from the employee in a separate action. *Subrogation* means that the employer can sue the employee for the amount of damages paid because of the employee's negligence.

Liability—being held legally responsible for negligent acts. *Rule or doctrine of personal liability* means that everyone is responsible for his/her own acts, even though someone else may also be held legally liable under another rule of law.

Vicarious liability—liability imposed without personal fault or without a caused relationship between the actions of the one held liable and the injury (usually a case of *respondeat superior*).

Locality rule or community rule—first enunciated in 1880 (*Small* vs. *Howard*), in which a small town doctor unsuccessfully performed complex surgery and was held not liable. The rationale was that a physician in a small or rural community lacks opportunity to keep abreast of professional advances. Gradually, courts took into account such facts as accessibility of medical facilities and experience. Beginning in the 1950s, various states' supreme courts abandoned the locality rule on the basis that modern communications, including availability of professional journals, TV, and rapid transportation made the rule outdated. The proper standard is seen as whether the practitioner is exercising the degree of care and skill of the average qualified practitioner, taking into account advances in the profession.

Long tail—the time lag between when an injury occurs and the claim is settled. Insurance companies say that because of this, it is difficult to determine reasonable premiums for a malpractice insurance risk.

Malpractice—"any *professional* misconduct, unreasonable lack of skill or fidelity in professional or judiciary duties, evil practice or invalid conduct"; also, as related to physicians, "bad, wrong, or injudicious treatment resulting in injury, unnecessary suffering, or death to the patient, and proceeding from carelessness, ignorance, lack of professional skill, disregard of established rules or principles, neglect, malicious or criminal intent."[5] (Note that malpractice refers only to professionals.)

Negligence—failing to conduct oneself in a prescribed manner, with due care, thereby doing harm to another. *Criminal negligence and gross negligence* are sometimes used interchangeably and refer to the commission or omission of an act, lawfully or unlawfully, in which such a degree of negligence exists as may cause a serious wrong to another. Almost any act of negligence resulting in the death of a patient would be considered criminal negligence.

Contributory negligence is a rather misleading expression used when the plaintiff has contributed to his own injury through his own negligence. This he may do accidentally or deliberately. Some authorities assert that a plaintiff who is guilty of contributory negligence cannot collect damages; others, that he may under certain conditions. As in most legal matters, decisions vary widely. Because contributory negligence must be proven by the defendant, as much written evidence as possible is needed.

Comparative negligence takes into consideration the degree of negligence of both defendant and plaintiff; this allows the possibility of the plaintiff having some redress, which is often not so if there has been contributory negligence.

Corporate negligence* means that the health care facility or an entity is negligent.

Outrageous Conduct Doctrine or Tort of Emotional Distress—allows plaintiff to base his case on intentional or negligent emotional distress caused by defendant (example: patient gave birth to premature stillborn child, and later when she asked about burial, nurse brought fetus floating in gallon jug of formaldehyde).[6]

Plaintiff—party bringing a civil suit, seeking damages or other legal relief.

Proximate cause—the immediate or direct cause of an injury in a malpractice case. Plaintiff must prove that defendant's malpractice caused, precipitated, or aggravated his/her condition.

Res Gestae—all of the related events in a particular legal situation, which may then be admitted into evidence.

Reasonably prudent man theory—standard that requires an individual to perform a task as any "reasonably prudent man of ordinary prudence, with comparable education, skills, and training under similar circumstances," would perform that same function.

Res Ipsa Loquitor—"The thing speaks for itself," a legal doctrine that gets around the need for expert testimony or the need for the plaintiff to prove the defendant's liability because the situation (harm) is self-evident to even a lay person. The defendant must prove, instead, that she/he is not responsible for the harm done. Before the rule of *res ipsa loquitor* can be applied, three conditions must be present: the injury would not ordinarily occur unless there were negligence; whatever caused the injury at the time was under the exclusive control of the defendant; the injured person had not contributed to the negligence or voluntarily assumed the risk.[7] A common example involving nurses is when sponges have been left inside an abdomen

---

*This is a new concept based on the landmark decision *Darling* v. *Charleston Community Memorial Hospital*, discussed later.

after surgery, and the nurse had made an inaccurate sponge count and did not alert the operating team.

Respondeat superior—"Let the master answer." The employer is responsible for what employees do within the scope of their employment. Independent contractors such as private duty nurses are not usually included.

Standard of care—simply defined as the skill and learning commonly possessed by members of the profession.

Standard of reasonableness—liability is based on conduct that is socially unreasonable. Although there is no exact answer, the standard of reasonableness for health care practitioners could be defined as "that degree of skill and knowledge customarily used by a competent health practitioner of similar education and experience in treating and caring for the sick and injured in the community in which the individual is practicing or learning his profession."[8]

Stare Decises—"Let the decision stand." The legal principle that previous decisions made by the court should be applied to new cases. Also called "precedent." The decisions cited are usually made at the appellate level, including the state supreme court or the Supreme Court of the United States, highest appellate court in the land.

Statute of limitations— legal limit on time a person has to file a suit in a civil matter. The statutory period usually begins when an injury occurs, but, in some cases, as with a sponge left in the abdomen, it starts when the injured person discovers the injury (*discovery*). In the case of an injury done to a minor, the statute usually will not "toll" (begin to run) until the child has reached age eighteen. The statute of limitations that relates to malpractice actions has commonly not been applied to nurses[9]; instead, the longer periods for statutes of limitations for negligence applied to them (thus not considering them as professionals). However, along with other new legislation related to the NP and PA, several states have revised their statutes of limita-

tions to include nurses.[10] Court decisions about the inclusion of nurses within malpractice statutes of limitations have varied, with a previous but changing tendency to hold them liable for negligence, not malpractice, because they were seen as performing under specific directions. The shorter time is intended to ensure a professional a "fair chance to defend on merit and not find his defenses eroded by lapse of time."[11] This apparently was not seen as necessary for anything less than "professional negligence." Although the length of time involved varies from state to state, it is about two years for malpractice, four years or more for negligence by "others."

Tort—civil wrong against an individual. In order to have a cause of action based on malpractice or negligence, four elements must be present:

1. There was a duty owed to the plaintiff by the defendant to use due care (reasonable care under the circumstances).
2. The duty was breached (defendant was negligent).
3. The plaintiff was injured or damaged in some way.
4. The plaintiff's injury was caused by the defendant's negligence (proximate cause).

No matter how negligent the health provider was, if there was no injury, there is no case. The plaintiff must also establish that a health practitioner/patient relationship existed and that the practitioner violated the standard of care. Most civil cases involving malpractice and negligence do not involve only one concept or legal doctrine. Some examples, based on real cases, follow.

A first-year student nurse was assigned by the instructor to care for a patient who later went into shock. Among other things, the student applied hot water bottles around the patient. The patient survived but was badly burned and sued the doctor, hospital, head nurse, faculty members, and school of nursing. This was a case of *res ipsa loquitor*. The student was clearly negligent, perhaps grossly negligent because she/he should have known the correct temperature and procedure for applying a hot water bottle to anyone and should have taken special precautions with an unconscious patient. (Whether the hot water bottle was ordered by the doctor or not was immaterial, for the action, properly carried out, was appropriate for a patient in shock.) The student is held to the standards of care *(standards of reasonableness)* of an RN, if performing RN functions. If the student is not capable of functioning safely unsupervised, she/he should not be carrying out those functions. The doctor may or may not be held liable, depending on that court's notion about the *captain of the ship doctrine*, or perhaps whether the doctor saw and/or felt the hot water bottles. The hospital will probably be held liable under *respondeat superior*, because students, even if not employed, are usually treated legally as employees. In addition, because the head nurse is responsible for all patients on the floor and presumably should have been involved in or should have assigned an RN in such an emergency, she too would be liable (and again, the hospital, under *respondeat superior*). The instructor might be found liable, not on the basis of *respondeat superior*— just as the head nurse or supervisor would not be liable if the student had been an RN, because none of these nurses are employers in the legal sense—but on the basis of inadequate supervision. The same would have been true of an RN who had assigned a new nurse's aide to apply the hot water bottles, unless she was sure that the aide knew how to do so and was capable of carrying out that function. If a supervisor or other nurse assigns a task to someone not competent to perform that task and a patient is injured because of that individual's incompetent performance, the supervising nurse can be held personally liable because it is part of her/his responsibility to know the competence and scope of practice of those being supervised. Although theoretically this nurse could rely on the subordinate's licensure, certification,

or registration, if any, as an indication of competence, if there is reason to believe that that individual would nevertheless perform carelessly or incompetently and the nurse still assigns that person to the task, the nurse is held accountable (as is the employer under the doctrine of *respondeat superior*).[12] The school might be found liable if the court believed the director had not used good judgment in employing or assigning the faculty member carrying out those teaching responsibilities. In another situation, the outcome would be different. A student gave an electric heating pad, per doctor's order, to a patient who was alert and mentally competent and demonstrated to the nurse her ability to adjust the temperature and her knowledge of the potential hazards. The patient fell asleep on the pad, set at a high temperature, and burned her abdomen. In this case, there would seem to be sufficient evidence of contributory negligence on the part of the patient, with the student having good reason to assume that the patient was capable of managing the heating pad. Therefore, even if the patient sued, her case would be weak. If the court used the doctrine of *comparative negligence*, some liability might be assigned to the student, if for instance she/he did not check on the patient in a reasonable time. If the heating pad were faulty, the hospital would probably be liable, not the nurse.

A particularly useful example from many points of view is the landmark decision of *Darling* v. *Charleston Community Memorial Hospital* (211 N.E. 2nd 53, Ill., 1965). A minor broke his leg playing football and was taken to Charleston Community Memorial Hospital, a JCAH-accredited hospital. There a cast was put on the leg in the emergency room, and he was sent to the floor. The nurses noted that the toes became cold and blue, charted this, and called the physician, who did not come. Over a period of days, they continued to note and chart deterioration of the condition of the exposed toes and continually notified the physician who came once but did not remedy the situation. The mother then took the boy to another hospital where an orthopedist was forced to amputate the leg because of advanced gangrene. The family sued the first doctor, the hospital, and the nurses involved. The physician settled out of court; he admitted he had set few legs and had not looked at a book on orthopedics in forty years. The hospital defense was that the care provided was in accordance with standard practice of like hospitals, that it had no control over the physician, and that it was not liable for the nurses' conduct because they were acting under the order of a physician. However, the appellate court, upholding the decision of the lower court, said that the hospital could be found liable either for breach of its own duty or for breach of duty of its nurses. The new hospital standards of care set by that ruling were reference to the hospital by-laws, regulations based on state statutes governing hospital licensure and criteria for JCAH accreditation. The court reasoned that these constituted a commitment that the hospital did not meet. In addition, the court held that the hospital had failed in its duties to review the work of the physician or to require consultation when the patient's condition clearly indicated the necessity for such action.

For nurses, the crucial point was the **newly defined duty to inform hospital admin-**istration of any deviation in proper medical care that poses a threat to the well-being of the patients. (The hospital was also expected to have a sufficient number of trained nurses capable of recognizing unattended problems in a patient's condition and reporting them) **Specifically, the court said:**

> the jury could reasonably have concluded that the nurses did not test for circulation in the leg as frequently as necessary, that skilled nurses would have promptly recognized the conditions that signalled a dangerous impairment of circulation in the plaintiff's leg, and would have known that the condition would become irreversible in a matter of hours. At that point, it became the nurses' duty to inform the attending physician, and if he failed to act, to advise the hospital authorities so that appropriate action might be taken (211 N.E. 2d at 258).[13]

Because Darling-type situations are not rare, it is vital for nurses to know their legal responsibilities (and rights) in such cases, so that they can act accordingly.

STANDARD OF CARE

The standard of care basically determines nurses' liability for negligent acts. If this standard is based on what the "reasonably prudent" nurse would do, who makes that judgment?[14] In litigation, it is the judge or jury, based on testimony that could include the following:

1. *Expert witness.* Did the nurse do what she/he should have? A nurse with special or appropriate knowledge testifies as to what would be expected of a nurse in the defendant's position in like circumstances. The expert witness would have the credentials to validate his/her expertise, but because the opposing side would also produce an equally prestigious expert witness to say what was useful to them, the credibility of that witness on testifying is critical.

2. *Professional literature.* Was the nurse's practice current? The *most current* nursing literature would be examined and perhaps quoted to validate (or not) that the nurse's practice in the situation was totally up to date.

3. *Hospital or agency policies.* Were hospital policies, especially nursing policies (in-house law), followed? Example: If side rails were or were not used, was what the nurse did according to hospital policy?*

4. *Manuals or procedure books.* Did the nurse follow accurately the usual procedure? Example: If the nurse gave an injection that was alleged to have injured

---

*On the other hand, if a nurse followed an outdated policy or followed policy without using nursing judgment (according to the expert witness), it could be held against her/him.

the patient, was it given correctly according to the procedure manual?

5. *Drug enclosures or drug reference books.* Did the nurse check for the latest information? Example: If the patient suffered from a drug reaction that the nurse did not perceive, was the information about the potential reaction in a drug reference book, such as the PDR (Physicians' Desk Reference) or drug insert?

6. *The profession's standards.* Did the nurse behave according to the published ANA standards, both general and in the specialty, if any?

7. *Licensure.* Did the nurse fulfill her responsibilities according to the legal definition of nursing in the licensure law or the law's rules and regulations? Example: Did she teach a diabetic patient about foot care?

If the judge or jury is satisfied that the standards were met satisfactorily, even if the patient has been injured, the injury that occurred would not be considered the result of the nurse's negligence. Different judgments in different jurisdictions must be expected. For instance, in one case, an occupational health nurse not recognizing the signs and symptoms of a coronary occlusion, sent the patient home unattended. When he died and she was sued, she was found not liable because having such knowledge was not seen as being a nursing responsibility. In an almost identical situation elsewhere, the nurse was found liable. Nevertheless, a nurse who knows the profession's standards and practices accordingly is in a much firmer position legally than one who does not.

Common Acts of Negligence

Among the acts of negligence a nurse is most likely to commit in the practice of nursing are the following:

1. *Careless attention to a patient's personal belongings,* resulting in the loss of valuable or necessary property, such as expensive jewelry, money, prostheses, or dentures.

2. *Failure to respond or to ask someone else to respond promptly to a patient's call light or signal* if, because of such failure, a patient attempts to take care of his own needs and is injured. This might happen when he attempts to get out of bed to go to the bathroom or reaches for a bedpan in the bedside stand.

3. *Failure to use adequate precautions to protect the patient against injury.* Every nurse knows that drugs or hot liquids or potentially harmful implements, such as scissors, must be kept out of reach of a young child or a delirious or confused patient. She/he knows the necessity of staying with—or having someone else stay with—a patient on a stretcher or narrow treatment table to keep him from falling, or with a helpless or irresponsible person at any time.

All students learn what to do to avoid harming the patient. They learn that the water used to fill a hot-water bottle must be a given temperature and no hotter; that certain patients' temperatures should not be taken by mouth lest they bite the thermometers and injure themselves with glass, mercury, or both; that every medicine must be given accurately to the right patient, whether it is five grains of aspirin or an injection of a highly potent drug; that a sponge count is a very important step in certain surgical operations and must never be neglected; that sterility of equipment is essential for safety in giving hypodermics or doing sterile dressings as well as for use during surgery; that particular care must be exercised when performing treatments such as an eye irrigation, bladder instillation, or others involving very delicate tissues; that strict precautions must be observed to prevent infections and cross-infections, such as diarrhea in the nursery for newborn babies; that injections and other procedures should be done with care.[15,16]

Nurses who are imprudent and take unsafe shortcuts or otherwise fail to adhere to what they know is competent nursing practice are being negligent, and if harm to a patient or co-worker can be traced to a nurse, she/he may be held liable. Negligence tends to involve carelessness as much as lack of knowledge.

4. *Failure to carry out orders* for treatments or medications. For example, if a patient dies because a nurse did not suction his tracheostomy tube at prescribed intervals, she/he could be held liable. Or if forgetting to give a medication to a patient with heart disease causes an attack, the nurse could be held liable for any suffering resulting from this negligence, although the court *might* hold that the patient would probably have had the attack anyway and refuse to allow damages.

5. *Failure to recognize and report a patient's untoward signs or symptoms*, the recognition and reporting of which could reasonably be expected from an intelligent and observant nurse. For example, a nurse doing a surgical dressing might overlook or fail to report to the charge nurse or physician that the patient's wound showed signs of infection; or might delay reporting excessive postoperative bleeding or an untoward reaction to a drug; or when admitting a patient, fail to note, report, and record injuries and mental confusion, information important to the patient's treatment.

6. *Failure to report one's own fatigue or illness* that might prevent the nurse from carrying out nursing responsibilities competently and safely, or that might conceivably spread infection—such as an intestinal ailment or influenza—to patients and other personnel.

7. *Irresponsible attention to a dying patient's requests* for medical attention or legal counsel.

8. *Failure to take whatever steps are necessary in certain emergencies to protect the victim* from further injury until medical care is available. This applies to any situation in which the nurse functions *as a nurse* or is known to be a nurse. It does not mean that the nurse must reveal himself or herself to be a nurse nor, so far as the law is concerned, is there any obligation or duty to render aid or assistance in an emergency. Only by statutory law can the rendering of such assistance be made obligatory. However, failure by the nurse or doctor to render aid not only may result in loss of human life but also violates every sense of decency.

As noted previously, the enactment of Good Samaritan laws in many states exempts doctors and nurses (and sometimes others) from civil liability when they give emergency care in "good faith" with "due care" or without "gross negligence." The first state to pass such a law was California in 1959; in 1963 California enacted such legislation specifically for nurses. By 1979 all states and the District of Columbia had Good Samaritan laws, not all including nurses in the coverage. No court has yet interpreted these statutes, and prior to their enactment, no case held a doctor or nurse liable for negligence in care at the site of an emergency. The law is intended to encourage assistance without fear of legal liability.

Registered nurses engaged in industrial or occupational health nursing are likely to be called upon to give first-aid treatment to patients with wounds and other injuries as part of their job responsibility. Such emergency treatment in a health care setting is not covered under the Good Samaritan laws. These nurses, just as nurses in an emergency room, should take every precaution to make sure they are operating within the bounds of legally authorized practice for ER nurses.

9. *Failure to see that faulty equipment is removed* from use, that crowded corridors or hallways adjacent to the nursing unit are cleared, that slippery or unclean floors are taken care of, that fire hazards are eliminated.

This is an area of negligence that, in most instances, would implicate others just as much as, or more than, the professional nurse. For example, the hospital administration would certainly share responsibility for fire hazards and dangerously crowded corridors, and the housekeeping and maintenance departments would not be blameless either. This does not lessen the nurse's responsibility for reporting unsafe conditions and following up on them.

It is wise to report persistent hazards in writing and to keep a copy for personal protection.

10. *Failure to recognize the dangers inherent in an order*, even if it is written by a physician who theoretically is better informed than the nurse about the potency and action of drugs. For example, if a written order calls for the administration of one-half grain of morphine sulfate to a six-month-old child, the nurse must question it—in fact refuse to give it—because she/he knows it is likely to kill an infant of that age. She/he likewise would never give bishydroxycoumarin (Dicumarol) or any other anticoagulant drug to a hemorrhaging patient, or penicillin to one who is known to be allergic to it. In each instance the nurse would be guilty of negligence because of failing to exercise the knowledge and judgment that could reasonably be expected of a registered nurse.

A nurse who follows a physician's orders is just as liable as that physician if the patient is injured because, for instance, a medication was the wrong dose, or given by the wrong route.[17] If she/he cannot read the order or it is incomplete, it is necessary to clarify that order with *that* physician. A nurse has a right to question the physician when in doubt about any aspect of an order, and the nursing service administration should support the nurse who does so. In fact, there should be a written policy as to the nurse's rights and responsibility in such matters, so that there is no confusion on anyone's part and no danger of retribution to a justifiably questioning nurse faced with an irate physician. The nurse should not simply refuse to carry out an order, for she/he might not have the most recent medical information and could injure the patient by *not* following the order (medical judgment versus nursing judgment). The key is what the reasonably prudent nurse would do. The supervisor often is expected to act as intermediary if there is a problem, but a good collegial relationship and mutual courtesy can prevent or ease a doctor-nurse confrontation.

Several other issues always arise in relation to "doctor's orders." What should be done about telephone orders? The dangers are evident, because in case of patient injury, either the doctor or nurse or both will be held responsible. There frequently are or should be hospital, sometimes legal, policies to serve as guides. If telephone orders are forbidden, and a patient is injured through confused orders, it could be termed negligence. If telephone orders are acceptable, precautions should be taken that they are clearly understood (and questioned if necessary), with the doctor required to confirm orders in writing as soon as possible. In states where PAs' written or telephone orders have been declared legal (as an extension of the physician), the same precautions must be taken, with the physician again confirming as quickly as possible.

Specialty Nursing

As nurses assume more responsibility in nursing, particularly in specialty areas, they often seek help in determining their legal status. Frequently their concern has to do with the scope of practice: are they performing within legal bounds? Negligence, whether in a highly specialized unit, an emergency, or a self-care unit, is still a question of what the reasonably prudent nurse would do. Therefore, although a nurse might look for a specific answer to a specific question, the legal dangers lie in the same set of instances described earlier, simply transposed to another setting.[18,19]

THE LEGAL IMPORTANCE
OF RECORDS

It would be almost impossible to overemphasize the importance of records in legal action, especially nurse's notes. They hold the only evidence that orders were carried out and what the results were; they are the only notes written with both time and date in chronological order; they offer the most detailed information on the patient.[20] Nurse's notes, like the rest of the chart, can be subpoenaed. No matter how skillfully a nurse practices her/his profession, if it is not documented accurately and completely, the jury can judge only by what is recorded. If the nurse is subpoenaed, comprehensive notes will not only give weight to the nurse's oral testimony, but will help him/her to remember what happened. A case may not come up for years, and, unless there was a severe problem at the time, it is difficult to remember exact details about one patient. General, broad phrases such as "resting comfortably," "good night," "feeling better," are totally inadequate. How could a jury interpret them? How could even another professional not knowing that patient interpret them?

The correct way to chart, with legal aspects in mind, is probably charting as one was taught and following good nursing practice: write what you see, hear, smell, feel; don't make flip or derogatory remarks.[21] Be as accurate as possible, but if a mistake is made, recopy or cross out with the original attached;[22] never alter a record in another way; this has been shown to influence a jury negatively.[23] Every good malpractice attorney calls on experts to examine charts for alterations, erasures, and additions. All too often, the nurse makes a change or an omission in the chart to protect a physician or the hospital. This can lead to criminal charges, such as the case of the OR nurse who did not record the illegal participation of an equipment salesman in surgery and who was cited for falsification of records.

Some of the most serious problems arising from poor charting concern lack of data, such as omission of a temperature reading or other vital signs, lack of observations about a patient's condition, no record of oxygen liter flow in a newborn infant; all these and others have resulted in liability judgments against nurses and hospitals, although in each it was contended that the "right" thing had been carried out.[24] Moreover, there are instances when a patient might be legally harmed by inaccurate reporting, as in child abuse or rape.[25]

Information in the patient's record that is particularly important from a legal point of view includes names and signatures of patient, nurses, and doctors; notations of the patient's condition on admission, with progress notes on changes for better or worse while in the hospital; accounts of injuries sustained accidentally while in the hospital, if any; a description of the patient's attitude toward his treatment and personnel; medications and other treatments given (what, when, how); vital signs; visits of doctors, consultants, and specialists; patient's permission for therapy and all special procedures such as surgery.

In case of patient injury, most hospitals and health agencies require completion of an "incident report." The purpose is to accurately document the incident for remedial and correctional use by the hospital or agency, for insurance information and sometimes for legal reasons. The wording should be chosen to avoid the implication of blame and should be totally objective and complete: what happened to the patient, what was done; what is his condition.[26] The incident report may or may not be discoverable, depending on the state's law; it is considered a business record, not part of the patient's chart. However, the incident *must* be just as accurately recorded in the patient's chart. This kind of omission casts a shadow of dishonesty over the nurse, if litigation occurs.

MALPRACTICE (LIABILITY) INSURANCE

Almost all lawyers in the health field now agree that nurses should carry their own malpractice or professional liability insurance, whether or not their employer's insurance includes them. The employer's insurance is intended primarily to protect the employer; the nurse is protected only to the extent that is needed for the primary purpose. It is quite conceivable that the employer might settle out of court, without consulting the nurse, to the nurse's disadvantage. The nurse has no control and no choice of lawyer.[27] There are a number of other limitations. The nurse would not be covered for anything beyond that job in that place of employment during the hours of employment. If the nurse alone is sued and the hospital is not, the hospital has no obligation to provide legal protection (and may choose not to). Moreover, if the nurse carries no personal liability insurance, there is the possibility of subrogation.[28] Should there be criminal charges, the employer or insurance carrier may choose to deny legal assistance, or the kind offered could be inadequate.[29] A nurse must remember that no matter how trivial, how unfounded a charge might be, a legal defense is necessary and often costly, aside from the possibility of being found liable and having to pay damages.

Malpractice insurance should be bought with some care so that adequate coverage is provided. The most important distinction to be made in selecting insurance is whether it is on an "occurrence" basis or a "claim made" basis. If the insurance policy is allowed to lapse, an incident that occurred at the time of coverage will be covered in an occurrence policy, but not on a claims made policy. The latter may be less expensive, but would almost require continuous coverage, which might be a problem for a nurse planning to take time out for child rearing or for one close to retirement. Benefits usually include paying any sum awarded as damages including medical costs, paying the cost of attorneys, and paying the bond required if appealing an adverse decision. Some also pay damages for injury arising out of acts of the insured as a member of an accreditation board or committee of a hospital or professional society, personal liability (such as slander, assault, libel), and personal injury and medical payments (not related to the individual's professional practice).[30]

Except for nurse anesthetists, who occasionally have difficulty in finding insurance and who pay higher premiums, nurses have had no problems getting malpractice insurance. Most carry the standard $200,000 per occurrence and $600,000 maximum liability per year, which is available to ANA members for about $30 a year. ANA now carries an occurrence policy; state associations vary in this, as well as in the additional benefits that might be offered. Insurance bought elsewhere is usually more costly. Even for the careful nurse, professional liability insurance is a good investment, as well as being tax-deductible.

IN COURT: THE DUE PROCESS OF LAW

What happens to a professional nurse who becomes involved in litigation? What steps should be taken to try to make sure that the case will be handled to the best advantage throughout? The answers to these questions will depend upon (1) whether the nurse is accused of committing the tort or crime; (2) whether she/he is an accessory either through actual participation or observance; (3) whether she/he is the person against whom the act was committed; or (4) whether she/he appears as an expert witness.*

Assuming that this is a civil case, five distinct steps are taken:

These are (1) the filing of a document called a complaint by a person called the plaintiff

---

*Springer gives a detailed explanation of the trial process; others give less detailed versions.

who contends that his legal rights have been infringed by the conduct of one or more other persons called *defendants;* (2) the written response of the defendants accused of having violated the legal rights of the plaintiff, termed an *answer;* (3) pretrial activities of both parties designed to elicit all the facts of the situation, termed *discovery;* (4) the *trial* of the case, in which all the relevant facts are presented to the judge or jury for decisions; and (5) *appeal* from a decision by a party who contends that the decision was wrongly made.[31]

The majority of persons who are asked to appear as witnesses during a hearing accept voluntarily. Others refuse and must be subpoenaed. A subpoena is a writ or order in the name of the court, referee, or other person authorized by law to issue the same, which requires the attendance of a witness at a trial or hearing under a penalty for failure. Cases involving the care of patients often necessitate the production of hospital records, X-rays, and photographs as evidence. A subpoena requiring a witness to bring this type of evidence with him contains a clause to that effect and is termed a *subpoena duces tecum.*

Plaintiff, defendant, and witnesses may be asked to make a *deposition,* an oral interrogation answering all kinds of questions about the issue concerned. It is given under oath and taken in writing before some judicial officer or attorney.[32] A witness has certain rights, including the right to refuse to testify as to privileged communication (extended to the nurse in only Arkansas and New York; partially in New Mexico and South Dakota), and the protection against self-incrimination afforded by the Fifth Amendment to the United States Constitution. The judge and jury usually do not expect a person on trial or serving as a witness to remember all of the minute details of a situation. Witnesses in malpractice suits are permitted to refer to the patient's record, which, of course, they should have reviewed with the attorney before the trial.

Only under serious circumstances is someone accused (and convicted) of perjury, which means making a false statement under oath or one that she/he neither knows nor believes to be true.

There are certain guidelines on testifying that are the same whether serving as an expert or other witness or if the nurse is the defendant:[33]

1. *Be prepared; review the deposition, the chart, technical and clinical knowledge of the disease or condition; discuss with the lawyer potential questions; educate the lawyer as to what points should be made. Trials are adversary procedures that are intended to probe, question, and explore all aspects of the issue.*
2. *Dress appropriately.*
3. *Behave appropriately: keep calm, be courteous, even if insulted; don't be sarcastic or angry; take your time (a cross-examiner attorney may try to put you in a poor light).*[34]
4. *Give adequate and appropriate information: if you can't remember, notes or the data source, such as the chart, can be checked. Answer fully, but don't volunteer additional information not asked for.*
5. *Don't use technical terminology, or, if use is necessary, translate it into lay terms.*
6. *Don't feel incompetent; don't get on the defensive; be decisive.*
7. *Don't be obviously partisan (unless you're the defendant).*
8. *Keep all materials; the decision may be appealed.*

In the expert witness role,[35] the same precepts hold, but in addition the nurse should present her/his credentials, degress, research, honors, whatever else is pertinent, without modesty; the opposing expert witness will certainly do so.

Expert witnesses are paid for preparation time, pretrial conferences, consultations, and testifying. Nurses are just beginning to act officially in this capacity, and at least one state nurses' association accepts applications for those interested in placement on an expert witness panel, screens applicants in a given field for a specific case, submits a choice of names to attorneys requesting such information, and has developed guidelines and continuing education for nurse expert witnesses.[36]

Other Torts and Crimes

The average nurse probably will not get involved in criminal offenses, although nurses, as anyone else, may steal, murder, or break other serious laws. Crimes most often committed are criminal assault and battery (striking or otherwise physically mistreating or threatening a patient); murder (in relation to right-to-live principles); and drug offenses. If found guilty of a felony, the nurse will probably also lose her/his license.

Sometimes nurses will be involved in litigation as *accessories;* that is, they are connected with the commission of a crime but did not actually do it themselves, although present and promoting the crime or near enough to assist if necessary.

An *abettor* encourages the commission of a crime but is absent when it is actually committed. The term *accomplice* is similar in meaning to both *accessory* and *abettor,* although a distinction may be made in some jurisdictions. A nurse (or anyone else for that matter) found guilty of any of these crimes may be held equally guilty with the person who commits the crime. However, whether the nurse is a perpetrator, a victim, or simply has to deal with people who are, it is useful to know the definition and scope of the most common criminal offenses.

Assault and Battery

Of all the legal terms appearing in the newspapers day after day, *assault* is seen most frequently, or so it seems. That is because, like *negligence,* it covers a wide range of violations against the rights of man. In general, every time that one person touches another in an angry, rude, or insolent manner and every blow or push with an intent to injure, or put the person in fear of injury, constitutes an assault and a battery. Legal action can result from any of these, unless the act can be justified or excused.

Also, every attempt to use force and violence with an intent to injure, or put one in fear of injury, constitutes an assault, such as striking at a person with or without a weapon; holding up a fist in a threatening attitude near enough to be able to strike; advancing with a hand uplifted in a threatening manner with intent to strike or put one in fear of being struck, even if the person is stopped before he gets near enough to carry the intention into effect.

A mere threat, unaccompanied by an offer to strike, is not an assault. Neither is touching a person, without force or violence, for the purpose of attracting his attention, unless it is done in a hostile or insulting manner.

A *battery,* as distinguished from an assault, is the actual striking or touching of the body of a man or woman in a violent, angry, rude, or insolent manner. But every laying on of hands is not a battery. The person's intention must be considered. If someone slaps a person on the back in fun or as an act of friendship, for example, it does not constitute a battery, for there is no intent to injure or put the person in fear of injury.

To constitute a battery, intent to injure or put one in fear must be accompanied by "unlawful violence." However, the slightest degree of force may constitute violence in the eyes of the law.

As in so many legal matters, the terms used to describe the acts are much less important than the acts themselves as far as the nonlegal public is concerned. In legal proceedings, however, terminology has a significant bearing on the outcome of a case. For example, should a nurse be either plaintiff or defendant in a case of assault or battery, or both, the terms used might influence considerably the conduct of the case and the settlement made. In day-to-day practice, however, the nurse need only be aware of the acts related to nursing that might conceivably be considered as assault or battery, or both, and therefore, subject to legal action. Assault and battery in the context of civil law is discussed in Chapter 22.

Embezzlement, Burglary, Larceny, Robbery

Suppose a nurse with access to the hospital pharmacy steals a bottle of morphine sulfate. Or a surgical resident breaks into the locked instrument room in the operating suite and helps himself to several surgical instruments for the private office he plans to have some day. Or a kitchen employee walks out of the hospital with a steak for his family's dinner. Or a cashier takes funds from the hospital's safe. Or a masked stranger stops a doctor's car, knocks him unconscious, and takes his wallet. Would these persons be guilty of crime, and would they be punishable by the law?

All of the offenders would have committed a crime, because taking another's property with intent to use it as one's own is forbidden by law and punishable under the law. Whether all would be brought to justice in a court of law or be meted out punishment by the persons or institutions they have injured would depend, of course, upon circumstances peculiar to each case. And if brought into court, the kind and degree of punishment would depend largely on decisions made in previous cases of a similar type in that community, as well as on the usual interpretation of the law made by the presiding judge. This in no way alters the fact the each of these persons did commit a crime, however. What would these crimes be called? There is a legal term for each, although there is, as usual, some overlapping in meaning and application.

The employee who took the steak committed *larceny*, or simply thievery, or stealing. In this case, it would be considered *petit larceny*, because the meat was of little value. Had he elected to take a carful of supplies amounting in value to approximately $100 or more, he would have entered the area of *grand larceny*. There are other considerations in some jurisdictions, but this distinction will usually suffice.

Anyone who, intending to commit a crime, breaks and enters a building or a room or any part of a building or who commits a crime in a building and breaks out of it is guilty of *burglary*, so the resident could be accused of burglary.

The cashier would be guilty of *embezzlement*, because he took another's property

that had been entrusted to his care. The holdup man committed *robbery* because he took the doctor's wallet by violence. Had he used force to snatch it from him or obtained it by threatening to injure him without actually doing it, he still would have effected robbery.

The nurse who took the morphine sulfate is guilty of larceny. Her crime is complicated greatly by the fact that she broke the narcotic law, because no one—not even a physician—is entitled to help himself to habit-forming drugs for his own consumption, even if he can acquire them legally. This nurse would be liable under the law to heavy fine, imprisonment, or both. She would surely be dismissed from her position, would probably lose her license, and her professional and personal future would be jeopardized.

Blackmail and Extortion

A person who attempts to get money or other valuable consideration from another through threat of public accusation, exposure, or censure is guilty of *blackmail*. Although nurses and physicians certainly have innumerable opportunities to use these intimidating tactics, one rarely hears of such instances. Punishment for proved blackmail is usually quite servere. Many threats are merely annoyances only and do not constitute blackmail; the law terms them *misdemeanors*.

Occasionally a case of extortion involving a nurse or doctor, or both, is reported in the news. *Extortion* is the illegal use of fear to obtain money, property, or something else of value from another with his consent. For example, a physician or nurse who threatens to discontinue caring for a wealthy patient unless she/he makes a will in his or her favor would be guilty of extortion. Fortunately, such cases are rare.

Defamation, Slander, Libel

As is true of so many legal terms, there is some overlapping of meaning and interpretation of the terms *defamation, slander,* and *libel.* In general, however, it is correct to consider *defamation* as the most inclusive because it covers any communication that is seriously detrimental to another person's reputation. If the communication is oral, it is technically called *slander;* if written or shown in pictures, effigies, or signs (without just cause or excuse), it is called *libel.* All three are considered wrongful acts (torts) under the law, and a person convicted of one or more of these in criminal or civil court is ordered to make amends, usually by paying the defamed person a compensatory fee.

In both slander and libel, a third person must be involved. For example, one person can make all kinds of derogatory statements directly to another without getting in trouble with the law *unless* overheard by a third person. Then the remarks become slanderous. Moreover, the third person must be able to understand what has been said. If it is spoken in unfamiliar language, for example, it is not slanderous under the law. Likewise a person can write anything she/he wishes to another, and the communication will not be considered libelous unless it is read and understood by a third person. A malicious and false statement made by one person to another about a third person also comprises slander.

Statements of a strong and uncomplimentary nature are not necessarily slanderous or libelous. They must be false, damaging to the offended person's reputation, and tending to subject him to public contempt and ridicule.

The best and often the only defense allowed for the person accused of slander or libel—under the law—is proof that she/he told the truth in whatever type of communication used. For example, if an employee tells an employer that another employee is untrustworthy because of having once served a prison sentence for grand larceny, the "injured" employee might sue for slander, but would be unlikely to do so if the story were true because it would not be difficult to prove its veracity in court. Furthermore, if the second employee did not lose his job or status in the community because of the revelation of his past life, he probably would get no more than an apology (ordered by the court) from the co-worker who attempted to get him in trouble.

If the defendant can prove that he divulged the information as part of a privileged communication, he is not guilty of slander or libel.

It is evident that there are many "if's," "and's," and "but's," associated with defamation, slander, and libel. Wise nurses avoid becoming embroiled in such litigations by being extremely careful in what they say or write about anyone. This is the only polite, professional, and legally safe way to behave. They also proceed with caution when they are the victims of slander and libel, knowing that litigation is expensive and time-consuming and, in many instances, hardly worth the trouble. On the other hand, they should not be overly meek in acceptance of unfair and untrue statements about them that are likely to adversely affect their reputations and future in nursing, as well as the good name of nursing in the community. There have been documented cases when nurses were slandered by a physician, for instance, in which they collected damages.

Homicide and Suicide

Homicide means killing a person by any means whatsoever. It is not necessarily a crime. If it is unquestionably an accident, it is called *excusable homicide.* If it is done in self-defense or in discharging a legal duty, such as in taking a prisoner, putting a condemned person to death, or preserving the peace, it is termed *justifiable homicide.* The accused must be able to prove justification, however.

Criminal homicide is either murder or manslaughter. *Murder* means the unlawful killing of one person by another of sound mind and with malice aforethought. It may be by direct violence, such as shooting or strangling, or by indirect violence, such as slow poisoning. Murder is usually divided into two degrees: *first degree* when it is premeditated and carried out deliberately; *second degree* when it is not planned beforehand but is nontheless performed with an intent to kill. In both, there must be a design to effect death.

Suicide is self-murder. It is considered criminal if the person is sane and of an age of discretion at the time of his action. An unsuccessful attempt to commit suicide is a misdemeanor under the law. If there is doubt as to whether a person has committed suicide, a court of law usually presumes that she/he has not, although this judgment may be reversed by evidence to the contrary. A person who encourages another to commit suicide is guilty if murder if the suicide is effected. Statutes vary from state to state.

As a professional person, it is not unusual for a nurse to become implicated in cases of murder and suicide, usually associated with patients. Following are a few suggestions for keeping as free of involvement as possible:

1. Any indication on the part of any patient or employee that she/he has suicidal tendencies should be taken seriously and reported to the appropriate person.
2. Generally, a patient with known suicidal inclinations should not be left alone, even for a second unless completely protected from self-harm by restraints or confinement.
3. Items that a depressed person might use for suicidal purposes should be kept away from him/her.
4. Observations should be accurately reported on the patient's chart.
5. Help should be sought for nurses or their families immediately upon becoming aware of suicidal tendencies.
6. Cooperation with the police and hospital authorities guarding a patient who is accused of homicide is important.
7. Unethical discussions of a homicide case involving a patient or employee should be avoided.
8. Complete and accurate records of all facts that might have bearing on the legal aspects of the case should be kept.

Among the more common other torts and crimes in which nurses occasionally are in-

volved in their professional lives are *forgery* —fraudulently making or altering a written document or item, such as a will, chart, or check; *kidnapping*—stealing and carrying off a human being, *rape*—illegal or forcible sexual intercourse; and *bribery*—an offer of a reward for doing wrong or for influencing conduct.

Drugs

The illness, crimes, and misery caused by the misuse of narcotics have made it imperative to have laws to control their purchase, possession, distribution, and sale. The problem of narcotic addiction is worldwide, and, since 1909, international meetings have been held at intervals to try to work out effective controls for the production, exportation, and importation of drugs. Their particular aim has been to limit the production of opiates to amounts needed for medical and scientific purposes, but efforts have been only partially successful; illicit traffic in narcotics is far from being fully controlled. However, the edicts of international agreements have placed an obligation on signatory nations to consider world regulations when developing national controls. The League of Nations sponsored efforts to control narcotics, and the United Nations is continually working on this problem:

> *With the establishment of the United Nations in 1945 and the creation by it in 1946 of a Commission on Narcotic Drugs, efforts to further international control of narcotics continued. The job of the commission, a policy-making body, is to advise the Economic and Social Council of the United Nations on ways to implement control of narcotics. The members of the commission consist of the principal narcotic-producing and narcotic-consuming nations of the world.*[37]

Every person who handles narcotics in any capacity—pharmacist, physician, nurse, and others—has a moral as well as a legal obligation to help further the international effort by conforming to all rules and regulations everywhere, always.

The United States, in 1914, adopted an an-

tinarcotic act—the Harrison Narcotic Act—
to be administered by a bureau of narcotics
within the Department of the Treasury. This
Act was so called because Francis Burton
Harrison, congressman from New York, was
chairman of the House Ways and Means
Committee, which favorably reported the
bill that became the narcotic law of 1914. It
has been amended frequently to meet the demands of changing times, and new legislation
is enacted as needed. For example, in 1956 a
strong Narcotic Control Act was passed, and
in 1961 a new law gave federal authorities
broader control of drug preparations containing small amounts of narcotics. This
came about largely because teen-agers were
reported to have become addicted through
taking such preparations as cough medicines, containing a small percentage of narcotics, which they could obtain without a
prescription.

The Harrison Narcotic Act regulates the
importation, manufacture, possession, sale,
purchase, prescription, and use of opium,
cocaine, and their derivatives within the United States and the imposition of federal
taxes on those who deal in narcotics, such as
importers or manufacturers of drugs, and
wholesale and retail dealers. Intrastate control of narcotics is accomplished through
state laws, most of which are very similar to
a Uniform Drug Act formulated by a national
committee in 1932. The latter also requires
records for receiving and administering
drugs, for which nurses are responsible
along with doctors and others.

Marijuana has been subject to changing legal patterns. In many states, its use but not
its sale has been decriminalized. Barbitu-
rates, principally used therapeutically as sed-
atives, but also a part of the illegal drug
scene, have been state-regulated through the
so-called lullaby laws—aimed originally at
the legitimate user, not the addict.

Among the other drugs subject to federal
or state control, or both, are poisons, caus-
tics, and corrosives, methyl or wood alcohol,
drugs for the treatment of venereal disease,
and amphetamines. Tranquilizers and other

relatively new drugs are also being given
closer scrutiny because of misuse and consequent dangerous effects.

Knowledge of the laws controlling the use
of drugs helps nurses to understand the reasons for the policies and procedures established by an institution or agency for the mutual welfare of the employer, employee, and
patient. It also helps them keep free of legal
involvements and prepares them to intelligently direct and advise others whom they
may supervise or who may look to them for
guidance in such matters. Nurses should also
be alert to changes in drug laws on either the
state or national level.*

LITIGATION TRENDS IN HEALTH CARE

Part of the doctrine of common law is that
anyone can sue anyone if she/he can get a
lawyer to take the case or is able to handle it
personally (such as is common in a small
claims court). This does not necessarily
mean that there is just cause or that the person suing (plaintiff) has a good chance of
winning; in fact, the defendant might be protected by law from being found liable, as
when someone, in good faith, reports child
abuse.

Most people are reasonably decent in their
dealings with others, and unless a person
sustains a serious injury or his property is
badly damaged or stolen, they will not institute legal proceedings. Sometimes this is because legal services are expensive, perhaps
more so than the cost of repairing the damage or paying the medical bills, and the offended person is realistic enough to know
this. Often the person inflicting the injury is
also realistic and prefers to settle the matter
out of court, knowing that it will be less
costly in the long run, or insurance may pay
for the damage inflicted. One or both parties
may settle their difficulties out of court be-

---

*Recent federal drug laws are discussed in Chapter
19.

cause one or the other or both wants to avoid publicity and does not want to have a court record of any kind.

People have been considered particularly reluctant to "make trouble" for nurses, doctors, or health agencies such as certain non-profit or voluntary hospitals, either out of respect for the services offered and/or because they presumably had so little money that it would seem unfair or pointless. The latter was probably always an inaccurate generality, but today patients and families who are or feel aggrieved are considerably more likely to sue any or all concerned, sometimes for enormous sums. Health care is big business. The number of claims and the severity of awards began to increase in the 1930s, declined during World War II, and then rose again.

A number of reasons have been cited: the "litigant spirit" of the general public, what seems to be a "sue if possible; I'm entitled" attitude;[38] changing medical technology that brought new risks, with a potential for exceptional severity of injury; sometimes high, unrealistic public expectations; the increase in specialization that has resulted in a deterioration of the physician/patient relationship; and patient resentment of depersonalized care and sometimes rude treatment in hospitals. At the height of the malpractice crisis, a specially appointed interdisciplinary committee reported that the prime factor in malpractice was malpractice. However, because there are so many more medical injuries than medical claims, a major factor might be interpersonal problems between provider and patient and frustration with the way specific complaints were handled or not handled.[39] The same report showed that in 1970, approximately 12,000 incidents triggered claim action. Claims leading to payment totaled more than $80 million. Hospitals and other institutions were named in 39 per cent of the claims and physicians in 49 per cent. Only 3 per cent were against allied health workers, but these figures are admittedly incomplete.[40] Other figures indicated that malpractice claims have doubled in some jurisdic-

tions in the past ten to fifteen years.[41] Most of these suits are settled out of court; few are actually paid. The dramatic multimillion dollar suits seldom result in awards anywhere near the original figure; sometimes they are not won at all. The largest awards have the largest elements of compensation for pain and suffering, almost exclusively occurring after some negligently caused catastrophic injury, such as severe brain damage, or paralysis, which obviously has an enormous effect on the victim's life-style.[42] The frequent suits and large awards were part of the reason for the mid-1970s' malpractice crisis, when many physicians could not get malpractice insurance, and neither hospitals nor physicians felt that they could afford it if they could get it.

The vast majority of malpractice cases are against physicians or hospitals. Don't nurses get sued? Absolutely. A good percentage of the hospital and physician suits include nurses and may be based on the nurse's negligence. Because of the various legal doctrines, explained earlier, the aggrieved patient has the option of suing multiple defendants. The *deep pocket* theory[43] of naming those who can pay has become traditional tort law strategy, as has the *fishnet theory* of suing every defendant available. Thus, the likelihood of recovery from one or more defendants is greater, and a favorite defense of admitting negligence but blaming an absent party is defeated.[44] Because, presumably, either or both the physician or hospital have more money than the nurse, either may have to pay the award even if it is the nurse who is clearly at fault. Particularly in the case of the hospital whose liability and responsibility may be only secondary (vicarious liability), it may recover damages from the employee primarily responsible for the loss.[45] The possibilities of pretrial arbitration and no-fault insurance have been considered. New York State, for instance, uses an arbitration procedure that makes preliminary recommendations as to the viability of a suit. The attraction of no-fault insurance is the increasing public tendency to believe that if someone is hurt, someone must pay, whether or not negligence is clearly evident. How costly this would be remains to be seen; no-fault auto insurance has been much more costly than ever contemplated. To get to the root of the problem, quality of care, government and health providers are looking at the impact of quality assurance techniques. It has also been noted that physicians, through self-owned insurance companies, are more stringently controlling the practices of their peers.[46] In addition, many hospitals have now adopted risk-management programs in which nurses are very much involved, focusing on the review and improvement of employee guidelines, personnel policies, incident reports, physician-nurse relationships, safety policies, patient records, research guidelines and anything else that might be a factor in legal suits.[47,48]

All of this is of concern to nurses. For individual nurses who have specific concerns about the legal aspects of their practice, it may be possible to get some information from the employing agency's legal counsel or state licensing board. Keeping abreast of legal trends is always necessary. Observing some basic principles will also help to avert problems:

1. Know your licensure law.
2. Don't do what you don't know how to do. (Learn how, if necessary.)
3. Keep your practice updated; continuing education is essential.
4. Use self-assessment, peer evaluation, audits, and supervisor's evaluations as guidelines for improving practice and follow up on criticisms and knowledge/skill gaps.
5. Don't be careless.
6. Practice interdependently; communicate with others.
7. Record accurately, objectively, and completely; don't erase.
8. Delegate safely and legally; know the preparation and abilities of those you supervise.
9. Help develop appropriate policies and procedures (in-house law).
10. Carry malpractice insurance.

Most of all, professional nurses can never forget that licensure is a privilege and a responsibility mandating accountability to the consumer it is intended to protect; therefore, nurses have a legal and moral obligation to practice safely.

REFERENCES

1. Mary Hemelt and Mary Ellen Mackert, *Dynamics of Law in Nursing and Health Care* (Reston, Va.: Reston Publishing Co., 1978), p. 3.
2. Ibid., p. 43.
3. Health Law Center, *Problems in Hospital Law* (Rockville, Md.: Aspen Systems Corp., 1974), pp. 47–54.
4. Irene Murchison and Thomas Nichols, *Legal Foundations of Nursing Practice* (New York: Macmillan Publishing Co., Inc., 1970), pp. 248–267.
5. Helen Creighton, *Law Every Nurse Should Know* (Philadelphia: W. B. Saunders Company, 1975), pp. 119–120, 185–186.
6. Hemelt and Mackert, op. cit., pp. 39–40.
7. Creighton, op. cit., pp. 249–250, reprinted from author's article, "Res Ipsa Loquitur," *Sup. Nurs.*, 3:8–14 (Sept. 1972).
8. Hemelt and Mackert, op. cit., pp. 10–11.
9. Charles Kramer, *Medical Malpractice*, 4th ed. (New York: Practicing Law Institute, 1976), p. 44.
10. Walter Eccard, "A Revolution in White —New Approaches to Treating Nurses as Professionals," *Vanderbilt Law Review*, 30:839–879 (1977).
11. *Swassing* v. *Baum*, 240 N.W. 2d 24; 195 Neb. 651 (1976).
12. Eric Springer, ed., *Nursing and the Law* (Pittsburgh, Pa.: Aspen Systems Corp., 1970), p. 11.
13. Murchison, op. cit., pp. 139–143.
14. Irene Murchison, Thomas Nichols, and Rachel Hanson, *Legal Accountability in the Nursing Process* (St. Louis: C. V. Mosby Company, 1977), pp. 55–64.
15. Helen Creighton, "Injections and the Law," *Sup. Nurse*, 10:64–68 (May 1979) and 10:68–71 (June 1979).
16. William Regan, "$30,000 Worth of Trou-

ble Over An Ice Pack," *RN,* **42**:81 (Apr. 1979).

17. Marguerite Mancini, "Proving Negligence in Nursing Practice," *Am. J. Nurs.,* **79**:337–338 (Feb. 1979).

18. Helen Creighton, "Your Legal Risks in Nursing Coronary Patients," *Nurs. 77,* **7**:65–71 (Jan. 1977).

19. Helen Creighton, "Your Legal Risks in Emergency Care," *Nurs. 78,* **8**:53–55 (Feb. 1978).

20. Avice Kerr, "Nurses' Notes: That's Where the Goodies Are," *Nurs. 75,* **5**:34 (Feb. 1975).

21. Marguerite Mancini, "Documenting Clinical Records," *Am. J. Nurs.,* **78**:1556, 1561 (Sept. 1978).

22. "Recopied Records," *Nurs. 75,* **5**:103 (May 1975).

23. Nathan Hershey and Roger Lawrence, "The Influence of Charting Upon Liability Determinations," *J. of Nurs. Admin.,* **6**:35–37 (Mar./Apr. 1976).

24. Ibid.

25. Ann Burgess and Anna Laszlo, "Courtroom Use of Hospital Records in Sexual Assault Cases," *Am. J. Nurs.,* **77**:64–68 (Jan. 1977).

26. Creighton, *Law Every Nurse Should Know,* op. cit., pp. 91–92.

27. Brooke Williams, "Malpractice: How Good Is Your Insurance Protection?" *Nurs. 76,* **6**:81–91 (Jan. 1976).

28. Marguerite Mancini, "What You Should Know About Malpractice Insurance," *Am. J. Nurse.,* **79**:729–730 (Apr. 1979).

29. "Facing a Grand Jury," *Am. J. Nurs.,* **76**:398–400 (Mar. 1976).

30. Williams, op. cit., pp. 90, 91.

31. Murchison and Nichols, op. cit., p. 20.

32. Hemelt and Mackert, op. cit., p. 225.

33. Marilyn McCartney, "In the Witness Box: How To Give Nursing Testimony," *Nurs. 77,* **7**:89–93 (Apr. 1977).

34. Charles Kramer, "Cross-Examination of the Medical Expert," *Trial,* **13**:26–30 Dec. 1977).

35. Rose Mary Shannon, "Testifying as an Expert Witness on Behalf of Your Patient," *MCN,* **4**:281–284 (Oct. 1977).

36. Arizona Nurses' Assn., *Guideline: the Nurse as an Expert Witness* (Phoenix, Az.: The Association, 1978).

37. William Pettit, *Manual of Pharmaceutical Law,* 3rd ed. (New York; Macmillan Publishing Co., Inc., 1962), p. 53.

38. Frank Trippet, "Of Hazards, Risks, and Culprits," *Time,* Aug. 28, 1978, p. 76.

39. Department of Health, Education and Welfare, *Medical Malpractice: Report of the Secretary's Commission on Medical Malpractice* (Washington, D.C.: The Department, 1973), pp. 24–25.

40. Department of Health, Education, and Welfare, *Appendix: Report of the Secretary's Commission on Medical Malpractice* (Washington, D.C.: The Department, 1973), pp. 1–2.

41. Trippett, op. cit.

42. William Schwartz and Neil Komesar, "Doctors, Damages and Deterrence: An Economic View of Medical Malpractice," *N. Engl. J. Med.,* **298**:1282–1289 (June 8, 1978).

43. Murchison and Nichols, op. cit., p. 234–236.

44. C. Dean Davis, "Why Aggrieved Patients Sue Multiple Defendants," *Hosp. Med. Staff,* **7**:16–21 (Mar. 1978).

45. Eric Springer, ed. *Nursing and the Law* (Pittsburgh, Pa.: Aspen Systems Corp., 1970), p. 71.

46. James Cooper and Sharman Stephens, "The Malpractice Crisis—What Was It All About?" *Inquiry,* **14**:243–253 (Sept. 1977).

47. Shannon Perry, "Managing to Avoid Malpractice," Parts I and II. *J. of Nurs. Admin.,* **8**:43–47 (Aug. 1978) and **8**:16–22 (Sept. 1978).

48. Barbara Rubin, "Medical Malpractice Suits Can Be Avoided," *Hospitals,* **52**:86 –88 (Nov. 1, 1978).

BIBLIOGRAPHY

Bromberg, Myron. "Legal Problems and Safeguards in the E.D." *RN,* **36** (May 1973) 49 ff. An overview of the pitfalls and safeguards in the emergency room. Includes such areas as cardiopulmonary resuscitation, consents, discharge.

Bell, Robert J. "Malpractice: The Nurse as a Defendant," *Nurs. Clin. North Am.,* **2** (Mar. 1967), 141–152. This article includes an introduction to the concept of malpractice and then examines a number of nursing functions and responsibilities in which malpractice may occur. The author stresses prevention of malpractice and offers suggestions to nurses who must defend themselves in a legal suit.

Bell, Melvin M., and Lois Prentice. "Patient v. Nurses," *Nurs. Clin. North Am.*, **2** (Mar. 1967), 129–140. Discusses liability and negligence in the context of patient care. Illustrated with case citations and numerous examples.

Carroll, Aileen L. "The Nurse on the Witness Stand," *Nurs. Clin. North Am.*, **2** (Mar. 1967), 153–159. A director of nursing who was called as a witness in a negligence and malpractice suit offers an account of her experiences in court.

Creighton, Helen. "Changes in the Legal Aspects of Nursing," *Hosp. Prog.*, **52** (Sept. 1971), 87–94. Changing concepts of patient care, the practice of nursing, and hospital liability laws are also changing the nurse's liability. Examples are given.

Creighton, Helen. "Legal Aspects of Nursing in the Operating Room," *AORN J.*, **15** (Mar. 1972), 48–53. Author describes types of negligence resulting in malpractice suits for OR nurses.

Creighton, Helen. "Malpractice and the Nurse," *Imprint*, **20** (Oct. 1973), 15, 29. A nurse-lawyer highlights situations that can cause malpractice suits for students.

Chapman, Matthew and Jane Record. "Defensibility of New Health Professionals at Law," *J. Health Politics, Policy and Law*, **4** (Spring, (1979), 30–47. Defines how tort law might define primary and secondary liability for NPs and PAs.

Demarco, Carl. "Breach of Duty," *Nurs. 76.*, **6** (Apr. 1976), 103–106. Discusses liability for drug-related injuries to patients.

Ede, Lorice, and Roger Nelson. "The 'Good Samaritan Law' and the Nurse's Immunity for Emergency Care," *Occup. Health Nurs.*, **20** (Sept. 1972), 10–15. Explains meaning and ramifications of these laws. Charts indicate in what states nurses are covered and the scope of coverage in all states.

Hershey, Nathan. "He Can't Take the Responsibility," *Am. J. Nurs.*, **66** (May 1966), 1053–1054. Emphasizes that a nurse cannot rely on assurances of a physician that he will take responsibility to provide protection from her own personal liability for negligence. Also clarifies doctrine of *respondeat superior*.

Hershey, Nathan. "Hospitals' Expanding Responsibility," *Am. J. Nurs.*, **66** (July 1966), 1546–1547. Discusses the responsibility of hospitals for the medical care given their patients, including nursing implications.

Hershey, Nathan. "Issues in the Care of Nursing Home Patients," *J. Nurs. Admin.*, **3** (Mar.–Apr. 1973), 43–46. Injuries to nursing home patients indicate the necessity to avoid unreasonable risks of harm, while still allowing patients to make such judgments as their condition allows.

Jahns, Marsha. "Court Decision Would Extend Liability," *Hospitals*, **48** (Jan. 16, 1974), 31–34. A judge extends hospital liability for adequacy of medical peer review system in case where physician overtly has practiced negligently for financial gain.

Lipman, Michel. "We Call as Our Next Witness," *RN*, **36** (Sept. 1973), 41 ff. Guidelines for the nurse who may be subpoenaed, including preparation for witnessing, pretrial witnessing, role in court, and cross-examination.

Murchison, Irene. "Role of Law in the Decision-Making Process in Occupational Health Nursing," *Occ. Health Nurs.* **21** (July 1973), 15–19. Gives examples of legal authority for OHNs and legal doctrines that influence conduct in decision making.

Nations, Wanda. "What Constitutes Abuse of Patients?" *Hospitals*, **47** (Dec. 1, 1973), 51–53. Legally defined and lesser abuse of patients, including both physical and verbal abuse are described to provide guidelines for hospital policies.

Porter, John. "Hospital Privileges for Nonphysicians Raise Hard Legal Questions," *Hosp. Med. Staff* **7** (Feb. 1978), 22–26. Cites problems of differing education, training, licensure and hospital's liability.

Regan, William. "Hospitals and Specials Share Legal Liability," *RN*, **30** (Mar. 1967), 50–56. The author identifies key areas of responsibility shared by private duty nurses and the hospitals in which they practice. Guidelines for preventing or relieving common problems are presented.

Regan, William. *The Regan Report on Nursing Law*. Providence, R.I.: Medical Press. Monthly report on current issues in the legal aspects of nursing. Variety of subjects in each issue with specific cases cited.

Rozovsky, Lorne. "Answers To The 15 Legal Questions Nurses Usually Ask," *Nurs. 78* **8** (July 1978), 73–77. Questions about doctor's orders, consents, patient records, and aspects of negligence.

Walker, A. Earl. "The Law and the Neurosurgi-

cal Nurse," *J. Neurosurg. Nurs.*, **3** (Dec. 1971),
83–92. Includes trends in neurosurgical nursing,
legal principles of responsibility and malpractice, court procedure, and prevention of damage claims.

Willig, Sidney. *Nurses's Guide to the Law.* New
York: McGraw-Hill Book Company, 1970. Author displays understanding of nursing today, in
terms of independent functions. Includes glossary and other useful data in appendix.

See also references following Chapter 21; references and bibliography of Chapters 17, 19, and 20.
The texts on nursing law cited in Chapter 17 all
include some aspect of the topics discussed in this
chapter. Books on hospital and medical law also have pertinent information. Parts of the Hemelt
and Mackert book are reprinted in *Nurs. 79,* **9**
(Oct. 1979) 57–64 (Nov. 1979) 57–64 and (Dec.
1979) 49–56.

In addition to these selected references, there
are monthly or bimonthly articles on legal aspects
of nursing and/or health care in *AJN, Nursing
Outlook, JONA, RN, Supervisor Nurse, Hospital
Progress, Hospitals,* and other health journals.
Some of these have been cited in the references to
show the style and content. Some of Creighton's
articles are reprinted in her book. Law journals
almost always have articles about health law. Examples of those exclusively devoted to health law
are *Medicolegal News* and *Journal of Law and
Medicine.*

Health Care and the Rights of People

Whether it is a consequence of the civil rights movement, the consumer movement,* or simply a new era in society, everyone now seems to be concerned with people's rights. As might be expected, health care has also been affected.

Until recently, people have felt helpless in their patient role—and small wonder. Stripped of their individuality as well as their belongings, they are thrust into an alien environment with little control over what happens to them. They are surrounded by unidentified faces and unidentifiable equipment. Their privacy is invaded. Their dignity is lost. They hesitate to complain or criticize for fear of reprisals from the staff. They are reluctant to press for answers to their questions because a "busy" message is communicated loud and clear. Underlying all is fear for their health, and even their life.

There is evidence, however, that consumers are no longer willing to put up with this state of affairs, will no longer accept the traditional role of "good" patient: the one who does as he's told and asks no awkward questions. The frequent denial of their fundamental rights—among them, to courtesy,

privacy, and, most of all, information—has brought about the ultimate form of patient rebellion—malpractice suits. As the HEW Secretary's Commission on Medical Malpractice has noted, the quality of the relationship between the patient, on the one hand, and the doctor or hospital, on the other, may make the difference between filing or not filing a malpractice suit. The Commission adds that it ". . . believes that to ignore these and other rights of the patient is both to betray simple humanity and to invite dissatisfaction that may lead to malpractice suits."[1]

PATIENTS' RIGHTS

Most of the rights about which patients are concerned are theirs legally as well as morally and have been so established by common law. They are also stated in the codes of ethics of both physicians and nurses (although, to be honest, much is by implication and thus open to considerable personal interpretation). And, since the well-publicized American Hospital Association's "A Patient's Bill of Rights" was presented in 1972, a spate of such "rights" statements has followed: for the disabled, the mentally ill, the

---

*See Chapter 6.

STATEMENT ON A PATIENT'S BILL OF RIGHTS
AMERICAN HOSPITAL ASSOCIATION, 1972.

The American Hospital Association presents a Patient's Bill of Rights with the expectation that observance of these rights will contribute to more effective patient care and greater satisfaction for the patient, his physician, and the hospital organization. Further, the Association presents these rights in the expectation that they will be supported by the hospital on behalf of its patients, as an integral part of the healing process. It is recognized that a personal relationship between the physician and the patient is essential for the provision of proper medical care. The traditional physician-patient relationship takes on a new dimension when care is rendered within an organizational structure. Legal precedent has established that the institution itself also has a responsibility to the patient. It is in recognition of these factors that these rights are affirmed.

1. The patient has the right to considerate and respectful care.

2. The patient has the right to obtain from his physician complete current information concerning his diagnosis, treatment, and prognosis in terms the patient can be reasonably expected to understand. When it is not medically advisable to give such information to the patient, the information should be made available to an appropriate person in his behalf. He has the right to know by name, the physician responsible for coordinating his care.

3. The patient has the right to receive from his physician information necessary to give informed consent prior to the start of any procedure and/or treatment. Except in emergencies, such information for informed consent, should include but not necessarily be limited to the specific procedure and/or treatment, the medically significant risks involved, and the probable duration of incapacitation. Where medically significant alternatives for care or treatment exist, or when the patient requests information concerning medical alternatives, the patient has the right to such information. The patient also has the right to know the name of the person responsible for the procedures and/or treatment.

4. The patient has the right to refuse treatment to the extent permitted by law, and to be informed of the medical consequences of his action.

5. The patient has the right to every consideration of his privacy concerning his own medical care program. Case discussion, consultation, examination, and treatment are confidential and should be conducted discreetly. Those not directly involved in his care must have the permission of the patient to be present.

6. The patient has the right to expect that all communications and records pertaining to his care should be treated as confidential.

7. The patient has the right to expect that within its capacity a hospital must make reasonable response to the request of a patient for services. The hospital must provide evaluation, service, and/or referral as indicated by the urgency of the case. When medically permissible a patient may be transferred to another facility only after he has received complete information and explanation concerning the needs for and alternatives to such a transfer. The institution to which the patient is to be transferred must first have accepted the patient for transfer.

8. The patient has the right to obtain information as to any relationship of his hospital to other health care and educational institutions insofar as his care is concerned. The patient has the right to obtain information as to the existence of any professional relationships among individuals, by name, who are treating him.

9. The patient has the right to be advised if the hospital proposes to engage in or perform human experimentation affecting his care or treatment. The patient has the right to refuse to participate in such research projects.

10. The patient has the right to expect reasonable continuity of care. He has the right to know in advance what appointment times and physicians are available and where. The patient has the right to expect that the hospital will provide a mechanism whereby he is informed by his physician or a delegate of the physician of the patient's continuing health care requirements following discharge.

11. The patient has the right to examine and receive an explanation of his bill regardless of source of payment.

12. The patient has the right to know what hospital rules and regulations apply to his conduct as a patient.

No catalogue of rights can guarantee for the patient the kind of treatment he has a right to expect. A hospital has many functions to perform, including the prevention and treatment of disease, the education of both health professionals and patients, and the conduct of clinical research. All these activities must be conducted with an overriding concern for the patient, and, above all, the recognition of his dignity as a human being. Success in achieving this recognition assures success in the defense of the rights of the patient.

retarded, the old, the young, the pregnant, the handicapped, the dying.

In some cases these statements have been the basis for new statutory law, as evidenced by the Minnesota legislature's adoption of a variation of the AHA Patient's Bill of Rights. A follow-up by the Minnesota Hospital Association on the effectiveness of this legislation one year later indicated that several of the hospitals and nursing homes surveyed reported that patients were receiving better explanations about care, that staff awareness of patients' rights and the importance of confidentiality had been heightened, and that in some cases patient advocates had been appointed. However, a major flouting of the law was noted in relation to patient consent to observation of care by nonessential personnel; more than half of the respondents did not obtain such consent.

The vagueness of the AHA statement and the inability to force compliance without legal intervention have made it a butt for some bitter humor. Annas, an attorney in the health field, quotes a commentator who likened the document to a fox telling the chickens what their rights are. Nevertheless, commenting on the required posting in hospitals of the Minnesota bill, Annas notes that the "trend toward publishing rights is important because it not only reminds people that they have rights, it also encourages them to assert them and to make further demands."[2] It might also remind the staff, for there is some evidence that they, too, are unaware of the patient's rights, even legal rights.

By the end of the 1970s, variations of the Patient's Bill of Rights became law in many states. Some legislatures passed specific bills incorporating either the AHA statements or a similar version; state or municipal hospital codes took similar action, sometimes including mental institutions and nursing homes. In 1974, new Medicare regulations for skilled nursing facilities included a section on patients' rights. Just how disgraceful the violation of rights of this captive group was might be judged when reviewing the rights: the right to send and receive mail; the right to

have spouses share rooms if both are patients, or allow privacy for visits; the right to have restraints used only if authorized by the physician and only for a limited time; the right to use one's own clothes and possessions, as space permits; and the right to require both written permission by the patient and accountings for management of his/her funds. And, as in other laws, the patient had to be told what his rights were.

Most patients had not known that they have any rights once they enter a health care institution. These rights are still being violated, but probably less so since there are legal sanctions. Now, patients or their advocates can prevent violations, remedy them, or seek civil redress in such cases as lack of informed consent.

Trends in Informed Consent

For years, when patients have been admitted to hospitals, they signed a frequently unread, universal consent form that almost literally gave the physician, his associates, and the hospital carte blanche in determining the patient's care. There was some rationale for this because civil suits for battery (unlawful touching) could theoretically be filed as a result of giving routine care such as baths. Patients undergoing surgery or some complex, dangerous treatment were asked to sign a separate form, usually stating something to the effect that permission was granted to the physician and/or his colleagues to perform the operation or treatment. Just how much the patient knew about the hows and whys of the surgery, the dangers and the alternatives, depended on the patient's assertiveness in asking questions and demanding answers and the physician's willingness to provide information. Nurses were taught *never* to answer those questions, or little else either, but to suggest, "Ask your doctor." Health professionals, and especially physicians, took the attitude, "We know best and will decide for you."

The majority of patients probably still enter treatment and undergo a variety of tests and even surgery without a clear understanding of the nature of the condition they have and what can be done about it. Although they may very well be receiving care that is medically acceptable, they have no real part in deciding what that care should be. Most physicians have believed that anything more than a superficial explanation is unnecessary, for the patient should "trust" the doctor. Kalisch has elaborated this point, calling it Aesculapian authority.[3] Yet the patient has always had the right to make decisions about his own body. A case was heard as early as 1905 on surgery without consent, and the classic legal decision is that of Judge Cardoza (*Schloendorff* v. *The Society of New York Hospital* (211 NY.125, 129–130, 105 NE 92, 93–1914): "Every human being of adult years and sound mind has a right to determine what shall be done with his own body."

A noted hospital law book also states:

> *It is an established principle of law that every human being of adult years and sound mind has the right to determine what shall be done with his own body. He may choose whether to be treated or not and to what extent, no matter how necessary the medical care, nor how imminent the danger to his life or health if he fails to submit to treatment.*[4]

The patient's need for and right to this kind of knowledge are highlighted by the increasing number of malpractice suits that involve an element of "informed consent."* For many years, in such suits, courts have tended to rule that the physician must provide only as much information as is general practice among his colleagues in the area, as determined by their expert testimony. Some recent decisions, however, are changing this attitude, most of them hinging on informed consent.

There was, for instance, the case of the physician who apparently repeatedly persuaded patients to have unnecessary laminectomies, and then performed them poorly.

One facet of the case against him and the hospital was lack of informed consent (actually, coerced consent). Both were found liable.[5] The landmark decisions, however, have involved situations in which the surgery was not done ineffectively, but where patients sued because of complications or results about which they had not been warned. In one such case, a patient, who had numerous complications after surgery for a duodenal ulcer, had been informed of the risks of the anesthesia but not the surgery. He received a verdict against both hospital and surgeon.[6] In another case, a woman of Korean ancestry won because the physician had not explained that with the dermabrasion she agreed to, the risk of hyperpigmentation (which she developed) was greater in those of Oriental background.[7]

In these and other cases, judges disallowed the right of the medical profession to determine how much the patient should be told; rather, they said, the patient should be told enough, in understandable lay language, to make a decision. The materiality of the risk or facts to be disclosed by the physician "is to be determined by applying the standards of a reasonable man, not a reasonable medical practitioner."[8]

There continue to be similar judgments and some legislation supporting the same concept. Annas states that the trend now is for the courts to view the doctor-patient relationship as a partnership in decision making rather than as a medical monopoly.[9] These trends have moved hospitals into reviewing and revising their consent forms. The catch-all admissions consent had already been ruled as "almost completely worthless" for anything other than avoiding battery complaints, because it does not designate the nature of the treatment to be given.[10] What has emerged are forms that contain all the required elements for the informed consent process, usually individualized by the physician for each patient, somewhat similar to those developed by Alfidi[11] and Hershey.[12] Often, they are available in the foreign languages most prevalent in the area.

---

*Some lawyers are advocating the use of the term *authorization for treatment*, implying patient control.

Consent is defined as a free, rational act which presupposes knowledge of the thing to which consent is given by a person who is legally capable of consent. *Informed consent* is not expected to include minutiae but to delineate the essential nature of the procedure and the consequences. The disclosure is to be "reasonable," without details which might unnecessarily frighten the patient. The patient may, of course, waive the right to such explanation. Consents are *not* needed for emergency care if there is an immediate threat to life and health, if experts agree that it is an emergency, if the patient is unable to consent and a legally authorized person can't be reached, and when the patient submits voluntarily. Criteria for a valid consent are written (unless oral consent can be proved in court); signed by the patient or person legally responsible for him/her (a person cannot give consent for his/her spouse in a nonemergency situation); procedure performed is the one consented to; and the presence of essential elements of an informed consent.[13] These include (1) an explanation of the condition; (2) a fair explanation of the procedures to be used and the consequences; (3) a description of alternative treatments or procedures; (4) a description of the benefits to be expected; (5) an offer to answer the patient's inquiries; and (6) freedom from coercion or unfair persuasions and inducements. The last has special significance, because the concept of informed consent really became viable with the Nuremberg Code, originating from the trials of Nazi physicians tho were convicted of experimenting on prisoners without their consent. The principles were then formalized in the Declaration of Helsinki, adopted by the Eighteenth World Medical Assembly in 1964, and revised in 1975. HHS accepts the same principles and requires their adherence in human research.[14]

The right to consent or not consent is one of the evolving issues in informed consent. The competent patient has the right to refuse consent, but a hospital can request under certain circumstances, a court order to act if the refusal endangers the patient's life. If a patient is considered physically unable, legally incompetent, or a minor, a guardian has the right to give or withhold consent. The trend in court decisions seems to be that the patient, unless proven totally incompetent, has the right to refuse. For example, a Jehovah's Witness refuses a blood transfusion, even though it might mean his life, because taking such transfusions are against his religion. The rulings have been in favor of allowing him to make his own decision; in fact, the Witnesses and AMA in 1979 agreed upon a consent form requesting that no blood or blood derivative be administered and releasing medical personnel and the hospital for responsibility for untoward results because of that refusal.[15] If a minor child of a Witness needs the blood and the parent refuses, a court order requested by the hospital usually permits the transfusion. This is based on a legal precedent when a judge ruled that parents had a right to be martyrs, if they wished, but had no right to make martyrs of their children. On the other hand, if the child is deemed a "mature minor," able to make an intelligent decision, regardless of chronological age, the child has been allowed to refuse the treatment. In another case, a seventy-nine-year-old diabetic refused to consent to a leg amputation. Her daughter petitioned to be her legal guardian so that she (the daughter) could sign the consent. The judge ruled that the woman was old but not senile, and had a right to make her own decision. In a slightly different situation, an alcoholic derelict was found unconscious on the street and taken to a hospital. When he became conscious, he refused to have his legs amputated for severe frostbite. The court order sought by the hospital was denied because, although the man was alcoholic, he was competent at the time of making his decision. (As it happened, he lost only a few toes from his frostbite.) In still another case, a young man on permanent kidney dialysis decided he did not want to live that way and refused continued treatment. He was allowed to do so and died within a short time. Other cases can also be cited.[16] The right of a competent patient to refuse treatment seems more firmly established than ever, but when the patient is unconscious, other legal questions arise.

The Nurse's Role in Informed Consent

Some physicians do not believe that it is feasible to obtain an informed consent because of such factors as lack of interest or education and high anxiety level, in which case a patient might refuse a "necessary treatment or operation."[17] There are physicians and others who believe that despite the increasing number of rulings favoring patients' full knowledge, most patients are not given information so that they really understand (and the courts really don't do enough about it.)[18] The physician may also use "therapeutic privilege" in which disclosure is not required because it might be detrimental to the patient. Or, information about certain alternatives may be withheld because the physician feels that they are too risky, unproven, or not appropriate.[19] Because it is generally agreed that nurses do not have the primary responsibility for getting the informed consent, what does the nurse do, if she/he believes that the patient has not been adequately informed? The nurse could take the initiative to question the patient about what she/he understands, as well as to be alert to signs that the patient is not clear about what is to be done. The physician should then be informed. The question most nurses have is how much can be told, especially if the physician chooses not to reveal further information. The Tuma case (Chapter 20) did not resolve the nurse's right to supply the missing information, and the nurse may be taking a personal risk. However, should the nurse decide to give further information, it should be totally accurate, carefully recorded, and the fact that it was given shared with the physician and others. Nurses have found ways to make the patient aware of knowledge gaps so that they ask the right questions, but it is unfortunate that most are still employed in situations where it could be detrimental to them to be the patient's advocate. More are taking the risk,

and changes may occur. Of course, if the patient is coaxed or coerced into signing without such an explanation, the consent is invalid. Moreover, if the patient withdraws consent, even verbally, the nurse is responsible for reporting this and seeing that the patient is not treated. This is a legal responsibility not only to the patient but also to the hospital, which can be held liable.

Hospitals are beginning to use a clerk to witness the consent form, after the physician makes his explanation, on the theory that only the signature is being witnessed, not the accuracy or depth of the explanation. Other hospitals ask the physician to bring another physician, presumably to validate the explanation. Where nurses still witness the form, it should be clear *what* they are witnessing— signature or explanation.[20] Hospital policy can clarify this.

The nurse's own and specific responsibility is to explain nursing care, including the whys and hows. Nurses are still reluctant to do so and feel threatened by a physician who demands that only limited or no explanations be given.

THE RIGHT TO DIE

Perhaps because improved technology has succeeded in artificially maintaining both respiratory and cardiac functions when a person can no longer do so, the definition of *clinical death* as the irrevocable cessation of heartbeat and breathing is no longer pertinent.* What of irreversible coma? In 1968, a faculty committee of the Harvard Medical School identified certain characteristics of a permanently nonfunctioning brain: (1) unreceptivity and unresponsivity, (2) no movements of breathing, (3) no reflexes, (4) flat electroencephalogram. Others developed variations of this definition.[21]

---

*Physicians have the authority and responsibility to pronounce a patient dead. Even though a nurse may quite accurately do so, the law, thus far, has not caught up with reality.

In common law, there has been a strongly entrenched cardiac definition of death until, in 1977, in Massachusetts, the Supreme Judicial Court officially recognized the use of brain death criteria.[22] In 1970, Kansas was the first state to adopt a brain death statute, using the same Harvard-type criteria, thus offering two "alternative" definitions of death to be used at the discretion of the attending physician. Other states have passed similar legislation. Various types of criteria have been adopted by state legislatures, but all are based on cessation of brain functioning.[23] Black notes an important aspect of brain death:

> Patients with brain death are not merely perpetually unresponsive: they are patients whose brain destruction, including loss of respiratory and cardiovascular control, means that life of all kind is soon to be lost as well.[24]

Still, there are many lay people and health professionals who do not feel that brain death is an adequate definition of physiological death. (On the other hand, a variety of surveys indicate that most people are beginning to favor euthanasia, if there is a terminal illness.) Thus, the majority of states still use the classic definition, and questions arise about the status of patients maintained on respirators.

Two rulings on the terminally ill, incompetent patient, made by two different state supreme courts, were the Saikewicz[25] and Quinlan[26] cases. In the first, the court upheld a decision not to give a severely retarded sixty-seven-year-old more chemotherapy that would be unpleasant for the sake of a short, extended life-span. (He died a month later of pneumonia.) However, such a decision was seen to be a court's responsibility, after an adjudicatory hearing. In the Quinlan case, a twenty-two-year-old woman received severe and irreversible brain damage that reduced her to a vegetative state, and the father petitioned the court to be made her guardian with the intention of having all extraordinary medical procedures sustaining her life re-moved. The New Jersey Supreme Court ruled that the father could be the guardian and have the life support systems discontinued with the concurrence of her family, the attending physicians, who might be chosen by the father, and the hospital ethics committee.[27] (After disconnection of the respirator, Karen Quinlan continued to live, sustained by fluids and other maintenance measures, and was transferred to a nursing home.) Health law experts debate the congruity of these and similar cases, and it is expected that other supreme courts faced by other unique circumstances will make separate rulings.[28]

Part of the judge's comments in the Quinlan case related to the belief that Karen Quinlan would have made a similar choice, if able. Until 1977, a person could not be assured that she/he would be allowed to die if brain death existed. The Euthanasia Educational Council (now called Concern for Dying) has made available "A Living Will" that directs family, physician, and friends to withhold artificial means in a case of inevitable death. Other versions also exist.[29] The "will," which can be revoked at any time, has no legal power, although, presumably, if the writer's intention were followed, those involved would not be judged guilty of murder. In 1977, California enacted a Natural Death Act, with carefully delineated and protective living will components. In the next year, Arkansas, Idaho, Nevada, New Mexico, North Carolina, Oregon, and Texas followed with similar statutes.[30,31] Later, Washington and other states did so. All granted civil and criminal immunity for those carrying out living will requests. Although there were no reported difficulties, some attorneys believe that because the right to refuse treatment already exists, such legislation only creates problems.[32]

The right-to-die issue is almost synonymous with *euthanasia*, a word of Greek origin meaning painless, easy, gentle, or good death. It is now commonly used to signify a killing that is promoted by some humanitarian motive, such as the relief of intolerable pain. There are two major categories of euthanasia: voluntary and involuntary. The first usually involves two parties, the competent adult patient and a doctor, nurse, or both, or an adult friend or relative. (The patient could commit suicide alone). It is voluntary euthanasia that the natural death laws seek to serve. Involuntary euthanasia, sometimes called mercy killing, is performed by someone other than the patient without the patient's consent, possibly because of unconsciousness. There are many pros and cons of euthanasia, with arguments usually falling into secular or religious categories.[33],[34] Nevertheless, according to the law, euthanasia is murder. In cases where a physician, nurse, or family have "pulled the plug" or otherwise carried out involuntary euthanasia, and there appeared to be no ulterior motive, the jury has usually freed the individual, often on the basis of temporary insanity. In 1979, however, a Maryland nurse was indicted for murder for discontinuing life support systems of brain dead patients. She did not deny that she had done so, but based her not guilty plea on the fact the patients were brain dead GORKs (God only really knows), according to local terminology.[35] She was acquitted. (Although she was termed compassionate by her nursing colleagues, they felt obligated to report her actions when she would not stop.)

Orders Not to Resuscitate

Patients in irreversible coma may have orders not to resuscitate (no-code, code blue, or other terms), with or without the consent and knowledge of the family. Are nurses in legal jeopardy if they obey? Are they in trouble if they choose not to? To a great extent these questions remain unanswered, because families may choose to let the patient die but do not want to say so, and many codes have been carried out with little discussion after the decision was made. Nurses who object on moral or religious grounds cannot be forced to participate (but for some people, it is just as wrong to resuscitate). However, without a specific hospital protocol, *not re-suscitating* could be considered malpractice. Nonwritten orders are a special problem for the nurse and should be questioned. If the orders are written, they should be in the context of the physician's judgment of the futility of resuscitation.[36] Some hospitals are following the Massachusetts General Hospital model, in which some critically ill patients are put into four categories from "maximal therapeutic effort" to "all therapy can be discontinued," with definitive protocols for each.[37] The arguments are strong that some policy should be set as a safeguard for all, including the patient.[38]

THE RIGHTS OF THE HELPLESS

Children, the mentally ill, the mentally retarded, and certain patients in nursing homes are often seen as relatively helpless, because they have been termed legally incompetent to make decisions about their health care for so many years. Often the rights overlap, as when a child or elderly person is mentally retarded (as in the Saikewicz case). Some of the rights of the elderly are being protected by the legalized bill of rights, and for mental patients, state laws and some high court decisions have served the same purpose. Both have focused on the mental patients' rights in the areas of voluntary and involuntary admissions; kind and length of restraints, including seclusion; informed consent to treatment, especially sterilization and psychosurgery; the rights of citizenship (voting); rights of privacy, especially as related to records; rights in research; and, especially, the right to treatment.[39],[40],[41],[42] Although rulings have varied, the trend is toward the protection of rights. The landmark decision of *Wyatt* v. *Stickney* (325 Federal Supplement, Alabama, 1972) clearly defined the purposes of commitment to a public hospital and the constitutional right to adequate treatment.[43] Other legal decisions relate to sterilization of the retarded, which came to a head when it was found that retarded adolescent Black girls were being sterilized without either they or their mothers apparently having a clear notion of what that meant. Restraints were increasingly put on sterilization until, in 1979, HEW tightened the regulations for federal participation in funding of sterilization procedures. Regulations included requirements of written and oral explanations of the operation, advice about alternate forms of birth control to be given in understandable language, and a waiting period. In addition, no federal funding was allowed for sterilization of those under twenty-one, mentally incompetent, or those institutionalized in correctional facilities or mental hospitals. However, this does not mean that a parent cannot have a retarded girl sterilized; it means that more precautions are being taken by the courts and the government to ensure that the child's rights are not violated. There is general concern for the rights of young people in the mental health system,[44] but parents maintain considerable control. In 1979, the Supreme Court upheld the constitutionality of state laws that allow parents to commit their minor children to state mental institutions; thirty-six states have such laws.

The other rights of young people and children relate primarily to consent for treatment or research and protection against abuse. It is a general rule that a parent or guardian must give consent for the medical or surgical treatment of a minor except in an emergency when it is imperative to give immediate care to save the minor's life. Legally, however, anyone who is capable of understanding what he is doing may give consent, because age is not always an exact criteria of maturity or intelligence. Many minors are perfectly capable of deciding for themselves whether to accept or reject recommended therapy and, in cases involving simple procedures, the courts have refused to invoke the rule requiring the consent of a parent or guardian. If the minor is married or has been otherwise emancipated from his/her parents, there is likely to be little question legally. In addition, states cite different ages and situations in which parental permission is needed for medical treatment. The

almost universal exception is allowing minors to consent to treatment for venereal disease, drug abuse, and pregnancy-related care.[45] Although it has been understood that health professionals have no legal obligation to report to parents that the minor has sought such treatment, a few states are beginning to add statutes that say that the minor doesn't need parental permission, but that parents must be notified.

The entire question of permission for contraception, abortion, and sterilization is in a state of flux. The key appears to be a designation of "mature minor"; emancipated minors are treated as adults. As recently as 1972, the U.S. Supreme Court ruled that state statutes prohibiting prescription of contraceptives to unmarried persons was unconstitutional because this would interfere with the right of privacy of those desiring them.[46] However, it did not rule on a minor's right to privacy in seeking or buying contraceptives. This was left to the states, and a number still set age limitations from fourteen to twenty-one. In many, however, doctors and other health professionals may provide birth control information and prescribe contraceptives to patients of any age without parental consent.[47] Changes in federal and state laws also frequently require welfare agencies to offer family planning services and supplies to sexually active minors. In general, there is a national trend toward granting minors the right to contraceptive advice and devices, and no case has been found where a doctor is liable for damage for prescribing contraceptives without parental consent.[48]

An even more dramatic change has occurred in relation to abortion. In 1976 the Supreme Court held that states may not constitutionally require the consent of a girl's parents as a condition for abortion during the first twelve weeks of pregnancy. In addition, parents cannot either prevent or force an abortion on the daughter who, in the eyes of the Court is now "a competent minor mature enough to have become pregnant." In the words of one federal court that overturned a parental consent statute:

It is not they (the parents) who have to bear the child. . . . It is difficult to think of any self-interest that a parent would have that compares with those significant interests of the pregnant minor.[49]

Should the young woman decide against an abortion and elect to bear the child, she can receive care related to her pregnancy without parental consent in almost every state. (That a pregnant teen-ager in some states can have an abortion without parental consent but not maternity services is one of the peculiarities of law in a rapidly changing society.) An unwed "mature minor" may also consent to treatment of her child.[50]

Groups, such as the American Academy of Pediatrics, the Society for Adolescent Medicine, and the National Association of Children's Hospitals and Related Institutions, have taken stands on protecting the rights of minors in health care. For example, the AAP Committee on Youth has presented a model act for consent of minors for health services, recommended for enactment in all states. It states that a minor may give consent for care if she/he was ever married, had a child, graduated from high school, is separated from parents, or supporting herself/himself. Specified are treatment for any communicable disease, drug abuse, pregnancy, and mental illness. In these cases the physician is obliged to inform the parents only in extreme circumstances. On the other hand, self-consent for abortion or sterilization is excepted.[51] An alternative model act offered by the State Committee on Legislation Concerning Adolescents' Medical Care of the Society for Adolescent Medicine is somewhat more succinct but similar in most points. It differentiates between anyone over eighteen (who is treated as having achieved majority) and emancipated minors. It does not mention abortion or sterilization. It also makes the minor liable for payment of health services. Model laws are hardly ever just that, nor are they generally accepted by every state, but they give direction, especially if developed by prestigious groups. The Pediatric Bill of Rights may also be a forerun-

ner to legal action, as was the AHA Patient's Bill of Rights. (Unless such a statement is incorporated into law, the effect is only moral, a guideline to encourage protection of rights, with no enforcement powers.) The Pediatric Bill of Rights addresses itself to the rights of young people in the areas of counseling and treatment for birth control, abortion, pregnancy, drug or alcohol dependency, venereal disease, confidentiality, and information about her/his condition, as well as protection if a parent refuses consent for needed treatment.[52]

Cases in which mature minors are being permitted to make life and death decisions are increasing. An example is the case of a thirteen-year-old who chose not to have a bone marrow transplant because of religious beliefs and potential danger to her donor sister. Another interesting trend is toward including very young children in making decisions about research in which they are asked to participate. In the past, as a rule, parents were asked whether they consented to their child's participation in research—medical, educational, psychological, or other. There has always been some concern as to whether the child should be subjected to such research if it was not a least potentially beneficial to him (such as the use of a new drug for a leukemic child). The child seldom was given the opportunity to decide whether or not to participate. New knowledge of the potential harm that could be done to the child, however innocuous the experiment, and appreciation of the child as a human being with individual rights have now resulted in recommendations that even a very young child be given a simple explanation about the proposed research and allowed to participate or not, or even withdraw later, without any form of coercion.[53,54,55] Given that choice, some children have decided not to participate.[56] Overall, though, the support for using healthy children in research or being volunteered for procedures not beneficial to themselves is eroding.[57,,58]

The question of whether parents may make a decision for a child, if the child's well-being is the parents' prime consideration, as in giving laetrile to a leukemic child, is not being decided with any consistency. (For that matter, neither has the legality of laetrile.)[59] Another unresolved issue is whether the grossly deformed neonate should be allowed to live. Few judges will rule to let it die, but often the decision is quietly made by parents and health personnel.[60] In other cases, the babies are used in research.[61] These situations are especially difficult for a nurse who may see the infant simply starve to death. More nurses and others are reporting such situations, but as in the right-to-die issue, ethical and moral considerations weigh strongly.

RIGHTS OF PATIENTS IN RESEARCH

The use of new, experimental drugs and treatments in hospitals, nursing homes, and other institutions that have a captive population—for example, prisons or homes for the mentally retarded—has been extensive. Nurses are often involved in giving the treatment or drugs. As noted earlier, HHS regulations now require specific informed consent for any human research carried out under HHS auspices, with strong emphasis on the need for a clear explanation of the experiment, possible dangers, and the subject's complete freedom to refuse or withdraw at any time.

In addition, the National Research Act of 1974 established a commission to, among other things, "identify the requirements for informed consent procedures for children, prisoners, and the mentally disabled and determine the need for a mechanism to assure that human subjects not covered by HEW regulations are protected."[62] (Part of that Commission report was cited previously.) Actually, nurses were in the forefront of this move, with a statement in the ANA Code of Ethics, "The nurse participates in research activities when assured that the rights of individual subjects are protected," as well as

an extensive ANA document on research guidelines.*

When the nurse is participating in research, at whatever level, seeing that the rights of patients are honored is both an ethical and legal responsibility. Nurses should know the patients' rights: self-determination to choose to participate; to have full information; to terminate participation without penalty; privacy and dignity; conservation of personal resources; freedom from arbitrary hurt and intrinsic risk of injury; as well as the special rights of minor and incompetent persons previously discussed.[63] For instance, nurses have been ordered to begin an experimental drug knowing that the patient has not given an informed consent. The nurse is then obligated to see that that patient does have the appropriate explanation. This is one more case when institutional policy that sets an administrative protocol for the nurse in such a situation is helpful. Creighton cites a number of instances where nurses were among those who participated in research that violated patients' rights, such as the disgraceful Tuskegee Syphilis Study, conducted by the U.S. Public Health Service over a forty-year period.[64] Moreover, today nurses themselves are likely to be the researchers. If the nurse is the investigator, she/he must observe all the usual requirements, such as informed consent and confidentiality. An interesting phenomenon that has been uncovered is that because nurses are generally trusted by patients, subjects will participate "for the nurse," but either refuse to sign the consent or not listen to an explanation, as not necessary.[65,66] The quality of research in which human subjects are involved is particularly important. Peer review, such as that offered by a hospital review board, can be helpful,[67] although sometimes there are no nurses on the board. Unfortunately, these boards, required if the research is HHS-funded, have been found to be not as protective of patients' rights as

---

*See Chapter 10.

they should be, especially in the areas of informed consent. There is usually no follow-up to determine whether the plans to preserve the subjects' rights that are presented in the proposals are really carried through.[68] The nurse, as primary investigator or participant, is in a position to see that these rights are not abrogated.

PATIENT RECORDS: CONFIDENTIALITY AND AVAILABILITY

All states have laws requiring hospitals, doctors, nurses, and sometimes other health workers to report on certain kinds of situations, because the patient may be unwilling or unable to do so. The nurse often has responsibility in these matters because, although it may be the physician's legal obligation, the nurse may be the only one actually aware of the situation. Even if such reporting is not required by a law per se, regulations of various state agencies may require such a report. Common reporting requirements are for communicable diseases, diseases in newborn babies, gunshot wounds, and criminal acts, including rape. More recently, reporting a physically abused or neglected child (battered child) has been given legal attention, and every state and the District of Columbia has such a law. Although other kinds of reporting are relatively objective, there are problems in reporting abused children because of the varying definitions of *child*, the question of whether there was abuse or an accident, with the consequent fear of parents suing. Usually, however, the person reporting is protected if "good faith" exists. In some states, there are penalties for *not* reporting such situations.

There is some evidence that in other than these legal requirements confidentiality of patients' records is frequently violated. Everyone has access except the patient.

'The tremendous growth of computerized health data, the development of huge data banks, and the advancements in record linkage pose an enormous threat to the privacy of medical information,' says a position paper on confidentiality adopted by the American Medical Records Association. 'The public is generally unaware of this threat or of the serious consequences of a loss of confidentiality in the health care system. Adequate measures to control medical privacy in the light of electronic information processing can and must be established. . . .[69]

A national study pointed out that from birth certificate to death certificate, the health and medical records of most Americans are part of a system that allows access by insurance companies, student researchers, and governmental agencies, to name a few, and that the information is often shared illegally with others such as employers. The report's author, Alan Westin, recommended that:

Health data systems should be created, altered and periodically audited through public rather than closed procedures.

Every health data system should put limits on relevance and social propriety of the personal information it collects and records.

Every health data system should have clear rules and procedures to insure citizen rights.

Health data system managers should take special measures to protect the accuracy and the security of the data they keep.

Managers should follow special procedures to allow medical research, health care evaluation and public oversight without impairing citizens' rights.[70]

Some thirty states have enacted laws to protect medical records, and the federal Freedom of Information Act (FOIA) denies access to an individual's medical record without that person's consent. Still, there are practical problems: if certain data is needed, as in following through on occupational health hazards;[71] can exceptions be made for research that would be beneficial to the well-being of people? The problem is not in aggregate figures, but when individual records must be scrutinized. Researchers were quite concerned with enactment of the 1974 Privacy Act* because HEW-funded research projects involving human subjects would be available to anyone, including participating subjects, by filing a request. Some of these cases are and will continue to go to court, but there seems to be a definite legislative and judicial trend toward safeguarding medical records and, in addition, giving patients access to their own records.

Most physicians and health administrators, however, have been hostile toward the concept of sharing the record with the patient. Some attorneys serving health care facilities tend to share the feeling, one group of authors writing that ". . . it is undesirable to allow patient or family to inspect the chart. (They) might find comments . . . which may be considered uncomplimentary or incorrect. The patient may then attempt to have the record changed or cause annoyance to the administration or the medical staff."[72] The writer was also concerned about the possibility of libel suits and suggested the omission of "characterizations or other remarks which may offend . . ." in the chart abstract (which could be given to the patient).

The time in which there is a choice in the matter of sharing the record may be ending. Whereas it is legally recognized that the patient's record is the property of the hospital or physician (in his office), the information that the record contains is not similarly protected. Both states and the federal government are legislating access—either direct patient access with or without a right to copy or indirect access (physician, attorney, or provision of summary only). In 1979, nineteen states allowed patients direct access to their records: Colorado, Connecticut, Florida, Hawaii, Illinois, Indiana, Massachusetts,[†] Minnesota, Nebraska, Nevada, New Jersey,[†] New York,[†] Ohio, Oklahoma, Oregon,

Tennessee, Texas,[†] Utah,[†] and Virginia,[†] either through statutory or case law. Those that give indirect access are Alabama,[†] Alaska,[†] California, District of Columbia,[†] Georgia,[†] Idaho,[†] Kansas,[†] Kentucky,[†] Louisiana,[†] Maine, Michigan,[†] Mississippi, North Carolina,[†] Pennsylvania,[†] Tennessee,[†] Utah, and Wisconsin. States may differentiate between doctor's and hospital records and have other idiosyncratic qualifications.[73] Of course, one certain way in which the patient can get access is through a malpractice suit in which the record is subpoenaed, a costly process for both provider and consumer.

The Commission on Medical Malpractice noted the relationship between closed records and malpractice suits, but the commission members were split in their desire to open records to patients. A compromise recommendation suggested making records available to the patient's attorney (which may be more beneficial for the attorney's income than the patient's enlightenment), but a vigorous minority report opposing this compromise was included.[74] Westin's study recommended giving patients access, and he anticipated that this was an inevitability.[75] The Privacy Protection Study Commission, created by the 1974 Privacy Act, also included recommendations on patient access. One federal step in this direction was the same FOIA and Privacy Act that prevented unauthorized access. Included are any records under the control of any agency of the federal government that contain an individual's name or any other identifying information. Medical records are specifically cited and would include those of patients in the Veterans Administration and other federal hospitals. Whether patients receiving medical care under Medicare are included is a subject of debate. Currently, the Professional Standards Review Organization (PSRO) regulations allow patients access under certain circumstances. The law is still somewhat controversial and interpretations are not altogether clear. For instance, there is some question as to whether contractors of a gov-

---

*See Chapter 19.

[†] Have mental health statutes that provide information to family, physician, attorney under certain circumstances, but not direct access.

ernment agency, such as hospitals receiving federal funds for medical care or research, are included. If so, considering the ubiquity of federal aid, almost all patient records would be open to the patient concerned. Meanwhile, there is federal legislation being introduced to specifically include Medicaid/Medicare records, leading to inclusion of *all* medical records.

Although perhaps the majority of physicians and hospitals still object to the open record concept because of the notion that patients wouldn't understand, would be frightened, or might choose to treat themselves, there is the beginning of a new philosophy to share the record with the patient so that both provider and consumer have an open relationship and decide on the needed care together. A health care center associated with the University of Vermont states in its "Principles of Practice":

> The best care of the patient is assured when the patient is part of the team and he shares his medical records with the providers of care. This is best effected by assuring that the record is complete, well organized, and available to the patient so that he can review the record for reliability, the subjective data and clarity of plans for treatment and education.[76]

Annas and others suggest that if the record is too technical, a knowledgeable patient advocate could be of assistance.[77] (Patient advocates are also recommended for other supportive purposes.) Does the nurse have any legal responsibility to be that intermediary? The answer is more complex than just a yes-no. Certainly, a nurse would not hand a patient the chart at request, for that would be inappropriate. Most states, as well as health care agencies, that permit access to records have a protocol to be followed. This usually involves providing both privacy and an opportunity for the physician and/or another person to explain the content. (Many hospitals are now willing to have the patient see the record, because the administration realizes that if the patient is concerned enough to demand his chart and it is withheld, the next

step is probably a malpractice suit; others agree that access is a right, or at least a trend, and are not waiting for legislation.) Both Annas[78] and Auerbach[79] give specific directions for obtaining records.

Privacy

Individuals who are in public life expect their every act will be of interest to the public, and they must, therefore, accept with good grace unfavorable news accounts and pictures as well as complimentary ones. Rarely can they successfully claim the citizen's right to privacy that is available to persons who are not of public interest.

Nurses who hold positions of importance may see unflattering pictures of themselves in newspapers and magazines that they might wish had never appeared in print. They would be unlikely to challenge the publication's right to carry them without permission, however, because the resulting publicity might turn out to be more unfavorable than the pictures. Under the law, they could instigate legal action if they wished because every citizen can withhold from the public any information about himself—verbal, written, or depicted—if he so desires.

Nurses and others who work with sick patients must be especially careful to avoid invading the patient's right to privacy, which is identical to that of any other person. Consent to treatment does not cover the use of a picture without specific permission, nor does it mean that the patient can be subjected to repeated examinations not necessary to his therapy without his express consent.

As noted previously, exceptions to respecting the patient's privacy are related to legal reporting obligations. The nurse may also be obligated to testify about otherwise confidential information in criminal cases.

Ethical practice prohibits the professional person from divulging any confidential information to anyone else, unless possibly to another physician or nurse who serves as a consultant. Neither does the ethical person engage in gossip based on this information, trivial and harmless though it may seem at the time. Moreover, the professional person has an obligation to set a good example for others in nonprofessional groups who may be less cognizant of their responsibilities in this respect.

Confidential information obtained through professional relationships is not the same as *privileged communication*, which is a legal concept providing that physician-patient, attorney-client, and priest-penitent have a special privilege. Should any court action arise in which the person (or persons) involved is called to testify, the law (in many states) will not require that such information be divulged. Not all states acknowledge that nurses can be recipients of privileged communications. The confidences exchanged between husband and wife are also considered privileged, and rarely is one spouse required to testify against another.

Assault and Battery

Assault and battery, although often considered with emphasis on the criminal interpretation, also has a patients' rights aspect that is related to everyday nursing practice, especially when dealing with certain types of patients. Grounds for civil action might include the following:

1. *Forcing a patient to submit to a treatment for which he has not given his consent either expressly in writing, orally, or by implication. Whether or not a consent was signed, a patient should not be forced, for resistance implies a withdrawal of consent.*
2. *Cutting a patient's hair or having it cut without his or her consent.*
3. *Lifting a protesting patient from his bed to a wheelchair or stretcher.*
4. *Threatening to strike or actually striking an unruly child or adult, except in self-defense.*
5. *Ejecting a visitor from a patient's room without the patient's consent.*
6. *In some states, performing alcohol, blood, urine, or health tests for presumed drunken driving without consent. There are some "implied consent" statutes in*

motor vehicle codes that provide that a person, for the privilege of being allowed to drive, gives an implied consent to furnishing a sample of blood, urine, or breath for chemical analysis when charged with driving while intoxicated. However, if the person objects and is forced, it might still be considered battery. Several states, acknowledging this, have enacted legislation to insulate hospital employees and health professionals from liability.[80]

False Imprisonment

As the term implies, *false imprisonment* means "restraining a person's liberty without the sanction of the law, or imprisonment of a person who is later found to be innocent of the crime for which he was imprisoned." The term also applies to many procedures that actually or conceivably are performed in hospital and nursing situations *if they are performed without the consent of the patient or his legal representative.* In most instances the nurse or other employee would not be held liable if it can be proved that what was done was necessary to protect others.

Among the most common nursing situations that might be considered false imprisonment are the following:

1. Restraining a patient by physical force or using appliances without written consent, especially in procedures where the use of restraints is not usually necessary. This is, or may be, a delicate situation because a nurse who does not use a restraint, such as side rails, to protect a patient may be accused of negligence, and if she/he does use them without consent, may be accused of false imprisonment. This would be a typical example of the need for prudent and reasonable action on the part of the nurse that a court of law would undoubtedly uphold.
2. Restraining a mentally ill patient who is neither dangerous to himself nor to others. For example, patients who wander about the hospital division making a nuisance of themselves, usually cannot le-

gally be locked in a room unless they show signs of violence.

3. Using arm, leg, or body restraints to keep a patient quiet while she/he is being administered an intravenous infusion may be considered false imprisonment. If this risk is involved—that is, if the patient objects to the treatment and refuses to consent to it—the physician should be called. Should the doctor order restraints for the patient, the nurse should make sure it is in writing before allowing anyone to proceed with the treatment. It is much better to assign someone to stay with the patient throughout a procedure than to restrain her/him without authorization.

4. Detaining a patient in the hospital against his will. If a patient insists on going home, or a parent or guardian insists on taking a minor or other dependent person out of the hospital before his condition warrants it, hospital authorities cannot legally require him to remain. In such instances the doctor should write an order permitting the hospital to allow the patient to go home "against advice," and the hospital's representative should see that the patient or guardian signs an official form absolving the hospital, medical staff, and nursing staff of all responsibility should the patient's early departure be detrimental to his health and welfare. If the patient refuses to sign, a record should be made on the chart of exactly what occurred and, probably, an incident report should be filed.

5. Detaining for an unreasonable period of time a patient who is medically ready to be discharged. The delay may be due to the patient's inability to pay his bill or it may be due to an inordinate wait, at his expense, for the delivery of an orthopedic appliance or other service. In such instances the nurse or nursing department may or may not be directly involved, but it is always wise to be cognizant of possible legal developments and to exercise sound judgment in order to be completely

fair to the patient and avoid trouble for all concerned.

ABORTION, STERILIZATION, CONTRACEPTION, AND TRANSPLANTS

Laws permitting abortion* have varied greatly from state to state over the years. In early 1973, the Supreme Court ruled that no state can interfere with a woman's right to obtain an abortion during the first trimester (twelve weeks) of pregnancy. During the second trimester, the state may interfere only to the extent of imposing regulations to safeguard the health of women seeking abortions. During the last trimester of pregnancy, a state may prohibit abortions except when the mother's life is at stake. (*Doe* v. *Bolton* and *Roe* v. *Wade*) Theoretically, all hospitals are required to perform abortions within these guidelines, and it is legal to assist with such a procedure; actually, the rights cannot be withheld. However, because of religious and moral reasons, some institutions are exempted from complying with the law, and individual doctors and nurses have refused to participate in abortions. An individual professional or other health worker may make that choice, and there is legal support for them (conscience clause).[81] (This does not preclude the right of the hospital to dismiss a nurse for refusing to carry out an assigned responsibility or to transfer her to another unit. There have been some suits by nurses objecting to transfer, but rulings have varied.)

The Supreme Court has also addressed the issue of the spouse's consent and found that such consent was not necessary. As mentioned earlier, the courts are also moving in the direction of not distinguishing between adult and minor females on abortion rights.

Sterilization means "termination of the

---

*Legislation relating to abortion is discussed in Chapter 19.

ability to produce offspring.'' Eugenic sterilization is the attempt to eliminate specific hereditary defects by sterilizing individuals who could pass on such defects to their offspring. Approximately half the states have authorized eugenic sterilization of the mentally deficient, mentally ill, and others.[82] Legality where no law exists is questionable. Civil or criminal liability for assault and battery may be imposed on anyone sterilizing another without following legal procedure or specific legal guidelines. Both laws and regulations have been in the process of change. If the life of a woman may be jeopardized if she becomes pregnant, a therapeutic sterilization may be performed with consent of the patient and sometimes her husband, although the latter is being challenged. If no statutes or judicial decisions state a policy against therapeutic sterilization, such operations may be considered as "medically necessary." If there is no medical necessity, the operation is termed *sterilization of convenience* or *contraceptive sterilization.* In some states, this is illegal; in others, arguable. (Seven states regulate therapeutic sterilization.) Here too, consents are often required from the individual and spouse and there may be a mandatory waiting period. The consequences of the operation must be made clear to all concerned, and often a special consent form is required. There seems to be little legal concern about male sterilization, the vasectomy, which is being done with increasing frequency. The legal consequences of unsuccessful sterilization, both male and female, have resulted in suits.[83]

Laws on family planning also vary greatly. Some laws read as though they are absolute prohibitions against information about contraceptive materials, but courts usually allow considerable freedom. The Economic Opportunity Amendments of 1967 made family planning one of the eight national emphasis efforts and funded it accordingly. Family planning programs are growing under federal, state, and private aegis, because many individuals and groups see family planning as a basic human right. Nurses are particularly

involved, for they do much of this counseling, either as specialists or as part of their general nursing role. Because there are still some state limitations, it is important for the nurse to keep up to date in this area.

Artificial insemination, the injection of seminal fluid by instrument into a female to induce pregnancy, is evolving into an acceptable medical procedure used by childless couples. (Consent by husband and wife is generally required.) Homologous artificial insemination (AIH) uses the semen of the husband and appears to present no legal dangers for doctors or nurses. Heterologous artificial insemination (AID) uses the semen of someone other than the husband and does raise the question of the child's legitimacy. On occasion, the question of adultery also arises in the courts if the husband's consent has not been obtained. Few states have enacted statutes to deal with the AID situation.

One relatively new legal aspect of human reproduction is the field of *genetics,* with which nurses, physicians, and lay genetic counselors must be concerned. Some of the issues have to do with AID, human genetic disease, genetic screening, *in vitro* fertilization (IVF), and genetic data banks. Confidentiality is of major importance. If a genetic disease is discovered, the counselor should not contact other relatives, even if it would benefit those relatives, without the screenee's consent. Informed consent that enables the patient to make such serious decisions as having abortions, sterilizations, or artificial inseminations are also vital. The furor caused by the 1978 English test-tube baby is evidence enough that the legal and ethical issues are far from resolved. In addition, legislation, such as the National Sickle Cell Anemia, Cooley's Anemia, Tay-Sachs, and Genetic Diseases Act, has encouraged or forced states to expand genetic screening to cover other disorders. Neonatal screening, for instance, will probably be expanded considerably and offers new opportunities and responsibilities for nurses. But with what is still a relatively new science, many legal questions will be evolving.[84]

Since Dr. Christian Barnard performed the first human heart transplant in 1967, the question of tissue and organ *transplants* has become a point of controversy. Tissue may be obtained from living persons or a dead body. With the living person, the major legal implications relate to negligence and informed consent.[85]

The greatest legal problems arise from procurement of tissue and organs from a dead body. The major question is, "When is an individual dead?" When the definition of death as brain death has not been clarified, there have been suits against doctors and hospitals concerning removal of organs before "death," as seen by the family, even if it was a desire of the patient.

Common law prevented the decedent from donating his own body or individual organs if the next of kin objected and statutes prohibited mutilation of bodies. However, now, forty-nine states have adopted, in one form or another, the Uniform Anatomical Gift Act, approved in 1968 by the National Conference of Commissioners on Uniform State Laws. The basic purposes are to permit an individual to control the disposition of his own body after death, to encourage such donations, to eliminate unnecessary and complicated formalities regarding the donation of human tissues and organs, to provide the necessary safeguards to protect the varied interests involved, and to define clearly the rights of the next of kin, the physician, the health institution, and the public (as represented by the medical examiner) in relation to the dead body. The Act provides that "any person who has attained majority may give all or any part of his body for research, transplantation, education, or for the general advancement of medical science, and may designate as the donee any hospital, surgeon, physician, medical or dental school or anatomical board."[86] The anatomical gift must be made in writing at least fifteen days prior to the donor's death. There is no obligation for the donee to accept the gift.

An autopsy (postmortem examination) by a licensed physician may be authorized by the deceased during his lifetime or after his death by the surviving spouse. In some states, the nearest living kin, who claims the body, may give the authorization. Physicians have the responsibility of getting the family's permission, although the nurses may be asked to witness the form. Sometimes they are also asked to encourage the family to agree to autopsy; there is no legal obligation one way or the other. In most states, an unclaimed body falls under the jurisdiction of the state's anatomical board and may be used for any legitimate purpose. Usually, unattended deaths or deaths of suspicious origin must be autopsied by a city (or other official) medical examiner.

NURSES' RIGHTS

Nurses may have more legal responsibilities because of their RN status, but they have the same rights as any other citizen. In relation to a nurse's profession, Fagin lists seven basic rights:

1. *The right to find dignity in self-expression and self-enhancement through the use of our special abilities and educational background.*
2. *The right to recognition for our contribution through the provision of an environment for its practice, and proper, professional economic rewards.*
3. *The right to a work environment which will minimize physical and emotional stress and health risks.*
4. *The right to control what is professional practice within the limits of the law.*
5. *The right to set standards for excellence in nursing.*
6. *The right to participate in policy making affecting nursing.*
7. *The right to social and political action in behalf of nursing and health care.*[87]

In addition are the human/professional rights to participate in professional decision making. Many of the legal rights of nurses are delineated in the nurse practice acts (Chapter 20), an indication of the power and privilege given by society. Nevertheless, some of the rights nurses may assume they have, such as being patient advocates, may conflict with the rights other professionals see as theirs or what employers see as inappropriate for employees.[88] There are those who believe that nurses should want no rights, because the concept of rights is interpreted as being given only to the powerless.[89] A nurse, acting as patient advocate, who speaks for the patient can have a problem; some nurses have been fired. At least one won a dramatic victory. She publicly criticized the care of patients in a state mental hospital, after leaving there in frustration because the administration neither listened to her nor made an effort to improve conditions. She was hired by another state institution, but dismissed shortly afterwards because of "incompetence." A newspaper had printed her complaints about the first hospital, and this caused "staff anxiety." There was no grievance procedure, so eventually she instituted a lawsuit. Both the American Civil Liberties Union and the Pennsylvania Nurses' Association joined as *amicus curiae*. The court ruled in her favor, noting that incompetence was unproven and also an afterthought in her discharge and that the employer simply wanted to get rid of an outspoken employee; the nurse's First Amendment rights had been violated. She was reinstated and awarded back pay.[90]

Other nurses have fought sex discrimination on the job: the Denver nurses,[91] for instance, and nursing faculty who have suffered rank and salary discrimination. An unusual case was that of two nurses who were fired for having "outside interests," their private practice carried on outside of their hospital working hours. The nurses knew that it was common practice for men employed by the hospital to have second jobs or private patients. Sixteen months later, an EEOC investigation found "reasonable cause" to believe that they were victims of sex discrimination. When the hospital would not accept this arbitration,

the nurses brought suit. Finally, the hospital settled out of court.[92]

It is clear that many nurses' rights issues are related to the individual nurse's employee status, and their resolution is the same as a similar situation with another employee, that is, hiring and firing incidents. One situation that has been gaining attention is fair treatment for nurses who cannot work on certain days because of religious reasons. Another is discrimination against male nurses. As might be expected, rulings have differed, so further EEOC and/or legal suits can be expected.

COLLECTIVE BARGAINING

Some employment issues are resolved by collective bargaining. Since the enactment of PL 93–360 in 1974, employees of nonprofit institutions join the ranks of other workers who have collective bargaining rights. Labor laws are discussed in Chapter 19 and major NLRB rulings in Chapter 25, but nurses' rights in the bargaining process are pertinent here.

The process of collective bargaining, because it is set by law, is similar regardless of who the bargaining agent is, and details can be found in any book on labor relations or in ANA Economic and General Welfare brochures.[93],[94] In the context of ANA, that is, state nurses' associations (SNAs) as collective bargaining agents, the following is presented as a brief overview. The process may be contested by the administration or be in competition with a union, which requires a number of additional steps.

1. The nurses (or group of nurses) in an institution, discontented with a situation or conditions, and having exhausted the usual channels for correction or improvement, ask the SNA for assistance.
2. A meeting is held outside the premises of the institution and always on off-duty time in which SNA staff and the nurses

explore the problems, and the nurses are guided as to what are reasonable, negotiable issues and how to proceed in forming a unit, for instance, who can be included in a unit. Administrative nurses are excluded, but the question of supervisors is still being debated in some places.

3. Authorization cards, which authorize the SNA to act as the nurses' bargaining representative, must be signed by at least 30 per cent of the group to be represented. Membership forms are also suggested because the SNA cannot provide service without funds. All collective bargaining activity must be done in nonwork areas where the employee is protected from employer interference. (There are a series of NLRB rules governing employee distribution and solicitation.)

4. If sufficient cards are signed, the SNA notifies the employer that organization is going on, calling attention to the fact that the activity is protected. Copies are distributed to the nurses so that they know they are protected.

5. An informational meeting is held for all nurses and SNA staff.

6. If it is agreed that the SNA shall represent the nurses, a bargaining unit is formed and officers elected.

7. To seek voluntary recognition of the unit by the employer, designation cards must be signed by a majority of the nurses; this will probably be checked by a mutually accepted third party.

8. If the employer chooses not to recognize the unit, or if the designation is challenged by another union, a series of actions takes place, including an NLRB-conducted election. To petition for election, any union must have designation cards signed by 30 per cent of the nurses in the proposed unit. The election is won or lost by the majority of nurses *voting*. They may vote for a particular union or specify none at all. The NLRB then certifies the winner as the exclusive bargaining agent. If the majority of nurses vote against *any* bargaining agent, the NLRB certifies this also.

9. Assuming that the SNA wins the election, the SNA representative, at the direction of the unit, attempts to settle the problems and complaints of the nurses by negotiating with administration. There are specific rules about what is negotiable. *Mandatory* subjects include salaries, fringe benefits, and conditions of employment, and both sides must bargain in good faith about these. *Voluntary* subjects can be almost anything else they *both* want to discuss, except for *prohibited* or illegal subjects such as a requirement that all workers become members of a union before being employed for thirty days.[95] It should be remembered that the director of nursing, both through position and law, is an administrator and, even though possibly in complete support of the nurses' demands, cannot join them. Quite often she/he has previously tried unsuccessfully to help them in achieving their goals.[96]

10. An agreement may or may not be reached, probably with some compromise on both sides. If there is agreement, a contract is signed outlining agreed upon conditions and the responsibilities of each group. Contracts are renegotiated at set time periods, usually several years. If no agreement can be reached, the dispute may be referred to binding or nonbinding arbitration by an outside group, or some job action such as picketing or a strike may occur. Picketing may be merely informational, to communicate the issues to the community, or it may be intended to prevent other employees or services from entering the institution. The latter, combined with a strike, is the very last resort, when all other efforts fail. If such action is decided upon, sufficient notice is given

to allow for disposition of patient care. Even if strikes are successful, there is often a lingering, unpleasant aftermath between participants and nonparticipants. However, as ANA members agreed as they gradually removed no-strike clauses from ANA and SNA policies, the strike is an ultimate weapon that may be necessary when the employer refuses any attempt to resolve the issues.

Once a contract is in place, there are times when individual nurses are in dispute with the employer. A grievance procedure is usually the vehicle to resolve the problem. A grievance may be caused by "an alleged violation of a contract provision, a change in a past practice, or an employer decision that is considered arbitrary, capricious, unreasonable, unfair, or discriminatory."[97] Simple complaints are not considered grievances. If informed discussion does not resolve the issue, a grievance procedure is followed. The steps include (1) written notice of grievance with written response within a set time; (2) if response is not satisfactory, an appeal to the director of nursing follows; (3) the employee, SNA representative, grievance chairman, and/or delegate, director of nursing, and director of personnel meet; (4) if no resolution, the final step is arbitration by a neutral third party selected by both parties involved.[98] The technique for carrying out the process involves interpersonal, adversary, and negotiating skills.[99]

Whether or not any union is the answer to some of the problems of nurse-employees,[100,101] the right to bargain is a valuable economic tool, as more nurses are beginning to realize.[102] There are alternatives to collective bargaining, and some have worked,[103] but there should be no notion on the part of nurses that collective bargaining is either unprofessional or unethical, if the rights of patients to safe care are preserved.[104] It is one way of controlling professional practice.[105]

Whether or not nurses are unionized, a good contract is useful in defining employer and employee and patient-nurse agreements. Fewer problems arise when both parties understand the rights and responsibilities of each. Although sometimes not realizing it, nurses are continually making contracts, whether as employees or as independent practitioners. A contract is defined as a legally enforceable promise between two or more persons to do or not to do something. The essential elements of a contract are mutual assent, promises or considerations, two or more parties of competent legal capacity, and an agreement that is a lawful act and not against public policy.[106] Contracts can be oral (verbally entered into) or written (all elements in writing). *Expressed contracts* are those in which specific terms have been agreed upon in writing or orally; *implied contracts* give rise to contractual obligations by some action or inaction without verbalization of terms. *A breach of contract* is the unjustified failure to fulfill the terms of the contract as agreed upon or when due. Three legal remedies are recognized: money damages, specific performance (what was promised must be carried out), and injunction (stopping a party from performing the act under other circumstances).

Several examples of nurse contracts can be given. A nurse seeks employment, and in the interview, employer and employee come to certain understandings. The nurse will perform his/her job safely, competently, and in accordance with the standards and policies of the institution (hours, dress, behavior). The employer will pay for those services (salary, fringes), will provide needed equipment to perform the services, and maintain the facilities and equipment properly.[107] (It might be noted at this point that if the nurse is hurt in an accident on the job, whether or not safe equipment or facilities were lacking, she/he is covered by Workmen's Compensation.) The contract may be oral, but is expressed. A written contract has many advantages; it prevents later misunderstandings about such common problems as rotations, shifts, and opportunities for transfer. If the nurse chose not to come to that institution after agreeing to do so, that is breach of contract, but probably the employer would not find it worthwhile to seek damages. If the employee had falsified references or other credentials, the contract would be void, because that is illegal. If the employee, with a written contract, found that the employer was violating it, she/he could seek redress, either damages or the fulfillment of the clause, for example, transfer to a specialty unit with the next vacancy. The ANA has prepared an employment contract that nurses can use as a model; the trend is toward written contracts at all levels of employment.

Written Contracts

A written contract ideally follows a more or less standard form, setting forth the terms of agreement in understandable language, in logical sequence, in readable type. Every written employment contract—both individual and group—should contain the following items. Some will be even more inclusive.

1. *Hours.* This refers to the length of the working day and week and preferably includes a statement about what will constitute overtime for which the employee will be entitled to extra pay at a higher rate.
2. *Salary.* The beginning salary should be set for the position the employee is accepting, as well as the amounts of periodic increases, when they are due, and the criteria for salary increase and/or promotion. Differentials for the evening and night shifts and rate and conditions of overtime pay should also be stipulated.
3. *Vacation.* The number of days or weeks allowed should be stated and the time when the employee will be entitled to take his or her first vacation. Any details of vacation "earnings" should be clearly stated such as: "Vacation for the first year of employment is given on the basis of one day per month. The nurse is entitled to take earned vacation days after she has completed six months of service. For the next two years, she is allowed two

weeks of vacation per calender year; three weeks thereafter."*

4. *Sick leave.* The number of days allowed should be stated and the basis on which they are "earned." The date on which the benefit begins should be included. If cumulative sick leave is allowed, this should be stated with any limitations clearly defined. Special regulations should be itemized, such as the necessity for presenting a health certificate from a physician when returning after sick leave. If a hospital requires nurses to carry hospitalization insurance, or takes care of them when they are ill or gives special rates, this should also be included. (The latter is seldom done now.)
5. *Holidays.* The holidays allowed should be listed and any fixed regulations regarding time off in lieu of a holiday should be stated as well as agreements related to tours of duty on holidays.
6. *Social Security coverage.* If the employing agency participates in the federal Social Security program, the nurses' contract should carry a statement to that effect and specify when salary deductions will be made.
7. *Pension plan.* If the employing agency has a retirement or pension plan, eligibility requirements should be mentioned in the contract, although details of the plan will not be included, of course.
8. *Duration of contract.* The contract should state the period of its duration and under what conditions it can be terminated by either employee or employer, and what the length of notice will be.

Information about rest periods or "breaks," meal hours, and so on, may be included in the contract if either the employing agency or the employee so desires.

Nurses wishing to pursue their education by taking collegiate courses while employed, might be wise to have the conditions under

---

*The figures given here are intended only as examples.

which they may do so stipulated in the contract or at least verified in a letter or memorandum; for example, whether they will be able to enroll in daytime courses or be excused from evening duty while taking an evening course. If the hospital offers an in-service education program, it is advisable for both the institution and the employed nurse to have a written agreement about obligations for attending sessions in on- or off-duty hours.

Regulations about extended leaves of absence for any reason whatsoever, including maternity leave, should be clearly spelled out.

Over and above the specific details of the contract and the way it is phrased is the fact that nurses should be sure they understand it and the terms to which they are agreeing. They should also be sure that the person with whom they make the contract has the authority to do so and should remember that, in most states, they cannot enter into a truly binding contract unless of legal age. If a formal contract is not used, the nurse may ask for a letter of appointment covering the most important points listed and others of importance in that particular situation.

Contracts between patients and an independent nurse practitioner might be just as clear-cut, if it is an employer-employee situation. Even if the patient comes to the primary care nurse, it is still a matter of service and a payment. More complex is the nurse and the patient in the therapeutic relationships. Assuming that their contract is related to improvement of the patient's health, is there also a patient responsibility? There are some doctors and nurses who now plan with their patient to develop a contract in which the responsibilities of each are spelled out. This is a new area in contractual relationships.

Another type of contract affects the education of nurses. The contract between schools and clinical facilities includes such important aspects as mutual agreements on autonomy and rights of each, as well as cooperation, nondiscrimination, staffing (not to be altered because of the presence of students), provision and reimbursement for equipment, responsibilities and rights of faculty and students, and faculty-student ratios.[108] Well thought-out contracts can not only improve learning opportunities, but help avoid legal problems.

Rights and Responsibilities of Students

When students of nursing begin their course of study, they, in effect if not in writing, enter into a contract with the school that does not expire until they graduate. It is understood that both the students and the school will assume certain responsibilities, many of which have legal implications. Most legal cases related to education have involved institutions of higher education (junior and senior colleges, universities) or general education. But once, students of a diploma program that closed threatened to sue for breach of contract because no arrangements had been made for continuation of their education, but the situation was resolved.[109] Most legislation and judicial decisions affecting education, however, probably can be interpreted to bear upon nursing education, as well. Every approved school of professional nursing must meet the criteria for approval set up by the state board of nursing, a legally appointed body found in every state, sometimes under a different name. The state-approved school must conduct an educational program that will prepare its graduates to take state board examinations and become licensed to practice as registered professional nurses. No matter where the students receive education and experience, the nursing school is still responsible for the content of the course of study. The board's minimum standards require the school to provide a faculty competent to teach students to practice nursing skillfully and safely and thus help to avoid injury to patients, co-workers, and themselves. Students are expected to be under the supervision of a faculty member who is also a registered nurse, and the school and the teacher are responsible with the student for the student's errors. As discussed in Chapter 21, most legal experts hold that when students give patient care, they are, for legal purposes, considered employees of the hospital. They are liable for their own negligence if injury results and the hospital will also be liable for the harm suffered under the doctrine of *respondeat superior*. This is certainly true if students are given assignments of a purely service nature, albeit with educational value. In this case, students are likely to work alone without direct supervision for more or less limited periods in a clinical division or as the senior member of a nursing team comprised of practical nurses and nursing aides. This is becoming less common.

In either case, the student nurse is held to the standard of a competent professional nurse in the performance of nursing duties. In several judicial decisions, it was determined that those performing duties customarily performed by professional nurses are held to those standards of care. Faculty supervising students are particularly liable if negligence occurs while the student is performing a task that he or she is not yet capable of performing in a manner consistent with standards of care. Such judgments are related not only to physical tasks or techniques performed, but also to knowledge and judgment in relation to the patient's care. If, for instance, a student does not take appropriate action, either personally or through correct reporting of an incipient injury to the patient, negligence is equally present.[110] Carrying malpractice insurance is a wise precaution, and many schools recommend or require its purchase by all students. Many state student nurses' associations offer low cost insurance with membership.

Whether it is wise educationally and practically for a nursing student to perform nursing functions as a regular, paid employee is debatable, because a student can legally function in only those capacities not restricted to licensed nursing personnel. State laws governing the practice of nursing vary widely and are subject to misinterpretation by the employing agency. Most laws classify students working part time, as employees. In this capacity students performing tasks requiring more judgment and skill than the position for which they are employed are subject not only to civil suits, but also to criminal charges for practicing without a license. An attorney's statement made ten years ago is still totally accurate:

> There can be no automatic agreement that the student will not be under pressure to operate beyond the level of employment she has been hired for. If the student does overstep her right to perform, it should be clearly recognized that the employer who may have encouraged the student to violate the law is not subject to any legal penalty. The individual who violates the law is required by the law to assume all responsibility. The situation is extremely complex for everyone concerned, including head nurses, supervisors, and administrators who have administrative responsibility for providing adequate care to patients, professional responsibility to uphold the standards of the profession, and legal responsibility assumed through delegation of duties. With all the problems we face in nursing today, the question of student employment may seem to be a relatively inconsequential one. But the involvements are most complex and the outcomes most serious for students and the profession. Decisions like this are important to professional advancement and must be based on knowledge, understanding and judgment.[111]

Because today's students usually have relatively limited clinical experience, although it is carefully selected for educational purposes, some students have chosen to seek positions in nursing settings in order to gain additional practice in technical skills. Hospitals and nursing homes tend to hire them as summer replacements for aides but may actually give them more advanced assignments. The dangers cited should be considered by employer and employee.

Traditionally, the relationship of institutions of higher education to a student under twenty-one years of age had been *in loco parentis*, which means that the school stands "in the place of the parent" and has the right to exercise similar authority over the student's physical, intellectual, and moral training. Since the early 1960s, courts have overturned this concept and it is no longer considered to have much legal validity. However, the student's enrollment in a particular college generally is an implied contract, which requires that the student live up to the reasonable academic and moral standards of the college,[112] with the school also having certain responsibitilies. For instance, if the student lives in a dormitory connected with the school, it must meet safety and sanitation standards established by local regulations. However, the school rarely assumes responsibility for the student's loss of personal property, and even if something of great value were stolen, the school would usually be obligated to do no more than try to help recover it, if that.

Undesirable student conduct may result in some discipline, including suspension or expulsion, and there has been considerable disagreement on the university's power in such circumstances. Generally, it is expected that the college's rules of conduct are made public and that the student has the right to a public hearing and due process. Legal rulings may be different as applied to private or public universities.[113] Private universities have greater power in many aspects. For instance, public universities cannot discipline students for exercising their constitutional right to protest (speeches, picketing, marching, leafleting, and so on) as long as the act itself is not illegal, but private institutions have no such legal obligation.[114]

Constitutional rights are most frequently cited by students in complaints: First Amendment (freedom of speech, religion, association, expression); Fourth Amendment (freedom from illegal search and seizure), and the Fifth and Fourteenth Amendments (due process of law). The courts recognize the student first as a citizen so that they will consider possible infrigements of these rights. Most commonly, First Amendment rights involve dress codes and personal appearance. Although schools do not pos-

sess absolute authority over students in this sense, some lower court rulings have approved establishment of dress codes necessary for cleanliness, safety, and health.[115] Beginning with *Dixon* v. *Alabama State Board of Education* in 1961, random, unannounced searches that schools had carried out previously are no longer allowed without student permission or a search warrant or evidence found is inadmissible in court. If material uncovered is proscribed by *written* institutional policy, it may be used in institutional proceedings.[116]

Due process has been a major issue of legal contention. In essence, the term means that the purpose of the rule or law be examined for fairness and reasonableness. Are the student and faculty understanding of the rule the same? Did the student have the opportunity to know about the rule and its implications? What is the relationship between the rule and the objectives of the school? Not too long ago, few schools had any grievance procedure, and this situation was believed by students to be a serious violation of rights. In 1975, the National Student Nurses' Association (NSNA) developed grievance procedure guidelines as part of a bill of rights for students.* Besides suggesting the makeup of the committee and general procedures, such issues as allowing sufficient time, access to information and appropriate records, presentation of evidence and use of witnesses were included.[117] The usual steps in any grievance process are followed for academic grievances also: an informal process first, written complaint and suggested remedy by the student grievant, written reply, hearing with presentation of evidence on both sides, a decision by the committee in a specific time, right of appeal, and sometimes, arbitration. With students, the right to continue with classwork during the total process is considered necessary.

Due process is considered crucial for students who are expelled or suspended for dis-

_____

*See Chapter 24.

ciplinary reasons or who feel that they are discriminated against in their extracurricular activities because of race, religion, sex, or sexual preference.[118] However, there seem to be an increasing number of grievances filed or legal complaints made because of academic concerns, especially grades. The courts have been reluctant to enter this arena of academic freedom. There has yet to be a definitive ruling on curriculum and degree requirements. The attitude is demonstrated by a highly significant statement made by one court (45 Federal Rules Decisions, 133(1968), 136):

> Education is the living and growing source of our progressive civilization, of our open repository of increasing knowledge, culture and our salutory democratic traditions. As such, education deserves the highest respect and the fullest protection of the courts in the performance of its lawful missions. . . . Only when erroneous and unwise actions in the field of education deprive students of federally protected rights or privileges does a federal court have power to intervene in the educational process. . . .[119]

This statement has a number of counterparts in other jurisdictions, such as the affirmation of a U.S. District Court (*Connelly* v. *University of Vermont and State Agricultural College*, 1965):

> in matters of scholarship, the school authorities are uniquely qualified by training and experience to judge the qualifications of a student. . . . The court is in a poor position indeed to substitute its judgments for that of the university. . . .[120]

The issue, instead, has almost always been due process; therefore, schools are developing grievance procedures to resolve academic disputes between student and school.[121] The process can create a number of tensions, but it may also bring to light school and teacher problems that should have and can be resolved to avoid serious student complaints.[122]

Now most colleges have grievance procedures for students who think that they have received unfair grades, and these procedures must first be followed before any lawsuit can be filed. It is generally advised that before waging such an all-out battle, the situation should be looked at practically. It must be proved that the grade is "arbitrary, capricious, and manifestly unjust," which is generally very difficult. Furthermore, unless that particular grade is extremely important to a student's career, the cost and time involved are greater than even a favorable result might warrant.[123]

The type of student records kept by schools varies and may consist of only the acdemic transcript or include extracurricular activities and problem situations, which are kept in an informal file. The enactment of the Buckley Amendment, described in Chapter 19, has clarified the issue of student access to records. The individual loses the right to confidentiality by waiving the right or by disclosing the information to a third person. A student's academic transcript is the most common document released, particularly to other schools and employers.

As more student activists, most of whom are now voting citizens, request or demand certain rights as part of the academic community, more legal decisions are made.* But, university rules that were once ironclad have become flexible, even without legal intervention. Students can often bring about desirable changes through participation in committees intended for this purpose. Nevertheless it is also helpful to know one's basic legal rights as individual and student.

The concept of rights need not be seen as an adversary proceeding. Both student and school have a new accountability.[124],[125] It might, in the long run, be more meaningful to look at certain student rights as freedoms

---

*One example is the "Truth in Testing" laws, the first of which was passed in New York state in 1979. It required manufacturers of standardized admission tests, such as the Scholastic Aptitude Test and Graduate Record Examination, to file test questions and correct answers with the New York Commissioner of Education after student scores are released. A federal version also allowed the students to see their answers and the correct answers after release of scores.

and responsibilities. The following have been suggested:

1. *Freedom to disagree.*
2. *Freedom to explore ideas.*
3. *Freedom to help choose educational goals.*
4. *Freedom to study independently.*
5. *Freedom to experiment.*
6. *Freedom to know faculty.*[126]

These freedoms are based on mutual respect and commitment by faculty and students and enhance not only the educational process, but nursing professionalism.

REFERENCES

1. U.S. Department of Health, Education and Welfare, *Secretary's Commission on Medical Malpractice* Report. DHEW Pub.No. (OS) 73–88 (Washington, D.C.: U.S. Government Printing Office, 1973), p. 71.
2. George Annas, "The Hospital: a Human Rights Wasteland," *Civil Liberties Rev.* (Fall 1974), p. 20.
3. Beatrice Kalisch, "Of Half Gods and Mortals: Aesculapian Authority," *Nurs. Outlook*, 23:22–28 (Jan. 1975).
4. Emanuel Hayt, Lillian Hayt and August Groeschel, *Law of Hospital, Physician and Patient* (Berwyn, Ill: Physicians' Record Co., 1972), p. 479.
5. J. H. Hedgepeth, "Trial Court Finds Hospital Strictly 'Liable' for Physician Negligence, *Hosp. Med. Staff* (Feb. 1974).
6. Helen Creighton, "Law for the Nurse Supervisor: Informed Consent," *Superv. Nurs.*, 6:9, 48–49 (Jan. 1975).
7. Ibid, p. 9.
8. Ibid, p. 48.
9. George Annas, *The Rights of Hospital Patients*, American Civil Liberties Union Handbook (New York: Avon Books, 1975), p. 64.
10. Nathan Hershey and S. H. Bushkoff, *Informed Consent Study* (Pittsburgh: Aspen Systems Corp., 1969), p. 3.
11. R. J. Alfidi, "Informed Consent: A Study of Patient Reaction." *JAMA*, 216: 1225–1329, (May 24, 1971).
12. Hershey and Bushkoff, op. cit.
13. David Warren, *Problems in Hospital Law*, 3rd ed. (Germantown, Md.: Aspen Systems Corp., 1978), pp. 95, 138–141, 178.
14. Linda Besch, "Informed Consent: A Patient's Right," *Nurs. Outlook*, 27:33 (Jan. 1979).
15. "Consent Form for Jehovah's Witnesses Agreed Upon," *Medicological News*, 7:12 (Summer 1979). Also in *Mod. Med.* (July 15–August 15, 1978).
16. Helen Creighton, "Refusal of Blood Transfusion," *Sup. Nurse*, 6:65–66 (Feb. 1975).
17. H. L. Hirsch, "Informed Consent—Fact or Fiction," *J. Leg. Med.*, 5:28 (Jan. 1977).
18. Jay Katz, "Informed Consent—A Fairy Tale? Law's Vision," *University of Pittsburgh Law Review*, 39:137–174 (Winter 1977).
19. Besch, op. cit., pp. 34–35.
20. Sue Reitz, "Signed Consent: Is It Really the Nurse's Responsibility?" Letter to the Editor, *Nurs. Outlook*, 27:154–155 (Mar. 1979).
21. Peter Black, "Criteria of Brain Death: Review and Comparison," *Nurs. Dig.*, 4:71–73 (Summer 1976). Condensed and reprinted from *Postgraduate Med.*, 57:69–74 (Feb. 1975).
22. Peter Black, "Brain Death," *N. Engl. J. Med.*, 299:398 (Aug. 24, 1978).
23. Ibid., pp. 398–399.
24. Ibid., p. 399.
25. *Belchertown State School* v. *Saikewicz*, 1977 Mass. Adv. Sh. 2461, 370 N.E. 2nd 417 (1977).
26. *In re Karen Quinlan* 69 N.J. 399 (1976).
27. Daniel Rothman and Nancy Rothman, *The Professional Nurse and the Law* (Boston: Little, Brown and Company, 1977), pp. 139–140.
28. George Annas, "Reconciling 'Quinlan' and 'Saikewicz': Decision Making for the Terminally Ill Incompetent," *Am. J. of Law & Med.*, 4:367–396 (Winter 1979).
29. Sissela Bok, "Personal Directions for Care at the End of Life," *N. Engl. J. Med.*, 295:367–369 (Aug. 12, 1976).
30. Jane Raible, "The Right To Refuse Treatment and Natural Death Legisla-

tion," *Medicological News*, **5**:6–8 (Fall 1977).

31. Emily Friedman, "'Natural Death' Laws Cause Hospitals Few Problems," *Hospitals*, **52**:124–148 (May 16, 1978).

32. Dennis Horan, "Right-To-Die Laws: Creating, Not Clarifying, Problems," *Hospital Progress*, **59**:62–78 (June 1978).

33. Joyce Beauchamp, "Euthanasia and the Nurse Practitioner," *Nurs. Dig.*, **4**:83–85 (Winter 1976). Condensed and reprinted from *Nurs. Forum*, **14**(1):56–73 (1975).

34. Marya Mannes, *Last Rights* (New York: William Morrow & Co., Inc., 1974).

35. "Nurse, on Trial for Murder, Called Compassionate," *New York Times*, Mar. 14, 1979, p. A17.

36. "Terminal Patient and No-code Orders," *Regan Report on Nursing Law*, **14**:1 (Nov. 1973).

37. "Optimum Care for Hopelessly Ill Patients," *N. Engl. J. Med.*, **295**:362–364 (Aug. 12, 1976).

38. Mitchell Rabkin, et al., "Orders Not to Resuscitate," *N. Engl. J. Med.*, **295**:364–366 (Aug. 12, 1976).

39. Robert Trotter, "Psychosurgery, the Courts and Congress," *Nurs. Dig.*, **2**:92–95 (Dec. 1973).

40. A. H. Bernstein, "Legal Rights of Mental Patients," *Hosp.*, **53**:49–52, 92 (Mar. 1979).

41. E. Parker and G. Tennent, "The 1959 Mental Health Act and Mentally Abnormal Offenders: A Comparative Study," *Med. Science and the Law*, **19**:29–38 (Jan. 1979).

42. Walter Barton and Charlotte Sandborn, *Law and the Mental Health Professions* (New York: International Universities Press, 1978).

43. Charles Prigmore and Paul Davis, "*Wyatt* v. *Stickney*: Rights of the Committed," *Nurs. Dig.*, **3**:70–77 (Summer 1974).

44. John Wilson, *The Rights of Adolescents in the Mental Health System* (Lexington, Ma.: Lexington Books, 1978).

45. Marguerite Mancini, "Nursing, Minors, and the Law," *Am. J. Nurs.*, **78**:124,126 (Jan. 1978).

46. Alan Sussman, *The Rights of Young People*, An American Civil Liberties Union Handbook (New York: Avon Books, 1977), p. 26.

47. Ibid., pp. 224–226.

48. Ibid., pp. 27–28.

49. Ibid., p. 29.

50. Ibid., pp. 30–31.

51. "A Model Act Providing For Consent of Minors For Health Services," *Pediatrics*, **59**:293–296 (Feb. 1973).

52. The National Association of Children's Hospitals and Related Institutions, Inc., *The Pediatric Bill of Rights*, 1974.

53. "Research with Children: The Rights of Children," (Editorial), *Child Psychiatry and Human Development*, **4**:67–70 (Winter 1973).

54. A. R. Jonesen, "Research Involving Children: Recommendations of the National Commission for the Protection of Human Subjects of Biomedical and Behavioral Research," *Pediatrics*, **62**:131–137 (1978).

55. "The Age of Consent," (Editorial), *Am. J. Public Health*, **68**:1071–1072 (Nov. 1978).

56. Charles Lewis, et al., "Informed Consent by Children and Participation in an Influenza Vaccine Trial," *Am. J. Public Health*, **68**:1079–1082.

57. Leonard Glantz, "Protecting Children and Society," *Medicolegal News*, **7**:2–3 (Summer 1979).

58. Edward Porcano, "Experimentation with Children: The Pawns of Medical Technology," *Medicolegal News*, **7**:4–9 (Summer 1979).

59. George Annas, "Legalizing Laetrile for the Terminally Ill," *Hastings Center Rep.*, **7**:19–20 (Dec. 1977).

60. John Kahring, "Conference Report: Seeking a Judicial Determination that Treatment May Be Withheld from a Seriously Ill Newborn," *Medicolegal News*, **7**:10–11 (Summer 1979).

61. Amatai Etzioni, "The Right to Know, to Decide, to Consent and to Donate," *Nurs. Res.*, **2**:43–50 (Oct. 1974).

62. R. S. Stone, "The Rights of Human Beings Participating as Subjects in Biochemical Research," (Guest Editorial), *J. Lab. Clin. Med.*, **85**:184 (Feb. 1975).

63. "Protecting Research Subjects," *Am. J. Nurs.*, **79**:1139–1140 (June 1979).

64. Helen Creighton, "Legal Concerns of Nursing Research," *Nurs. Res.*, **26**:337–341 (Sept./Oct. 1977).

65. Katharyn May. "The Nurse as Researcher: Impediment to Informed Consent," *Nurs. Outlook*, **27**:36–39 (Jan. 1979).

66. Kathleen Kelly and Eleanor McClelland, "Signed Consent: Protection or Constraint?" *Nurs. Outlook*, **27**:40–42 (Jan. 1979).

67. Ruth MacKay and John Soule, "Nurses as Investigators: Some Ethical and Legal Issues," *Nurs Digest*, **5**:7–9 (Spring 1977).

68. Bradford Gray, "An Assessment of Institutional Review Committees in Human Experimentation," *Med. Care*, **13**:318–328 (Apr. 1975).

69. Marcia Opp, "The Confidentiality Dilemma," *Nurs. Digest*, **4**:17–19 (Fall 1976).

70. Harold Schmeck, Jr., "Medical Records Privacy Violated, Goverment-Backed Study Finds," *New York Times*, Jan. 13, 1977, p. 42. (The Westin report is cited in the bibliography of this chapter).

71. Carol Levine, "Sharing Secrets: Health Records and Health Hazards," *Hastings Center Rep.*, **7**:13–15 (Dec. 1977).

72. Hayt, et al., op. cit., p. 1094.

73. Melissa Auerbach and Ted Bogue, *Getting Yours: A Consumer's Guide to Obtaining Your Medical Record* (Washington, D.C.: Public Citizen's Health Research Group, 1978).

74. U. S. Department of Health, Education and Welfare, op. cit., pp. 76, 77, 109, 110, 127, 134.

75. Alan Westin, "New Era in Medical Records," *Hastings Center Rep.*, **7**:23–28 (Dec. 1977).

76. Given Health Care Center, *Principles of Practice* (Burlington, Vt.: University of Vermont, mimeographed), p. 1.

77. George Annas and Joseph Healey, "The Patient's Rights Advocate," *J. Nurs. Admin.*, **4**:25–31 (May/June 1974).

78. *The Rights of Hospital Patients*, op. cit., pp. 112–120.

79. Auerbach and Bogue, op. cit., pp. 10–17.

80. Health Law Center, *Problems in Hospital Law* (Rockville, Md.: Aspen Systems Corp., 1972), pp. 95–96.

81. Mary Hemelt and Mary Ellen Mackert, *Dynamics of Law in Nursing and Health Care* (Reston, Va.: Reston Publishing Co., 1978), pp. 68–71.

82. Helen Creighton, *Law Every Nurse Should Know*, 3rd ed. (Philadelphia: W. B. Saunders Company, 1975), pp. 166–167.

83. Helen Creighton, "The Unplanned Child," *Sup. Nurse*, **3**:7–8 (June 1972).

84. Philip Reilly, *Genetics, Law and Social Policy* (Cambridge, Ma.: Harvard University Press, 1977).

85. Helen Creighton, "Legal Problems Related to Transplant Management," *J. Renal Tech.*, **4**:35–39 (Dec./Jan. 1975). Also in *Law Every Nurse Should Know*, pp. 291–292.

86. Daniel Rothman and Nancy Rothman, *The Professional Nurse and the Law* (Boston: Little, Brown and Company, 1977).

87. Claire Fagin, "Nurses' Rights," *Am. J. Nurs.*, **75**:84 (Jan. 1975).

88. Elsie Bandman, "Do Nurses Have Rights? Yes," *Am. J. Nurs.*, **78**:84–86 (Jan. 1978).

89. Bertram Bandman, "Do Nurses Have Rights? No," *Am. J. Nurs.*, **78**:84–86 (Jan. 1978).

90. Helen Creighton, "A Nurse's Freedom of Speech," *Sup. Nurs.*, **5**:45–48 (Apr. 1974).

91. Bonnie Bullough, "The Struggle for Women's Rights in Denver: A Personal Account," *Nurs. Outlook*, **26**:535–536 (Sept. 1978).

92. "Two Tenacious RNs Fight Hospital Over Sex Discrimination and Make It Pay," *RN*, **42**:15–16 (Mar. 1979).

93. American Nurses' Association, *Organizing the Local Unit* (Kansas City: The Association, 1975).

94. American Nurses' Association, *Dynamics of a Local Unit* (Kansas City: The Association, 1975).

95. "Collective Bargaining: What Is Negotiable?" *Am. J. Nurs.*, **69**:1892–1895 (Sept. 1969).

96. Pamela Atkinson and Linda Goodwin, "The Role of the Nursing Administrator

in Collective Bargaining," *Nurs. Cl. of North America*, **13**:111–118 (Mar. 1978).

97. Elaine Beletz and Mary Meng, "The Grievance Process," *Am. J. Nurs.*, **77**:265 (Feb. 1977).

98. Ibid., pp. 257–260.

99. Elaine Beletz, "Some Pointers for Grievance Handlers," *Sup. Nurs.*, **8**:12–14 (Aug. 1977).

100. Debra Wynne, "A Union Contract Was the Only Language Our Hospital Would Understand," *RN*, **41**:66–68 (May 1978).

101. Jan Natonski, "Why a Union Contract Didn't Work at Our Hospital," *RN*, **41**:69–71 (May 1978).

102. Lynn Donovan, "Is Nursing Ripe for a Union Explosion?" *RN*, **41**:63–65 (May 1978).

103. Michael Miller, "Nurses' Right to Strike," *Nurs. Digest*, **4**:47–51 (Fall 1976).

104. Leone Conta, "Bargaining by Professionals," *Am. J. Nurs.*, **72**:309–312 (Feb. 1972).

105. Ada Jaycox, "Who Defines and Controls Nursing Practice?" *Am. J. Nurs.*, **69**:977–982 (May 1969).

106. Hemelt and Mackert, op. cit., p. 45.

107. Ibid., pp. 49–52.

108. Rosemary Dale, "Contracting for Student Clinical Experience," *Nurse Educator*, **1**:22–25 (May/June 1976).

109. "Students Accuse Hospital of Breach of Promise," *Am. J. Nurs.*, **73**:1314 (Aug. 1973).

110. Eric Springer, *Nursing and the Law* (Pittsburgh: Aspen Systems Corp., 1970), pp. 8–10.

111. Bernice E. Anderson, "The Question of Student Employment," *Am. J. Nurs.*, **59**:1579 (Nov. 1959).

112. Michael Nussbaum, *Students' Legal Rights: What They Are and How to Protect Them* (New York: Harper & Row, Publishers, 1970), pp. 1–3.

113. Ibid., pp. 11–14, 44–65.

114. Ibid., pp. 25–34.

115. Clementine Pollok, et al., "Students' Rights," *Am. J. Nurs.*, **76**:601 (Apr. 1976).

116. Ibid., p. 601.

117. *The Bill of Rights for Students of Nursing* (New York: National Student Nurses' Association, 1975).

118. *Law Every Nurse Should Know*, pp. 66–68.

119. Clementine Pollok, et al., "Faculties Have Rights, Too," *Am. J. Nurs.*, **77**:636 (Apr. 1977).

120. Ibid., p. 637.

121. Jann Logsdon, et al., "The Development of an Academic Grievance Procedure," *Nurs. Outlook*, **27**:184–190 (Mar. 1979).

122. Karen Robinson and Sharon Bridgewater, "Named in a Grievance: It Happened to Us," *Nurs. Outlook*, **27**:191–194 (Mar. 1979).

123. Nussbaum, op. cit., pp. 76–78.

124. Richard Millard, "The New Accountability," *Nurs. Outlook*, **23**:496–500 (Aug. 1975).

125. Dorothy McMullan, "Accountability and Nursing Education," *Nurs. Outlook*, **23**:501–503 (Aug. 1975).

126. Rothman, op. cit., pp. 90–91.

BIBLIOGRAPHY

Andrews, Lois. "The Last Night." *Am. J. Nurs.*, **74** (July 1974), 1305–1306. Two nurses let a man die rather than let him endure more "heroic" measures.

Annas, George. "Problems of Informed Consent and Confidentiality in Genetic Counseling." In Milunsky and Annas, eds., *Genetics and the Law*. New York: Plenum Press, 1976, pp. 111–122. Good source for these issues.

Annas, George. "Rights of the Terminally Ill Patient." *J. Nurs. Admin.*, **4** (Mar./Apr. 1974), 40–44. Excellent discussion of right to confidentiality, privacy, consent, choice of place and time of death.

Annas, George. *The Rights of Hospital Patients*. American Civil Liberties Handbook. New York: Avon Books, 1975. Intended for general public. Gives explicit directions for obtaining rights. Includes section on medical terminology.

Brown, Robert, et al. *The Rights of Older Persons*. American Civil Liberties Handbook. New York: Discus Books, 1979.

Carnegie, Elizabeth. "The Patient's Bill of Rights and the Nurse." *Nurs. Clinics of N. Am.* **9** (Sept. 1974), 557–562. Responsibilities of the nurse.

Creighton, Helen. "More About Informal Consent." *Sup. Nurs.* **9** (Mar. 1978), 84–86. Good review of role of nurse in getting patient's informed consent and reasons for litigation against physicians.

"Control Over Conditions of Practice." *Nurs. Forum*, **10** (Summer 1971), 229–331. An entire issue is devoted to the controversy of the use of collective bargaining techniques by nurses, with individual articles by I. Mauksch, A. Jacox, B. Bullough, N. Grand, E. Erickson, A. Zimmerman, and K. Klassen covering pro's and cons, the ANA Economic Security Program, and some historical background.

Dodge, Joan S. "What Patients Should Be Told: Patients' and Nurses' Beliefs." *Am. J. Nurs.*, **72** (Oct. 1972), 1852–1854. Differences are shown, but point is that patients do want information.

Kelly, Lucie Young. "The Patient's Right To Know." *Nurs. Outlook*, **24** (Jan. 1976), 26–32. An overview of major issues; references at end of article are useful.

Kelly, Lucie Y. "The Rights of Young People in Health Care." *Nurs. Pract.*, **2** (Nov./Dec. 1977), 10–12. A thorough review of trends and legal issues; useful references.

Levine, Alan, and Eve Cary. *Rights of Students.* American Civil Liberties Handbook. New York: Discus Books, 1977. A revised edition that covers all major aspects of student rights; most emphasis on public schools.

Lipman, Michel. " 'Informed Consent' and the Nurse's Role." *RN*, **35** (Sept. 1972), 50–51ff. Discusses requirements of informed consent and special aspects of the nurse's role.

Neuhaus, Evelyn, et al. "Patient Responses to Request for Written Permission to Review Medical Records." *Am. J. Pub. Health*, **66** (Nov. 1976), 1090–1092. A study asking MDs to allow review of patient records shows that permission varies with type of specialties, diagnosis, and individual physician.

Nussbaum, Michael. *Student Legal Rights: What They Are and How to Protect Them.* New York: Harper & Row, Publishers, 1970. A small paperback containing a description of student rights and practical suggestions on how to protect them. A comprehensive list of significant student legal rights cases in the appendix.

Quinn, Nancy, and A.R. Somers. "The Patient's Bill of Rights: A Significant Aspect of the Consumer Revolution." *Nurs. Outlook*, **22** (Apr. 1974), 243. Consumers discuss meaning of patient's rights bill, giving some history and predictions for future.

Ritz, Arlene, and Rose Marie McMahon.

"Commitment to Standards Ends in the Courts." *Nurs. Educator*, **1** (Sept./Oct. 1976), 22–24. Students challenged right of AD program to upgrade its standards by raising grade required for admission. Court decision favors program's right.

Saxton, Dolores. "Collective Bargaining in Academe: A Personal Approach." *Nurs. Outlook*, **21** (Nov. 1973), 704–707. A faculty member describes the situation that precipitated job action, the results, and the advantages and disadvantages of a group contract.

Sussman, Alan. *The Rights of Young People.* American Civil Liberties Handbook. New York: Avon Books, 1977. Includes all major issues; specific section on health care.

"The Patient's Right to Know." *Briefs*, **38** (Feb. 1974), 25–28 ff. Reviews various aspects of informed consent and problems of access to medical records.

Werther, William, and Carol Lockhart. *Labor Relations in the Health Professions.* Boston: Little, Brown and Company, 1976). Excellent. Good legal background, as well as clear review of rights and process.

Westin, Alan. *Computers, Health Records and Citizens' Rights.* NBS Monograph 157 (Washington, D.C.: U. S. Dept. of Commerce, National Bureau of Standards, 1977). Comprehensive study of the issues with extensive bibliography. Recommendations made.

See also references at end of Chapter 22 and references and bibliography, Chapters 6, 10, 11, 16, 17, 19, 24, 25. Public Affairs Pamphlets No. 480 (Rights of Teenagers as Patients, 1972), No. 492 (Rights of Retarded Persons, 1973) and No. 535 (Rights of Patients): Public Affairs Pamphlets, 381 Park Avenue, South, New York, N.Y. 10016. *Children's Rights Report* is issued by the Juvenile Rights Project of the ACLU Foundation in New York and usually includes health-related items. The Summer 1979 issue of *Medicolegal News* has a series of articles on legal rights of children. The May 1978 issue of *AJN*, section on ethics includes articles that consider legal rights, as well. The nursing and hospital law books cited in this and preceding chapters vary in the depth in which various topics ae explored; Creighton has large section on contracts; Hemelt and Mackert, on child abuse; Springer, on legal reporting requirements. References and bibliographies in books and journals are frequently extensive.

PROFESSIONAL COMPONENTS AND CAREER DEVELOPMENT

ORGANIZATIONS
AND
PUBLICATIONS

Organizational Procedures and Issues

The more complex and highly organized society becomes, the harder it is for a single individual to exert any significant influence or power. There are exceptions to this rule, of course. There will always be pioneers and crusaders—individuals who, through sheer force of personality, conviction, and determination succeed in making an impact. But by and large the concerted effort of a group of people working in an organized manner is necessary today to accomplish a given purpose, to effect a change in the status quo.

This is as true in nursing as in any other field, on both student and graduate levels. One student alone, for instance, can do little to change what may seem to be the out-of-date or autocratic practices of the nursing school administration; but, working through the student association in the school or through the state unit of the National Student Nurses' Association, she/he may very well be enabled to bring about the desired improvements. Similarly, one nurse, no matter how dedicated or determined, would never have been able to make it easier and less expensive for our older citizens to obtain needed hospital and medical care. Yet the strong voice of the American Nurses' Association speaking out in favor of health insurance coverage for the aging under the Social Security system was one of the factors that brought about what is now known as Medicare. And it must be remembered that the American Nurses' Association took this stand because the majority of its members indicated that this was what *they* wanted. So, working through the professional organization, the individual *was* heard, *did* have influence, *did* help to bring about change.

There are many persons who are inclined to do nothing more than grumble to themselves and their colleagues about what they don't like or, on the other hand, what they would like to see accomplished. But so long as these individuals do no more than complain and unless they join with their colleagues to act in an organized, effective way, they will in all probability have to continue to be powerless and dissatisfied. This is not to say that a person should simply become a ''joiner''—someone who seems to become a member of almost any organization for which she/he is eligible. Such a process only scatters one's interests and energies in many directions and provides no focus. But there are many organizations concerned with health and nursing that a nursing student or RN will want to either join, support, or at least be familiar with. By membership in some of them, the nurse will be able to work with colleagues in advancing their own nursing interests or those of nursing as a whole; in others, they will find the companionship of those with the same, perhaps more specific, concerns; and in still others, they will be enabled to keep abreast of the many forces that are influencing nursing and health care today.

The nature and purpose of these nursing and health organizations will be discussed in succeeding chapters. Of concern here, however, is the nurse's role—or anyone's role, for that matter—as an organization member. Presumably, an individual will have joined the organization because its concerns and goals are the same as one's own. Joining is not enough, however; full realization of one's own and the organization's objectives demands active and informed participation. For whatever an association's purposes may be, its success depends on intelligent, industrious, and conscientious leadership; a willing, enthusiastic, and well-informed membership; adequate financial support; and sound business organization and administration. It is the responsibility of each member to help make all of these things realities.

MEMBERSHIP RESPONSIBILITIES

Members of any organization should feel responsible for learning as much as possible about it—its history, purposes, the number and composition of its membership, and its principal activities. They should study the constitution and bylaws, the code of ethics if there is one, and subscribe to its offical publication. They should learn the names of the organization's principal current officers and preferably their background. When attending meetings, they should listen carefully to the discussion and become familiar with the most important issues under consideration and the conditions and facts that influence the decisions to be taken. This will take time, but just a few hours a week spent on such matters can eventually prepare new members for productive and personally rewarding participation in the organization's work.

As soon as the individual is ready to take a more active part in the meetings, he or she can enter into discussions, ask relevant questions, help clarify issues by presenting a fresh and knowledgeable point of view, accept appointments to committees, and volunteer to help as time and ability dictate. Restraint, diplomacy, and a sense of good timing should guide new members as they find their place in any group.

Individuals who hold or aspire to hold office should have a copy of authoritative rules of order for organizing and conducting an organization's business and should become familiar enough with the publication so they can readily find the information needed. The individual who holds the president's office or presides over formal business meetings in any other capacity must know how to do so efficiently without recourse to the book of rules except for an answer to unusually difficult questions. The rules of order used by a particular association are usually named in its bylaws.

The average member does not need to be as conversant as an officer with the minute details of parliamentary procedure, but should know how to address the presiding officer; formulate, present, and vote on a motion; and be familiar with other basic procedures that facilitate the progress of the meeting. This knowledge will enhance his/her ability to express views and contribute to the discussion without embarrassment or lack of confidence. On the other hand, it would be naive not to recognize that parliamentary procedure can be used as a manipulative tool to bring about certain action or lack of action. For instance, if an item is not placed on the agenda by the presider, other officers or members, it is not likely to be discussed and certainly not acted on. If the item is placed in an unfavorable position—at the end of a long session when people are less alert, at a point when a certain voting constituency is present for a short time (some bylaws allow any member present to vote), or at a point when certain information is not yet available, or after a controversial, emotional, related item—the action taken might be quite different than if the topic were discussed at another time. There are also those who misuse the intricacies of parliamentary procedure by complex motions to amend, substitute, or amend the amendment of a motion repeatedly so that the members may be totally confused about the real issue in the motion to be voted on. Those speaking to a motion may also be deliberately or inadvertently obscure, incorrect, or inappropriate in their statements which, if the usual procedure in speaking from the floor is observed, may make the point difficult to correct and clarify. (And then there are always those who like to be heard whether or not what they say is pertinent.) Therefore, the "average" member should be alert to these machinations and learn how to combat them. If a motion seems to have been railroaded through, it is particularly useful to know how that action can be reversed before the final adjournment.* Because any organization has its political aspects, those who are interested in seeing that certain action is taken seldom take a chance on this simply occurring during a business meeting. There is an effort to sell individuals or subgroups within the organization on the idea before formal action is taken; that is, lobbying. The formal action can be orchestrated: who makes the motion, who speaks to it, what supporting information must be introduced, is it best referred to a task force or committee and, most important of all, are the votes there. A politically astute member tries to estimate at what point the issue is most likely to be voted in the desired direction, delaying the vote by some form of postponement if necessary.

WHO DOES THE WORK?

Even the most careful plans and the finest constitution and bylaws do not ensure a

healthy, productive organization. The plans and directions must be implemented. Who does this? Every officer, every committee member, every member at large shares the responsibility for knowing what that person as an individual can do for the good of the entire membership and for doing it—unless health or some other serious handicap is a deterrent.

An incapacitated officer should tender his or her resignation promptly and give the organization the opportunity and privilege of deciding whether or not the organization needs and wants him or her to continue in office in spite of the handicap. Members who accept an appointment to a committee and later find themselves unable to assist with its work should withdraw, leaving the chairman or other authorized person free to appoint another, more productive member.

The ideal members of any organization unquestionably are those who pay their dues promptly, attend meetings whenever possible, keep abreast of developments, support and help advance the association's programs, speak intelligently at meetings, offer constructive suggestions, volunteer their services and talents, accept committee appointments, and promote the goals that have been adopted by the association, even though they may occasionally have some personal reservations about them.

Such paragons, of course, do not come in large numbers but most of an association's active members have at least some of these attributes. Even the members who do no more than pay their dues regularly make some contribution, because by so doing, they provide both moral and financial support for the organization's programs. The general rule, however, is that the more actively individuals participate in the functioning of their association, the more benefit and satisfaction they will derive from their membership. By the same token, the more active, articulate, and informed members an association has, the better its chances of accomplishing the objectives for which it was formed.

*See later section on motions.

President, Chairperson,* Moderator

Although the elected or appointed head of an association does a great deal of work behind the scenes day after day throughout a term of office, the membership thinks of this person most frequently as the one who presides at meetings. This is one of the most important responsibilities for which a leader needs particular skills, talents, and personality assets.

The individual should be in complete control of emotions; avoid distracting mannerisms and loquacity; speak in a clear, well-modulated voice; be discreet, impartial, and courteous; have considerable stamina and be businesslike. However, a good sense of humor and the ability to laugh at oneself is a decided asset. A good leader should be able to sense the atmosphere of a meeting and prevent it from becoming explosive or detrimental to productive progress. It is even important to be sensitive to the physical comfort of the assembly and to do what is possible to improve ventilation, lighting, seating arrangements, or whatever else is indicated to keep everyone alert and interested. The presiding officer should be prompt for every meeting, ready to function at the appointed time, and, as soon as a quorum is present, call the meeting to order. This encourages habitual latecomers to be on time and helps to assure prompt adjournment also.

The president must have a thorough knowledge of the history of the organization, what it has done in the past, and what it plans to do in the future. Rarely should a question find the president completely unprepared; if she/he does not know the answer, she/he should know on whom to call for it or where it can be found. Sometimes, of course, the questions are referred to someone else even if the chair knows the answer. This might happen when a query is raised about the organization's finances, and the president asks the treasurer to answer. Any officer must know when it is appropriate to withhold information as well as when to disclose it. It is important always to be in control of the situation and to keep the assembled audience informed about the discussion before the house to avoid the confusion that results when members do not understand the issue.

Rarely should the presiding officer express a personal opinion on an issue. This is because of the need to maintain a neutral attitude and because one of the chief duties of a leader is to encourage others to participate. It is a good policy to subtly encourage the less assertive member to speak up and discourage the individuals who always want to express their views at length. In all this the presiding head must be eminently fair and unbiased, allowing all the right to air their views.

The chair must be thoroughly familiar with the agenda of every meeting over which she/he presides and know how to complete it expeditiously and in accordance with the rules of procedure adopted by the organization. This is learned through study of the rules, observing other presiding officers in action, and experience. Every meeting will bring confidence and learning from successes and failures.

A president may have exhibited considerable ability to lead discussions, but may not have had extensive practice in handling motions, one of the major responsibilities of a presiding officer. Sometimes this is a simple procedure, but it can become involved. The chairman who understands the intricacies guides the action deftly and gains the respect of the group; the one who gets confused about what step takes precedence over another, for example, may create a chaotic situation that will leave the members dissatisfied and possibly highly critical.

It is vital to be acquainted with as many members of the organization as possible and to become familiar with their interests and abilities. This will help in making appointments to committees and selecting members

---

*The current trend is to use the term *chairperson* instead of *chairman*. However, some organizations may use chairman or chairwoman, or simply, chair.

for other assignments. If the organization is widespread, visits to several different areas or constituent associations each year, giving necessary help, often stimulate the members in their work. On social occasions the president should mingle with members; this will establish rapport with the various groups and will tend to promote interest and enthusiasm.

The president must keep in touch with the work and progress of other officers and the committees in the organization and cooperate amicably and constructively with them. Democratic principles must be observed, allowing each person to use the initiative and authority necessary to discharge assigned duties and responsibilities without interference while, at the same time, demanding first-rate performance. If the organization has a paid executive secretary or director and a headquarters staff, the officers must observe the same principles and practices, carrying the appropriate responsibilities but never usurping prerogatives that are rightfully those of the staff.

It is clear that the head of any organization needs leadership qualities in large measure. Although every individual elected to such an office probably will not possess all of them, there will be innumerable opportunities to develop them.

Vice President

Although, theoretically, a vice president—particularly a first vice president—is as capable as the president, because she/he must be prepared to function in the president's absence or in an emergency, the qualifications tend to be less exacting. Many persons with outstanding leadership ability are unwilling to accept the relatively inactive post of the vice presidency. This happens in organizations of all sizes and types, from a local volunteer group, to the federal government.

To make the office more challenging, some associations declare in their bylaws that the vice presidents shall also be heads of committees or assume other responsibilities. Among the most common are chairperson of the program, policy development, or bylaws committees. Vice presidents may also represent the organization in meetings or interorganizational committees or task forces. This gives the vice president an opportunity to make a specific contribution to the organization and also gives visibility.

One trend that seems to be occurring is to include a president-elect on the board, preparing that person for assumption of the presidential office with minimal orientation. There are some disadvantages: a double-term commitment on the part of that individual and probable inability to prevent that person from succeeding to the presidency if she/he proves to be ineffectual at the board level.

Secretary

Some organizations have two secretaries: the recording secretary who takes the minutes and the corresponding secretary who deals with the correspondence. There is also the secretary-treasurer option. If the organization is large enough to have a professional staff, the actual taking of detailed minutes and handling correspondence is done by staff, but both are checked and sometimes signed by the secretary, president, or other appropriate person. Nevertheless, the functions of the secretary as spelled out in the bylaws are the responsibility of the elected person.

In a smaller organization, the secretary who thinks and writes clearly, is well informed about the association's business, and has the necessary knowledge and skill to write appropriate minutes is invaluable.[1] The secretary must be able to keep alert throughout meetings that can be both tedious and frustrating, and maintain an outward attitude of equanimity, neutrality, and cooperation regardless of inner conflicts. She/he must be objective and impartial in all reports in spite of the fact that at times it is necessary to "interpret the interpretations" of others when transcribing the notes taken at a meeting. It is important to be methodical, reliable, and prompt in getting out all reports and memoranda. The corresponding secretary needs to be a master of the courteous and appropriate phrase, because these responsibilities have important public relations connotations. Neatness and promptness of response in correspondence are highly desirable.

Treasurer

It is not unusual for the treasurer of an organization to be selected with greater care than the president, and almost as much is expected. The principal qualifications should be honesty, accuracy, and conscientiousness in keeping records, and knowledge of bookkeeping procedures, budgeting, and financial reporting. Business experience is a decided asset. The membership, even when it knows better, often judges the treasurer's ability by the balance on hand in the treasury.

The treasurer of any organization is often chairman of its committee on finance. This post requires the usual skills necessary to conduct a committee meeting well plus additional ability to discuss facts and figures intelligently, often before board members who may not be well-versed in financial matters but are vitally interested in the organization's purse strings. The president's work is also facilitated by a competent treasurer because so many of the organization's activities depend on its financial status. Even if the details of the financial management of the organization are carried out by skilled employees, the board has fiduciary responsibility for the association. Budgets cannot be properly developed or adhered to and intelligent financial decisions cannot be made if accurate information is not available. Therefore, board members and especially the treasurer must have at least a basic understanding of financial management.

Councils and Committees

An organization's bylaws usually call for the inclusion of permanent councils and standing committees, with the number depending more on the scope of the activities than on the volume.

The quantity and quality of work done by each special group greatly influence the status and progress of the organization, although sometimes so indirectly that the general membership is unaware of its extent. For example, the nominating committee is responsible for finding persons who are willing and eligible to fill elected offices and who have the qualifications for them. This requires diligence and excellent salesmanship, especially if the prospective candidate is initially reluctant to serve. In large or widely scattered organizations, a great many members do not know the candidates personally. They must depend on the nominating committee to select the best available people; they then base their voting decisions on whatever information about them is released through official channels.

Members of the nominating committee, therefore, must always seek the best person or persons regardless of friendships, school ties, personal obligations, or any other influential factor. And it follows logically that the persons responsible for appointing or electing members of this committee must consider integrity to be one of their most important personal qualifications. Their influence on the future of the organization is considerable, for a ballot can be set up in such a way that a certain individual or someone representing a particular constituency is sure to win that election. This is especially true with a mail ballot, where a strong write-in vote is almost impossible to achieve unless it is highly organized.

The work of other permanent councils and committees often is equally important. Some aspects of it may be obvious; others may need definition and delineation of responsibilities.[2]

PARLIAMENTARY PROCEDURES

The purpose of the business meetings of any organization is to transact business with the greatest possible dispatch while recognizing the rights of individual members present and absent, giving minority and opposing groups ample opportunity to air their views, yet assuring that the wishes of the majority prevail. To achieve this purpose, a methodical order of conducting the meetings is essential.

When early American congresses first organized, they naturally borrowed from the British Parliament many practices, which they adapted for their own use. Further changes were made from time to time until a distinctive American system evolved. The terms *parliamentary procedure* and (incorrectly) *parliamentary law* are used, however, in referring to both the American and British systems, which still have a good deal in common.

The procedures that have been used for many years by the United States Senate and House of Representatives developed from four sources:

1. The Constitution of the United States of America.
2. Jefferson's *Manual of Parliamentary Procedure*, which he prepared while he was vice president and presided over the Senate.
3. Rules that have been adopted by the House since its beginning and that may be changed with each Congress; these rules are sometimes called the "legislative manual."
4. Decisions rendered by the presiding officer and the chairman of the Committee of the whole House.

The transactions of less imposing bodies than the United States Congress are governed similarly. Each usually has a constitution and bylaws citing the officers and their duties in general, the order of business, voting regulations, and other matters related to the conduct of business meetings. The presiding officer makes decisions consistent with his authority, often with the advice of a parliamentarian employed by the organization; each major meeting of the membership or house of delegates may produce changes in rules or the formulation of new ones needed to expedite its own activities; and each organization adopts a manual of parliamentary procedure to guide the business transactions.

The most popular guide for formal business procedure is *Robert's Rules of Order Revised*. This reference work, written by General Henry M. Robert of the United States Army and published originally in 1876, is based upon the rules and practices of Congress. It is generally considered the most authoritative book of its kind, and some organizations attempt to follow it to the letter. Others use it only as a final authority to settle a controversial point. Still others select simpler but equally reliable rules of order to guide their transactions, such as *Sturgis' Standard Code of Parliamentary Procedure* by Alice F. Sturgis, and *Parliamentary Law* by F. M. Gregg.

As stated in *Robert's Rules of Order, Revised:*

> *Parliamentary procedure, properly used, provides the means whereby the affairs of an organization or club can be controlled by the general will within the whole membership. The "general will" in this sense does not always imply even near unanimity or 'consensus' but rather the right of the deliberate majority to decide. Complementary to this is the right of the minority—at least a strong minority—to require the majority to be deliberate—that is—to act according to its considered judgment after a full and fair "working through" of the issues involved.* [3]

Although Robert's and other such publications include duties of officers and committees and other information, the discussion here will be concerned with the conduct of a business meeting because duties of officers and other details are defined in an organization's constitution and bylaws, which supersede any other rules.

Some of the principles and techniques of parliamentary procedure can perhaps be best presented by following an imaginary annual meeting of the National Student Nurses' Association from beginning to end. This organization, described in the next chapter, is the membership organization for nursing students. When the NSNA bylaws do not specify a procedure, *Robert's Rules of Order, Revised* is used as a guide.

Most formal meetings have an order of business. A classic example follows.

1. Call to order.
2. Minutes of previous meetings.
3. Reports of officers, boards, standing committees.
   Executive reports.
   Executive announcements.
   Order and procedure of reports.
     President.
     Vice president.
     Secretary.
     Treasurer.
     Board of directors.
   Standing committees.
4. Reports of special committees.
5. Announcements.
6. Unfinished business.
7. New business.
8. Adjournment.

In this meeting, these steps will be considered one at a time and others, which are often included in the order of business, interpolated.

Although the following discussion implies that the NSNA's business is completed in one session, it usually takes several sessions to finish it. This is usual at convention meetings and may be required in the bylaws by certain wording such as the need for the nominating committee to report the ticket at a certain time.

An order of business must be flexible enough to be realistic. For example, if there is good reason for having the reports of special committees given ahead of the standing committees, the president is privileged to make that change simply by announcing it from the chair. The president also is privileged to make announcements or have others make them and to invite the headquarters staff members and guests to address the assembly whenever it appears prudent, proper, and helpful to so do. A major reordering of the agenda by the presiding officer or another member may require approval of the total group.

Call to Order

The president calls the meeting to order by rapping a gavel for attention if necessary and saying, "Will the meeting please come to order?" or words to that effect. It may be customary to have someone give an invocation after which the secretary presents the agenda for the meeting and the parliamentarian explains the basic rules of parliamentary procedure that will be followed.

To make sure that a quorum (as defined in the NSNA bylaws) is present, the president asks the secretary to call a roll of delegates. If a quorum is present, the president so states; if not, she/he may declare a recess or fill in the time with matters of a nonbusiness nature until sufficient members arrive.

Minutes of the Preceding Meeting

Although the NSNA's secretary keeps accurate and complete files on all business transacted at every meeting of the association, it is highly improbable that minutes of the association's last meeting will be read, because these would be long, detailed, and time-consuming. So, in lieu of reading the minutes, most large membership organizations distribute mimeographed copies of the previous meeting.

However, in meetings of smaller groups within the NSNA, such as the executive board or one of the committees, the second step in the order of business is the reading of the minutes of the preceding meeting. This is done by the secretary at the request of the chairman or silently by the members. It is also possible that minutes will have been distributed and read before the meeting. When this is finished, the chair asks the members if they wish to make any additions or corrections. A member wishing to make a change rises and after being recognized makes a statement that might be something like this: "Madame (or Mister) Chairman, my name is Helen Gibson [or simply "Helen Gibson"], Kentucky. The secretary reported that the president of the New Jersey association moved that the executive board investigate the feasibility of promoting a national student nurse week. The motion was actually made by the president of the New York State association.''

Small groups in which members know each other may not need to identify themselves. Nonetheless, it is correct parliamentary procedure. The chairman and the recording secretary *must* know who is speaking and other members *like* to know.

The president says "Thank you" to the member and asks the secretary to change the record, unless the correction is contradicted by someone. When all requests for additions or corrections have been made, the president states, "The minutes will be accepted as corrected." If no changes are indicated, she says, "The minutes will be accepted as read."

Report of the President

The president usually reads his or her own report, but has the privilege of asking the secretary or someone else to read it. If reading it personally, she/he will ask the first vice-president to "take the chair" until the report is completed. This is because correct parliamentary procedure requires that a meeting must always have a presiding officer and the president cannot preside and read a report at the same time.

Although the president's report may contain some facts and figures, it is not usually a business report. Rather it is of a general nature and greatly influenced by the president's personality. Included will be an account of the progress made by the association during the past year, the satisfactions and perhaps the disappointments; some of the things done while president, such as visiting state nurses' associations and speaking at meetings; plans and ambitions for the future with implied and possibly formulated recommendations based on needs as he or she sees them; and expressions of appreciation to others for their support and assistance.

No formal acceptance procedure of the

president's report is indicated. After concluding this address the president gives a copy of it to the secretary for the record and resumes the chair.

Everyone who makes a formal report before the house of delegates will follow the president's example and give the secretary a copy either before or immediately after presenting it to the assembly.

Report of the Secretary

The secretary's report includes information about his or her personal activities in the office, stressing the broad scope of official duties. When the report has been completed, the president "accepts it as read" without asking for a vote by the delegates.

Report of the Treasurer

The treasurer's report is a statement showing the income and expenses of the association during the past year and its financial status at the end of the fiscal year. When the treasurer has finished reading the report, the president says, "The treasurer's report is accepted as read," and may add, "And it is filed for audit."

Any questions about the treasurer's report should be asked at this time. The president may reply or may ask the treasurer to do so. General discussion is permitted at the president's discretion.

Report of the Committee on Nominations

Much of the work of the nominating committee—deciding upon appropriate candidates for office, securing their permission to be nominated, and compiling their biographies—is done prior to the annual meeting. At the meeting the chairman of the nominating committee, when called upon by the president, reads the slate of officers to the assembly. When finished, she/he says, "Madame Chairman, I move the adoption of this slate of officers." The president then asks the house if there are other nominations. If there are none, a delegate will move that the nominations be closed. This motion will be seconded and voted promptly.

A *nomination from the floor* can be made by any delegate by addressing the chair, naming the proposed candidate, and giving briefly the proposed nominees' qualifications for the post. A special form supplied by the nominating committee, containing detailed information about the candidate, is submitted to the nominating committee if the nomination is seconded. Nominations from the floor are closed by house vote.

Following the meeting, the nominating committee reviews the information about candidates who were nominated from the floor and may post their names and the offices for which they are candidates near the voting place where balloting is done. It is also possible that a convention paper or other form of written communication will be distributed to members with election information and the nominees' names and qualifications. If may or may not be possible to have the new names printed on the ballot in time for the election. If not, the names may be written in by the delegates wishing to vote for them.

Voting is done at a time and place designated by the executive board. Delegates must present credentials before they are allowed to vote. When voting is completed—usually within a few hours—the tellers who were appointed by the president at the first meeting count the ballots and prepare a report to be given at the NSNA's closing business session. A plurality vote (more votes than any other candidate for the same office) is required for election by the NSNA. If a majority vote were required, a candidate would need at least one more than half the votes cast to be elected.

Reports of Other Committees

As the NSNA president calls for reports of the association's other committees, the chairman of each goes to the platform—if invited by the president—or to a microphone or other place where she/he can be seen and heard easily by the entire assembly, addresses the chair, and reads the report. If any action is to be taken (usually recommen-

dations), the committee chairman or someone else says, "Madame (Mister) Chairman (or President), I move the acceptance of this report" or "adoption of the recommendation". A delegate may second the motion, and the motion is handled like any other. If no action is required on any sections of the report, the preceding step may be omitted and the president will thank the reporting person. At times, reports are presented in a book of reports and are not read if the business of the committee does not appear controversial or call for action. They can still be discussed, however, if members desire.

Unfinished Business

At this point the president makes sure that any items of business left incomplete because of time limitations, absent persons, and so on, are satisfactorily completed.

New Business

New business is often the most interesting and exciting part of the agenda. If the issues are controversial, debate may be heated and lengthy. Even if they're not, the topics discussed indicate the course the association will take during the months ahead.

Resolutions

Resolutions may be one of the most important parts of a major meeting, because they are indications of the organization's position on key issues. Resolutions are submitted by individual members, groups, or committees within the organization to a resolutions committee and/or the board of directors. A resolutions committee, may, usually with the permission of the originators, combine similar resolutions or change some aspect of a resolution.

The board has the privilege of supporting or not supporting the resolution, and in some organizations it can withhold it from the voting body. Some organizations hold preliminary hearings to expedite action and/or agreement without the formality of strict parliamentary procedure. This often clarifies misunderstandings and saves time during the business meeting. Generally, a member whose resolution has been rejected for presentation has the right to introduce it from the floor.

Resolutions, except courtesy resolutions, often are meant to be acted upon by the organization after the meeting. For instance, a resolution may call for a letter to the President of the United States calling for better federal funding of nursing education, or it could direct long-term activities of the organization. Although the wording is often formal, with one or more *whereas* clauses giving the reasons for the resolution preceding the resolution, there is no reason why the wording cannot be clear and concise, so that the message is understood by all. Reviewing the past resolutions of an organization gives an excellent picture of its philosophy and goals and is one means of judging its quality. Therefore, although resolutions frequently come toward the end of a meeting, they should be given careful thought before voting.

Adjournment

After the amenities have been observed, such as the passing of other resolutions expressing appreciation for services and courtesies, and perhaps introduction of the new officers, the meeting is adjourned by motion and vote.

THE MATTER OF MOTIONS

The work of a business session is greatly facilitated if officers and members know and practice the proper methods of handling motions according to parliamentary procedure. A motion is a proposal or suggestion intended to initiate action, effect progress, or allow the assembly to express itself as holding certain views. It is through these motions —made, seconded, discussed, and approved by a majority of the delegates—that the association is enabled to transact its business, make decisions, and move forward.

Uncomplicated motions may be passed very quickly by *silent assent*, such as accepting the secretary's report as read; or by *viva voce*, which means responding "aye" or "no" ("yea" or "nay") in response to a request from the presiding officer; *viva voce* may also be used in voting on involved issues. However, if the vote is, or is likely to be, close, the chair will ask for a *show of hands* or a *standing vote*, because they permit an actual count. A *written vote*, or *ballot*, may be indicated and is usually required for elections.

To Make a Motion

A member who wishes to make a motion always:

1. Stands and goes to a microphone when indicated.
2. Waits, if necessary, until a speaker ahead has stopped talking. In general, it is advisable to remain seated until the previous speaker has finished, but if several members have motions to present, it is well to "get in line."
3. Waits for the chair's signal to go ahead. This may be done with a nod of the head or verbally.
4. Addresses the presiding officer as Madame (or Mister) Chairman, Chairperson, President, or Speaker.
5. Identifies oneself by name and state, as indicated.
6. States the motion clearly and succinctly. When time permits, it is a good idea to write out a motion before rising to make it. This helps the individual to be sure she/ he will say what is intended and also repeat it verbatim, if requested. Frequently, a written motion is given to the secretary to be sure it will be recorded accurately in the minutes.

Most motions require seconding before action. The chair will call for a second, if indicated, particularly when there is likely to be discussion of the motion. The member who does the seconding rises, addresses the chair, and after identification, says, "I second the motion." If no one seconds a motion calling for seconding, the motion is automatically lost and the president so states. No mention of it is made in the official records.

Discussion

Assuming that a motion is seconded, the chair next says, "It has been moved and seconded that . . . Is there any discussion?" If there is none, she/he asks for a vote by one of the methods previously mentioned. A member wishing to ask a question or make a comment follows the usual procedure for recognition.

Sometimes discussion is prolonged, heated, and confused, involving proposed amendments to the original motion and perhaps even amendments to the amendment, known as subsidiary amendments. The presiding officer must be fair and skillful to permit all persons to express their views and yet not seriously impede the progress of the meeting. The action must then be guided back to the original motion, disposing of the last-mentioned items first.

Discussion of a motion may be terminated if a member calls for "the question." This means that the member feels that the matter has been discussed sufficiently for the members to vote intelligently on it.

Because to terminate the discussion without the approval of the assembly would infringe on the privilege of unlimited debate, the chairman then asks, "Are you ready for the question?" If a sufficient number, as predetermined by the association's rules of order, vote in the affirmative, the motion is put to a vote. Otherwise, debate must be reopened or some other method must be used to handle the motion before the house.

Decision

The ultimate disposition of a motion depends on the majority decision of the delegates.* If more than half of them vote in fa-

vor of it, it is passed; if the majority vote "no," the motion is, of course, defeated. Sometimes a motion is passed "as amended", that is, not in its original form, but with one or more changes in it, or additions to it, as proposed from the floor during the discussion.

When there is obvious conflict or confusion about a particular motion, especially when it may have become complicated or unclear as a result of several proposed amendments, a motion to *refer it to a committee* may be made. This motion in itself may be debated. If it is passed, then the original motion goes to an appropriate committee for further study and possible presentation at some later date.

It is also possible to vote to *table* a motion; this means that it is set aside temporarily, permitting the chair to progress with the agenda, but will be taken up again later in the same session or meeting. A vote to *postpone* action on the motion until some other time may also be taken. Decisions to table or postpone action on a motion are most likely to be made when the matter at hand is a complicated or hotly debated issue. Any of these actions gives the members more time to clarify their thinking about it. It also permits more time to marshal arguments pro and con and, finally, permits the president, possibly aided by the parliamentarian, to study the motion so that at some later date it may be reviewed lucidly for the delegates.

Occasionally, members pass a motion that they later regret, either because the decision was made hastily, with incomplete information, or in a state of confusion. To bring that same motion before the assembly again, an individual voting on the prevailing side may move to "reconsider." Anyone can second. The motion to reconsider takes precedence over other motions, and therefore is acted on at once, regardless of what else is being discussed. It is debatable, and if passed, the entire issue of the previously passed motion is open for discussion, with the opportunity to clarify or to introduce needed information. It is then handled in the usual manner.

---

*Some organizations require a two-thirds vote for passage of a motion, or of motions in certain areas. These requirements are spelled out in the association's bylaws.

The responsible member and, especially, officer of any organization will not want to depend on this necessarily brief presentation of parliamentary procedure as the sole guide to informed action. If a meeting is not run expeditiously and fairly, members become rapidly disenchanted with the entire organization. Meetings may be the only way in which members participate in the decision-making process of the organization, and if they see it as disorganized or a setup, many withdraw completely. It requires the knowledge and skill of both officers and members to see that meetings are conducted as they should be, so that the voice of the members prevails.

MEMBER-STAFF
INTERRELATIONSHIPS

As nursing organizations grow larger, many acquire professional staff, supported by clerical and sometimes technical assistants. Not too long ago, an executive secretary was a retired member of some nursing association, untutored in association management, who learned on the job. Today, the professional executive, still scarce, is seen as essential, for she/he deals with large amounts of money, a complex organization, and, frequently, thousands of volunteers.

Although the professional staff of nursing associations may consist of nurses, members of the same organization, with voting and officeholding rights, the *job* role is different. The members make policy through the volunteer board and officers; the staff carries out policy. Because volunteers are transient —a board of directors inevitably changes after each election—it is often only the staff who have continuity. Yet, should their opinions as to a certain action be in direct opposition to the board's or committee's, unless they can sell their point of view, it is the staff's responsibility to do what the volunteers decide. Staff may try very hard, directly or indirectly, to influence the key members of the organization. Many mem-

bers do not have a clear concept of the careful balance needed between board and staff lines of authority and responsibility. Just as volunteers should expect to devote an adequate amount of time to the association and bring to it the same amount of intellectual commitment and judgment used in their professional pursuits, staff members are expected to provide not just services but leadership, and must create confidence in their judgment and in the program. Staff are expected to prepare guidelines and backup material so that volunteers' time is not wasted and they can react to specifics, not generalities. Staff and volunteers should regard each other as valuable colleagues with whom bad news as well as good news is shared. Staff must learn to identify the special abilities of volunteers so that they are put to use.[4]

It is also important that staff identify their roles, responsibilities, and activities, so that expectations are real. Volunteers should not get involved in what is not their responsibility. An executive director (ED) manages the office and personnel. When volunteers attempt to interfere in personnel matters, problems inevitably result. If the ED is incompetent, she/he should be terminated by the board.

Selection of an executive director in a large nursing association may be made by an appointed search committee. Criteria for selection should be carefully thought through to meet the needs of that organization. In a study done by the Foundation of the American Society of Association Executives, the qualities considered most important for a successful association executive were listed by both EDs and voluntary leaders. Agreed on by both as most important were (1) interpersonal relationships, empathy, rapport, and (2) dedication, commitment, energy, and hard work. EDs then listed, in order (1) integrity; (2) organizational/administrative abilities; (3) creativity, innovativeness, and vision; the volunteers preferred (1) organizational/administrative abilities; (2) intelligence, planning; (3) knowledge of industry or profession and of association management.[5] The heavy emphasis on management skills by the volunteer leaders is not unexpected when the importance of having a well-run organization is considered. However, perhaps the most significant point to remember in staff-volunteer relationships is that both are presumably working toward the same goals, and when there are unusual tensions between the two, it is often the result of misunderstanding or disagreement on how these goals are to be achieved. As in any other professional and human relationship, good communication is essential.

Issues and Concerns

Probably because of the proliferation of professional associations, there are many more concerns about them. If at one time an organization was run by volunteers in spare time, typing notices with two fingers or with the help of somebody's sister, now organizations are a form of big business; they include powerful unions and well-funded professional organizations. In 1979, 5,000 major trade and professional associations were identified, with the figure jumping to 40,000 if state and local constituent groups are included. There is, on the average, one nonprofit association for every two or three for profit corporations.[6] All seek economic and other advantages for their members, and they seek the power necessary to succeed. Politicians do not want a strong, organized group against them, and there is no doubt that organizational lobbying gets action, especially if associations cooperate with each other.[7] Still, there is also concern that the power of such organizations is not good for the public, and trade associations and professional organizations have been found subject to the Sherman Act and the Federal Trade Commission Act, which relate to price fixing and restraint of trade.[8] In nursing, this has stopped the setting of fees for private duty nurses and raised questions about certification and accreditation by the professional organizations.

But more critical are the issues of what the president of one professional organization calls the internal crisis of identity and mission.[9] The key question asked about this professional organization for university professors is also pertinent to nursing's professional organization: recognizing that the heterogeneity of the professional generates threatening tensions and divisions within the organization, is there a sufficient residue of *common* concern to justify the creation of one body to bring together all who call themselves professional nurses?

One problem in nursing is that so many nurses do not understand what the functions of a professional association are and therefore have inappropriate expectations. Sociologist Robert Merton has delineated the functions in three categories: functions for individual practitioners, for the profession, and for society. For individuals, the association (1) gives social and moral support to help them perform their roles, especially in terms of economic and general welfare (salary, conditions of work, opportunities for advancement), continuing education, and working toward legally enforced standards of competence; and (2) develops social and moral ties among its members so that each becomes his brother's keeper. For the profession, the organization must set rigorous standards and help enforce them (quality of those recruited, of education, practice, and research.) The profession must always press for higher standards. For society, the organization helps furnish the social bonds through which society coheres, providing unity in action.

The association mediates between the practitioner and profession on the one hand, and on the other, their social environment, of which the most important parts are allied occupations and professions, the universities, the local community, and the government.[10]

The conclusion for the American Association of University Professors (AAUP) was that it did indeed have common purposes for all, but that it was necessary to work at maintaining and gaining membership and to be selective in the issues and roles that can be reasonably undertaken. Membership of most organizations, however, is and probably always will be made up of people with varying degrees of commitment, with at least half indifferent, and the others ranging from the ambitous to the ambivalent/dissident.[11] No association can please them all. But one president concluded, "We are what we are because we are a voice of and for the profession. Without that, we are nothing."[12]

Peplau addressed the same problems: the dilemmas of diversity versus consensus; part versus the whole; wishes of members versus public interest.[13] Both presidents, like Merton, concluded that unless there is one voice for a profession, no one will listen. Adequate numbers of participating members are crucial. "To be able to speak for the profession, the association must be representative of as many of the profession as possible."[14]

In the following chapters, it will be seen how the increasing numbers of organizations that nurses can and do join overlap, compete, and frequently disagree. Add to that the trade unions that some nurses are choosing to represent them, and it is small wonder that the public asks, "Which is nursing's real association? Who speaks for nursing?"

REFERENCES

1. "Meeting Minutes: What They Should Contain," *Leadership.* 1:59–60 (May 1979).
2. "Learning the Ropes As A Committee Chairman," *Leadership.* 1:57–58 (Nov. 1978).
3. Henry Robert. *Robert's Rules of Order.* Revised (New York: William Morrow and Co., Inc., 1971), p. iii.
4. "What Should You Expect From Staff and Staff From You?" *Leadership.* 1:63–64 (Nov. 1978).
5. "Qualities Needed for a Successful Chief Staff Executive," *Leadership,* 1: 54–55 (Nov. 1978).
6. "What Is An Association?" *Leadership,* 1:51–52 (May 1979).
7. Debra Stratton. "A Winning Combination: Associations Work Together for Legislative Victory," *Leadership.* 1:39–45 (Nov. 1978).
8. Basil Mezines and Steven Fillman. "Antitrust Guide for Association Members," *Leadership.* 1:47–49 (Nov. 1978).
9. Peter Steiner. "The Current Crisis of the Association," *AAUP Bull.,* **64**:135–141 (Sept. 1978).
10. Robert Merton. "The Functions of the Professional Association," *Am. J. Nurs.,* **58**:50–54 (Jan. 1958).
11. James Low. "The Public, Your Members, Your Staff: Forces That Shape Your Professional Organization," *Leadership.* 1:9–13 (May 1979).
12. Steiner, op. cit. p. 138.
13. Hildegard Peplau. "Dilemmas of Organizing Nurses," *Image,* **4**(3): 4–8 (1970–1971).
14. Merton, op. cit., p. 54.

BIBLIOGRAPHY

Grumme, Marguerite. *Basic Principles of Parliamentary Law and Protocol.* St. Louis, Mo.: The author, 1973. A small pamphlet citing some of the key points in parliamentary procedure.

Hegarty, Edward J. *How to Run Better Meetings.* New York: McGraw-Hill Book Company, 1957. Humorous and entertaining, this book points out the typical problems encountered in almost any meeting and suggests ways of dealing with them effectively.

Merton, Robert K. "Dilemmas of Democracy in the Voluntary Associations," *Am. J. Nurs.,* **66** (May 1966), 1055–1061. Thought-provoking examination of the democratic voluntary association, including the theories upon which it is based, its functional requirements and structural parts, and the characteristics of its members and nonmembers. The main conflict facing such an organization is the division of group energies between activities aimed either at achieving goals or maintaining the organization. The author recommends the thoughtful alternation of these two activities as one method of minimizing such conflict.

Merton, Robert K. "The Functions of the Professional Association," *Am. J. Nurs.,* **58** (Jan. 1958), 50–54. A now classic analysis of the functions, purposes, services, and *raison d'etre* of professional organizations. Required reading.

McGuire, Mary J. "Mr. Robert, Please—," *Nurs. Outlook,* **4** (Apr. 1955), 194–195. A helpful discussion of how amendments to bylaws can be acted upon at an organization's business meeting without tiring and boring the delegates.

Pepalu, Hildegard. "Dilemmas of Organizing Nurses," *Image*, **4** (1970–71), 4–8, No. 3. Fromer ANA president explains various options for developing the organization to serve nurses.

Robert, Sarah Corbin. "Rules of Right and Reason," *Am. J. Nurs.*, **60** (Apr. 1960), 526–529. The author explains some of the principles on which parliamentary rules and practices are based and applies them to typical situations. Points out some of the common errors made at meetings.

Smith, David, and Richard Reddy. "Improving Participation in Voluntary Action," *J. Nurs. Admin.*, **3** (May–June 1973), 36–42. Practical guidelines for taking advantage of the probabilities of human behavior to encourage voluntary group action.

See also references at end of Chapter 23 and bibliography and references of following chapters on the various organizations, as well as those related to Chapter 16. *Leadership*, "a publication for the effective association volunteer," was first published in 1978 and its articles are invaluable for both volunteers and staff. Included are short, pertinent how-to-do-it articles, as well as more thoughtful analyses of issues. Merton and other sociologists frequently write about associations and provide an in-depth understanding of the sociological implications.

National Student Nurses' Association

The National Student Nurses' Association, Inc. (NSNA), established in 1953, is the national organization for nursing students in the United States and its territories, possessions, and dependencies. NSNA's purpose is "to assume responsibility for contributing to nursing education in order to provide for the highest quality health care; to provide programs representative of fundamental and current professional interests and concerns; and to aid in the development of the whole person, his/her professional role, and his/her responsibility for the health care of people in all walks of life."[1] The functions of the organization, as listed in the bylaws, are as follows:

1. To have direct input into standards of nursing education and influence the educational process.
2. To influence health care, nursing education, and practice through legislative activities, as appropriate.
3. To promote and encourage participation in community affairs and activities toward improved health care and the resolution of related social issues.
4. To represent nursing students to the consumer, to institutions, and other organizations.

5. To promote and encourage students' participation in interdisciplinary activities.
6. To promote and encourage recruitment efforts, participation in student activities, and educational opportunities regardless of person's race, color, creed, sex, age, life-style, national origin, or economic status.
7. To promote and encourage collaborative relationships with the American Nurses' Association, the National League for Nursing, the International Council of Nurses, as well as the other nursing and related health organizations.

The NSNA is autonomous, student-financed, and student-run. It is the voice of all nursing students speaking out on issues of concern to nursing students and nursing.

MEMBERSHIP

Students are eligible for active membership in NSNA if they are undergraduate students enrolled in state-approved programs leading to licensure as a registered nurse or registered nurses enrolled in undergraduate programs in nursing. Students are eligible for associate membership if they are prenursing students enrolled in college or university programs designed as preparation for entrance into an undergraduate program leading to an associate degree, diploma, or baccalaureate degree in nursing. Associate members have all of the privileges of membership except the right to hold office as president and vice president at state and national levels.

Application for membership is made directly to NSNA. Dues* paid are combined national and those levied by the school and/or state association; the latter vary from state to state. The dues structure is decided by vote of membership.

NSNA also has two categories of membership not open to students. Sustaining membership is open at the national level to any individual or organization interested in furthering the development and growth of NSNA, upon approval by the board of directors. Sustaining members receive literature and other information from the NSNA office. Dues vary for sustaining members, which may include NSNA alumni, other individuals, local organizations, and national organizations. Honorary membership is conferred by a two-thirds vote of the House of Delegates upon recommendation by the board of directors to persons who have rendered distinguished service or valuable assistance to NSNA. This is the highest honor NSNA can bestow upon an individual.

History

Just when or where the idea of a national association of nursing students had its origin will probably never be known. But, for many years and in increasing numbers, students had been attending the national conventions of ANA and NLN, eager to learn of the activities of these two associations that would soon be affecting them as graduate nurses. Special sessions were arranged at these conventions so that students could meet together and discuss mutual problems. At the same time, some student nurses' organizations had been formed on a state level, giving students an awareness of both the strength and the values of group association and action. It was inevitable, of course, that the idea of a national association would arise sooner or later. Once it did, nursing students throughout the United States began to work enthusiastically in that direction.

In June 1952, approximately 1,000 students attending a national nursing convention in Atlantic City voted to start preparations for the formal organization in 1953 of a national student nurses' association under the sponsorship of the Coordinating Council of the ANA and NLN. In the intervening year a committee of nursing students and representatives of ANA and NLN worked on organization plans, and in June 1953, the National Student Nurses' association was officially launched. Bylaws were adopted and NSNA's first officers were elected.

In its first few years, NSNA had little money, a small membership, no real headquarters of its own, and no headquarters staff. Its main assets at the time were the persistence, determination, and dedication of its members plus financial and moral assistance from ANA and NLN. A year after NSNA's founding, these two organizations appointed (and paid) a coordinator to help NSNA function; much of the association's activities were transacted through correspondence. Each organization also provided a staff consultant to NSNA and helped finance the association's necessary expenses and publications. Among the latter were the bylaws and a newsletter. The next step was a headquarters office. Today NSNA rents its own office at 10 Columbus Circle, New York, New York 10019.

Even in its early years NSNA was able to help finance itself. And year after year, NSNA's share of the costs increased. Membership grew and annual dues, which had originally been fifteen cents per year, were raised to fifty cents in 1957. Finally in 1958— only five years after its inception—NSNA

---

*Because dues change, the current figure should be checked with the organization.

became financially independent. The original coordinator appointed in 1954, Frances Tompkins, became the executive secretary (later changed to executive director) and headed a staff of two. In 1959, NSNA became legally incorporated as the National Student Nurses' Association, Inc., a nonprofit association. Today the association pays for headquarters offices, a staff of twelve, and all the other expenses incidental to running the business of a large membership association. It holds and finances its own annual convention. And, at the same time, it has initiated and financed several important projects in the interests not only of its members but of the nursing profession as a whole.

General Plan of Organization

The policy and program of NSNA are determined by its House of Delegates, whose membership consists of elected representatives from the school and state associations. The delegates at each annual convention elect NSNA's three officers, five nonofficer directors, one of whom will become editor of *Imprint*, the official journal of NSNA, and a four-member nominating committee. Officers serve for one year or until their respective successors are elected.

Two consultants are appointed, one each by the ANA and NLN, in consultation with the NSNA board of directors. They serve for a two-year period, or until their respective successor is appointed. According to the bylaws, these consultants are charged with providing an interchange of information between their boards and the NSNA. All consultants are expected to serve only as resource persons, consulting with officers, members, and staff, and attending meetings of the association. In *Guidelines for Consultants/Advisors of Nursing Student Organizations*, published by NSNA, a summary of responsibilities states:

> It is truly the consultant's role to stand and wait for the student organization to grow by providing background information and encouragement, but not by providing decisions.

The decisions must come from the students themselves.[2]

The board of directors manages the affairs of the association between the annual meetings of the membership, and an executive committee, consisting of the president and two other officers, transacts business of an emergency nature between board meetings. There is only one standing committee (nominations), but the board has the authority to establish other committees as needed.

Constituent organizations may or may not function in a similar manner; their bylaws must be submitted to NSNA for review.

In 1976, the NSNA House of Delegates mandated a change in the structure of the association, giving school chapters the eligibility for constituency status and delegate representation. Under this system, school chapters must submit their bylaws to NSNA for review, and have fifteen members. Delegate representation is based upon the number of students in the school who are members. State associations who have two recognized school chapters and their own bylaws in conformity are recognized as NSNA constituents and are entitled to one voting delegate.

Projects, Activities, Services

NSNA carries on a wide variety of activities, services, and projects to carry out its purpose and functions. Even in its early years, the association sought participation in ANA and NLN committees and sent representatives to the National Conference on Citizenship and the International Council of Nurses (ICN).

Early projects were the Minority Group Recruitment project, (which has developed into Project Breakthrough) and the Taiwan Project.

The latter project, carried out in cooperation with the American Bureau for Medical Aid to China, grew out of NSNA members' interest in nursing students in other countries, coupled with a desire to assist whenever possible. After a firsthand report about the inadequate, overcrowded living accommodations for nursing students at the National Defense Medical Center, Taiwan, Delegates to the 1961 NSNA convention voted to raise $25,000 to build and equip a new dormitory for this group. By 1965, through vigorous fund-raising drives carried out on all levels of NSNA, the larger sum of $37,000 had been accumulated.

The completed fifty-student residence, named the NSNA Dormitory, was officially dedicated in March 1966, with American government officials cutting the traditional ribbon and representing both NSNA and the United States government at the ceremony.

Today, NSNA representatives sit on many committees of ANA and other health organizations. NSNA is also a leading participant in the recently organized student assembly of the ICN, and the NSNA president served as its chairperson during the 1977 ICN in Tokyo.

NSNA members are involved in community health activities, such as hypertension screening, health fairs, child abuse, teen-age pregnancy, and education in death and dying. Some of these activities are carried out in cooperation with other student health groups.

Project Tomorrow

Project Tomorrow is NSNA's career planning service for students of nursing. Since 1975, Project Tomorrow has been held each fall in selected sites across the country. Topics have included reality shock, decision making, self-assessment, and career planning. In conjunction with Project Tomorrow, NSNA has published resource materials on career planning.

Breakthrough to Nursing

NSNA has always been involved in recruitment activities directed toward interesting qualified men and women in undertaking nursing careers. In 1965, however, NSNA launched a nationwide project directed toward the recruitment of blacks, Indians, Spanish-surnamed, Hispanic, and other minority groups into the nursing profession.

Known as the National Recruitment Project, this long-term effort grew out of an increasing awareness on the part of nursing students of their collective responsibility for supporting the civil rights movement, for recruiting for nursing, for alerting young men and women in minority groups to the opportunities in a nursing career, and out of the recognition of the value of ethnic minority nurses in improving the care of their own ethnic groups.[3]

The national project was proposed at the 1965 NSNA convention by the 1964–1965 NSNA Nursing Recruitment Committee, whose recommendations were based on results of pilot projects conducted in Colorado, Minnesota, and Washington, D.C. The delegates voted to undertake the project on a national scale.

The project was officially defined as

focusing on the recruitment of Negroes and other minority groups into the nursing profession. Also, this project takes into account that nursing students have a vital interest in improving the position of Negroes and other minority groups in our society. Especially valuable volunteers in this project would be those students of minority groups. Not only would these students help in establishing rapport, but also would serve as an example that the nursing profession is attainable for all. This is truly a project for every NSNA member.[4]

By early 1967 the project was well underway in many different areas of the country, with the different state associations tackling the problem in various ways. In collaboration with other appropriate community groups—the Urban League, those associated with Head Start or other antipoverty programs, and civil rights groups—nursing students throughout the United States worked diligently not only to interest minority group members in nursing but also to help them financially, morally, and educationally to undertake such a career.

In 1971 NSNA set the Breakthrough to Nursing Project,[5] as it is now called, as a priority and sought funds to strengthen and expand the existing program. Later that year, NSNA was awarded a contract for $100,000 by the Division of Nursing, HEW. In 1974, a three-year grant was recieved from DHEW that expanded Breakthrough to forty funded target areas. The grant ended in June 1977, but students are still involved in Breakthrough to Nursing on a nonfunded basis.

The objectives of the project were (1) to develop and implement a publicity campaign to inform and interest potential nursing candidates in a nursing career; (2) to coordinate nursing student recruitment efforts with community organizations and schools of nursing in support of the program to reach more minority students; (3) to participate in recruitment program activities such as conferences, workshops, and career days focused on increasing the number of minority students recruited into nursing; (4) to work with public school counselors, teachers, school nurses, and other secondary school personnel to assist with the identification, motivation, and encouragement of disadvantaged and/or minority group students interested in a career in nursing; and (5) to inform the public and nursing community of the goals of the project.

In order to carry out these objectives, the involvement and support of nursing student volunteers, faculty, and heads of schools of nursing were essential. Student volunteers in Breakthrough areas carried out such activities as career fairs, education of school counselors, work with schools and community groups to provide tutorial and counseling services, development and distribution of brochures, help with the application and registration procedures in colleges, and provision of information about financial resources.

To raise the level of awareness of the need for minority nurses, a publicity campaign was developed using various media. A number of brochures, booklets, and posters are available for distribution nationally. Although there are still problems such as racial polarization, increasingly competitive en-

trance into crowded nursing programs, and retention of students after recruitment, there is no doubt that the project has had an impact on nursing, on NSNA members and the community.

Legislation

One of the most impressive NSNA developments in recent years is the active and knowledgeable participation of NSNA members in legislation. Excellent resources on the legislative activities on a national level and assistance and support in legislation provided by NSNA to constituent associations resulted in legislative committees in most states. During the crises of federal funding for health during the 1970s, students testified before congressional committees and supported the passage of the Nurse Training Act by active participation in the political process. They have also urged passage of the ERA and national health insurance. Students are also encouraged to work with state nurses' associations, state political action committees, and other groups on health legislation on the local and state level, and to educate members in such areas as state nurse practice acts and political activism.

Interdisciplinary Activities

NSNA has shown a forward-looking interest in the health and social problems of society, often combined with like interest in interdisciplinary cooperation. With the Student American Medical Association (SAMA), Student American Pharmaceutical Association (SAPhA), and the American Student Dental Association (ASDA), individual nursing students have participated in Head Start, Appalachian and Indian health, migrant health, and Job Corps projects. Unfortunately, federal cutbacks have reduced these nationally sponsored summer projects considerably. However, on the local level, involvement in Student Professionals Engaged in Education on Drugs (SPEED) and the OTC (Over-the-counter) Drug Project to educate the public to the dangers of over-the-counter drugs continues. NSNA was also one of the sixteen original sponsors of the well-received television film "VD Blues," carried by Public Broadcasting Service, and members helped answer phones at the local "VD hotline" the night of the broadcast.

Although NSNA members' involvement in interdisciplinary projects tapered off at the end of the 1970s, they are still actively involved in working with other health care professionals. NSNA is a member of the National Coalition of Student Professionals, which provides interdisciplinary communication and activities on the national level. The major joint student activity in 1979 and 1980, for instance, was the Student Coordinating Committee that worked in cooperation with Concern for Dying, formerly the Euthanasia Educational Council. Nursing, medical, and law students joined forces to educate professional students and others on death and dying. Programs were presented at each convention, with a major emphasis on the role of the nurse.

Other Professional Activities

Almost since the inception of NSNA, members have been invited to participate in the committees of ANA and NLN. Such participation has increased as NSNA has sought to take an active part in the debates, discussions, and decisions concerning nursing. Usually the resolutions of NSNA support the goals of the ANA and NLN, and, at times, they move ahead of the others in their acceptance of change. The support of both organizations is often asked on issues that require the support of nurse administrators, educators, or others. Some of the issues involved have been in relation to curriculum change, clinical experience opportunities, responsibilities of men students, education for practice, career mobility, and accreditation.

Scholarship Funds

NSNA administers its own scholarship program, giving scholarships ranging from $500 to $2,000 to its members. The Frances Tompkins Educational Opportunity Fund was established in 1969 to enable individuals and organizations to contribute funds to educate nursing students and others to study and understand the scope of present and future community health needs with a view to developing innovative programs. The fund is incorporated and has obtained federal tax exemption. Before funding for projects can be requested, however, a sufficient amount of money must be accumulated in the fund. Other scholarship monies are obtained from various organizations, and contributors have included both commercial enterprises and professional organizations. Scholarships available are the PRN scholarships, open to all NSNA members; special PRN scholarships, which may have criteria specified by the donor; and the Breakthrough to Nursing scholarships for ethnic persons who are NSNA members. Scholarship applications become available in the fall of each year.

Also under the aegis of NSNA is the Laura D. Smith Scholarship Fund. Each year the NSNA has awarded a $600 scholarship to a registered nurse who plans to matriculate for either a bachelor's or master's degree. The nurse may be a graduate of a diploma, associate degree, or baccalaureate degree program but must have been a member of the NSNA while in nursing school. This scholarship was established in 1962 in honor of Laura D. Smith, former senior editor of the *American Journal of Nursing* and NSNA adviser, who died in 1961. Application for the scholarship should be made to its administrator: Nurses' Educational Funds, AJN Company, 10 Columbus Circle, New York, N.Y. 10019.

Publications and Resources

Imprint, the official NSNA magazine, came into existence in 1968, and a subscription is given to members. Subscriptions are also available to other interested groups, schools, and individuals. Published four times during the academic year, as of 1979, a fifth issue will be devoted to career planning, the only publication of the kind geared specifically toward students. *Imprint* is the only nursing magazine edited by a nursing student, and students are encouraged to contribute articles and letters. Students may also take advantage of the annual Johnson & Johnson Baby Products Writing Contest, which offers cash prizes.

Other publications include the *NSNA News*, a newsletter that keeps organization leaders at state and school levels informed of pertinent issues and activities; the Business Book, which serves as an annual report and is printed for the annual convention; and informational, supportive materials on students' rights, guidelines for faculty evaluation, and guidelines for clinical evaluation. Most states and some schools also publish newsletters.

At the tenth anniversary of its founding, NSNA had accomplished a great deal.[6] At its twenty-fifth, it had become an involved group whose activities demonstrated committed professionalism.[7] Gone were the stunt nights and uniform nights of the early days. "Students learned to conduct meetings and to use parliamentary procedure, they showed concern about their education and their future practice, and they showed concern for others."[8] They were involved in many of the same issues as ANA and NLN and often seemed to show more foresight.

Education was of prime interest, and among the issues discussed were curriculum planning, accreditation and entry into practice, and student rights. Perhaps the last two were the most controversial. Since 1963, entry into practice has been discussed at conventions, and in 1967 the NSNA House of Delegates, comprised largely of diploma graduates, made the historic decision to support ANA's first position paper on education for nursing, calling for a minimum of a baccalaureate degree for entry into practice. This position was reinforced in 1976 and 1979, but, as early as 1969, NSNA delegates also encouraged the development and demonstration of nursing education programs that would recognize an individual's previously acquired knowledge and skill. For the next decade, convention resolutions called for pathways for career mobility for AD and diploma nurses.

As in other fields, nursing students have also fought for their own rights, and NSNA has maintained a commitment to student rights. In 1970, a guideline for a student bill of rights was distributed to all constituents, a mandate of the 1969 delegates. In 1975, a comprehensive bill of rights and grievance procedures were accepted and published.[9] The statement was adopted in schools throughout the country.

In the area of practice, students have taken positive stands on the concept of mandatory licensure, maldistribution of nursing manpower, national standards for practice, substitution of unlicensed personnel for nurses, and use of student nurses as a substitute for nurses. They have also supported economic security and in 1966 and 1975 supported the ANA position that in the event of a non-RN strike, students would not substitute for striking workers unless patients were endangered.

Finally, NSNA members have been involved in issues affecting the public's health, for instance, participation in projects to educate the public about the dangers of smoking. NSNA offers the opportunity for nursing students to be heard, becomes a forum for debate of health and social issues as well as nursing issues, provides opportunity for interdisciplinary contacts, and is a testing ground for leadership skills. Participation and involvement can be a meaningful and valuable part of the nursing student's education.

NSNA members, and students in general, have become more and more aware of their responsibilities and of the impact they can have. As new issues have arisen, especially during the past decade, they have not been afraid to face them and take a stand. They have not only spoken words, they have acted to carry out their beliefs. They have come a long way from the silent generation of the fifties.[10]

REFERENCES

1. National Student Nurses' Association, Inc., *Bylaws* (New York: The Association, 1978).
2. National Student Nurses' Association, *Guidelines for Consultants/Advisors of Nursing Student Organizations* (New York: The Association, 1972), p. 8.
3. Nancy Johnson, "Recruitment of Minority Groups—A Priority for NSNA," *Nurs. Outlook*, **14**:29–30 (Apr. 1966).
4. "Needed for Nursing: The Best Talents," *NSNA Newsletter*, **12**:1 (Dec. 1965).
5. National Student Nurses' Association, *Breakthrough to Nursing* (New York: The Association, 1973).
6. *NSNA's Ten Tall Years* (New York: National Student Nurses' Association, Inc., 1963).
7. "NSNA Today," *Am. J. Nurs.*, **77**:624–626 (Apr. 1977).
8. *NSNA '77: A Retrospective* (New York: National Student Nurses' Association, Inc., 1977), p. 12.
9. *The Bill of Rights for Students of Nursing* (New York: National Student Nurses' Association, Inc., 1975).
10. Robin Kriegel, "From the Silent Generation to the Involved Generation," *Imprint* (April 1978). Reprinted in *NSNA '77: A Retrospective*, op. cit., p. 15.

BIBLIOGRAPHY

Imprint is the best reference for reports of past and ongoing activities of NSNA, but both *AJN* and *Nursing Outlook* usually report on the annual NSNA convention in addition to news items and pertinent articles. Various publications of NSNA may be requested from NSNA headquarters. Some of these are cited at the end of Chapter 24.

American Nurses' Association

The American Nurses' Association (ANA) is nursing's professional organization, with membership open only to registered professional nurses. As such, it is the most significant of all organizations to which nurses may belong, because it is the one through which nurses decide upon the functions, activities, and goals of their profession.* The ANA serves as spokesman and agent for nurses and nursing, acting in accordance with the expressed wishes of its membership. ANA membership is voluntary and in 1980 totaled more than 170,000 nurses.

The ANA was established in 1897 by a group of nurses who, even then, recognized the need for a membership association within which nurses could work together in concerted action. Its original name was the Nurses' Associated Alumnae of the United States and Canada, but in order to incorporate under the laws of the state of New York, it was necessary to drop reference to another country in the organization's title. This was done in 1901; however, the name remained Nurses' Associated Alumnae of the United States until 1911 when it became the Ameri-

can Nurses' Association. The Canadian nurses formed their own membership association.

History shows the ANA's primary concern has always been individual nurses and the public they serve. Thus, in its early years ANA worked diligently for improved and uniform standards of nursing education, for registration and licensure of all nurses educated according to these standards, and toward improving the welfare of nurses. The need for such actions, and the difficulties involved, become apparent if one remembers that in the early 1900s many hospitals opened schools for economic reasons only, with no real interest in the education or employment of the nurses, and the public had no guarantee that any nurse gave safe care.[1] The ANA's efforts served to protect the public from unsafe nursing care provided by those who might call themselves nurses but who had little or no preparation. In recent years, the ANA has continued to give major attention to setting standards of practice and education, although the National League for Nursing has retained the accreditation functions for nursing education programs.

The ANA is now giving increasing attention to the welfare of the nurse, recognizing that the best nursing care can only be given

---

*For a comprehensive history of ANA, the best source is *One Strong Voice*, cited in the bibliography.

by nurses who find their working conditions a source of satisfaction, not of frustration.

Purposes and Functions

Throughout its existence, the ANA's functions and activities[2] have been adapted or expanded in accordance with the changing needs of the profession and the public. As a changed or changing major function becomes crystallized, it is incorporated in the bylaws by vote of the ANA House of Delegates. Thus, the purposes of ANA, as stated in the current bylaws, are to:

1. Work for the improvement of health standards and the availability of health care services for all people.
2. Foster high standards of nursing.
3. Stimulate and promote the professional development of nurses and advance their economic and general welfare.

These purposes are unrestricted by considerations of nationality, race, creed, life-style, color, sex, or age.

ANA's current functions, also as outlined in the bylaws, are further to:

1. Establish and enunciate standards of nursing practice, nursing education, and nursing service and to implement them through appropriate channels.
2. Establish a code of ethical conduct for nurses.
3. Stimulate and promote research in nursing, disseminate research findings, and encourage the utilization of new knowledge as a basis for nursing.
4. Provide for continuing education for nurses.
5. Promote and protect the economic and general welfare of nurses.
6. Assume an active role as consumer advocate in health.
7. Analyze, predict, and influence new dimensions of health practices and the delivery of health care.
8. Act and speak for the nursing profession in regard to legislation, governmental programs, and national health policy.

9. Represent and speak for the nursing profession with allied health, national and international organizations, governmental bodies, and the public.
10. Serve as the official representative of the United States nurses as a member of the International Council of Nurses.
11. Promote relationships and collaboration with the National Student Nurses' Association.
12. Ensure a national archive for the collection and preservation of documents and other materials which have contributed and continue to contribute to the historical and cultural development of nursing.

Membership and Dues[3]

The ANA is made up of state and territorial associations. The former are made up of district nurses' associations, the number within each state varying with its geography, population distribution, and other factors. The state or territorial associations are known as "constituent units" of which there are at present fifty-three: one in each of the fifty states plus the District of Columbia, the Virgin Islands, and Guam. These, in turn, have a total of 860 district associations. (State associations are frequently referred to as SNAs; districts, as DNAs.)

To become a member of the ANA, a nurse usually joins at the local level and automatically becomes a member of the state association and the ANA. However, there have been a number of membership projects allowing individuals to join at any level, not necessarily including the national. Some SNAs believe that this increases membership.

Direct membership in the ANA is open only to nurses residing in foreign countries or in United States territories or possessions where there is no constituent association. The basic membership requirement at all levels of the association is licensure as a registered nurse in at least one state (not under revocation for professional misconduct in any state). A graduate nurse from any for-

AMERICAN NURSES' ASSOCIATION
STRUCTURAL UNITS, NATIONAL LEVEL

1980

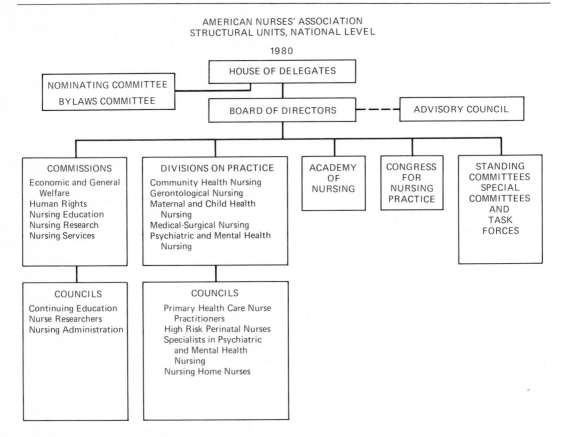

eign country who has been granted RN licensure is also eligible for membership.

Dues at a national level are set by the House of Delegates; a small amount goes to the International Council of Nurses (ICN). In some states or local areas, there is provision for installment payments or payroll deductions in the place of employment. (The latter is particularly common if the nurses are under a contract negotiated by the state association.) For those members in states on central billing, a bank credit card may be used to pay dues. Inasmuch as both the district and state associations levy dues for their support, the dues paid by the nurse with tri-level membership is a total of national, state, and district. The last two vary from state to state. Members in the special membership project states paid only for the levels to which they belonged.

Nurses not actively employed in nursing, registered nurse students in full-time study, new graduates for a first year of membership, and those sixty-two years of age or over who are not earning more than the Social Security system allows without loss of Social Security payments may elect to pay 50 per cent of the annual dues.

After due process, as described in the bylaws, members may be censured or expelled by the association and its constituents for violation of the ANA Code for Nurses or of the organization's bylaws.

General Plan of Organization

From time to time ANA's organizational structure undergoes some minor or major changes to enable the association to function more efficiently in the light of changing circumstances or needs. Some major changes were made in 1976 by the House of Delegates meeting in convention and are included in the following description of how ANA is organized and how it functions. Changes made in 1980 are added.

House of Delegates, Officers, Board[4]

The business of the association is carried on by its House of Delegates and board of directors. The House of Delegates, made up of a designated number of membership representatives elected by the state associations, is the highest authority in the association. It meets in convention every two (even-numbered) years to transact the association's business and to establish policies and programs. It also elects ANA's board of directors and officers, the majority of the members of its nominating committee, and some members of its commissions (to be described later). Thus, control of the association remains always in the hands of its membership.

Throughout the years ANA's House of Delegates has made many important decisions related to nursing and nurses. At many successive conventions, for instance, it went on record as supporting the principle underlying the legislation that eventually brought Medicare into being. As far back as 1946, it made several decisions designed to discourage discriminatory policies, in regard to nationality, race, religion, or color, within the nursing profession. In 1964 it voted to revise the bylaws so that ANA's responsibility for nursing education and nursing services might be more explicitly stated. In 1966 it adopted a national salary goal with a differential for nurses with a baccalaureate degree. In 1968 the Congress on Practice was created, re-emphasizing ANA's concern with practice. In 1970 even with the news that ANA was in a financial crisis because of mismanagement of funds and a consequent cutback of programs, the delegates resolved to recruit more of the disadvantaged into nursing, to help reduce the many threats to the environment, to become more deeply involved in health plan-

ning, and to develop closer working relationships with consumers of health care.

In 1972 some of the priorities set were directed toward defining requirements for high-quality nursing services, clarifying the scope of nursing practice, providing for continuing peer review, recognizing excellence and continued competence among practitioners of nursing, expanding and improving all aspects of education, and assisting SNAs with their economic security activities. Also adopted was an affirmative action program, which called for appointing an ombudsman to the ANA staff.

In 1974, convention action gave major emphasis to national health insurance, nurses' participation in PSROs, implementation of standards for nursing practice, certification for excellence in practice, reaffirmation of support of individual licensure (as opposed to institutional licensure), support of continuing education programs and a mandate to the ANA board of directors to establish a system of accreditation of CE programs and to study the possibility of accrediting other nursing education programs, efforts to effect direct fee-for-service reimbursement for nursing practitioners, the role of the ANA in collective bargaining, and a series of activities related to foreign nurses to eradicate their exploitation and assist in their becoming qualified to practice.

In 1976, the bicentennial convention year had a distinct historical focus in its non-House activities; fifteen nurse pioneers were named to the new ANA Hall of Fame. The House also approved a number of bylaws changes and passed resolutions on nurse advocacy for the elderly, responsibilities of nurses in nursing homes, alternatives to hospitalization for the mentally disabled and retarded, and involvement of nurses in health planning. The 1978 and 1980 Houses set as priorities for the next biennium: improving the quality of care provided to the public; advancing the profession so that the health care needs of people are met; enlarging the influence of the nursing profession in the determination and execution of public policy and strengthening the ANA so that it may better serve the needs and interests of the profession. Also approved were major resolutions on national health insurance, quality assurance, human rights, career mobility, and identifying, titling, and developing competency statements for two categories of nursing practice. These are all illustrations of the wide scope of House of Delegates' decisions and ANA activities and the directions in which the efforts of the organization are pointed.

In the intervals between the biennial conventions, the board of directors transacts the general business of the association. This is a fifteen-member body, consisting of ten directors and the association's officers; a president, two vice presidents, secretary and treasurer. Terms of office are planned on a staggered basis to prevent a complete turnover at any one time and to provide for continuity of program and action.

Serving to implement ANA policies and programs is the headquarters staff of more than 100, most of them nurses, and a supporting clerical and secretarial staff. They carry out the day-by-day activities of the association in accordance with the policies adopted by the House of Delegates and ANA's general functions. ANA headquarters, since 1972, is at 2420 Pershing Road, Kansas City, Missouri 64108.

Standing Committees[5]

Similar to other large organizations, the ANA has its standing committees, those that are written into the bylaws and that continue from year to year to assist with specific, continuing programs and functions of the association. As adopted in 1976, there are four such committees of the House of Delegates: bylaws, nominating, chairpersons, and ethics. These standing committees differ from what are called special committees, which are appointed from time to time on an ad hoc basis to accomplish special purposes. Special committees may be board committees or House of Delegates committees.

Except for the nominating committee

(elected by the House) and the Committee on Chairpersons* (consisting of the chairpersons of the Commissions Divisions and the Congress and chaired by a member of the ANA board executive committee), and committees of the Commissions and divisions, committee members are appointed by the board. Board committees include committee on committees, which makes recommendations for appointments on committees and task forces, finance, planning and budget, employee relations and membership committees.

Divisions on Practice[6]

Also established in 1966 were the five divisions on practice: community health, gerontological, maternal and child health, medical-surgical, and psychiatric and mental health nursing practice. ANA members may affiliate with one or two of these divisions, according to individual interests and in relation to the type of nursing practice they are doing. For affiliation with more than two, additional annual fees must be paid.

The purpose of these divisions is to enable nurses practicing within the same general clinical area to work together for continuing improvement of that practice. For instance, public health, occupational health, school, and outpatient department nurses could combine their skills and knowledge to advance practice within the comprehensive area covered by the Division on Community Health Nursing Practice.

The general functions of the divisions are that each one within its own clinical area will develop, evaluate, and revise standards for practice; conduct clinical and scientific sessions; stimulate research and disseminate relevant information to its membership; maintain working relationships and communication with other groups both within and outside the association; provide for recognition of professional achievement and excellence within each clinical area; and provide

---

*Eliminated by 1980 House vote.

for certification in nursing practice in the area of the division's concern.

Within each division, an executive board of expert clinicians is responsible for programs that assist the individual practitioner by conducting and participating in conference and study projects and by disseminating current information about clinical practice. A standards committee within each division develops and implements written standards for practice in the area of concern. A certification board is also appointed to develop the division's specialized criteria for certification.

The Congress for Nursing Practice[7]

The Congress for Nursing Practice consists of ten members, five elected by the House of Delegates and one member appointed by each of the five divisions. According to 1980 House action, the Congress for Nursing Practice created in 1976 was to be eliminated. Instead, a new Commission of Nursing Practice was to be added to the bylaws for a 1982 vote. Functions were intended to be similar to those of other commissions (as related to practice). Under the commission would be clinical practice councils.

Commissions[8]

Important in ANA's structure are five commissions: Nursing Education, Nursing Services, and Economic and General Welfare, created in 1966; Research, added in 1970; and Human Rights, added in 1976. The commissions, through their members, are responsible for the educational and delivery systems for practice, the enlargement of the knowledge base for practice, the economics of practice and health care, and the rights of nurses and recipients of nursing services. All establish the scope of the associations' responsibility in their particular area, act as consultant to other ANA/SNA groups, formulate policy and devise causes of action related to legislation. The general purpose of each is to develop and implement a program of activity designed to carry out its functions

and obtain recognition and acceptance of the extent of the association's concern, action, and influence in its respective area of responsibility. Each commission is composed of nine members, all of them with expertise in the field represented by their commission. The majority of the commissions' members are elected by the House of Delegates, with a lesser number appointed by the respective commission.

The Commission on Nursing Education is primarily responsible for evaluating relevant scientific and educational developments, changes in health needs and practice as they apply to nursing education, promoting research and implementing findings in all areas of nursing education, developing standards of nursing education, and devising methods for implementation and evaluation. The Commission on Nursing Services has similar responsibilities in relation to nursing services, as well as providing for recognition of excellence in practice in nursing service administration.

The Commission on Economic and General Welfare develops and implements general economic and employment standards, carries on economic education programs, and studies and evaluates the economics of health care and of nursing.

The Commission on Nursing Research participates in setting standards for protection of human subjects and assists in devising methods for implementation and evaluation, recommends priorities for the profession's research concerns, encourages and stimulates research in all areas of nursing, develops and implements a program to assist in the dissemination of research findings, and develops and provides for dissemination of research-related documents needed by the association.

Some of the responsibilities of the Commission on Human Rights are to develop the means by which the association can systematically focus on human rights as an integral component of comprehensive nursing care to all consumers; develop and implement affirmative action programs with structural units and constituent associations; devise and implement means to maximize both the involvement and viewpoints of minority members in association activities, standards, and publications; and determine priorities relevant to human rights and recommend appropriate actions to structural units and constituent associations.

Although the commissions must report to and are accountable to the board and the House of Delegates, the tendency of some to publish statements and positions considered controversial without board or House approval has periodically caused concern.

Special Councils

When the divisions on practice were first established by the House of Delegates, it was noted that further specialization was likely to occur, and it did. In 1971, the Council of Nurse Researchers was established; in 1972, the Council on Continuing Education; and in 1973, the Council of Nurse Practitioners in the Nursing of Children. In November 1977, the Councils of Pediatric Nurse Practitioners and Family Nurse Practitioners and Clinicians merged to form the Council of Primary Health Care Nurse Practitioners, and by 1980, the councils consisted of Continuing Education, Nurse Researchers, Nursing Administration, Primary Health Care Nurse Practitioners, High-Risk Perinatal Nursing Care, Advanced Practitioners in Medical-Surgical Nursing, Specialists in Psychiatric and Mental Health Nursing, and Nursing Home Nurses. Others are still evolving. It is hoped that by meeting the interest needs of nurses in ANA, they will continue their ANA participation even if choosing to join also one of the many other specialty organizations now available.

The decision to establish a council is made by the structural unit (division on practice or commission) to which the council will be accountable. Criteria, besides ANA membership, are determined by the new council's interim executive committee, with approval of the sponsoring unit's executive committee. Membership in the councils gives nurses

opportunities to explore common issues and concerns in their specialty, set standards of practice, and participate in scientific sessions and other educational meetings.

Other Councils

There are two additional councils designed especially for the purpose of facilitating communications and working relationships between ANA and constituent or related groups.

The Advisory Council* serves as a direct channel of communication between ANA and its constituent (state) associations.[9] This council is composed of two members from each state association and the NSNA (the president or an alternate must be one of them.) An executive committee, elected from among its ANA members, serves during the biennium to plan its activities, which are funded by a budget submitted to the ANA board. Meetings with the ANA board are held at least annually at a time and place determined by the executive committees of the council and the ANA board. The Advisory Council has no executive authority; it serves primarily as a communications medium and consulting body. At its meetings, state representatives have an opportunity to hear detailed and firsthand reports of ANA activities, present and projected, and an equal opportunity to present the views and opinions of the state associations in relation to these activities.

The Coordinating Council of the American Nurses' Association and the National League for Nursing is an important means of communication between these two closely related organizations. The council, comprised of the boards of directors of both associations, serves as a forum for discussion of different points of view, as a clearinghouse for activities of concern to both groups, and as an opportunity to consider and plan interrelated activities.

At one time the Council of State Boards of

---

*If the House meets yearly, as proposed in 1980, the council will be eliminated.

Nursing was also within the aegis of ANA. The Council had consisted of one representative from each state board of nursing authorized by law to license practitioners of nursing in jurisdictions where SNAs existed and was accountable to and funded by the ANA board. Among its major responsibilities were the development and regulation of the use of the State Board Test Pool examinations for RN and PN licensure. In 1978, however, the Council removed itself from the ANA and became a separate entity. (See Chapter 20 for current status and functions.) In part, this was due to the several rulings of the Federal Trade Commission citing restraint of trade when the professional organization of a group also has influence over the licensing of the practitioners or the accreditation of the educational programs. Although there was great resistance and dismay about this action on the part of the delegates at the 1978 convention, the separation was a fait accompli at that time. A liaison committee was then established between the two organizations.

Constituent Associations[10]

ANA's fifty-three constituent units are concerned with the same overall purposes as the national association but do not necessarily carry out the same functions.

Sometimes the efforts of the national and state associations are complementary to each other. In the field of economic security, the majority of state associations are prepared to serve as bargaining agents for the nurses within that state. But they do this against a background of guidelines, policies, and principles developed by ANA and learned through workshops and institutes sponsored by the national association.

State associations are also becoming more aggressively involved in state legislation, as well as responding to proposed legislation at the national level.

The district associations are the real grass roots of ANA. These units represent the association level that comes closest to the nursing practitioners, the people, and the

community. It is in the districts that the total membership of ANA works, serves its community, and finds both its satisfactions and its problems.

A nurse joining ANA should not underestimate the power of the district. The district is directly concerned with the local nurse's problems, both as an individual and as a nurse serving the community. The interested member has an opportunity to work toward solving those problems with nurse colleagues and other professionals in the area. Equally important, all the districts together make up the broad base of ANA structure. What is done at this level makes its way to the top and determines the major functions of the association. The nurse who cares about the profession will most certainly want to share in this process.

Academy of Nursing

A significant action taken by the 1966 House of Delegates was the creation of an Academy of Nursing to provide for recognition of professional achievement and excellence. Because of the financial problems of ANA in 1970, the Academy was not established until early 1973. At that time, thirty-six nationally prominent nurses were selected as charter fellows of the Academy by the ANA board of directors. Included were practitioners, researchers, academicians, and administrators from thirty-four states. Criteria for selection of the charter fellows took into account:

1. *Evidence of ability to contribute creatively to the advancement of nursing education, administration, clinical practice, or research.*
2. *Evidence of ability to perceive nursing in its broadest social and cultural aspects.*
3. *Evidence of ability to analyze facts, ideas, trends, and problems, to generalize and draw conclusions.*
4. *Evidence of ability to develop, evolve, and test theory.*[11]

Within its first year, the Academy members developed bylaws, elected a ten-member governing council, set criteria for admission of additional fellows, initiated a publication, took a stand on the differences between medical care and health care, explored the roles of nursing and other professions in health care delivery, the political influence of nursing, female identity, patient rights versus professional rights and power, and also urged that the effects of the ANA Standards of Nursing Practice be spelled out in quantifiable terms.[12]

The objectives of the AAN are to

Advance new concepts in nursing and health care.

Identify and explore issues in health, in the professions, and in society as they affect and are affected by nurses and nursing.

Examine the dynamics within nursing, the interrelationships among the segments within nursing, and examine the interaction among nurses as all these affect the development of the nursing profession.

Identify and propose resolutions to issues and problems confronting nursing and health.[13]

The members, designated as Fellows of the American Academy of Nursing, are entitled to use the initials F.A.A.N. following their names.

Potential fellows may be self nominated or nominated by a fellow in good standing (except during service on the governing council). After screening by the elected AAN Governing Council, a confidential ballot of names of candidates judged to fulfill the membership criteria is sent to all fellows. The Governing Council then lists the candidates according to votes cast and declares as newly elected Fellows those receiving affirmative votes from at least two thirds of the Fellows voting.

Criteria for selection of Fellows are as follows:

1. Member in good standing in the American Nurses' Association.
2. Five years of professional experience exclusive of educational preparation.

3. Evidence of outstanding contributions to nursing, such as:
   a. Pioneering efforts that contribute information useful in surmounting barriers to effective nursing practice of facilitating excellence in nursing practice.
   b. Successful implementation of creative approaches to curriculum development, definition of specialized areas for practice, or development of specialized training programs.
   c. Research or demonstration projects that contribute to improvement in nursing and health service delivery.
   d. Creative development, utilization, or evaluation of specific concepts or principles in nursing education, nursing practice, or health services.
   e. Authorship of books, papers, or other communication media that have significant implications for nursing.
4. Evidence of potential to continue contributions to nursing, such as:
   a. Efforts and projects that relate to contemporary problems.
   b. Efforts and projects that reflect broad perspective on nursing including social, cultural and political considerations.

The Governing Council may also recommend and the Academy approve the admission of Honorary Fellows in recognition of outstanding past contributions to nursing. There is a limit to the number of Fellows that comprise the Academy. Those who attain the age of 65 or 68 may elect emeritus status which allows for participation but not election to the Governing Council. Since 1973, the Academy has held a yearly Scientific Session combined with business meetings. The focus of these sessions has been on such topics as models for health care delivery, long-term care, primary care, and nursing's influence on health policy. The published papers are available from ANA and are included in the ANA Publications List.

MAJOR ANA PROGRAMS AND SERVICES

The programs and services of ANA represent the total results of the efforts of members and staff, elected officers, committees, commissions, divisions, and councils. These include meeting with members of other groups and disciplines; planning or attending institutes, workshops, conventions, or committee meetings; developing and writing brochures, manuals, position papers, standards, or testimony to be presented to Congress; implementing ongoing programs, planning new ones, or trying to solve the problem of how to serve the members best within the limitations of the budget. Every issue of the *American Journal of Nursing* and of *The American Nurse* carries reports of these many and varied activities. Presented here are brief descriptions of some (but not all) of the major ANA programs and services.

Nursing Services

The ANA works continually and in many ways to improve the quality of nursing care available to the public. In its role as the professional association for registered nurses, it assumes responsibility for the competence of its members and defines and interprets principles and standards of nursing practice and education. In 1965, through its Committee on Nursing Service, ANA issued its *Standards for Organized Nursing Services,* intended to serve both as a guide to the development of efficient nursing services and as a yardstick against which these services can be measured. In 1973 this publication was replaced by *Standards for Nursing Services,* developed by the Commission on Nursing Services.* The preamble states, "These standards are intended for use in any health care system to serve as guidelines for nursing service. The standards must be implemented with the understanding that there

will be ongoing evaluation and revision of the nursing service objectives and functions to meet the health care needs of society."[14] In addition, there are a number of other publications related to nursing services in general and to allied nursing personnel. Some of these are planned for revision, but are still basically pertinent.

An important paper that responded to concerns on nursing manpower was the 1978 report of a Commission Task Force on Development of a Policy for Nursing Resources, which identified five levels of nursing practice in the current nursing work force. In 1979 another task force developed a useful statement, "Characteristics of a Professional Climate of Administration and Practice in a Nursing Department," later added to the new (1978) *Roles, Responsibilities and Qualifications for Nurse Administrators.**

The formation of the Council of Nurse Administrators, first called the Council of Nursing Service Facilitators, increased the ability of ANA to serve the needs of this key group. (Because of ANA's involvement in collective bargaining through the SNAs, some nurse administrators have felt a conflict of interest and have chosen to belong to the NLN or AHA administrator groups.) In 1979, a two-level certification program for nurse administrators was initiated—one for those at the executive level and the other for those in middle management nursing positions.

ANA's concern for quality nursing care is clearly manifested by the practice standards with their implications for peer review, and the consequent action of ANA and many state associations to assist nurses to implement the standards. The *General Standards of Nursing Practice*[†] and standards in geriatrics, community health, maternal and child health, psychiatric and mental health, and

---

*It was revised again in 1979–1980.

---

*See section on nursing administration in Chapter 15.

[†]See Chapter 9.

medical-surgical nursing practice, published in 1973 and 1974, were the results of the work of divisional committees on standards. These standards, general enough to encompass the variety of practitioners within each division, are intended as models to measure the quality of nursing performance, another assurance to the public that quality care will be delivered. As the need for standards in highly specialized areas of practice were identified, various ANA divisions cooperated with specialty organizations to formulate standards. Examples are *Standards of Pediatric Oncology Nursing Practice*, 1978, developed by the ANA Division of Maternal and Child Health Nursing Practice and the Association of Pediatric Oncology Nurses, and *Outcome Standards for Cancer Nursing Practice*, 1979, developed by ANA's Division of Medical-Surgical Nursing Practice and the Oncology Nursing Society. The divisions and ANA councils also work together in setting standards.

Two of the key publications from the Congress of Nursing Practice are the *Quality Assurance Workbook*, 1976, and *A Plan for Implementation of the Standards of Nursing Practice*, 1977. These are part of the overall plan to asist SNAs and individuals in the utilization of the standards of practice. Many workshops, seminars, and other programs were also held to provide nurses with new knowledge to facilitate implementation and thereby improve nursing care. Major papers and/or the proceedings of these conferences were made available, particularly for national conferences, so that nurses who could not attend might still have access to the information.

Certification

Probably the most exciting development in recent years is the ANA certification program. This program was originally intended to recognize professional achievement and excellence in practice, both to help practitioners maintain motivation for superior performance and to provide another means to

establish and maintain standards of professional practice "to the end that all citizens will have quality nursing care."[15]

This concern for control of standards and improvement of nursing practice was manifested in the adoption by the 1958 House of Delegates of Goal Two: "To establish ways within the ANA to provide formal recognition of personal achievement and superior performance in nursing." In 1968, Interim Certification Boards began work with the Congress for Nursing Practice to establish criteria for certification. Action slowed during the period of financial crisis, but by 1973 ANA was completing arrangements for its certification program. Included was an arrangement with the Educational Testing Service of Princeton, New Jersey, to provide technical support in the development of systems for certification, including appropriate examinations. (ANA-appointed groups provided the content for these tests and ETS, the test development expertise.) By 1974, criteria had been fully delineated for geriatric nursing, psychiatric and mental health nursing, pediatric nurse practitioners in ambulatory care, and community health nursing. Any currently licensed registered nurse who could demonstrate currency of knowledge and excellence in practice, regardless of the basic program from which the nurse graduated, was eligible to take the examinations.

The first examinations were taken by approximately 300 pediatric and geriatric nurses in May 1973, but more than 5,000 applications had been received, attesting to the significance members attached to the program. Until then, the nurse had rarely been recognized or rewarded for excellent patient care; monetary rewards, prestige, and promotion had been via the administrative route or through educational achievement.

However, almost immediately several problems arose. Not everyone agreed that ANA was the best group to certify nurses. For example, both the American Association of Nurse Anesthetists and American College of Nurse Midwives expected to continue to certify in their specialties (although this is for admission into the specialty field). Other specialty nursing organizations also planned their own certification program. Most of these certifications were for a different purpose from that of ANA's, which was for excellence in practice. After several years of cooperation with the ANA in development of nurse practitioner programs and roles, the American Academy of Pediatrics in 1974 withdrew as an official participant in the certification of nurse practitioners because, "the academy's proposal of a pediatric nurse associate to work under physician direction in performance of both nursing services and delegated medical tasks is not supported by the ANA."[16] In addition, AAP proposed to begin its own certification program. Under the aegis of the new National Association of Pediatric Nurse Associates and Practitioners (NAPNAP), certification of pediatric nurse practitioners was initiated, this certification indicating that certain criteria had been met for entry into a nursing specialty. (This type of certification was more in line with the standard interpretation of certification, which is discussed in Chapter 20.) Some NPs already favored certification of this kind because it set a standard for specialty practice which was particularly important where the NP's legal status was unclear. It was also favored by employers over certification for excellence. In 1976, the ANA announced that it would certify at two levels: (1) certification for *competence* in specialized areas of practice with distinctive eligibility requirements, and (2) certification for excellence in practice, with diplomate status in a proposed American College of Nursing Practice for certified nurses who met additional criteria.[17] This proposal was given a hostile reception at that year's convention, largely because the new diplomate status called for a master's degree and many of those certified for excellence had no degree at all and little hope of acquiring a master's in the near future. With protest mounting, the diplomate proposal was put in abeyance and although those nurses who were already certified for

excellence maintained that certification, emphasis for the new clinical certification programs was on advanced specialty practice. Certification, then, was described as based on assessment of knowledge, demonstration of current clinical practice, and endorsement of colleagues, and was seen as a tangible acknowledgement of achievement in a specific area of nursing practice.

By 1980, certification examinations were being offered in thirteen specialty areas: adult nurse practitioner; clinical specialist in adult psychiatric and mental health nursing; clinical specialist in child and adolescent psychiatric and mental health nursing; clinical specialist in medical-surgical nursing; family nurse practitioner; gerontological nurse; gerontological nurse practitioner; medical-surgical nurse; nursing of the child/adolescent with acute or chronic illness or disabling condition; pediatric nurse practitioner; psychiatric and mental health nurse; community health nurse; school nurse practitioner. Exams for nursing administration were given for the first time in 1979. Examinations were and are given in various part of the country.

Criteria for certification vary to some extent for the various specialties but may include an examination and evaluation of specified documents submitted by the nurse such as pilot studies, projects, case studies, abstracts representing the candidate's case load, other evidence of continuing growth as a practitioner, statement of a philosophy of practice, references, and biographical data. In all cases, currency in practice beyond the requirements of licensure must be shown and the candidate must be licensed in the United States. Past practice experience is no longer required. (There must have been a practice component in the program of study.) Specific details on each certification, including eligibility criteria and cost, are available from ANA. Certification is granted for five years, at the end of which time the individual has the option of submitting evidence and credentials for renewal.

As of 1979, ANA and some of the specialty nursing organizations were making special efforts to cooperate in the certification process. Because certification is intended as a protection of the public, certification of the same type by several organizations is confusing. Various alternatives include joint sponsorship of a certification process or endorsement of each other's certification. Internally, the ANA Interdivisional Council on Certification works with all divisional certification boards to move toward agreement on certain commonalities in the entire certification process.

Nursing Education

The important ANA function of setting standards and policies for nursing education has been demonstrated in many ways. The 1965 "Position Paper" was the beginning of a series of specific actions toward implementing the position that education for entry into professional nursing practice should be at the baccalaureate level.* Because this will probably remain an issue for some time, one of the ongoing activities of the Commission on Nursing Education is to educate both the profession and others about the reasoning behind this position. Hearings, workshops, and various kinds of publications assist in the process. In 1979, for instance, the Commission held a series of regional hearings for dialogue with members and nonmembers.

The Commission has made a number of other important educational statements in the last few years; among them, the statements on graduate education, discussed in Chapter 13, and the statement *Flexible Patterns of Nursing Education*, which supports and gives a brief overview of innovative changes in nursing education at all levels. Of major significance is *Standards for Nursing Education* (1974), which delineates goals and standards (institutions, students, faculty, programs, facilities and resources, organization and administration) for AD, diploma and

baccalaureate education, as well as for continuing education.

The topic of continuing education has also been given considerable attention by ANA, gaining impetus in 1971 with the establishment of the Council on Continuing Education and the awarding of a grant for a project entitled, "Identification of Need for Continuing Education for Nurses by the National Professional Organization."* A series of publications on continuing education followed. Published in 1974 were ANA's *Statement on Continuing Education* and the *Standards for Continuing Education Guidelines* for State Nurses' Associations, which provided the rationale and responsibilities of the ANA and SNAs for continuing education. ANA endorsed the concept of continuing education for all nurses as one of the means by which they can maintain competence. ANA believes that maintaining competence is primarily the responsibility of the practitioner. Because of a practical and philosophical reluctance to transfer this responsibility to government, the association, by vote of its 1972 House of Delegates, opposed mandatory continuing education as a condition for renewal of a license to practice. This was reversed by the ANA House in 1974, and particular emphasis was put on SNA control rather than government control. The House directed ANA to provide support to those states that choose to establish continuing education as one prerequisite for relicensure, as well as to those states that choose to encourage continuing education through a voluntary program. Recognizing the need to assist nurses to improve practice, a list of responsibilities of both ANA and SNA and guidelines for carrying them out, as well as other related publications, were issued.[18,19,20,21,22] It was the responsibility of the Council on Continuing Education, under the Commission on Education, to aid in ac-

---

*This is discussed in some detail in Chapter 12.

*See Chapters 12 and 13 for discussion of issues in continuing education as well as information on continuing education units and accreditation.

ceptance and implementation. By 1979, most SNAs had some sort of continuing education approved programs. However, as nurse practitioner programs continued to proliferate on a continuing education basis, some type of accreditation of these educational programs was also adjudged essential. Therefore, the Council on Continuing Education and the (then) Council of Pediatric Nurse Practitioners held their first business meetings in 1973 to explore these concerns. In 1975, the Commission on Nursing Education completed details on a mechanism to approve nurse practitioner programs that are nondegree granting. Also formed was the National Accreditation Board for Continuing Education Programs and a National Review Committee for Expanded Role Programs. Then, acting on a 1974 House of Delegates directive, the ANA board of directors approved a fee schedule for accreditation of continuing education activities of state nurses' associations, organizations with approval processes, colleges and universities.

The system that was eventually set up in 1975 consisted of the National Accrediting Board (NAB) for Continuing Education, which established Regional Accrediting Committees and the National Review Committee. The latter at first accredited continuing education programs preparing nurses for expanded roles, but in 1980 the regional committees assumed this responsibility as well as continuing to accredit SNAs, university and college continuing education programs, and programs of national nursing and other organizations and state boards. The purpose of this comprehensive accreditation system was to allow such "accredited" organizations to approve the continuing education programs or offerings of applying sponsors and constituents, which would create some uniformity of standards since the ANA continuing education standards would be the baseline criteria.[23] The NAB has overall authority and responsibility for implementing, regulating and evaluating the accreditation system.

The process worked to some extent, with various groups seeking approval. A major breakthrough was the Federation's first position statement (unanimously approved by all organizations involved, as was policy), which endorsed the ANA accreditation mechanism. The variety of programs using the service can be seen in the most recent official listing of accredited programs/offerings, organizations, and expanded role programs.[24] However, because of the cost of the accreditation, the complexity of the process, and the amount of lead time required, some groups are seeking direct approval of the state boards in states requiring mandatory licensure, and some university/college programs are using their own continuing education accreditation, especially if the nursing program is NLN-accredited, which includes continuing education. The ANA or its divisions and commissions that give programs must seek provider status to meet the requirements of the state boards and of the National Accreditation Board. The issue of mandatory continuing education is on shifting ground, but the need for high quality in continuing education will always be important. In the next few years, the role of the ANA may expand greatly, especially because the Credentialing Study* has made some strong recommendations in that direction. The specific process for accreditation will inevitably change as needs indicate.

Legislation and Legal Activities

ANA's legislative program is an important one that often affects, both directly and indirectly, the welfare of both nurses and the public.† The association's legislative endeavors are concentrated on matters affecting nurses, nursing, and health, but in today's society these matters represent an

---

*The Credentialing Study, funded by ANA, is discussed in Chapter 5.

† For more information regarding legislation, see Chapters 18 and 19.

extremely broad area of activity, ranging from child care to gun control.[25]

ANA's legislative program comprises three main endeavors: (1) to help state nurses' associations promote effective nursing practice acts in their states in order to protect the public and the nursing profession from unqualified practitioners; (2) to offer consultation on other legislative measures that affect nurses; and (3) to speak for nursing in relation to federal legislation for health, education, labor, and welfare, and for social programs such as civil rights.

The first ANA Committee on Legislation was established in 1923 with the responsibility of watching federal legislation affecting nursing, representing the ANA in such matters. The ANA board also determined at that time to confine the association legislatively to matters of health, nurses, and nursing. Until 1970, when it was disbanded by House action, the committee formulated policy and recommended action. Since that time, the various commissions and divisions of practice have developed legislative policies, which are then referred to the staff of the Government Relations Program for consideration, and finally referred to the board for action. Legislative decisions are based on these policy statements, House resolutions, and, of course, on the ANA platform.

The major responsibility for coordinating legislative information and action lies with the ANA Government Relations Program. It was not until late 1951 that ANA opened an office in Washington, with one staff person to act as full-time lobbyist, and even then direction for the legislative program emanated from ANA headquarters in New York. From that time the Washington staff has expanded considerably, and their responsibilities have increased and broadened to include: lobbying (through its registered lobbyists); development of relationships with congressional members and their staffs and committee staffs; contacts with key figures in the administrative branch of government; maintaining relations with other national organizations; preparing most of the statements and infor-

mation presented to congressional committees; drafting letters to government officials; presenting testimony; acting as backup for members presenting testimony; and representing ANA in many capacities.[26]

Over the years ANA has represented nursing in the Capital on a number of major issues: funds for nursing education, social security amendments to cover nurses, national health insurance, quality of care in nursing homes, collective bargaining rights, civil rights, problems of nurses in the federal service, tax revision, higher education, problems of health manpower, and general support for improvement of health care. In addition, ANA lobbies for or against legislation that may affect nursing directly and immediately, such as funding for nursing education, collective bargaining, and reimbursement for nurses. For instance, ANA has always monitored the status of the Nurse Training Act (NTA), which has funded so much of nursing education and research. In 1973, ANA joined with NLN and other groups to gain release of impounded funds that had been committed to various health purposes, including nursing education. They won. In 1978–79, when President Carter, after pocket-vetoing the NTA, also attempted to rescind funds that had been assigned to various health professional educational programs, the ANA and other nursing groups led the battle against rescission. Despite many pressures from the White House, in a period of tight economy, the Congress was convinced that nursing education needed support, and nursing lost a smaller percentage of funds than any other health occupation or profession. Major newspapers and journals commented on "nursing's clout." It is important to note that as invaluable as the ANA Washington staff was with both its behind-the-scenes and visible lobbying activities, there would have been no success without the active backup of nurses, as well as consumers, labor, and other health groups. In this case, the largest volume of mail was from nurses, nursing organizations, and schools; some also visited or called home offices of congressional members.[27] Participation in the legislative process, as described in Chapter 18, is essential for nurses if the profession is to have any impact in influencing health policy.

ANA has often cooperated and coordinated with other health disciplines but also faced areas of disagreement (such as early opposition of the AMA and others to funding for nurse education). Such philosophical differences still occur, but there has been increasing cooperation with both health and social groups to achieve mutual legislative goals.

Communication about legislative matters is particularly important to help members keep abreast of key legislative issues. Beginning in 1955, *Capital Commentary*, first called *Legislation News*, was sent to state associations, schools of nursing, state boards of nursing, state boards of health, chief nurses in federal services, and selected individuals. The demand and the need became so great that now it is incorporated in the *American Nurse*. Prepared monthly while Congress is in session, *Capital Commentary* highlights major legislative and related developments.

Legislative information is also provided in the *American Journal of Nursing*, and special communications are sent out from the Washington office when membership support is needed for legislative programs. Periodically, discussion guides and manuals have been developed for the use of SNAs, and the Government Relations staff frequently participate in state and national conventions and other meetings. For many nurses, the real excitement is on a state level, particularly in the last few years, when issues of health care, health education, and especially new nurse practice acts have been the focus of legislative attention. State nurses' associations have a vital role in providing information and assistance to members on pertinent legislative issues, and, when funds allow, there is often a legislative staff, a lobbyist, and perhaps a separate legislative newsletter at the state level.

In addition to specific legislative action, ANA also becomes involved in various legal matters directed toward the welfare of nurses. In some cases, ANA acts as friend of the court, providing information about the issue involved, as in the Denver nurses[28] and the Manhart cases.[29] The latter has affected ANA's long-standing fight for equal pension rights for women employees. Since the Supreme Court ruled that the employer in the Manhart case has shown bias in requiring its women employees to contribute larger amounts to its pension fund than men, pending cases of a similar nature by ANA against certain pension plans were settled favorably. Since 1973 ANA has filed charges of discrimination in various district offices of the Equal Employment Opportunity Commission (EEOC), some of which it won and some of which are still unsettled. ANA has also presented oral arguments and briefs on various National Labor Relations Board (NLRB) hearings. The attorneys of SNAs also become involved in collective bargaining litigation or, at times, provide support for nurse practitioners cited by a medical board for practice of medicine without a license. Because of the increasing number and expense of such cases, in 1979, ANA established a legal defense fund to assist nurses involved in litigation concerning professional or sex discrimination issues, and donations are being solicited. The number of such services that ANA offers expands yearly.

Nurses' Coalition for Action in Politics

Important components of nursing lobbying efforts are the nursing political action groups. Most professional organizations have such groups, which are independent of the organization but related to it. This is because a tax exempt, incorporated professional organization such as ANA (or AMA) is under definite legal constraints as far as partisan political action is concerned. In 1971, a small group of nurses in New York formed the Nurses for Political Action (NPA) to serve as a political arm for ANA by providing financial support for candidates and engaging in other political activities, as well as providing political education to nurses. In 1973, ANA directed an ad hoc committee to explore the possibility of a political action committee. For various reasons, a new organization evolved: Nurses' Coalition for Action in Politics (N-CAP), which was officially organized in 1974 with a $50,000 ANA grant, as a voluntary, unincorporated, nonpartisan political action group. Since the initial grant, ANA does not fund N-CAP, but does appoint some members of the board of trustees. N-CAP has a single purpose: to promote the improvement of the health care of the people through the political route. Its two major functions are education and support. Education is directed toward encouraging nurses and others to take a more active part in governmental affairs and to educate them on the political process and political issues relevant to health care and to assist them in organizing themselves for effective political action. For this purpose, N-CAP has sponsored workshops and prepared educational materials, including a handbook called *Clout!* N-CAP has also encouraged and assisted political action coalitions (PACs) on the state level. Many states now have active PACs that primarily give attention to state issues but are also able to coordinate collective action on national legislation.

Support is offered to political candidates (regardless of political affiliation) whose acts demonstrate dedication to constructive health care legislation. This support may be in the form of endorsement or include monetary contributions. The first 189 candidates were endorsed by N-CAP in 1976 with contributions to fifty-eight totaling $30,000. Results were encouraging, both in terms of election of the candidates and awareness on their part of nursing's interests and influence. For the 1978 elections, 231 national candidates were endorsed, with $85,000 in campaign contributions going to 121, an indication of a broader base of political interest on the part of nursing. Endorsements were made in consultation with state PACs when-

ever possible.[30] Of the thirty-one active state PACs, about 90 per cent also endorsed state candidates. The fact that nurses, or at least ANA members, are perhaps more politically active than other citizens was shown by an N-CAP sponsored survey: 91 percent are registered to vote, 75 per cent have written a letter to an officeholder expressing an opinion, 58 per cent have attended a political meeting or rally, and about 58 per cent have contributed money to a candidate.[31]

To support these activities, N-CAP accepts donations. Nurses and others can become active members through contributions of $10 to $99, or sustaining members with contributions of $100 or more. N-CAP is headquartered at ANA's Washington Office: 1030 15th Street, N.W., Suite 108, Washington, D.C. 20005.

Economic and General Welfare

The ways in which ANA has worked to promote the welfare of its membership have varied with the times. When it was first incorporated, it gave as one of its purposes: "To distribute relief among such nurses as may become ill, disabled, or destitute." Today, thanks to an economic security program adopted in 1946 and steadily expanded and strengthened since that time, it works actively to ensure that nurses have a voice in determining their employment conditions, that nursing salaries are appropriate to nursing responsibilities, and that employment conditions are of the kind to enable nurses to give a high quality of care.

ANA's economic security program promotes the concept that nurses have a right to form a group to choose a representative to negotiate for them with their employer, and to have the mutually agreed-upon provisions put into writing. It endorses the constructive use of collective bargaining techniques in nurses' negotiations with their employers. Although ANA does not as a rule serve as bargaining agent for groups of nurses, except for some federal institutions, many state nurses' associations do so. ANA helps to develop the principles and techniques for such employer-employee negotiations and advises and assists the state associations with their economic security activities as much as possible. In addition, a major role of the ANA and the Economic and General Welfare Commission on the national level is to develop policy positions such as the 1974 statement on third party reimbursement for services of independent nurse practitioners and the 1979 statement on hospital cost containment. Because of its status as a collective bargaining organization, ANA must follow the requirements of the Labor-Management Reporting Act of 1959 (Landrum-Griffin Law) which affects voting rights and elections of officers.

ANA has been providing the state associations with varying degrees of assistance over the years, sometimes to the extent of supporting staff especially employed to work in state economic security programs, but this kind of help tends to be eliminated when the overall budget is limited. However, in November 1973, the president of ANA announced, "The association will commit substantial financial resources to support the constituent nurses' associations to bring about collective bargaining in each health care facility."[32] It was noted that ANA's previous collective bargaining efforts had been focused primarily on improving salaries, fringe benefits, and working conditions, but that now the thrust would be broadened "to improve the quality of nursing care, to assure the public of the individual and collective accountability of qualified professional nurses, and to increase accessibility of health care services for the public."[33] This was to be accomplished by nurses achieving the right to make decisions affecting them, their practice, and the quality of care.

Although this approach to collective bargaining might be considered new to individuals who think of economic security only in terms of salaries, fringe benefits, and working conditions, job action by nurses has often been in protest of inadequate patient care, which has not been improved by the employer.

The ANA economic security program is often misunderstood by members, nonmembers, and others. Seeing that the economic security of its members is maintained is one of the classic roles of a professional association, and, especially in recent years, economic security has been seen as extending beyond purely monetary matters and conditions of employment, to involving nurses in the decision-making aspects of nursing care. An example might be that, through an agreed-upon process, perhaps including a formal committee structure, nurses' objections to inadequate staffing or illegal or inappropriate job assignments would be instrumental in bringing about changes that would provide improved care.

In the last few years, the nurse's right to adequate monetary compensation has been recognized almost universally, although in many places, salaries and benefits are still abysmal, and there is still a struggle involved for improvement, with or without ANA representation as bargaining agents. However, there is even more employer resistance to allowing nurses a voice in policy making, both because of the possible financial impact and because of fear of loss of control, as well as on the basis of general philosophic disagreement.

One major advantage that employers in nonprofit health care institutions and government agencies had is that the National Labor Relations Act (NLRA), which provides the legal basis for collective bargaining activities, did not extend its protection to employees of these institutions. This means, basically, that the employer did not need to engage in collective bargaining activities or acknowledge the rights of workers to organize and elect representatives. If employees did organize, they could be dismissed; only if the individual state had passed legislation including these workers would they be protected. Since 1946, when ANA first called on its state constituents to represent nurses in collective bargaining, states have been active in varied degrees, often concentrating first on gaining legal protection.[34] Even so, the degree of SNA activity has varied depending on finances, staff, and the acceptance of the collective bargaining concept in specific communities. From 1963 to 1973, the number of state nurses' associations that have negotiated contracts increased from eight to thirty-two, and the number of nurses covered increased fivefold to 60,000.[35] Also in that time period, the ANA House made several major decisions in relation to economic security issues. In 1968, the ANA's eighteen-year-old no-strike policy was rescinded, and in 1970, the twenty-year-old neutrality policy (that nurses maintain a neutral position in labor-management disputes between their employers and non-nurse employees) was also rescinded.

The 1974 passage of the NLRA amendment to include employees of nonprofit health care institutions created a flurry of activity. In 1975, as the result of a legal brief presented by ANA, the NLRA ruled that a separate unit of professional registered nurses is appropriate under the normal unit determination criteria, and by early 1980, the professional organization was the largest collective bargaining representative of registered nurses employed in the nation. Also in 1975, the ANA board of directors established the Shirley Titus Award in recognition of individual nurses' contributions to the association's economic and general welfare program. Finally, the formation of the Commission of Economic and General Welfare in 1976 was a further indication of increased ANA membership interest and commitment in economic and general welfare issues.

The fact that unions, which have been successful in organizing nonprofessional health workers and a number of professionals, will inevitably look toward including nurses in a bargaining package brings some impetus to ANA/SNA activities. There is serious concern that unions, with strong economic backing and single purpose goals to increasing monetary and working benefits, may prove competitive, for nurses frequently do not see the professional organization as a strong, or even appropriate, bargaining agent. Because

past experience shows that unions have taken little action to negotiate contracts involving nurses in decisions that could improve patient care, and many nurses are not even aware that such participation is possible, one of the most worthwhile purposes of collective bargaining could be lost.

This trend for unions to organize nurses was accelerated in 1979 when the American Federation of Teachers started an all-out campaign to organize nurses and other health workers. At the same time, both the Wisconsin and Texas SNAs elected to discontinue their collective bargaining activities, both because of the cost and the fact that in Texas the conservative tenor of politics made organizing difficult and less than fruitful. How many states would follow suit was of great concern to ANA. Although ANA is designated as a union in terms of its collective bargaining role, it is a multipurpose organization, and funds must be divided among the programs according to the House of Delegates' set priorities. In the economic crunch of the late 1970s and early 1980s, it was difficult to serve all programs to the satisfaction of members—and economic security was one of the more expensive. Yet, given the lack of interest of most nurses in joining their professional organization, if they should choose a trade union instead of ANA to represent them, it is doubtful that they would pay ANA dues as well—a point that has already been demonstrated by those nurses making the switch. In that case, how could there be a unified voice for nursing?

In the years following the 1974 NLRA amendments, ANA and SNAs were frequently involved in legal actions regarding various aspects of collective bargaining that are unique to nursing: whether nurses could be in separate units, the status of head nurses and supervisors as management, and whether the fact that supervisors and directors of nursing may sit on the board of directors of an SNA means that the collective bargaining agent (the SNA) is controlled by management. As noted earlier, in action taken in 1975, the NLRB ruled in favor of professional nursing, stating that professional nurses possessed interests separate from those of other professional employees in the health industry and could form separate units.[36] The supervisor problem was met in one way by language in the newly passed Civil Service Reform Act in 1978 in which nurses were excluded from the classic supervisor definition—hiring, directing, assigning promoting, disciplining or removing employees—unless it was the preponderance of their job.[37]

On the negative side, however, in the Anne Arundel Hospital case (Maryland), a United States Court of Appeals for the Fourth Circuit ruled that the NLRB had exceeded its legal powers by certifying the Maryland Nurses' Association as the bargaining representative for a unit of RNs, because the local unit was subject to fiscal, policy, and administrative control of MNA (and thus the board).[38] In early 1979, in the Sierra Vista (California) case, the NLRB reached a decision stating that certification of a nurses' association as collective bargaining agent was not contingent on delegation of their authority to autonomous chapters of local bargaining units, which might mean that the CNA could serve as bargaining agent. These cases are not settled with one ruling, and frequently further action is taken through appeal mechanisms or legislation. For instance, in 1978, a bill was introduced that would define the term *supervisor* in a way similar to the Civil Service definition so that those nurses have the same rights as others to form collective bargaining units. Litigation on key issues can be long and expensive, but the carefully structured process of forming a unit also takes knowledge, effort, and sometimes legal consultation.*

Because ANA recognizes that other employed groups also have the right to organize, some guidlines have been developed in the event of a dispute between the employer and these groups. Nurses are urged to continue to perform their distinctive nursing duties; press for action in the interest of safe patient care to reduce the patient census; refuse to assume duties normally discharged by other personnel unless a clear and present danger to patients exists; and coordinate their activities and efforts through their local unit organizations and SNA, using established channels for intercommunications with management and the other employee groups.[39]

It should be noted that concern for the economic security of nurses is not limited to the American scene. In 1973 an unprecedented committee meeting was held jointly by the World Health Organization and the International Labor Organization to discuss urgent and radical measures to alleviate international problems of shortage, maldistribution, and poor utilization of nurses. A major objective of the meeting of health care experts from nineteen nations was to set viable recommendations for an international labor instrument covering factors influencing conditions of life and work in the nursing profession. Among the proposals presented were the right of collective bargaining, a forty-hour basic week, payment for overtime, two consecutive days of rest, and four weeks compulsory paid leave per year. There is belief that the meeting, initiated by the International Council of Nurses, will have positive long-range effects on nursing around the world.[40]

In 1975, International Women's Year, ICN also endorsed equal work, equal pay laws. But the issues are not easily resolved. At the 1977 ICN meeting, economic issues were discussed extensively, and in the 1979 meeting of the Council of National Representatives in Kenya, the subject of social and economic welfare affecting nurses was given top priority. Reports in the CNR meeting indicated that unions in many countries were attempting to represent nursing and control the profession.

Although the economic benefits gained through collective bargaining are obvious, the test of nurses' commitment to patient

---

*The steps in forming a collective bargaining unit are presented in Chapter 22.

care will come as they acquire the right to become joint decision makers in improvement of patient care—in how well and how fully they participate.

Human Rights Activities

ANA works toward integrating qualified members of all racial and ethnic groups into the nursing profession and tries to achieve sound human rights practices. From the time of its founding, ANA as a national organization has never had any discriminatory policies for membership in the association. Until 1964, however, a few of its constituent associations denied membership to black nurses. In these instances, ANA made provision for black nurses to bypass district and state associations and become members of ANA directly. At that point (1950) the National Association for Colored Graduate Nurses (NACGN) voluntarily went out of existence, on the basis that there was no longer a need for such a specialized membership association. At the same time strong pressure from ANA and the other state associations was exerted until now all state and district associations have discontinued such discriminatory practices, and minority group nurses are appointed and elected to committees and offices at district, state, and national levels. ANA has also strongly supported every major civil rights bill affecting health, education, public accommodations, nursing, and equal employment opportunities. In 1956, long before most health and professional associations had taken a positive stance on civil rights, ANA's board of directors adopted a statement supporting the principle that health and education should not be supported by tax funds if there are any discriminatory practices. Testimony along these lines was presented at federal hearings.

Even so, there was some feeling that more effort was necessary, and in 1972 the House of Delegates passed the Affirmative Action Resolution, calling for a task force to develop and implement a program to correct inequities. The program was defined as "a positive ongoing effort which is results-oriented and specifically designed to transcend neutrality. It was aimed at not only nondiscriminatory programming but action to correct past deficiencies at all levels and in all segments of an organization.[41] The overall objectives were similar to those of the current Commission on Human Rights. An ombudsman was also provided for and appointed.

The program went into action in 1973, and a task force of minority and nonminority members met with ANA units to identify problems and make plans. A minority position statement was developed, recommending methodology for change on such issues as problems of recruitment and retention of minority students, lack of data on career patterns of minority group registered nurses, and the need to include information in nursing education of the health needs of minority groups.[42] In the years that followed, several regional conferences were held on quality care for ethnic minority clients, and the papers were published.[43] A bibliography, *Minority Groups in Nursing*,[44] was also published by the Task Force in 1973, and an updated bibliography was published in 1976 after the establishment of the Commission on Human Rights. Both were a compilation of the literature on ethnic people of color, men, and people with different life-styles, in nursing, as well as other pertinent topics relating to minorities and the provision of health care to minorities.[45]

In 1974, ANA was awarded a six-year grant by the Center for Minority Group Mental Health Programs of the National Institute of Mental Health to establish and administer the Registered Nurse Fellowship Program for Ethnic/Racial Minorities. The program supported thirty-five minority nurses in doctoral study in psychiatric mental health nursing or a related behavioral or social science. A second fellowship program funded by NIMH in 1977 complemented the first program and supported thirty-five more minority nurses in obtaining doctorates in clinical psychiatric mental health nursing. These programs were sponsored by the ANA Commission on Human Rights and the Division of Psychiatric and Mental Health Nursing, respectively.

ANA's Human Rights Commission has been extremely active since its formation. Among its activities are human rights conferences and the initiation of a plan to produce monographs on historical and contemporary minority/ethnic nursing leaders. The Commission in general is alert to, and makes statements about, potential or actual problems in human rights, especially as related to minority groups. For instance, programmatic activities for the 1980 convention were developed around a unit assessment of all structural units and SNAs to determine the extent to which the goals and promises of the integration of the National Association of Colored Graduate Nurses (NACGN) and ANA had been achieved. The Commission also selects the candidates for the Mary Mahoney Medal previously awarded by the NACGN, for outstanding contributions to the cause of integration in nursing. The award has been presented at the ANA convention since the NACGN was dissolved.

ANA has taken positive legal action on minority rights, such as the Bakke case, and women's rights (salary and pension discrepancies). Since 1974 the ANA has taken a position in support of ERA passage and participates in various women's rights programs and activities. In 1978, the decision was made not to hold any major ANA meetings in states that had not ratified the ERA. This decision required a shift of the 1981 ICN meeting to Los Angeles instead of Kansas City, Missouri, for which Kansas City and the state unsuccessfully filed charges against ANA and NOW. There is no doubt that activities related to human rights will continue. It is important that the valuable services of all nurses are fully utilized and the nursing needs of the American pluralistic society met.

Research and Studies

In 1979 an ANA Department of Research and Policy Analysis was established to include the former Department of Research, the Human Rights Unit, the position of man-

power economist, and the Department of Statistics. The purpose was to provide a sound development of the research and information base to effect policy development for the entire organization and to continue to provide important informational services to members, the public, and ongoing projects and programs. This staff continually collects data about nurses, nursing, and nursing resources. One result of this effort is *Facts About Nursing*, published periodically, a statistical summary of information about nurses, nursing, and related health services and groups. The staff also carries out special surveys—of salaries and employment conditions, for instance—and through a contract with the U.S. Public Health Service, conducts a periodic inventory or manpower study of all registered nurses in the United States. Various governmental contracts may also be awarded. One major grant was a national survey of nurse-doctorates, awarded in 1978.

ANA is also the recipient of contracts to carry out specific programs, such as one funded by HEW for a continuing education program for registered nurses giving patient care in nursing homes, and another to develop criteria for measuring quality and effectiveness of nursing care in relation to participation in PSROs. These activities allow nurses to share input into the health care picture with other health practitioners. In addition, ANA, with financial assistance from the U.S. Public Health Service, Division of Nursing, has sponsored since 1965 national conferences for nurse researchers, a valuable means for the exchange and critique of nursing studies. As noted previously, the activities of the ANA Commission on Nursing Research are also geared toward identification of research needs and support of research in all areas of nursing. Liaison is maintained with appropriate groups, including the American Nurses' Foundation, separate from but closely allied with ANA.

The American Nurses' Foundation

The American Nurses' Foundation was created by ANA to meet the need for an independent, permanent nonprofit organization devoted to nursing research. It was an outgrowth of the ANA's expanding research activities, particularly the five-year *Studies of Nursing Function*, which was undertaken by ANA after the 1950 convention, both because of a mandate by membership nationally and as an assumption of the profession's responsibility to determine its own functions.

Initial financing of this project was provided by the state nurses' associations, but by the third year the ANA board of directors decided to finance the program from the association's budget. Between 1950 and 1955, twenty-seven studies were funded. *Nurses Invest in Patient Care*, a preliminary report, was prepared and published by ANA in 1956. *20,000 Nurses Tell Their Story*, by Everett C. Hughes, Helen MacGill Hughes, and Irwin Deutscher, was published in 1958; it was a synthesis of the findings of the studies.

So that such research could be continued and expanded, the ANA board recommended that the 1954 House of Delegates "authorize the incoming board of directors to secure information and to develop a foundation or trust for receiving tax-free funds for desirable charitable, scientific, literary or educational projects in line with the aims and purposes of the American Nurses' Association." After six months of committee study, the establishment of the American Nurses' Foundation was approved by the new board. It was incorporated in 1955 and tax-exempt status was approved in 1956. The foundation was organized exclusively for charitable, scientific, literary, and educational purposes. During the first three years, grants totaling $105,834 were awarded by ANF to nine institutions. These grants supported studies of the work of nurses in general and private duty, psychiatric nursing, outpatient nursing, and industrial nursing, as well as student nurses. The ninety-seven subsequent grants covered the subject areas of patient care, administration, education, and clinical research. Between 1955 and 1965, ANF received $617,000 from the Public Health Service and $156,000 from other foundations in support of specific nursing research and projects. Between 1955 and 1973, the foundation approved more than sixty-nine proposals, most of which were developmental grants, often awarded to doctoral candidates for implementation of their research projects. Almost half a million dollars was awarded for all the research grants supported.

During that time, the major objectives to which ANF gave attention were to provide financial support for research and to disseminate and to promote dissemination of research findings through publications, conferences, and other communications media. Through the developmental grant program, ANF encouraged and supported exploration of promising research ideas, development of research methodology, pilot studies, or perfection of specific research designs. Funds up to approximately $4,000 for one year were awarded for these purposes. Research grants were awarded for well-designed systematic studies not limited as to amount or time.[46]

Subjects selected for investigation ranged from basic science research with indirect applications to nursing to applied research in clinical nursing practice. Whereas role and function studies characterized earlier research, a shift gradually occurred toward study of nursing practice. It was also evident that over the years nurses were becoming more sophisticated in research. More than 70 per cent of the grants given were to nurses; in all studies, the majority of principal investigators were nurses. Criteria for review of proposals were scientific merit of the proposal, significance and relevance of the research to nursing, review of literature with knowledge of previous research in the area of study, qualifications of the researcher, appropriate research design and methodology, adequate facilities and instrumentation for conducting the research, appropriate budget for enactment of the research with provision for consultation if needed, and provision for publication of research findings.[47] Between 1962 and 1974, ANF also prepared research abstracts, usually published in *Nursing Re-*

search, and carried out studies at headquarters through grants received from other funding sources. In 1976, ANF received support from two large companies for support of a conference on nursing and health care administration. This conference was directed toward assessing the issues facing the organized delivery of health care and developing recommendations for educational and research policies in nursing service administration. The Robert Wood Johnson Foundation made a grant to ANF in support of the 1976 American Academy of Nursing's conference on primary care. The year 1976 also saw the initiation of two major programs. In the first of these, the U.S. Department of State awarded what became three-year funding for the establishment of an international communications network. Purposes of the network were to establish links among nursing leaders in foreign countries and to facilitate services that nurses in the United States can provide their counterparts in third-world countries. The third year of the grant supported three crosscultural studies, three regional workshops in this country, and participation of ANF representatives in a conference of European nurse researchers in the Netherlands and in a conference on health care in Togo, West Africa. In the second program, begun in 1976, nurses in Kansas City implemented the "Know Your Body" project of the American Health Foundation in four local school districts, working with 2,100 junior high school students. This project, which includes education, screening, and intervention, will yield epidemiological and clinical research data for further exploration. The intervention aspects of the program are also yielding opportunities to expand the role of nursing and to implement wellness concepts.

In 1979, the ANF board established major new objectives focusing on analysis of health policy issues of priority to nursing, support for the career development of nurses, and assistance to the educational and research activities of ANA. Within the context of the first objective, ANF planned to raise the necessary funding by preparing grant proposals for public and private sources of funding. Within the second, small grant funding was to be continued, with an enlargment of research activities to include both clinical and nonclinical studies. (The same selection criteria would apply.) The third objective was seen as enabling the ANF staff to obtain funding and providing consultation to groups within the association that wished to initiate research projects. These could result in publications leading to greater visibility for nursing.[48]

Most of the foundation's publications are reports of studies it has supported or conducted. A major publication for the time was the *International Directory of Nurses with Earned Doctoral Degrees*, published in 1973 and listing 1,019 nurses from nineteen countries. This directory contains updated information from the first 1969 directory and the three supplements published in *Nursing Research*, as well as several hundred new names. *Nursing Research Report*, published periodically since 1966, usually features reports on studies supported or conducted by the foundation.

Obviously, funding is of vital concern to ANF. Unfortunately, the foundation never attained a stable financial base. In 1959, in order to establish a strong base upon which to operate, the foundation launched a nationwide drive for funds, enlisting support from the nursing community, the business community, and the general public. When the campaign closed officially in 1964, three quarters of a million dollars had been raised. Since then, there have been a number of efforts to reach potential donors, including others in the health field. Many individuals, nursing institutions, and other groups give spontaneously, sometimes in the form of memorial gifts or as bequests. All are tax deductible. However, increased funding is necessary to maintain and expand programs, and in 1979, another major fund drive was initiated, spurred by a matching fund offer of the American Journal of Nursing Company.

ANF is governed by its bylaws and directed by a nine-member board of trustees. All trustees are registered nurses. A finance committee and a research advisory committee report to the board of trustees. The finance committee monitors budget preparation, the investment portfolio, and fundraising activities. The research advisory committee establishes guidelines for administering the small grant program and recommends recipients to the board for final approval. In 1978, the executive director of ANA was appointed as part-time executive director of ANF. There is also a professional headquarters staff involved in carrying out certain research projects.

Requests for information about completed ANF research projects or applications for grants (which should include an outline of the research question and the proposed design) may be sent to ANF headquarters at 2420 Pershing Road, Kansas City, Missouri 64108.

Communications

The ANA's professional journal, the *American Journal of Nursing*, published monthly by the American Journal of Nursing Company, which is owned by ANA, is available to ANA members at a reduced rate. Because ANA is the sole stockholder of the AJN Company (see Chapter 29), the ANA board of directors "votes the stock" to choose the directors of the board of the AJN Company. The association publishes *The American Nurse*, a free newspaper and ANA's official organ, which reports ANA activities and happenings important to nursing. Divisions, councils, and commissions may also publish newsletters as funds permit.

Other publications include *Facts About Nursing;* various surveys, such as the *1977 National Sample Survey of Registered Nurses;* major reports, such as *The Study of Credentialing in Nursing: A New Approach;* its biennial *Reports to the ANA House of Delegates* and *Summary Convention Proceedings;* papers presented at meetings; and certain publications of the AAN and ANF. The association also publishes position statements, guidelines for practice, bulletins,

manuals, and brochures for specialized groups within the organization and sends out news releases and announcements concerning activities of interest to the public. Available from the ANA upon request is its periodically revised *Publications*. This listing includes ANA's own publications, reprints of *American Journal of Nursing* articles pertinent to ANA programs, and other publications.

ANA's communications department carries a large share of the responsibility for many of these publications. This department also conducts a continuing educational and informational service to interpret ANA's activities, programs, and goals to nurses, allied groups, government, special agencies, and the public, and monitors news and public opinion trends affecting the profession.

The ANA-sponsored "Year of the Nurse," April 1977 to June 1978, with the slogan, "Qualified to Care," received national attention with acknowledgement by President Carter, the Congress, and state and local governments, as well as the media. It was intended to show the American public the new image of the nurse. In 1979, the International Year of the Child, ANA hearings across the country on the needs of children and youth also received favorable national attention.

ANA Participation with Other Groups

Cooperation and coordination with other groups is an important part of the function of ANA. Conferences, programs, workshops, task forces, and other meetings to share information and learning, or work on mutual problems are ongoing with other nursing, medical, and health organizations, hospital and health professional groups, and many others.

Participation of nurses, usually ANA members, in governmental planning and action groups is the result of concerted ANA efforts and carefully developed relationships with other groups and organizations. Examples of some of these activities are the joint conferences between the ANA and the National Foundation, March of Dimes, in 1975; joint statements, such as that by the Inter-professional Task Force on Health Care of Women and Children (including other nursing organizations and medical groups) on family-centered birthing (1978); the establishment of a Nursing Practice Advisory Panel in 1979 by the United States Pharmacopeial Convention and the ANA Congress for Nursing Practice; and, also in 1979, a larger conference on Rural Health, sponsored by twelve groups.

An especially useful participative activity was the National Joint Practice Committee, described in Chapter 27. Interaction with other organizations or consultation requests by government or other groups brings considerable visibility to nurses. For instance, the final report of the U.S. Senate subcommittee dealing with long-term care needs (1975) spotlighted the ANA recommendations.

One breakthrough that has not yet been forthcoming is ANA membership in the Joint Commission for the Accreditation of Hospitals (JCAH). In 1977, for the sixth time in eight years, ANA was denied membership on the Accreditation Council for Long-Term Care Facilities. It was opposed by two of the four members of the council, the American Medical Association, and the American Health Care Association (consisting primarily of proprietary nursing home owners). The American Hospital Association and the American Association of Homes for the Aging supported ANA membership, but unanimous agreement was necessary.[49] ANA has participated, through individually appointed members, in various aspects of JCAH accreditation, but has never succeeded in getting membership on either the commission board or on any council.[50]

The JCAH situation demonstrates a somewhat universal reluctance to share power, but coordination of activities and sharing of information are seen by others as ways to increase power and to function more effectively, particularly in legislative activities. Much misunderstanding between groups oc-

curs because of a lack of clear understanding of the goals and attitudes of each. ANA has spent considerable effort in fostering relationships. Besides such formally established communicating/coordinating groups as those between the Council of State Boards, the AMA,* the NSNA,* the NLN,* the NFLPN,* and the AACN,* ANA staff and members relate to or meet with some 200 organizations and groups.

International Activities

ANA was one of the three charter members of the International Council of Nurses (ICN) and is an active participant in the work of this international nursing organization. Essentially, ICN is a federation of national associations of professional nurses (one from each country), and ANA is the member association for the United States (see Chapter 28). ANA also supports United Nations' programs.

ANA is particularly interested in seeing that nurses who come to the United States to work are qualified by education and experience to take and pass a licensing examination in this country and that they do not come in response to misleading advertisements or unethical employment inducements. ANA attempts to establish safeguards to be sure that nurses from other countries meet minimum qualifications for employment in this country to forestall lowering of standards of nursing care in American hospitals. In light of an increased influx of foreign nurses into the United States, the tighter economic situation for American nurses, an increased demand for nurses with advanced education, and the tendency of some state legislatures to lower qualifications standards for foreign nurses, a resolution was passed at the 1974 convention for ANA to work with the federal agencies to develop screening tests for foreign nurses, to work to eradicate unethical, exploitive recruitment, to encourage international standards for licensure, and to

---

*These oranizations are described in Chapters 24, 26, and 27.

assist unlicensed nurses to become qualified for licensure. (At one time, ANA had developed guidelines for agencies that had exchange visitor programs to avoid exploitation of foreign nurses coming for educational purposes. The association is no longer involved in these programs, in part because exploitation was almost impossible to control.) Earlier ANA was requested by the Bureau of Health Manpower Education to obtain statistical and descriptive data on foreign nurse graduate applicants for RN licensure in the United States. The problems were reaffirmed. One of the results was the formation of the Commission on Graduates of Foreign Nursing Schools (CGFNS),* which set up a system of qualifying examinations for foreign nurses. Some of these actions have met resistance from certain employers, although ANA and AHA representatives, meeting in joint session concerning the foreign nurse issue, agreed on the necessity to maintain standards. A group of Filipino nurses in 1979 filed a suit charging discrimination against them because of the new demand by state boards for the foreign nurse to take the CGFNS examinations.

ANA continues to encourage international contacts and activities, such as the first ANA Trans-Pacific Nursing Conference held in Australia in 1976 and the formation of the Advisory Committee on Vietnamese Nursing Personnel in 1975, requested by the White House and the U.S. Department of State.

Other Activities and Services

Among other ANA benefits for nurses, insurance of various kinds, such as disability income protection, life, hospital supplemental, dental, cancer, major medical, and professional liability protection (malpractice), is available at favorable group rates at national and state levels. Vacation tours or seminar-vacation tours provide not only budget rates but the companionship of other nurses.

*See Chapter 27.

Some state or local associations have group discount purchasing arrangements.

Many educational programs, seminars, workshops, clinical conferences, scientific sessions, and so on, are available at all levels at reduced rates for ANA members. They are geared to current issues and new developments in health and nursing and are available without cost or for minimum fees.

The Individual Nurse and ANA

A classic article by sociologist Robert Merton cites the functions of any professional organization as including social and moral support for the individual practitioner to help him perform his role as a professional, to set rigorous standards for the profession and help enforce them, to advance and disseminate research and professional knowledge, to help furnish the social bonds through which society coheres, and to speak for the profession.[51] In carrying out some of these functions, the association is seen as a "kind of organizational gadfly, stinging the profession into new and more demanding formulations of purpose."[52] Not all members agree with their organization's goals, and the difficult task of achieving a flexible consensus of values and policies must be accomplished, with full two-way communication between the constituences and the organizational top. However, the key to success of any organization is the participation of its actual and potential members. This review of the American Nurses' Association and its activities is at best an overview. As needs of members and demands of society require, changes occur, rapidly, inevitably, and, it is hoped, appropriately—but not always easily. The best way for a nurse to keep up with, and share in, the changes taking place is through active ANA membership. The American Nurses' Association speaks for nurses; nonmembers have no part in that voice and have no right to complain if it is not representing them. The strength in the organization and in nursing lies in thinking, communicating nurses committed to the goal of improving nursing care for the public and working together in an organized fashion to achieve this goal.

REFERENCES

1. Teresa Christy, "The First Fifty Years," *Am. J. Nurs.*, 71:1788 (Sept. 1971).
2. American Nurses' Association, *Bylaws* (Kansas City, Mo.: The Association, 1978), pp. 5, 6.
3. Ibid., pp. 6–8.
4. Ibid., pp. 9–13.
5. Ibid., pp. 13–15.
6. Ibid., pp. 15–18.
7. Ibid., pp. 18–19.
8. Ibid., pp. 19–23.
9. Ibid., p. 27.
10. Ibid., pp. 26–27.
11. Press release, ANA, "National Academy of Nursing Launched by ANA," Feb. 6, 1973.
12. "Academy President Says Medical, Health Care Differ," *Am. Nurse*, 5:3 (Dec. 1973).
13. American Academy of Nursing, *Bylaws* (Kansas City, Mo.: The Academy, 1978), p. 1.
14. American Nurses' Association, *Standards for Nursing Services* (Kansas City, Mo.: The Association, 1973).
15. American Nurses' Association, *ANA Certification* (Kansas City, Mo.: The Association, 1973).
16. "Pediatricians Withdraw Unilaterally from ANA Certification Program," *Am. J. Nurs.*, 74:387–389 (Mar. 1974).
17. "New Certification Approach to be Initiated," *Am. Nurse*, 8:1 (June 1, 1976).
18. American Nurses' Association, *Standards for Continuing Education in Nursing* (Kansas City, Mo.: The Association, 1975).
19. American Nurses' Association, *Continuing Education in Nursing: Guidelines for State Voluntary and Mandatory Systems* (Kansas City, Mo.: The Association, 1975).
20. American Nurses' Association, *Self-Directed Continuing Education in Nursing* (Kansas City, Mo.: The Association, 1978).
21. American Nurses' Association, *Guidelines for Continuing Education in Developmental Disabilities* (Kansas City, Mo.: The Association, 1978).
22. American Nurses' Association, *Continuing Education in Nursing: An Overview* (Kansas City, Mo.: The Association, 1979).
23. American Nurses' Association, *Accreditation of Continuing Education in Nursing* (Kansas City, Mo.: The Association, 1975).
24. American Nurses' Association, *Directory of Accredited Organizations, Approved Programs/Offerings, and Accredited Continuing Education Certificate Programs Preparing Nurse Practitioners* (Kansas City, Mo.: The Association, 1980).
25. Julia Thompson, *ANA in Washington* (Kansas City, Mo.: American Nurses' Association, 1972).
26. Ibid., pp. 7–8.
27. "Magazine Cites ANA Lobbying," *Am. Nurse*, 11:2 (Apr. 20, 1979).
28. "Denver RNs Appeal Judicial Decision on Pay-Scale Suit," *Am. J. Nurs.*, 78:957–964 (June 1978).
29. "Manhart Decision May Affect ANA Fight To Eliminate Sex Bias in Pensions," *Am. J. Nurs.*, 78:962 (June 1978).
30. "231 N-CAP Endorsements for November 7 Election," *Am. Nurse*, 10:1, 16 (Oct. 15, 1978).
31. "Nurses Politically Concerned and Active, Study of Voting Habits Reveals," *Am. J. Nurs.*, 79:1181, 1194 (July 1979).
32. "Campaign Launched to Organize RNs," *Am. Nurse*, 5:1 (Dec. 1973).
33. Ibid., p. 10.
34. Barbara Schutt, "Collective Action for Professional Security," *Am. J. Nurs.*, 73:1947 (Nov. 1973).
35. Ibid., pp. 1946–1947.
36. "NLRB Rules on Nursing's Community of Interest," *Am. Nurse*, 7:1 (June 1975).
37. " 'Supervisor' Language is Clarified in Civil Service Act," *Am. J. Nurs.*, 78:2001 (Dec. 1978).
38. "Fourth Circuit Court Rules on Anne Arundel Hospital Case," *Am. Nurse*, 9:1 (Nov 15, 1977).
39. American Nurses' Association, *ANA's*

Economic and General Welfare Program: Philosophy, Goals, Policies, Positions (Kansas City, Mo.: The Association, 1975).

40. "International Guidelines for Nurses Urged," *Am. Nurse,* 6:6 (Feb. 1974).

41. "Affirmative Action Projects Launched," *Am. Nurse,* 5:1 (May 1973).

42. Ibid.

43. American Nurses' Association, *Affirmative Action: Toward Quality Nursing Care for a Multiracial Society* (Kansas City, Mo.: The Association, 1976).

44. American Nurses' Association, *Minority Groups in Nursing: A Selected Bibliography* (Kansas City, Mo.: The Association, 1973).

45. American Nurses' Association, *Minority Groups in Nursing, 1976: A Bibliography* (Kansas City, Mo.: The Association, 1976).

46. Susan Taylor, "American Nurses' Foundation, 1955–1970," *Nurs. Res. Rep.,* 5: 1–3 (Dec. 1970).

47. Martha Pitel, "An Overview of ANF-Supported Research 1955–1971," *Nurs. Res. Rep.,* 7:1, 4 (Mar. 1972).

48. "ANF Board Adopts New Focus for Programming," *Am. Nurse,* 10:1, 9 (Aug. 15, 1978).

49. "ANA Denied Membership on JCAH Council," *Am. Nurse,* 9:1,5 (Jan. 15, 1977).

50. "ANA Pursues Membership on JCAH Board," *Am. Nurse,* 8:3,10 (Oct. 15, 1976).

51. Robert Merton, "The Functions of the Professional Association," *Am. J. Nurs.,* 58:50–54 (Jan. 1958).

52. Ibid.

BIBLIOGRAPHY

"A Working Day for ANA's Washington Lobbyists," *Am. J. Nurs.,* 78 (Sept. 1978), 1434–1435. Pictures and text of how these lobbyists work.

"American Nurses' Association's First Position on Education for Nursing," *Am. J. Nurs.,* 65 (Dec. 1965), 106–111. Definitive statement on education for professional and technical nursing, including rationale, implications, and conclusions.

Erickson, Eva. "Collective Bargaining: An Inappropriate Technique for Professionals." *J. Nurs. Admin.,* 3 (Mar./Apr. 1973), 54–58. Reprinted from *Nurs. Forum,* 10(3) (1971). Argues that in a profession, decisions for action are placed on the individual; in collective bargaining, they are designated by the contract.

Flanagan, Lyndia. *One Strong Voice: The Story of the American Nurses' Association.* Kansas City, Mo.: American Nurses' Association, 1976. The best available reference on ANA. Includes historical data not easily found elsewhere, a brief account of ANA in relation to other significant activities between 1896 and 1976, the various proposals for joint or interrelated organizations, and major addresses of all ANA presidents through 1979.

Grand, Norma. "Nursing Ideologies and Collective Bargaining." *J. Nurs. Admin.,* 3 (Mar./Apr. 1973), 29–32. Explains the ANA rationale for the economic and general welfare program.

Hopping, Betty. "Professionalism and Unionism: Conflicting Ideologies." *Nurs. Forum,* 15(4) (1976), 373–383. Compares the two ideologies, concluding that they are in contradiction. Good references and bibliography.

"Illustrious Past, Challenging Future," *Am. J. Nurs.,* 71 (Sept. 1971), 1773–1775. Illustrated article on history of ANA and predictions for the future.

Jacox, Ada. "Who Defines and Controls Nursing Practice?" *Am. J. Nurs.,* 69 (May 1969), 977–982. Study has become a classic of one mass resignation, the attitudes of nurse administrators, those who resigned and those who did not. Author urges collective action by nurses for control of their profession.

La Monica, Elaine, and Fanny Siegel. "A Professional Organization That Helps All of Us." Barbara Nichols. "ANA: A Multipurpose, Representative Professional Organization." *J. Nurs. Admin.,* 9 (May 1979), 16–21. First authors suggest change in services to include consultation to individuals and groups; rebuttal by ANA president reaffirms role and effectiveness of ANA but leaves door open for initiation of structural changes.

Minor, Irene, and Ethelrine Shaw. "ANA and Affirmative Action." *Am. J. Nurs.,* 73 (Oct. 1973), 1738–1739. Report of how ANA is moving to fulfill its promises of equal opportunity for minority group nurses and development of programs relevant to the health care of minority groups.

"Nurses, Nursing, and the ANA." *Am. J. Nurs.*, **70** (Apr. 1970), 808–815. An ANA survey describes some of the AJN subscribers' feelings about nursing, nurses, and the ANA.

Schutt, Barbara. "Collective Action for Professional Security," *Am. J. Nurs.*, **73** (Nov. 1973), 1946–1951. A survey of the status of economic security activity in nursing. Good background information.

Scott, William C., Elizabeth K. Porter, and Donald W. Smith. "The Long Shadow," *Am. J. Nurs.*, **66** (Mar. 1966), 538–543. The clause in the Taft-Hartley Act exempting nonprofit hospitals from the obligation to bargain collectively with their employees has seriously impeded progress of ANA economic security program. The efforts of ANA to repeal this provision are chronicled.

Thompson, Julia. *The ANA in Washington.* Kansas City, Mo.: American Nurses' Association, 1972. A brief history of the federal legislative concerns and activities of the ANA during the last twenty years. Includes summary of various other federal legislative activities of interest to nurses.

See also references in Chapter 25 and all issues of *AJN,* which report on ANA activities, including a report of each biennial convention. *American Nurse* is invaluable to keep abreast of major nursing issues and current legislation, as well as ANA activities and positions. Position statements, standards, guidelines and other ANA related publications can be ordered from ANA Publications; some are free for single copies, and others vary in price. The history of the ANA may be found in any history of nursing text, and the September 1971 issue of the *American Journal of Nursing* has a number of key articles relating to the origin and development of the ANA, at the point of its seventy-fifth anniversary. Also see the section on "Issues in Nursing Organization" in Michael Miller and Beverly Flynn, ed., *Current Perspectives in Nursing: Social Issues and Trends.* Vol. 1. St. Louis, Mo.: C. V. Mosby Company, 1977, which discusses the pros and cons of joining ANA or another organization and the role of collective bargaining.

26

National League for Nursing

The main purpose of the National League for Nursing (usually referred to as NLN or the League) is best expressed in this phrase from its Certificate of Incorporation, ". . . that the nursing needs of the people will be met."[1] The ANA is concerned with this same goal, but these two major nursing organizations approach this objective in different ways. ANA, as the membership organization for registered nurses, works primarily through nurses and within the profession. NLN, whose membership includes not only nurses but other members of the health team, interested lay people, and agencies concerned with nursing education and service, works within the community and in association with individuals and groups outside of, but interested in, nursing. In pursuit of the same general end of better nursing care, each of the two organizations carries its own programs, responsibilities, and functions.

HISTORY

It will be easier, perhaps, to understand the distinction between NLN and ANA if events that led up to the establishment of the NLN in 1952 are reviewed. In many ways, the NLN is older than the date suggests, be-

cause it grew out of several pre-existing nursing organizations and absorbed many of the functions they had carried.*

In the mid-1940s the nursing profession decided to take a long hard look at its entire organizational structure. At this time there were six national nursing organizations and a host of jointly sponsored committees, activities, and services. This somewhat cumbersome arrangement resulted not only in an overlapping expenditure of time, effort, and resources, but also in confusion in the minds of both nurses and the public as to the purpose and functions of each organization.

Starting in 1944, nurses, under the leadership of the Committee on Structure of National Nursing Organizations, began to study the way in which their profession was organized. The culmination of this long and painstaking self-examination came in 1952. At that time, nurses voted in favor of having two major organizations: a strengthened and reorganized ANA, which would continue to serve as the membership association for registered nurses, and a new organization, the National League for Nursing, through which nurses and others interested in nursing,

---

*See Chapters 3 and 4.

along with institutions (both education and service), could work together to strengthen nursing education and nursing services.

The six organizations prior to the 1952 decision were ANA, the National League of Nursing Education (NLNE), the National Organization for Public Health Nursing (NOPHN), the Association of Collegiate Schools of Nursing (ACSN), the National Association of Colored Graduate Nurses (NACGN), and the American Association of Industrial Nurses (AAIN). The NACGN voluntarily went out of existence in 1951, because the ANA required all its constituents to admit to membership registered nurses without discrimination on the basis of color. The AAIN decided to continue as a separate organization. The newly created NLN, however, inherited the major functions of the other three organizations—excluding, of course, ANA.

The National League of Nursing Education was the first nursing organization in the United States. Established in 1893 under the formidable title of the American Society of Superintendents of Training Schools for Nurses of the United States and Canada (it became the NLNE in 1912), its purpose was to standardize and improve the education of nurses. Originally for nurses only, it broadened its membership policies in 1943 to admit lay members.

The National Organization for Public Health Nursing was established in 1912. As its title implies, it was an organization concerned not only with public health nurses but also with the development of public health nursing services. It provided for both agency and individual membership—the latter, except in NOPHN's very early years, open to non-nurses as well as nurses.

The prime objective of the Association of Collegiate Schools of Nursing, started in 1933 when baccalaureate degree education for nurses was just beginning to make headway, was to develop nursing education on a professional and collegiate basis. Membership was open principally to accredited programs offering college degrees in nursing;

each institution was represented by one or more persons from its faculty.

The newly created NLN also absorbed many of the functions of three major committees—Joint Committee on Practical Nurses and Auxiliary Workers in Nursing Services (1945); Joint Committee on Careers in Nursing (1948); National Committee for the Improvement of Nursing Services (1949) —and assumed administration of the National Nursing Accrediting Service, which had been started in 1949 under joint organizational sponsorship. Inheriting what might be called the "community-centeredness" of these seven predecessor nursing groups, NLN was formally established in 1952.

As the years went on, however, it became evident that some clearer distinction needed to be made between ANA and NLN functions, intended from the beginning to be distinct but complementary. The first major statement to delineate the roles of the two organizations was issued in 1966. A new statement was published in 1970 and was reaffirmed in 1973. Because this statement spells out clearly and officially the current roles of the ANA and NLN, it is presented in full:

> *The American Nurses' Association and the National League for Nursing as cooperating organizations in the field of nursing have the need to examine periodically the fundamental premises on which they will work together and serve society. While they are totally different organizations in both responsibilities and structure, they are complementary in purpose and function.*
>
> *The American Nurses' Association, as the professional organization of registered nurses, sets standards for nursing education, nursing practice, and organized nursing services. In the development and modification of standards, ANA secures consultation and advice from NLN and other sources, but retains responsibility for deciding the final content. The ANA works to implement these standards through its members and its constituents, with the NLN and with a variety of other organizations and governmental bodies.*

ANA represents the official voice of American nurses with other professions, community organizations, and the International Council of Nurses. ANA speaks for registered nurses on legislative matters concerning health, education, and the general welfare of people. ANA protects the economic and general welfare of nurses and promotes their professional development.

The National League for Nursing links the interests of organized nursing with those of the community through its membership of individuals, drawn from all ranks of nursing personnel, the allied professions, and the community, and agencies, which are educational institutions and providers of nursing service. NLN works to help communities improve the nursing services and education programs they need by offering services in accreditation, consultation, testing, research, and publications. The programs carried out by its constituent leagues foster community planning for nursing as a primary component of comprehensive health care. NLN observes nursing in action and shares its findings with ANA.

The needs of the profession and the needs of the public for nursing service are different from those of 1952, when a design for function and structure of both organizations was adopted. Change in the demands upon both organizations has caused each to examine its own functions and structure, and its relationship with the other. It is essential that ANA and NLN work cooperatively in areas of common concern as each builds its program in full recognition of the role of the other.

PURPOSES AND FUNCTIONS

The NLN's original purpose, as described in its certificate of incorporation, remains unchanged: "to foster the development and improvement of hospital, industrial, public health, and other organized nursing service and of nursing education through the coordinated action of nurses, allied professional groups, citizens, agencies, and schools to the end that the nursing needs of the people will be met."[1]

In 1978, a revised statement on the mission

of NLN was developed by the membership structure committee and approved by the NLN board.

The mission of the National League for Nursing is to

1. Assess on a continuing basis the present and future needs of people.
2. Foster the development of programs designed to meet the emerging and projected nursing needs of people.
3. Develop and support services for the improvement of nursing service and nursing education through accreditation, consultation, continuing education, evaluation, public information, research, and other activities.
4. Foster the development of leadership in nursing education and practice.
5. Work with consumer, voluntary, governmental, and other agencies, groups, and organizations for the advancement of nursing and the achievement of comprehensive health care.

In carrying out its mission, the National League for Nursing:

1. Promotes quality educational programs that prepare nurses for practice.
2. Promotes quality educational programs that prepares nurses for major administrative and leadership positions in institutions, organizations, and agencies.
3. Provides within NLN a unified system of accreditation that collaborates with other nursing agencies, organizations, groups, and institutions as well as those that interface with nursing.
4. Provides within NLN a unified system of consultation for each of its educational and service constituencies.
5. Provides within NLN a unified system of continuing education for its constituencies.
6. Conducts continually updated testing and evaluation programs for nursing practice and for nursing education, including life experiences.
7. Conducts surveys related to NLN functions and interests.

8. Conducts and promotes research which focuses on nursing education and nursing practice as they have an impact on health care delivery systems.

9. Maintains a program of public information by which NLN shares the results of its surveys, research, deliberations, actions, and other pertinent information.

10. Exercises active responsibility in the planning and formation of public policy in the areas of health, education, and welfare.

11. Promotes joint program planning between leaders of nursing education and nursing practice in order to foster closer working relationships.

12. Fosters consumer involvement so that NLN may respond appropriately to consumer needs.

13. Provides appropriate mechanisms and programs to anticipate and respond to changes in health care delivery systems and nursing's impact on them.

These principles were reiterated in a slightly different format in a final revision as the NLN Statement of Purpose, published in December, 1978.

MEMBERSHIP

There are two major classes of membership within the NLN, individual and agency. *Individual* membership is open to anyone interested in fostering the development and improvement of nursing service and education. This might include professional nurses, student nurses, licensed practical nurses, other workers in nursing, members of allied professions, and lay persons interested in nursing. Top echelon administrators (directors of nursing) and those persons next in line bearing the title "associate" or "assistant" may join the National Forum for Administrators of Nursing Services (NFANS), formed in 1977 as the first special

NLN ORGANIZATION CHART (1979)

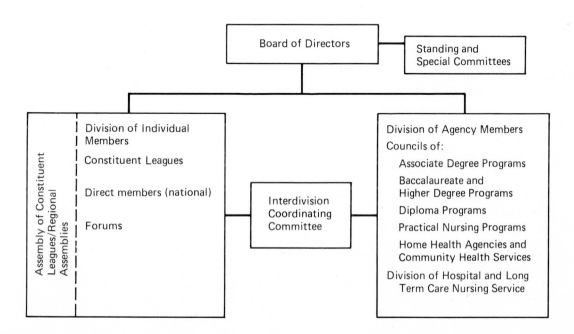

interest forum for individual members. *Agency* membership is for organizations or groups providing community nursing services and for the various schools conducting approved educational programs in nursing. Each member agency designates two individuals, with voting rights, to serve as its representatives within NLN.

There is another category of agency membership (allied) for agencies interested in the work of the NLN but not qualifying within the preceding categories. These agencies do not have voting power.

Until 1967, NLN, like ANA, was structured on a local-state-national level. At that time, however, it was decided that the "constituent units" (formerly state leagues) of NLN need not necessarily follow state lines. A constituent league may now take in only part of a state (a large metropolitan center, for instance), a whole state, parts of several different states, or several different states as a whole. The emphasis is on organization according to interests and needs in given regions or areas rather than in given states. (This change reflects the emphasis now given in many other fields to regional organization or planning.) Forty-five constituent leagues for nursing implement national goals and objectives through statewide programming. Many have local units (about ninety-five in 1979) to stimulate community interest in cooperative planning for nursing and health care services and present programs at the local level. In 1979 there were more than 17,000 individual members, and almost 1,800 agency members, mostly nursing education programs.

Individual members join the NLN and the constituent league in the area in which they reside or work. If there is no league in that area, they may join NLN directly at the national level. Annual dues for each individual member combine the national and the constituent league dues. Retiree fees are correspondingly lower.

Agency members join NLN directly, not through its constituent units. Dues for NLN member agencies vary with many factors, including available services.

GENERAL PLAN OF ORGANIZATION

Although both individual and agency members are concerned with the "further development and improvement of nursing services and education,"[2] the groups approach this task through different channels.

Accordingly, in NLN's organizational pattern, these two large membership groups are divided into the Division of Individual Members and the Division of Agency Members. The Division of Individual Members is expected to work through the constituent leagues for nursing, the forums, and the Assembly of Constituent Leagues for Nursing. The latter is composed of the president of each constituent league and other individuals who may be designated by the Assembly. Among the purposes of the Assembly is to plan and facilitate ways by which the NLN program may be implemented, to serve as a forum for exchange and discussion of ideas, problems, and recommendations, to serve in an advisory capacity to the League, and to present recommendations for action to the board of directors—usually through the executive committee of the Assembly. The Assembly meets annually. There are also four regional assemblies meeting annually and sponsoring forums, conferences, and workshops. Individual members may join any one of the councils in the Division of Agency Members.

Councils of Agency Members

Agency members are expected to work through their respective councils, although, of course, their two representatives also have votes in the general affairs of the organization. There are five councils: Associate Degree Programs (CADP), Baccalaureate and Higher Degree Programs (CBHDP), Diploma Programs (CDP), Practical Nursing

Programs (CPNP), and Home Health Agencies and Community Health Services (CHHA/CHS). The first four fall into one of the two large categories of agencies represented in NLN membership, programs of nursing education, whereas, CHHA/CHS represents the other, institutions or organizations providing community nursing services. Councils may be dissolved, or new ones created, in the light of changing circumstances.

Each council works within its own readily identifiable field of interest, but there are certain activities in which all engage. All are involved in consultation, and all have accreditation functions. Workshops and programs are held regionally and nationally. Councils may also have joint committees with other organizations or groups. A number of examples can be given of the varying focus of each council. For example, CBHDP and CHHA/CHS have been particularly interested in legislative matters. The CBHDP Legislative Advisory Committee has been empowered to formulate positions on health care legislation pertinent to baccalaureate and higher degree education. It has also maintained a survey of state legislation affecting their areas of interest. CHHA/CHS members and staff have worked with congressional staff on legislative proposals and with HEW groups concerned with such programs as Medicare, Medicaid, and Social Security.

Council committees vary according to each council's needs. Each has an executive committee, which guides and administers the affairs of the council under the direction of the board of directors. The executive committee also determines what other meetings are held besides the biennial meeting (there are usually one or two more a year).

Forums

In 1979, forums were added to the organizational structure. As defined by the bylaws, the word means any group of individual members of the League with an identified interest that has been authorized by the board of directors. Forums have executive committees to administer forum affairs. The chairman is included in the Inter-Division Coordinating Council.

Board of Directors, Officers, Committees

The NLN's board of directors consists of its five elected officers (president, president elect, first and second vice presidents, and treasurer), the secretary, the chairmen of the councils, twelve elected directors, the executive committee (four members) of the Assembly of Constituent Leagues for Nursing, and two board-appointed directors.

The council chairmen and the executive committee of the Assembly of Constituent Leagues are elected by their respective groups. The officers, twelve directors, and three members of the committee on nominations are elected by the membership every two years.

Balloting is done by mail, with both individual and agency members entitled to vote. All of these offices and elected positions are open to both nurse and non-nurse NLN members. In the 1979-1981 biennium, the first non-nurse president served.

At NLN business sessions held at the biennial conventions, decisions are made by the individual and agency members present, provided there are enough to meet the League's quorum requirements. Each individual member has one vote, and each member agency has two.

The NLN has two types of committees—standing and special—and these may be elected or appointed. The composition and methods of election or appointment and the term of office of committees are spelled out in the bylaws. The Committee on Nominations is currently the only elected committee of the overall organization.

In the appointed category are five standing committees: executive, constitution and bylaws, finance, perspectives, and pension. The executive committee, composed of NLN's elected officers, other board members appointed to the committee as representatives of NLN's broad services and programs, and NLN's executive director (without vote), act for the entire board between meetings of that group.

The perspectives committee predicts the societal changes that affect nursing, analyzes issues in the delivery of health services, and examines trends in professional and technical education. It also identifies goals for each biennium. The 1979 Biennial Convention approved the following program goals delineated by the perspectives committee.

1. Establish mechanisms to analyze manpower resources in the nursing profession and advise on the recruitment of nursing students.
2. Create greater understanding of and support for care that must be rendered over the long term, particularly for the mentally ill, the developmentally disabled, the handicapped, and the elderly.
3. Assist nursing education and service to teach and implement methods for achieving cost effectiveness and cost containment.
4. Encourage nurses to expand their role in health promotion, illness prevention, and self-care.
5. Promote nursing research and its utilization.
6. Continue to evaluate preparation for beginning practice in nursing.
7. Seek to identify mutual responsibilities among health professionals.
8. Initiate methods to assure that continuing education fulfills its purpose of improving, extending, and updating nursing practice.
9. Encourage nursing representation on policy-making bodies.
10. Continue to provide leadership in improving nursing education and nursing service.

Also considered standing committees are the Council Executive Committees, the Forum Executive Committees, and the Executive Committee of the Assembly of Constituent Leagues for Nursing, mentioned

previously, and the Interdivision Coordinating Committee, which consists of the chairman or appointed alternate of the council executive committees and assembly executive committee. The major purposes of this last committee are primarily communication and coordination.

From time to time the League appoints other special committees to deal with matters of general, and often continuing, concern to the organization as a whole. One of the newest and potentially most active special committees is the Public Affairs Committee appointed in 1972. The main focus of this committee is to study current significant issues relating to the nation's health care delivery, identify those in which the NLN should take a stand, and prepare position statements on these issues for approval by the board of directors.

SERVICES AND PROGRAMS

More or less permanent components within the League are a variety of services and programs carried out through its organized staff divisions.

Accreditation*

The NLN accrediting service has been a stimulant to the improvement of nursing education since its inception in 1949 under the name of the National Nursing Accrediting Service. Related to nursing education, it is a service that reviews and evaluates nursing education programs of various types such as those preparing practical nurses; diploma, associate degree, and baccalaureate degree programs for registered nurses; and programs leading to a master's degree in nursing. Those meeting NLN criteria within each category are granted NLN accreditation.

To operate legally, of course, each school of nursing must have the approval of the state government, as represented by its

---

*See Chapter 12 for controversial issues in accreditation.

board of nurse examiners. But standards vary from state to state, despite efforts to standardize them as much as possible; in some, the requirements for school approval are minimal. Criteria for NLN accreditation, however, are nationally determined; they represent the combined thinking of experts in the various kinds of programs. League accreditation, therefore, symbolizes a nursing education program of high quality in all respects—admission and achievement standards, curriculum, faculty preparation, library, laboratory and other facilities, and the like.

NLN accreditation is voluntary. The school requests this service and pays for the evaluation. There is no guarantee that the end result will be accreditation.

The published criteria for evaluation of each type of program, determined by the appropriate council, are basic guides, as is the booklet on policies and procedures of accreditation. Most schools conduct a thorough evaluation of all aspects of their program through committees of faculty and students, use of studies, and review of other data. The results of the evaluation are incorporated in a self-evaluation report, which is sent to NLN (previously notified as to the program's intent to seek evaluation). NLN accreditation is a peer evaluation and the visitors who come to the program to verify and clarify the data and explore ramifications of the report are faculty and/or faculty administrators of like programs, who have been selected for and especially trained by NLN to review programs. Often NLN visits are made cooperatively with regional or specialty accrediting associations or state board visits. NLN visitors may be able to point out weaknesses in the report, which can be corrected and also give supplementary information to the Board of Review, which meets in New York several times a year to review the materials for accreditation that have been sent from the schools and the visitors' reports.

Recommendations for improvement are sent to the school, with or without the granting of accreditation. If a program is ac-

credited, interim reports of the status of the program are sent to NLN at specified intervals before another major accreditation visit. If the program is not accredited, there is an appeal procedure, and, of course, the opportunity to correct the deficiencies and reapply for accreditation. Within recent years there has been greater flexibility in the acceptance of ways to meet accreditation standards so that programs of greatly varying educational approaches are being accredited. The common denominator is quality. Increasingly, NLN accreditation is sought and worked toward, because of the significance of this accreditation to the prospective student, the faculty member, and the community. In addition, only NLN-accredited schools are eligible for the nursing education funds made available through the Nurse Training Act of 1964 and later amendments. NLN is officially recognized by the Council on Post-Secondary Accreditation and the U.S. Office of Education as the accrediting agency for master's, baccalaureate, associate degree, diploma, and practical nurse programs. A deterring factor has been the resistance to NLN accreditation by some junior colleges that feared requests for accreditation from all other specialty programs. Even so, the number of accredited AD programs has risen to more than one half of the total number operating. Continuing education programs within the total nursing program seeking accreditation are also accredited.

Each year a list of NLN-accredited programs of nursing is published in the NLN journal. There are also pamphlets issued listing all state-approved and accredited nursing programs. By 1980, more than 1100 educational programs held NLN accreditation; over 70 percent of the total of basic RN programs were accredited by the League.

Early in 1966 the NLN inaugurated a second type of accreditation program, in conjunction with the American Public Health Association, this one for community nursing services. (Although the NLN does not accredit nursing services in other institutions, it has developed criteria and other tools for hospitals and nursing homes to use in self-evaluation.) It was initiated because of the interest expressed by the membership of both organizations in a method of evaluating the services being provided by them in the community. The program was made available to all organizations offering nursing services to people outside of hospitals, extended-care facilities, and nursing homes. From 1966 through 1968 agencies applied for and received preliminary accreditation. In 1968, as agencies began to meet the criteria required, the program moved into its second phase of full accreditation. Policies were developed by a joint NLN-APHA policy committee, but the program is administered by the NLN.

In 1971 consideration was given to the possibility of expanding the program to include other disciplines that provide out-of-institution personal care service. Therefore, the American Dietetic Association, American Occupational Therapy Association, American Physical Therapy Association, American Speech and Hearing Association, National Association of Social Workers, and National Council of Homemaker-Home Health Services, Inc., now work with the Accreditation Standards and Review Committee. Public health medicine is represented by a member of the Medical Care Section, APHA. Agencies seeking NLN-APHA accreditation receive a *Guide for Preparing Accreditation Reports*, which is used in the extensive self-study necessary. A site visit is then made by a consultant from the NLN staff and an administrator from a comparable agency in another state. The agency's report and site visitors' report are then studied by a peer member Board of Review. There is a process of appeal, if the Board of Review decision is not acceptable to the agency. A brief interim report is required two years after accreditation and another report and a site visit at least every five years. The program has expanded to include home health agency and community nursing services. More than seventy-five of these services were accredited in 1974. This number had grown to over one hundred in 1980 and is increasing. A list of accredited agencies has appeared yearly in the May issue of *Nursing Outlook* and is now reported in various NLN publications.

Consultation Services (Divisions of Nursing, Measurement, and Constituent League Services)

In connection with its accreditation services, the NLN offers consultation to any school of nursing seeking help with its educational program; thus a school failing to meet accreditation standards may be helped to achieve them, or one just starting or seeking to improve its program can be helped by NLN expertise. Consultation may be given through personal visits to the schools or through regional meetings such as workshops and institutes. Paid staff and appointed NLN members work steadily on this NLN program. It offers similar assistance to community health agencies searching for better and more efficient ways to serve their communities. And, with new attention being given to evaluation techniques in all fields of nursing, the testing service offers valuable assistance.

Consultation services to NLN constituencies and other community groups embrace a wide range of interests such as organization and management, financial development, establishing new community health service and education programs, evaluating programs, improving administrative practices, and areas of research and testing.

Test Services (Division of Measurement)

NLN conducts one of the largest professional testing services in the country. Test batteries have been developed in NLN's Department of Test Development by experts in tests and educational measurements and in nursing. The tests available through NLN fall into several categories: guidance and placement of students for schools of professional and practical nursing, and achievement of professional and practical nursing students while in nursing school, and, since 1978-1979, the pre-immigration screening examination and nursing tests prepared for the Commission on Graduates of Foreign Nursing Schools.* All are objective tests that are machine-scored under the direction of the NLN Department of Evaluation Services. There are separate sets of tests for practical nursing and for professional nursing. Also included are achievement tests for baccalaureate students. In addition, the Division of Measurement acts as the test service agency for the State Board Test Pool Examination for RN and PN licensure of the National Council of State Boards of Nursing.

Depending on the nature and purpose of the tests, they may be given at central locations within a state or the nation, or at individual schools. They are all returned to NLN headquarters for scoring, and the scores are then released to the schools or state boards of nursing. Pre-admission test results are available directly to the examinees. Almost three million tests were processed in the 1977-79 biennium. The League does not make the decision as to whether an individual's score means that she/he is qualified for admission to a school, has a satisfactory achievement in the subjects tested, or has met the requirements for licensure in a given state. This judgment is left to the individual schools or state boards, although NLN provides national standards as a guide.

The League's testing services are offered on a voluntary basis; no school or state is required to use them. In addition, every state now uses the State Board Test Pool Examinations for professional nurse licensure. All states but one use the tests for practical nurse licensure, and hundreds of nursing schools, both professional and practical, use the others. Costs to individual nurses and schools are minimal. The tests undergo almost continual evaluation and revision to maintain their validity and ensure appropriateness of content. New tests are added from time to time and others are discarded and replaced. Nursing is the only profession

*See Chapter 27.

to have developed such a national testing service.

Information Services (Division of Public Information)

If the NLN is to achieve its objective of improving nursing education and service, it must keep a constant flow of information going to both its membership and the general public. It accomplishes this primarily through the staff of its Division of Public Information, which distributes a wide variety of informative materials.

Some of this material is of a promotional character, explaining the nature and purpose of League programs and activities. Other publications are statistical or highly factual, such as school directories, lists of accredited schools of nursing, or reports of conferences and workshops. Still other material available through the League include accreditation criteria, management guides, evaluation aids, and career guidance materials.

Each year the NLN issues a publications catalog that is available on request from its headquarters office and is also sent to all members. More than 300 publications are listed in the 1980 catalog.

The League also publishes *NLN News,* a newsletter sent to all members ten times a year, along with various specialized bulletins —*Data Digest,* summaries of NLN research studies; *Public Affairs Advisory,* updates on key health issues and legislation; *NLN Bookshelf,* listings of new publications; *Speak Out!,* reports on membership opinion surveys; *Insider Letter,* reports on board meetings; and *NLN Meeting Calendar.* The councils prepare and distribute material of interest to their members through memos and newsletters. In 1980, a new official journal, *Nursing and Health Care* was published, after termination of this relationship with *Nursing Outlook,* by mutual consent.

The public affairs activities of the League are also conducted within the Division of Public Information. Members are kept informed of current federal and state legislation and health care issues through some of the publications cited as well as position papers on controversial topics.

NLN's Summer Study Fellowships in Public Policy Program has also been a high priority public affairs activity. The program, sponsored by the Robert Wood Johnson Foundation, was the first in the nation to provide opportunities for nursing students to participate in health policy making. Annual fellowships were awarded to ten outstanding nursing students from NLN-accredited baccalaureate, master's, and doctoral programs. Selected on a competitive basis, the fellows worked as professional staff in congressional, executive branch, and other legislative offices under the guidance of government staff preceptors. If new funding is available, it is expected that the fellowships will continue.

Research and Studies (Division of Research)

The activities of the Division of Research include data collection (as well as development of the data-gathering instruments), research studies, and special projects. Annually, for instance, the NLN collects information on admissions, graduations, and enrollments in programs of practical and professional nursing education. Aspects of this data have been published in *Nursing Outlook* and are now reported in various NLN publications. The *NLN Nursing Data Book*, first published in 1978, is a compilation of statistical information on nursing education and newly licensed nurses. Also published are booklets and directories on state-approved programs preparing students for licensure as RNs or LPNs. The directories indicate types of program, accreditation status, administrative control, financial support, and data on admissions, enrollments, and graduation. In 1973, a new directory was added, the *Directory of Career Mobility Opportunities in Nursing,* listing programs with open curriculum practices. A bienniel Nurse–Faculty Census is published also.

The NLN, as need and resources permit,

surveys or studies other selected aspects of nursing education or nursing service programs. In addition, it carries on both short-term and long-term research projects through its Division of Research. Some of these projects are financed by the League itself; some are financed through grants from other agencies. (The NLN, unlike ANA, enjoys tax-exempt status, and funds granted to it are not considered taxable income.)

One long-range study, the Nurse Career-Pattern Study,* designed to identify the characteristics of nurses in various educational programs in order to provide clues for recruitment, guidance, and employment of nurses, was funded by the U.S. Public Health Service. The first report, published in 1972, was the first comprehensive report provided of nursing students in baccalaureate, diploma, and associate degree programs. The Open Curriculum Study, first funded by the Exxon Education Foundation, surveyed current practices in open curriculum, and their evaluation. The State Board Test Pool Examination Validation Study evaluated the SBTPE as a means of establishing a minimum for safe and effective practice. The final report resulted in the development of a new type of examination, although the SBTPEs were found valid. Other HEW-funded projects were related to employment opportunities for new graduates and an investigation and evaluation of ways in which students are selected for nursing education programs, in order to determine specific factors that may act as barriers to admission or successful completion of programs.

Interorganizational Relationships

The NLN works closely with the ANA and NSNA. However, throughout its entire program NLN also maintains active liaison with many other national agencies, both governmental and voluntary. Among them are the American Public Health Association, the National Federation of Licensed Practical

---

*See Chapter 11.

Nurses, the National Association for Practical Nurse Education and Service, the United States Public Health Service, the American Nursing Homes Association, the American Association of Junior Colleges, the American Dietetic Association, the American Hospital Association, the American Medical Association, and the National Lung Association.

The NLN is also a member of the American Council on Education, the National Health Council, and the National Interagency Council on Smoking and Health.

Other Services and Activities

Because of its tax exempt status as an educational and charitable organization, the League (and its constituent leagues) is prohibited from participating in any political campaign on behalf of or in opposition to any particular candidate, and no substantial part of its activities may consist of influencing legislation. Therefore, the League has no lobbyist. However, this prohibition does not extend to dealing with administrative agencies or the executive branch of the government. Hence the NLN's successful suit on behalf of nursing schools against the HEW secretary and the federal budget director in 1973 to release impounded funds (see Chapter 18), although precedent-breaking, was a suitable activity. The League is also permitted to inform members fully of proposed legislation, engage in non-partisan analysis or study and disseminate results, and give factual testimony and information. Preferably these presentations are made on request of the legislators. Within this framework the NLN has been involved in legislation affecting nursing and has been helpful in its implementation.

When the ANA moved to Kansas City, Missouri, a joint careers program, in which ANA and NLN exchanged daily requests from the public for information about nursing, was terminated. However, the decision was made for the NLN to fulfill its obligation to the public with information and materials about nursing, nursing careers, and nursing education. In late 1973, NLN's Nursing Information Service was granted funds by the National Fund for Graduate Nursing Education to produce two leaflets on nursing careers. Since that time, new brochures have been developed, and NLN's Careers Information Service sends packets of information about nursing as a career to high school counselors each year.

Also in 1973, the NLN chose the National Library of Medicine in Bethesda, Maryland, home of the world's largest collection of health sciences literature, as the official repository of NLN's historical documents and records. These include the history of NLN, old photographs of American nurses, correspondence by Florence Nightingale and other nursing leaders, and the history of NOPHN. League officials also plan to join in a campaign to identify and acquire other nursing memorabilia for the library.[3]

The impact of NLN on nursing does not lie only in the services and activities of the organization and its component groups. It is equally important to look at some of the major pronouncements made by the NLN, in taking stands on nursing issues. Among these is a 1965 resolution on nursing education that recommended community planning to "implement the orderly movement of nursing education into institutions of higher learning in such a way that the flow of nurses into the community will not be interrupted." A 1970 statement on open curriculum urged changes in programs to aid mobility in nursing without lowering standards, and in 1976, a new and stronger version was approved by the board of directors. A 1971 statement (revised 1976) about degree programs with no major in nursing was intended, in part, to help RNs who were seeking degrees to make informed choices. In 1972 *Nursing Education in the Seventies* spelled out needed characteristics of an effective system of nursing education and the actions needed to attain these characteristics. A 1966 statement encouraged continuity of nursing care, and in 1973, the statement on *Quality Review of*

Health Care Services urged intra- and inter-professional review of care standards; the updated 1979 version urged greater participation of nurses in PSROs. Other position papers are on national health insurance, nursing's responsibility to minorities and disadvantaged groups, and NLN's role in continuing education in nursing. A controversial NLN statement was made in 1979, "Preparation for Beginning Practice in Nursing," in which support for all four types of nursing education programs was reiterated, "for the present." Because the League accredits all four types of programs, this position was not surprising to some, although the 1965 NLN resolution that was never rescinded seems to present a contradictory view. A report of the NLN Task Force on Competencies of Graduates of Nursing Programs, also released in 1979, identified differences in the knowledge base and in minimal expectations of the new graduate of the four types of nursing programs studied (practical, AD, diploma, and baccalaureate), as well as differences in the practice role in terms of structured/unstructured settings, focus of care and accountability.

One of the most successful NLN projects was a service to the community, the League's childhood immunization project, funded for two years by HEW's Center for Disease Control. NLN coordinated the nation's voluntary sector to join the federal government to immunize 20 million children by October 1, 1979 and to establish a permanent maintenance system to ensure routine protection for all newborns. In addition, at the grass roots level, NLN's constituent leagues worked closely with all kinds of community groups to solve special health and education problems, thus helping to fulfill the ultimate goal of NLN to improve the health of the people.

The NLN headquarters, with its staff of more than 200, over half of whom are non-nurses, is located at 10 Columbus Circle, New York, N.Y. 10019. Regional offices are located in Chicago, Atlanta, and San Bruno, California.

REFERENCES

1. National League for Nursing. *Bylaws* (New York: The League, 1977).
2. Ibid., p. 12.
3. "Historical Records Go to Archives." *NLN News.* **21**:2–3 (Nov. 1973).

BIBLIOGRAPHY

Beal, Wayne. "This I Believe—About the National League for Nursing." *Nurs. Outlook.* **19** (Feb. 1971), 99 ff. Concepts of the NLN as it is and might be.

Filimore, Anna, Marion W. Sheahan, and Julia M. Miller. "The NLN Is Everybody's Business." *Nurs. Outlook.* **1** (Jan. 1953), 22–27. This, the first article in the first issue of NLN's official publication, describes the purposes, programs, aspirations, and plans of the organization that had been formed less than a year before.

Haynes, Inez. "NLN at Ten." *Nurs. Outlook.* **10** (June 1962), 372–377. NLN's general director reviews NLN's progress during its first decade of existence and projects future activities and goals.

Kibrick, Anne. "NLN: Nursing's Voice in Community Health." *Nurs. Outlook.* **19** (July 1971). 435. The then president of NLN discusses the role of NLN in community health.

Mauksch, Ingeborg. "This I Believe—About the National League for Nursing." *Nurs. Outlook.* **19** (Feb. 1971), 98 ff. Some concepts of NLN and suggestions for the future, including that the organization become even more oriented to health.

NLN at Twenty. Reprinted from *Nursing Outlook* (June 1972). An article on the challenges to NLN and changes taking place in the organization, and an accompanying editorial. Available free from NLN Publications Order unit.

Walsh, Margaret E. "NLN: Twenty-Five Years of Nursing Leadership." *Nurs. Outlook.* **25** (Apr. 1977), 248–249. NLN executive director briefly reviews its history and projects its future.

Walsh, Margaret E. "The Role of NLN in Continuing Education in Nursing." *J. Contin. Educ. Nurs.*, **3** (May/June 1972). 44–48. Executive director of NLN explains how the organization supports continuing education.

Additional news and information can be found in the various NLN publications, including data from many of the research projects.

Other Nursing and Related Organizations in the United States

Within the last ten years an increasing number of specialty organizations for nurses have been added to those already well established. Although all nurses can find a place for themselves within the American Nurses' Association, some, particularly those in clinical or occupational specialties, have elected to join one of the other nursing organizations instead of, or in addition to, the ANA. The aegis of these organizations varies. Some are totally independent; others are part of a medical or educational organization. Some restrict membership to nurses; others include medical-technical personnel employed in the same clinical specialty.

Although there have always been other nursing organizations, ANA has generally been accepted as *the* professional organization that speaks for nursing. Some of the earlier groups later merged into ANA. The first of the specialty organizations that still exists was the American Association of Nurse Anesthetists (1931). In the 1940s and 1950s, AAIN, (now AAOHN,) AORN, and ACNM followed, but beginning in 1968, literally dozens of others were organized. They were either splinter groups that broke off from ANA and formed their own association or evolved

as the profession became more specialized. Nurses who switched membership often said that ANA did not meet their needs, particularly after ANA directed more of its resources to the economic security program. Few maintained dual membership, either because they could not or would not spare the time or dues money. Special interest groups seem to have several things in common: they state that they do not intend to get involved in the economic security concerns of their members, and their major concern is to provide a forum for sharing ideas, experiences, and problems related to a particular specialty or interest, including continuing education and standard setting. Most indicate that they plan to remain autonomous organizations.

The proliferation of nursing organizations, although meeting the special needs of some nurses, has also caused some confusion among nurses, other health workers, and the public. Do these organizations speak for nursing in addition to the ANA? In place of the ANA? Members of the nursing organizations were also concerned. A lack of unity in common health care interests can be disastrous to successful achievement of desired goals. Therefore, in November 1972, the

ANA hosted a meeting of ten specialty groups and NSNA to "explore how the organizations can work toward more coordination in areas of common interest." It was found that concerns were similar and that such a meeting was generally considered long overdue.

In its second meeting, hosted by the Critical Care Nurses and held at the Western White House in San Clemente, California, in January 1973, federal nurses and representatives from the National Commission on Nursing and Nursing Education were also invited, and the group was asked to consider forming a National Nurses Congress. Although this suggestion was rejected, the participants accepted the importance of the specialty groups, at the same time recognizing the unique role of the ANA. They agreed in principle to statements on institutional licensure and continuing education and reaffirmed that practice was the basic purpose of the nursing profession.[2]

At the third meeting of presidents and executive secretaries of the specialty nursing organizations, ANA, and NSNA, held in June 1973, this group adopted a name—The Federation of Specialty Nursing Organizations and American Nurses' Association. They identified a specialty nursing organization as a "national organization of registered nurses governed by an elected body with by-laws defining purpose and functions for improvement of health care; and a body of knowledge and skill in a defined area of clinical practice." Those attending expressed mutual support and agreed on some of the issues of the times.[3] As of 1980, there were 21 specialty organizations in the Federation besides ANA. They are American Association of Critical-Care Nurses, American Association of Nephrology Nurses and Technicians, American Association of Neurosurgical Nurses, American Association of Nurse Anesthetists, American Association of Occupational Health Nurses Inc., American College of Nurse-Midwives, American Public Health Association, American

Urological Association, Allied, The Association of Operating Room Nurses, Inc., Association for Practitioners in Infection Control, Association of Rehabilitation Nurses, Emergency Department Nurses Association, International Association for Enterostomal Therapy, Inc., National Association of Pediatric Nurse Associates and Practitioners, National Association of School Nurses, Inc., National Intravenous Therapy Association, Inc., The Nurses' Association of the American College of Obstetricians and Gynecologists, National Nurses' Society on Alcoholism, Oncology Nursing Society, with the last admitted being the American Society of Plastic and Reconstructive Surgical Nurses and the American Society of Opthalmic Registered Nurses, Inc.

Within the same year, the ANA and NLN developed closer working relationships with the relatively new American Association of Colleges of Nursing. Many of their mutual interests were in the area of federal legislation for health care, and their first major joint statement noted the need for a system of health maintenance that would allow people to benefit fully from nursing's contributions. Representatives of the three organizations then met to draft plans to implement the proposals in the statement.[4] In January 1974, the ANA and AACN formed the Alliance of the American Nurses' Association and the American Association of Colleges of Nursing.[5]

Such collaborative activities among nursing organizations show a new maturity in nursing that not only recognizes the importance of joining together on major health issues, but also takes positive cooperative action. Such action will enable nurses to be a stronger force in the planning and delivery of health care services. The nursing organizations noted in this chapter are not all clinical specialty groups; some exist to serve other needs of nurses, educationally, socially, or spiritually. It is entirely possible that still more nursing organizations will evolve through the years as nurses assume new health care roles. Those discussed in this chapter appear to be most firmly established and active at this time.

ALPHA TAU DELTA

The Alpha Tau Delta Nursing Fraternity, Incorporated, is a professional fraternity that was founded on February 15, 1921, at the University of California, Berkeley. Chapters are established only in schools of nursing where the baccalaureate or higher degree programs are fully accredited by the National League for Nursing. In 1979, it had twenty-one active collegiate chapters and nine alumnae chapters. Membership is based upon scholarship, personality, and character and has no restriction as to race, color, or creed.

The purposes of Alpha Tau Delta are to further higher professional and educational standards, to develop character and leadership, to encourage excellence of individual performance, and to organize and maintain an interfraternity spirit of cooperation. Besides the chapter scholarships, financial aid is given annually through the Miriam Fay Furlong National Grant Awards. Other awards are the Efficiency Rating Performance Award to a chapter and award keys and merit awards to individuals for outstanding accomplishments.

The governing body of ATD is its biennial national convention. It is composed of elected delegates from each college and alumnae chapter, and the seven national council officers.

The national paper, *Cap'tions of Alpha Tau Delta*, is published in the spring and fall of each year. Alpha Tau Delta is a member of Professional Panhellenic Association, and through this organization is represented in the Interfraternity Research and Advisory Council. National headquarters for ATD is at 489 Serento Circle, Thousand Oaks, California 90805.

AMERICAN ASSOCIATION OF COLLEGES OF NURSING

The American Association of Colleges of Nursing (AACN) was formed in May 1969, at a meeting attended by forty-four deans and directors of nursing programs located in institutions of higher education. For approximately two years prior to this time, a group of deans of the National League for Nursing accredited graduate programs in nursing had been meeting together informally to explore the kind of organizational arrangement needed to focus on significant issues influencing higher education in nursing, and to provide a forum for the deans and directors to meet together to debate these issues and to take rapid and concerted action with respect to them. These early meetings culminated in the vote in 1969 to establish an independent Conference of Deans of College and University Schools of Nursing, composed of the deans and directors of the National League for Nursing accredited baccalaureate and higher degree programs in the United States, and directed toward the purpose of providing knowledgeable leadership in nursing.

The first general meeting of the newly organized group was held in Chicago during October 1969. The association has undergone several changes in names since the initial meeting; its present name, the American Association of Colleges of Nursing, was accepted by the membership at the meeting held in February 1973. AACN meets regularly twice yearly. A headquarters office was established in Washington, D.C., early in 1973, and the association became legally incorporated in Washington, D.C., in March of that same year.

The central purpose of the association is to improve necessary care and its delivery in the public interest through advancing the quality of academic nursing education and strategic leadership in nursing. Membership in the Association is of two kinds: institutional regular, represented by the key nurse administrative person in an NLN-accredited baccalaureate and/or graduate program in nursing, and institutional provisional, represented by the key nurse administrative person in a baccalaureate and/or graduate program with a goal of achieving NLN accreditation in no less than four years.

The objectives of the American Association of Colleges of Nursing are (1) studying the effectiveness of education in providing a high quality of nursing service to the public; (2) exchanging and disseminating ideas and information about the value of nursing education at the baccalaureate and graduate levels as related to the quality of nursing service to the public; (3) promoting understanding of the scope of nursing and its relationships for the health and well-being of individuals, families, and society in general; (4) influencing governmental policy with respect to the advancement of education, research, and service in nursing and to the improvement of health care for all people; (5) working cooperatively and collaboratively with other professional nursing organizations, with professional organizations in other health professions, and in higher education to the end that health care for all citizens may be continually re-evaluated and improved; and (6) serving in an advisory and/or advocacy role to administrators of baccalaureate and graduate programs in nursing.

The American Association of Colleges of Nursing, through its membership, has been involved actively in strengthening and extending the position of collegiate nursing education within institutions of higher learning. Since its inception, the association has been involved in legislation, socialization of deans, and issues pertinent to higher education for nurses. AACN has grown rapidly in membership and has given active and vigorous leadership for higher education in nursing. As an association and through action by individual deans, the association has taken a strong position in influencing legislation for the improvement of health care delivery and for support of health manpower education.

The association works closely with both the ANA and the NLN to translate into action the recommendations that are a part of the position paper accepted by the American Association of Colleges of Nursing, American Nurses' Association, and National League for Nursing, entitled "Nursing's Contribution and Commitment." AACN is located at Eleven Dupont Circle, Suite 430, Washington, D.C. 20036.

AMERICAN ASSOCIATION OF CRITICAL-CARE NURSES

The American Association of Critical-Care Nurses (AACN) was founded in 1969 as the American Association of Cardiovascular Nurses. It was re-incorporated in California in 1972 under its present name so that it could serve the RN in the entire spectrum of critical-care management. Present membership now totals 32,000 with 202 chapters located throughout the United States and internationally. Its major purpose is to provide continuing education for the critical-care nurse and potential critical-care nurse. The philosophy of AACN is that each critically ill person has the right to expect nursing care provided by a critical-care nurse. Printed nursing care guides, critical-care course curricula, lesson plans, regional symposia, and tutorial services are available to members. Other objectives are to emphasize and promote understanding of the critical-care concept, to maintain a central bureau for information about critical-care nursing, and to maintain liaison with other professional nursing and health-related organizations and agencies.

Membership is available to registered nurses who provide specialized care to the critically ill patient whether in a critical-care unit (such as coronary care, intensive-shock unit, respiratory, burn, neonatal, pediatric intensive care, emergency room, mobile ambulance, cardiopulmonary laboratory), or wherever a critically ill patient may be found. Associate membership is available to licensed practical nurses, licensed vocational nurses, graduate nurses, and student nurses who are involved with or interested in the care of the critically ill. Teachers of critical-care nurses, whether in hospitals, academic institutions, or health agencies are a vital part of the association. International memberships are available to nurses who submit proof of RN licensure and/or registration in their country.

As a means of providing peer recognition, AACN offers a certification program through its affiliate organization, the AACN Certification Board. The CCRN certification program was developed to formally recognize professional competency of critical-care nurses. Levels of practice have been identified as critical-care nurse I (C-CRNI), the knowledgeable nurse specialist, and critical-care nurse II (C-CRNII), the clinician with expertise. Examinations, which began in 1973, are given in various parts of the country. A nurse who completes the examinations successfully is given a Certificate of Achievement. A statement of this achievement is sent to the nurse's employer upon the written request of the nurse.

Other benefits of membership are reduced rates for malpractice insurance and free copies of the official publication, *Heart and Lung: The Journal of Critical Care.* Conventions are held yearly, and include a Teaching Institute. Membership information may be obtained by writing to AACN, P.O. Box C-19528, Irvine, CA 92713. Information concerning CCRN certification may be obtained by writing to AACN Certification Board, P.O. Box C-19519, Irvine, CA 92713.

THE AMERICAN ASSOCIATION FOR NEPHROLOGY NURSES AND TECHNICIANS

The American Association for Nephrology Nurses and Technicians (AANNT) was founded in 1969 as an organization of nurses, technicians, social workers, and dietitians interested in the care of patients with renal disease. The purpose is primarily educational through numerous national, regional, and local programs, seminars, and conferences. Other major activities include the study of and preparation for specialty certification, a registry for continuing education credit, and provision of standards of nursing practice in the hemodialysis and transplantation areas. The objectives of the AANNT are to develop and update standards for the practice of nephrology nursing and technology, provide the mechanisms to promote individual professional growth, support a certification process that identifies various levels of competence and excellence in practice, and promotes research, development, and demonstration of advances in nephrology nursing and technology.

There are approximately 3,800 members of the national organization, a large majority of whom are registered nurses. AANNT began as a nationally based association and established five regional groups the following year. Several chapters have been established within each region. A few local groups are not recognized. Any RN, LPN, or technician interested in the care of patients with renal disease is eligible for regular membership. Dietitians and social workers may participate as associate members. AANNT's major publications consist of the proceedings of the annual program meeting each April (in conjunction with the American Society for Artificial Internal Organs), *Standards of Clinical Practice*, and a quarterly journal entitled, *The Journal of the American Association of Nephrology Nurses and Technicians.*

Careers related to the organization are usually highly specialized and related to either dialysis (hemo- or peritoneal) or transplantation. This field is rather young among specialty practice groups, but continuing expansion is anticipated, particularly with the implementation of HR 1, which provides federal funding for all forms of therapy for end-stage kidney disease. AANNT headquarters is located at Two Talcott Road, Suite 8, Park Ridge, Illinois 60068.

AMERICAN ASSOCIATION OF NEUROSURGICAL NURSES

The American Association of Neurosurgical Nurses (AANN), which is associated with the American Association of Neurological Surgeons, was founded in 1968. The purposes of the organization are to foster and promote interest, education, and high standards of practice in neurosurgical nursing. The major functions are to provide for continuing growth in the field and to provide a medium for direct communication between nurses in neurosurgery in the United States and Canada.

Criteria for membership include graduation from a state- or provincial-accredited school of nursing and RN licensure, two letters of reference from persons actively engaged in neurosurgery or neurosurgical nursing, and citizenship in the United States or Canada. RNs from the neurological nursing, rehabilitation, and paramedical fields may be considered for associate membership within certain numerical limits. All members (active or associate) of AANN are automatically members of the World Federation of Neurosurgical Nurses. Currently there are more than 900 members.

Major publications include the *Journal of Neurosurgical Nursing*, published quarterly; *Synapse*, the Association newsletter; *Standards of Neurological and Neurosurgical Nursing Practice*, and the *Speaker's Bureau List*, available on request from the Educational Resource Committee. Continuing education programs are provided on a regional and national level.

Certification examinations are offered twice a year at various locations throughout the country. Information regarding the examination may be obtained by writing the American Board of Neurosurgical Nursing, 304 East 45th Street, New York, New York 10017.

The association meets annually in conjunction with the AANS. The address of the business office of the AANN is 625 N. Michigan Avenue, Chicago, Illinois 60611.

AMERICAN ASSOCIATION OF NURSE ANESTHETISTS

Organized in 1931, the American Association of Nurse Anesthetists (AANA) is for professional nurses who are qualified by training and experience to give anesthesia. Nurses wishing to join AANA as active members must meet the standards of education and experience set forth in the organization's bylaws; this includes taking a qualifying examination administered by the association.

The objectives of the AANA, in general, are to advance the science and art of anesthesiology, to develop standards and techniques in the administration of anesthetics, to promote cooperation between nurse anesthetists and members of allied professions, to publish materials to aid in the association's activities and keep members informed, and to conduct an educational program stressing the importance of proper administration of anesthetics.*

Local associations of nurse anesthetists may organize as constituent units of AANA in states or other geographical areas acceptable to the board of trustees of AANA. Nurses in areas without local associations apply for membership directly to the national office.

With the assistance and encouragement of the American Hospital Association, AANA developed an accreditation program for schools for nurse anesthetists that went into effect in 1952. Only graduates of AANA-approved schools are now eligible to take the qualifying examination for association membership.

---

*Originally, the objectives of AANA included program accreditation and certification of practitioners. These activities are now carried out by autonomous councils.

The association holds an annual convention. The sessions are open to AANA members, as well as others in the health care field.

The *Journal of the American Association of Nurse Anesthetists* is published bimonthly. The headquarters office is at 216 West Higgins, Park Ridge, Ill. 60068.

AMERICAN ASSOCIATION OF OCCUPATIONAL HEALTH NURSES

The American Association of Occupational Health Nurses (AAOHN), organized in 1942, is an association of registered professional nurses employed in occupational health. The purposes of the association are to constitute a professional association of nurses engaged in the practice of occupational health nursing, to maintain the honor and character of the nursing profession, to improve community health by bettering nursing service to workers, to develop and promote standards for nurses and occupational health nursing services, to stimulate interest in and provide a forum for the discussion of problems in the field of industrial nursing, and to stimulate occupational health nurse participation in all nursing activities at local, state, and national levels. AAOHN's major activities are to formulate and develop principles and standards of occupational health nursing practice in order that the nurse in occupational health may utilize more fully her professional knowledge and training in her service to workers and management and to the community; to promote, by means of publications, conferences, workshops, and symposia, both formal and informal programs of education designed specifically for the nurse in occupational health; to identify the rightful place of nursing in the occupational health program and to encourage cooperation among all groups engaged in protecting the health and welfare of the worker; to impress upon management, physicians, and allied groups the importance of integrating into the activities of industry the services to be rendered by the occupational health nurse.

AAOHN is built upon its 115 local, state, and regional constituent associations, which have more than 9,000 members. A nonprofit organization, AAOHN derives its operating income from membership dues.

AAOHN may represent occupational health nurses in public policy discussions that affect their day-to-day practice. It also studies and attempts to influence legislative actions. However, the organization believes that increased professional competency, not collective bargaining, is the method for the occupational health nurse to achieve economic opportunity and security. Its goal is to promote the occupational health nurse as an impartial professional worker.

AAOHN's annual meeting is held in conjunction with that of the Occupational Medical Association, the combined meeting being called the American Occupational Health Conference. Symposia and workshops are also held on other occasions.

In addition to its official monthly magazine, *Occupational Health Nursing*, AAOHN also issues special manuals, brochures, and guides for promoting nursing excellence in occupational health, including practice standards and occupational nursing service objectives. The organization's headquarters are located at 575 Lexington Avenue, New York, N.Y. 10022.

AMERICAN COLLEGE OF NURSE-MIDWIVES

The philosophy of the American College of Nurse-Midwives (ACNM) is based on the beliefs that every child-bearing family has a right to a safe, satisfying experience with respect for human dignity and worth; for variety in cultural forms; and for the parents' right to self-determination. The American College of Nurse-Midwives defines a certified nurse-midwife (CNM) as an individual educated in the two disciplines of nursing and midwifery, who possesses evidence of certification according to the requirements of the organization. In pursuit of its goals, and working frequently in cooperation with other groups, ACNM identifies areas of appropriate nurse-midwifery practice, studies the activities of the nurse-midwife, establishes qualifications for those activities, administers a national program for certification of nurse-midwives,* approves educational programs in nurse-midwifery,* sponsors research and develops literature in this field, and serves as a channel for communication and interpretation about nurse-midwifery on regional, national, and international levels.

The American College of Nurse-Midwifery was established in 1955; it merged in 1969 with the American Association of Nurse-Midwives, founded in 1929, to become the American College of Nurse-Midwives. Membership is limited to ACNM-certified nurse-midwives, although they do not have to live in the United States.

ACNM is governed by an elected board. The president, vice president, secretary, treasurer, and the six regional representatives serve two-year terms. A national convention is held annually.

ACNM and its members conduct or take part in conferences, institutes, and workshops concerned with the practice of nurse-midwifery and with the improvement of services in the maternal and child health field. The official bimonthly newsletter of the college is *Quickening;* the official publication is *The Journal of Nurse-Midwifery.* The American College of Nurse-Midwives is located at Suite 801, 1012 Fourteenth Street, N.W., Washington, D.C. 20005.

AMERICAN INDIAN/ALASKAN NATIVE NURSES' ASSOCIATION

Established in 1972, as the American Indian Nurses' Association, the American Indian/Alaskan Native Nurses' Association

---

*Certification and accreditation activities are being transferred to autonomous groups.

(AIANNA) is a professional association of American Indian and Alaskan Native registered nurses. The purposes of the association are to promote optimum health among these people, to promote a more equitable number within the nursing profession, to educate all populations about the specific health needs of Indian and Alaskan Native people, and to recommend proper solutions to their health needs.[6]

To achieve these purposes, the AIANNA aims toward developing awareness of the true history and cultural differences of the Indian/Native people, promoting and evaluating research of these groups, encouraging and assisting Indian/Alaskan Native consumers in becoming more involved in the delivery of health care services, and recommending various governmental and private agencies in developing programs designed to improve the total health of these people.

In order to promote a more equitable number of American Indians within the nursing profession, the AIANNA works with schools of nursing, Indian and Alaskan Native communities, and federal and private agencies. The AIANNA/Allstate Scholarship is administered by the AIANNA staff. This particular scholarship is for Associate Degree programs primarily, although it has been used for partial baccalaureate funding recently. In addition, American Indian nursing students are eligible to apply for loans from the Dr. Ethel E. Wortis Emergency Fund on a loan-at-no-interest basis. In 1975, the Association initiated a directory of Indian nurses. In 1978, the organization's name was changed to include the Alaskan Native nurses. The national office address is P.O. Box 1588, Norman, Oklahoma 73070.

AMERICAN UROLOGICAL ASSOCIATION, ALLIED

Organized in 1972, the American Urological Association Allied (AUAA), is an organization dedicated to advancing the cause of professionalism and better patient care in the field of urology and to encouraging others in the health care field to adopt urology as a full-time nursing specialty. At the present time, there are 1,066 members. The AUAA is divided into eight geographical sections with a total of thirty-one chapters.

It is the purpose of the AUAA to serve as a vehicle for the distribution of all available information in the field of urology and to continually point the way to advanced nursing techniques and new equipment, and to assist those who wish to commit themselves to become urology specialists.

The AUAA Council is working towards the planning of national, regional, and local meetings. An annual national meeting is held in conjunction with the American Urological Association.

Active membership is open to those in health care professions who have completed an approved course of instruction or its equivalent and are actively engaged in the field of urology. Associate membership is available. The AUAA provides certification for members on three levels. The certification board is separate from the organization and consists of members from both the AUAA and the American Urological Association. Certification is based on assessment of knowledge, demonstration of current clinical practice, and endorsement by colleagues. A newsletter, *Uro-Gram*, is published six times a year. The administrative offices are located at 21510 South Main Street, Carson, California 90745.

ASSOCIATION OF OPERATING ROOM NURSES

The Association of Operating Room Nurses (AORN) is an organization of professional operating room nurses with both national and international members and a universal interest in encouraging cooperative action by registered nurses to improve the quality of operating room nursing. Although a group of operating room nurses first formed in 1949 with the intention of affiliat-

ing with either ANA or NLN, and was actively a part of ANA for some years, the member operating room nurses gradually came to believe that their educational, organizational, and interest needs could only be met by an independent organization devoted specifically to operating room nursing. Therefore, they incorporated in 1957 and officially named the organization the Association of Operating Room Nurses. Current membership is almost 26,000 with a total of 257 chapters.

The stated objectives of AORN are to motivate and encourage operating room (OR) nurses to accept personal responsibility for their continuing education, which can help them provide quality care to surgical patients; increase the understanding, knowledge, and skills of OR nursing personnel; foster leadership qualities in the professional operating room RN; promote and encourage effective communications and interpersonal relationships between OR personnel and their patients and related medical workers; promote increased nurse interest and participation in professional organizations; maintain cooperative relationships with other professional organizations; study existing practices and new developments in the fields of OR nursing and education; encourage RNs and students of nursing to specialize in OR nursing; and be an effective voice in the ever-changing functions of nursing in general and OR nursing in particular.

Any registered professional nurse directly associated with OR nursing, full-time or part-time, is eligible for active membership. Associate membership is offered to any RN inactive in nursing but who was qualified to be an active member prior to becoming inactive. Other RNs involved in anesthesia, recovery room, emergency room, OB labor and delivery, nursing service administration, intensive-care or coronary-care units, central supply, and industry may also be eligible for associate memberships.

AORN has a full-time nurse executive director and a nurse director of education and has established a National Committee on Education, which supervises educational matters of concern to members and other OR personnel. Local chapters plan regional institutes with NCE guidance, and educational programs are also held during the annual convention. AORN awards continuing education units for noncredit educational programs, in line with the recommendations of the National Task Force on the Continuing Education Unit.

The official AORN organ is the monthly *AORN Journal,* which publishes original articles on operating room nursing and key nursing issues as well as local chapter news and reports of national activities. Other publications include information about OR nursing and a manual, "What Every OR Supervisor Should Know." A list of publications currently available may be obtained from AORN headquarters.

AORN has worked with ANA, NLN, and the American College of Surgeons on various issues, particularly the training of ancillary personnel for the operating room. A special AORN committee developed comprehensive guidelines for the selection, training, and certification of OR technicians. In 1968, the board of directors structured an allied association, the Association of Operating Room Technicians (AORT). An AORN-AORT advisory board developed educational activities, including the implementation of a certifying examination, and was responsible for granting that certification as well as accrediting ORT education programs. AORN withdrew from this board in mid-1973 because of various disagreements between the two organizations. The program accreditation process was turned over to AMA's Council on Medical Education, but certification responsibilities were retained by AORT. AORN headquarters is at 10170 E. Mississippi Avenue, Denver, Colorado 80231.

ASSOCIATION FOR PRACTITIONERS IN INFECTION CONTROL

The Association for Practitioners in Infection Control (APIC) grew out of a need for an organization to provide communication and education to those persons involved in infection control activities. In 1972, a steering committee met, at which time APIC was established. In 1973, the first international elections were held to elect members of the board of directors and officers.

The purpose of APIC is to improve patient care by serving the needs and aims of all disciplines who are united by infection control activities. Specific objectives are developing communication, supporting educational programs that assist the practitioner in gaining proficiency, encouraging the development of effective infection control programs, encouraging the standardization of infection control programs, and promoting quality of research.

Membership is open to all individuals involved in infection control activities. Further information may be obtained by writing to 1557 North Pinecrest, Wichita, Kansas 67208.

ASSOCIATION OF REHABILITATION NURSES

The Association of Rehabilitation Nurses (ARN) was founded in 1974 to advance the quality of rehabilitation nursing service by offering educational opportunities to promote an awareness and interest in rehabilitation nursing and to facilitate the exchange of ideas in rehabilitation programs.

Local workshops, regional seminars, and annual educational conferences are held throughout the country yearly. The ARN also has conducted a needs assessment survey of its members and is working on a basis for core curriculum. The association has established itself as a representative organization for professional rehabilitation nurses and has become involved in legislative and professional issues affecting the specialty of rehabilitation nursing. ARN is structured to provide for chapters on a state or area basis and for seven regions in North America.

Current membership is approximately 1,300. Regular membership in ARN is open to RNs concerned with or engaged in the active practice of rehabilitation nursing. Associate (nonvoting) membership is available to those in other health care disciplines, and any others interested in rehabilitation and in the activities of ARN. Chapter membership is also available.

The *ARN Journal* is the official publication of the Association of Rehabilitation Nurses and is designed to reflect the thought, trends, policies, and research in rehabilitative nursing. Standards of Rehabilitation Nursing have been published jointly by the ANA and ARN. The organization's headquarters is located at Suite 470, 1701 Lake Avenue, Glenview, Illinois 60025.

DEPARTMENT OF SCHOOL NURSES, AN AFFILIATE OF THE NATIONAL EDUCATION ASSOCIATION

The Department of School Nurses, an affiliate of the National Education Association (DSN/NEA) was established by the NEA Representative Assembly in July 1968. Active membership is open to all registered professional school nurses employed by a board of education, governing board of a private school, or board of trustees of an institution of higher education. Membership in NEA is a prerequisite. Currently there are approximately 1,900 nurse members.

The purpose of DSN/NEA is "to strengthen the nation's educational process through improvement of the health status of children and youth." Among the activities and advantages are supporting legislative efforts for better health for students and adults, providing educational travel opportunities, making efforts toward improved financing of schools, and providing consultative services in cases of unfair dismissal practices.

The official journal of DSN/NEA is *The School Nurse*. Other publications are informational for both school nurses and the public, including standards for school nurse services and their evaluation, studies of school nurse practices, and definitions of function.

The organization is located at NEA headquarters, 1201 Sixteenth St., N.W., Washington, D.C. 20036.

EMERGENCY DEPARTMENT NURSES' ASSOCIATION

The Emergency Department Nurses' Association (EDNA) was incorporated in December 1970, and since that time has grown to an active membership in excess of 11,000. It was founded to represent nurses faced with all the problems of providing emergency care so that these nurses could pool their knowledge and seek solutions to these problems, set standards, and develop improved methods for practicing efficient emergency medicine. Eligible for membership are registered nurses and licensed practical-vocational nurses actively engaged in the activities of an emergency department and its policies and procedures, or engaged in an occupation requiring the need for knowledge of such policies or procedures (school nurse, industrial nurse).

The major objective of EDNA is to provide optimum emergency care to patients in emergency departments. Members are urged to promote a positive attitude toward education on all levels within the emergency department by continuing study through the EDNA organization, to support formal programs of instruction for emergency techniques and for postgraduate courses on the professional level, and to participate in community planning of total emergency care.

Since 1975, EDNA has published *The Journal of Emergency Nursing*, which provides articles on all aspects of emergency nursing. The association has published a *Continuing Education Curriculum* with teaching guidelines for twenty-six areas of emergency nursing. During the Annual EDNA Scientific Assembly, both business and clinical programs are presented as well as postgraduate courses. Instructor certification courses for participants who have the responsibility of training both medical personnel and the community, are also offered.

The EDNA national office is located at 666 N. Lake Shore Drive, Suite 1729, Chicago, Illinois 60611.

NATIONAL ASSOCIATION OF HISPANIC NURSES

The National Association of Hispanic Nurses (NAHN) was formed in June 1976 in Atlantic City under the name National Association of Spanish Speaking/Spanish Surnamed Nurses (NASSSSN). Evolving from an ad hoc committee of the Spanish Speaking/Spanish Surnamed caucus formed at the 1974 ANA convention, it brought together for the first time Hispanic nurses from all Hispanic subgroups—Mexican-American, Puerto Rican, Cuban, and Latin American—to provide a forum for exchange of information and experiences about health care services to the Hispanic community. Its name was changed in 1979.

The objectives of NAHN are to provide a forum in which Hispanic nurses can analyze, research, and evaluate the health care needs of the Hispanic community; to disseminate research findings and policy perspectives dealing with Hispanic health care needs to local, state, and federal agencies so as to impact policy making and the allocation of resources; to identify Hispanic nurses throughout the nation to ascertain the size of this work force available to provide culturally sensitive nursing care to Hispanic consumers; to identify Hispanic nurses throughout the nation so as to monitor the size and growth of this group of health care professionals; to collaborate, assist, and provide technical assistance to other Hispanic health-oriented professionals; to identify barriers to the delivery of health services for Hispanic consumers and recommend to local, state, and federal agencies appropriate solutions; to identify barriers to quality education for Hispanic nursing students and recommend to local, state, and federal agencies appropriate solutions; to assess the safety and quality of health care delivery services

for the Hispanic community; to work for the recruitment and retention of Hispanic students in nursing educational programs, so as to increase the number of bilingual and bicultural nurses who can provide culturally sensitive nursing care to Hispanic consumers; to develop, test, and promote culturally sensitive models of intervention and approaches that will provide effective nursing care for Hispanic consumers; to ensure that Hispanic nurses have equal access to educational, professional, and economic opportunities; and to provide an opportunity for Hispanic nurses from all over the United States and Puerto Rico to share information dealing with their professional concerns, experiences, and research.

Membership is open to any Hispanic nurse in the United States, the Commonwealth of Puerto Rico, or other jurisdiction of the United States. Non-Hispanic nurses interested and concerned about the health delivery needs of the Hispanic community as well as the professional needs of Hispanic nurses are welcome to apply for associate membership.

The NAHN publishes a newsletter and is compiling a Directory of Hispanic Nurses in the United States. The organization holds biennial national conferences (even years). NAHN's mailing address is 12044 Seventh Avenue, N.W., Seattle, Washington 98177.

NATIONAL ASSOCIATION OF PEDIATRIC NURSE ASSOCIATES AND PRACTITIONERS

The National Association of Pediatric Nurse Associates and Practitioners (NAPNAP) was organized in 1973. To achieve its goal of the delivery of the highest quality health care to children, NAPNAP works closely with the American Academy of Pediatrics (AAP), which has supported joint ventures with NAPNAP such as the development of the National Qualifying Examination for Pediatric Nurse Practitioners and Pediatric Nurse Associates (PNP/As).

The objectives of NAPNAP are to make available continuing education for its members, work toward standardization and accreditation of programs to prepare the Pediatric Nurse Associate or Practitioner, work toward certification of PNP/As in conjunction with other certifying bodies, facilitate and support appropriate changes in legislation to formalize the PNA-PNP role, and to arrange a central employment file.

Active members must be RNs who have completed a course following the guidelines developed by the AAP/AMA Liaison Committee for PNA-PNPs, RNs who are practicing as PNA-PNPs and were trained prior to the guidelines, RNs who were prepared as Family Nurse Practitioners or School Nurse Practitioners, RNs who are faculty members who prepare such Nurse Practitioners, and RNs who otherwise qualify for active membership but live outside the United States and who submit proof of licensure or registration in the nurse's native country or state. Associate, student, and chapter memberships are also available.

There are currently approximately 1,500 PNP/As certified through examination by the National Board of PNP/As. The association has been in the process of incorporating the NAPNAP Foundation to promote research and educational activities related to the primary health care of children and their families.

The official journal of NAPNAP is *Pediatric Nursing*, which is distributed to all members and published bimonthly. The "Pediatric Nurse Practitioner Newsletter" is also published bimonthly and distributed without charge to all pediatric nurse practitioners. In an effort to provide guidance for PNP/As and those who employ them, "The Scope of Practice Statement" for Pediatric Nurse Practitioners/Associates was published jointly by NAPNAP and the American Academy of Pediatrics in 1975.

Educational opportunities are available to all members through seminars, regional conferences, and joint participation at the AAP meetings. NAPNAP headquarters is located at North Woodbury Road, Box 56, Pitman, New Jersey 08071.

NATIONAL BLACK NURSES' ASSOCIATION

The National Black Nurses' Association (NBNA) was formed at the end of 1971 as an outgrowth of the Black Nurses' Caucus held during the 1970 ANA convention. These nurses believed that black Americans and other minority groups "are by design or neglect excluded from the means to achieve access to the health mainstream of America" and that black nurses have the "understanding, knowledge, interest, concern, and experience to make a significant difference in the health care status of the Black Community." The group's leaders have also cited failure of the integration of NACGN into ANA as a reason for beginning a new organization and state that such lack of integration is evidenced by the absence of black nurses in leadership positions, limited opportunities in policy making, failure to recognize quality of performance of black nurses, loss of identity of black nurses, tokenism, and failure to increase significantly the percentage of black RNs.[7]

The purpose and objectives of NBNA, as stated in the membership brochure, are to

> *Define and determine nursing care for Black consumers for optimum quality of care by acting as their advocates.*
> *Act as change agent in restructuring existing institutions and/or helping to establish institutions to suit our needs.*
> *Serve as the national nursing body to influence legislation and policies that affect Black people and work cooperatively and collaboratively with other health workers to this end.*
> *Conduct, analyze, and publish research to increase the body of knowledge about health needs of Blacks.*
> *Compile and maintain a National Directory of Black Nurses to assist with the dissemination of information regarding Black nurses and nursing on national and local levels by the use of all media.*

Set standards and guidelines for quality education of Black nurses on all levels by providing consultation to nursing faculties and by monitoring for proper utilization and placement of Black nurses.

Recruit, counsel, and assist Black persons interested in nursing to ensure a constant procession of Blacks into the field.

Be the vehicle for unification of Black nurses of varied age groups, educational levels, and geographic locations to endure continuity and flow of our common heritage.

Collaborate with other Black groups to compile archives relevant to the historical, current, and future activities of Black nurses.

Provide the impetus and means for Black nurses to write and publish on an individual or collaborative basis.

Membership is open to RNs, LPNs, and student nurses. The first national conference was held in 1973, and yearly conferences are planned. Further information may be obtained from National Black Nurses' Association, 318 The Ohio Building, 175 South Main St., Akron, Ohio 44308.

NATIONAL INTRAVENOUS THERAPY ASSOCIATION, INC.

The National Intravenous Therapy Association, Inc. (NITA) was established primarily to promote education and encourage high-quality practice for intravenous (IV) nurses. The objectives of NITA are to provide the benefits and protection of a qualified IV nurse to the patient, encourage high-quality professional practice through the establishment of standards and controls, and disseminate knowledge by providing for interchange of information among its members.

Membership is offered on an active, associate, or inactive basis. Active members must be registered nurses, working full- or part-time in the field of IV therapy, and in good standing with the licensing agency of the state or country in which the member resides or works. There are currently 1,150 members. The association has an annual convention, and there are sixteen chapters with regular meetings and seminars. Benefits that may be obtained through the association include professional and personal liability insurance. Members receive the official bimonthly publication entitled, *NITA*. The NITA business office is located at 850 Third Avenue, New York, N.Y. 10022.

NATIONAL MALE NURSE ASSOCIATION

The National Male Nurse Association (NMNA) evolved from the Michigan Male Nurses' Association, which was founded in the early 1970s as a forum for discussion of the problems and concerns of men nurses. The major objectives are to provide men nurses an opportunity to:

1. Join together in order to help eliminate prejudice in nursing.
2. Interest men in the nursing profession.
3. Encourage education and promote further professional growth.
4. Provide opportunity to discuss common problems.
5. Advise and assist in areas of professional inequities.
6. Help develop sensitivities to various social needs.
7. Promote the principles and practices of positive health care.

The group has established a Luther Christman Award for contributions to the development of the nursing profession. President Ford was the first awardee and Myrtle Aydelotte, then executive director of ANA, was another. Conventions are usually held annually. Headquarters are at 2309 State Street, Saginaw, Michigan 48602.

NATIONAL NURSES' SOCIETY ON ALCOHOLISM

The National Nurses' Society on Alcoholism (NNSA), a component of the National Council on Alcoholism, is an association of nurses interested in that problem. The purposes are to extend knowledge, to disseminate information, to promote quality nursing care for the alcoholic patient and his family, and to become involved with public policy and social issues concerning alcohol use and alcoholism. This organization serves as a forum for those nurses interested in alcoholism to share their knowledge and experience and to continue their education. As a component of the National Council on Alcoholism, the NNSA has the primary responsibility in the field of nursing.

Membership is available to all currently licensed nurses in any of the fifty states, the District of Columbia, Puerto Rico, territories of the United States, and other countries of North America. All members of the NNSA are automatically members of the National Council on Alcoholism. Candidate membership may be given to student nurses in their senior year.

NNSA meets annually, and the National Forum proceedings, other than the business meetings, are open to nonmembers. NNSA participates in conferences, panel discussions, and teaching sessions. The Society is governed by an elected board whose members serve for three years.

The NNSA publishes the *NNSA Newsletter* quarterly for distribution to its members. The Society is located at 733 Third Avenue, New York, N.Y. 10017.

THE NURSES' ASSOCIATION OF THE AMERICAN COLLEGE OF OBSTETRICIANS AND GYNECOLOGISTS

The Nurses' Association of the American College of Obstetricians and Gynecologists (NAACOG) was organized in 1969. The purposes of NAACOG are to promote, in conjunction with the American College of Obstetricians and Gynecologists, the highest standards of obstetrical, gynecological, and neonatal nursing practice, education, and research; to cooperate at all levels with members of the health team; and to stimulate interest in obstetrical, gynecological, and neonatal nursing. There are currently 17,000 members.

The organization is structured into eight districts or regions and further divided into sections, comprised of states, the District of Columbia, and provinces in Canada. Members elect section, district, and national officers. Membership qualifications include graduation from a state (or province) accredited school of nursing; current licensure as a registered nurse; active participation or interest in obstetric, gynecologic, or neonatal nursing; and demonstration of high ethical standards and professional standing. Election to membership is by action of the executive board. Associate membership is offered to allied health workers whose primary job responsibility is patient care in OGN nursing and who function under the supervision of a registered nurse or physician. Election to membership is by action of the association executive board.

Major activities are related to continuing education through conferences, seminars, workshops, and continuing education courses. The association has developed a manual of standards for OGN nursing and criteria for certification of excellence in OGN nursing practice. Members serve on various College committees, and Fellows of the College serve on association committees. The association works with a number of allied professional organizations on items of mutual interest. National meetings of the association are held every other year, either in conjunction with College meetings or separately.

The official publication of NAACOG is the *Journal of Obstetric, Gynecologic and Neonatal Nursing*, which reflects current ideas, trends, policy, and research in this area of specialty nursing. The *Bulletin* contains news of section, district, and national association activities, as do various newsletters at the local level. The administrative office of NAACOG is located at 1 E. Wacker Drive, Suite 2700, Chicago, Illinois 60601.

NURSES' CHRISTIAN FELLOWSHIP

The Nurses' Christian Fellowship (NCF), established in 1948, is affiliated with the Inter-Varsity Christian Fellowship, a nonprofit religious organization. It exists to help both students and nurses to grow spiritually as they mature professionally. Its focus is on ministering to the whole person—physically, psychosocially, and spiritually—in health and illness or in the face of death. Training, including crisis intervention and the spiritual dimension of care, is provided through nursing-oriented Bible studies, fellowship groups, summer conferences, workshops, and seminars. The Nurses' Christian Fellowship is a member of NCF International.

The *Nurse's Lamp*, its bimonthly publication, and other materials are available from Nurses' Christian Fellowship, 233 Langdon Street, Madison, Wisconsin 53703.

ONCOLOGY NURSING SOCIETY

The Oncology Nursing Society (ONS) was founded in 1975. The purposes of the organization are to develop new knowledge leading to the earlier detection and improvement of care of persons at risk for, or diagnosed with, cancer; to disseminate knowledge and information to nurses involved in the care of such patients; to encourage nurses to specialize in the care of cancer patients; and to establish guidelines of nursing care for patients with cancer. There are approximately 1,200 members in ONS. All registered nurses engaged in or interested in oncology are eligible to petition for membership.

The *Oncology Nursing Forum*, published quarterly, is the official publication of the ONS. The first board of directors was elected in 1977 and consists of four officers. The Oncology Nursing Society has completed the first set of standards for oncology nursing care, which was published by ANA in 1978. Additional information may be obtained by writing to P.O. Box 33, Oakmont, Pennsylvania 15139.

SIGMA THETA TAU

Sigma Theta Tau, Inc., is the national honor society of nursing in the United States, comparable to the national honor societies in other professions. Organized in 1922,[8] Sigma Theta Tau (the initials of the Greek words meaning "love," "courage," and "honor") had grown in 1980 to 128 chapters in colleges and universities offering baccalaureate and higher degree programs in nursing.

Members are chosen from students enrolled in NLN-accredited nursing programs leading to a baccalaureate or higher degree. Criteria for selection are high scholastic achievement, leadership qualities, and capacity for personal and professional growth. Graduate nurses who hold a baccalaureate or higher degree may also be selected on the basis of having shown marked achievement in the field of nursing. The overall purposes of the society are to recognize superior achievement and the development of leadership qualities, to foster high professional standards, to encourage creative work, and to strengthen commitment to the ideals and purposes of the profession.

The National Council, which is composed of Sigma Theta Tau's five elected national officers, meets three times a year. The House of Delegates, composed of two delegates from each local chapter, plus the National Council, is the governing body of the society. It meets biennially. Local chapters hold at least four meetings during the academic year, usually of an educational nature. Many local chapters grant scholarships and research funds. A research fund has been established on the national level from which grants are made to nurses engaged in research.

Image, a scholarly peer-review journal, is published three times annually; and *Reflections*, the society's newsletter, is published five times annually. Research presentations are scheduled at national meetings of the National League for Nursing and the American Nurses' Association. Regional meetings to promote scholarly nursing are also sponsored. The national headquarters is located at 1100 West Michigan Street, Indianapolis, Indiana 46223.

HEALTH-RELATED ORGANIZATIONS

Many health-related organizations, both governmental and nongovernmental, frequently provide opportunities for participation by nurses through some form of membership, consultation, or inclusion on committees or programs. A number provide services specifically for nurses, such as workshops, conferences, publications, and audio-visual materials. Nurses may also be invited to attend other program sessions, present papers, or serve on panels. Some examples include the American Cancer Society, the American Heart Association, the American Medical Association, and the Catholic Hospital Association.

There are also organizations in which there are large, active nursing components. Some of the most visible of these are described here, as well as the two practical nurse organizations.

THE AMERICAN HOSPITAL ASSOCIATION

The American Hospital Association (AHA) includes a number of groups and activities involving nursing. The purpose of the Assembly of Hospital Schools of Nursing is to represent and express the views of the members of the Assembly and to assist the House of Delegates and Board of Trustees in the development and implementation of policies and programs designed to promote recognition, support, and improvement of hospital schools of nursing as part of the general education system. Membership is open to hospital schools of nursing of AHA institutional members.

The *American Society for Health Manpower Education and Training* was founded in 1970. Hospital-based educators and trainers are eligible for individual membership. About 40 per cent of the group are nurses. A national meeting and concurrent conferences are held annually. Other conferences are held regionally, according to the needs cited by those in a particular area. *Cross Reference on Human Resources Management* is published for members.

The primary functions of the Division of general Nursing at the American Hospital Association include consultation, education, and information services on such topics as nurse recruitment, nurse manpower utilization, performance appraisals, collective bargaining, and quality assurance; responding to concerns on mandatory continuing education; monitoring foreign nurse issues; interpreting nursing education levels and competency; and maintaining relationships with other organizations. The Division of Nursing is headed by a director of nursing. The staff members supportive of the division include RNs with expertise in the areas described.

The *American Society for Nursing Service Administrators* (ASNSA) is an affiliated society of the American Hospital Association. The objectives of ASNSA are to provide a medium for the interchange of ideas and dissemination of information relative to nursing service administration, provide consultation and direction on all matters relating to nursing and health care issues, promote educational programs and activities to strengthen nursing service administration, and to develop a recognition program for professional excellence in the field of nursing service administration.

ASNSA is organized into the board of directors, committees, members, and associates. To qualify as a member of ASNSA, a registered nurse must be the nurse administrator holding the highest level management position in the organization of nursing service in a health care institution. Associate membership is available to nurses holding line management positions who are directly accountable to the top nurse administrator.

Members have full use of AHA library facilities. In addition, members also receive publications such as *Hospitals*, a weekly newsletter of health care news, the *AHA Guide to the Health Care Field*, and position papers published by the ASNSA and AHA. Members may attend the annual business and program meeting of the ASNSA; national, regional, and local institutes and workshops; the annual AHA convention; and the annual meeting of the AHA. The organization is located at 840 North Lake Shore Drive, Chicago, Illinois 60611.

THE AMERICAN PUBLIC HEALTH ASSOCIATION

The American Public Health Association (APHA), established in 1872, is the largest organization of its kind in the world, with a membership of more than 30,231, in addition to the approximately 30,000 members of its affiliates. As a professional organization, it represents workers of forty-four health-related fields in the shaping of national and local public health policies; as a communications network, it circulates new knowledge through the internationally respected *American Journal of Public Health* and a publishing house operation of major proportions. The *Nation's Health* is the official monthly newspaper of the association.

Of the twenty-three specialized sections that comprise APHA, the Public Health Nursing Section is the third largest, with more than 3,000 members, and one of the oldest, having celebrated its fiftieth anniversary in 1972. Highly active and influential, the Public Health Nursing Section provides a voice for nursing interests within the APHA structure, and nationally through that structure. Section members participate on APHA's program development board, action board, task forces and committees and with other sections of the association. Through cooperative relationships with other nursing groups, such as the American Nurses' Association, Federation of Specialty Nursing Organizations, and the National League for

Nursing, it strives for improvement of nursing and education services within the broad perspective of public health.

In the last ten years, the section has studied numerous aspects and issues of public health nursing, including organization and administration, relationships between hospitals and public health agencies, population planning, services for unwed mothers, team nursing, salaries, educational and professional qualifications, quality assurance and staffing issues. Recently, a primary concern of the section, as voiced in policy resolutions presented to the APHA program development board, has been the further study of the expanded role of the nurse in health care. In its investigation of these issues, the Public Health Nursing Section has continuously been in the organizational forefront of the APHA structure. In the past thirty-five years, more than forty nurses have been elected members of APHA's Governing Council including the executive board, for a total of nearly 150 years of service. Nurses Marion Sheahan and Margaret Dolan have served as president of the APHA in 1960 and 1973, respectively, and several nurses have held the office of vice president. In addition, Marion Sheahan and Margaret Arnstein have both won the Sedgwick Memorial Medal, one of APHA's highest citations; the Albert Lasker and Martha May Eliot Awards have been won by nurses several times; and the prestigious Bronfman Prize was given to Ruth B. Freeman, RN, in 1971.

The APHA annual meeting provides an excellent forum for the Public Health Nurses' scientific and business exchanges and social events, but meetings of the various section councils and committees are also held throughout the year. Two awards are given by the section at each annual meeting to recognize nurses who have made outstanding contributions to public health nursing. A fascinating and detailed *History of the Public Health Nursing Section, 1922–1972*, by Ella E. McNeil, is now out of print but on file in the APHA archives. In 1977, the Margaret B. Dolan Lectureship Fund was established by the PHN Section, and at the 1978 APHA convention, the first lecture was presented as the convention keynote address. APHA headquarters address is 1015 15th Street, N.W., Washington, D.C. 20005.

AMERICAN RED CROSS

Founded in 1881 by Clara Barton, who had ministered to the sick and wounded on the battlefields of the Civil War, the American Red Cross operates under a Congressional Charter granted in 1905. The President of the United States serves as honorary chairman and appoints the chairman and seven other members of the volunteer fifty-member Board of Governors. To administer its activities, there are four field offices, sixty-one divisions, and more than 3,000 local chapters. Internationally, the American Red Cross is a member of the League of Red Cross Societies and supports the International Committee of the Red Cross, which is the guardian of the four Geneva Conventions.

The aims of the American Red Cross are to improve the quality of human life and enhance individual self-reliance and concern for others. It works toward these aims through national and chapter services governed and directed by volunteers. American Red Cross services help people avoid emergencies, prepare for emergencies, and cope with them when they occur.

To accomplish its aims, the Red Cross provides volunteer blood services to a large segment of the nation, conducts community services and, as mandated by its Congressional Charter, serves as an independent medium of voluntary relief and communication between the American people and their armed forces; maintains a system of local, national, and international disaster preparedness and relief; and assists the government of the United States to meet humanitarian treaty commitments. The Red Cross has a number of publications describing its programs.

Ever since the Red Cross was founded,

Nursing and Health Services has been one of the important units in many Red Cross societies. In the United States, a Division of Nursing Services was established in the American Red Cross in 1909, with Jane A. Delano as its first director. The maintenance of a reserve of qualified professional nurses who could be mobilized quickly in emergencies such as disaster or war was the initial purpose of the Red Cross Nursing Services. During World Wars I and II, the Red Cross Nursing Services recruited and certified the majority of the nurses assigned to the military nurse corps. In 1947, legislation was passed by the Congress of the United States establishing a permanent nurse corps for the armed forces, including the maintenance of a nurse reserve, thus relieving the Red Cross of maintaining this service. However, the need for nurses to volunteer in community services remains as great as it ever was, and nurses are urged to enroll in the Red Cross for this purpose.

Red Cross Nursing and Health Services today are designed to extend community resources in helping to meet the health needs of people at home and in the community. Policies and standards for all Red Cross services are determined at the national level. At the local level, the chapter Nursing and Health Services committees are responsible for planning and implementing the nursing services. Not all chapters have identical services because community needs, resources, and interests vary. However, standardized educational courses are available throughout the nation. Although the services may vary, Nursing and Health Services maintains a reserve of volunteer nurses who become enrolled as Red Cross nurses for the following activities:

Disaster Health Services. One of the charter-mandated services provided by Red Cross is to meet the human needs of the victims of disaster. Nurses are prepared through a series of training courses to adapt their nursing skills to meet nursing needs brought about by disasters and to serve at the time of local and national disasters. The basic training includes skills in providing health services in disaster areas as well as meeting other immediate needs of disaster victims. Through advanced training and experience on disaster operations, nurses can be prepared to serve at the Disaster Health Services supervisory and director level on national disasters.

Educational Courses. In order to assist the population to assume the responsibility for their own health maintenance, encourage preventive health care, and increase self-reliance, Red Cross Nursing and Health Services courses are available to the general public, elementary and secondary schools, colleges and schools of nursing, military dependents on United States military establishments at home and abroad, and other special groups. These courses include Providing Health Services in Disaster; Home Nursing; Preparation for Parenthood; Parenting; Vital Signs; Cardiopulmonary Resuscitation; Multiple Sclerosis (ARC-MS) Home Care; Good Grooming; and Mother's Aide. New courses are developed to meet specific needs. As an example, Nursing and Health Services is presently working with other agencies to provide a course in Respite Care. This course will prepare individuals to give respite to family members responsible for the long-term care of someone handicapped or with a chronic illness. Nursing and Health Services also works with other agencies in the development of training material for the preparation of home health aides and other courses. Continuing Education Units have been approved in many states for the instructor preparation for the courses mentioned.

Direct Services. In providing direct services for individuals and community groups, Nursing and Health Services volunteers are involved in activities such as assisting in blood services; immunization, vision, and hearing clinics; hypertension detection and follow-up programs; testing for sickle cell anemia, diabetes, and lead poison; emergency aid stations; counseling and school health programs. These services are provided in cooperation with state and local public and private agencies.

The American Red Cross Nursing and Health Services and Red Cross Blood Services Nursing work closely with all local, state, and federal nursing services and national organizations in the advancement of nursing education and nursing services in general, as well as for Red Cross nursing in particular.

Nurses participating in any of the Red Cross activities are provided recognition as part of a humanitarian organization through nurse enrollment. The basic requirements for enrolling as a Red Cross nurse are the following:

1. Graduation from a state-approved school of professional nursing.
2. Registration following graduation and current registration where it is required by law for the type of work the nurse expects to do for the American Red Cross.
3. Satisfactory personal, educational, and professional qualifications, and a state of health consistent with the work the nurse plans to do.

In addition to these basic requirements, the nurse will be asked to give some Red Cross service as evidence of his or her willingness and desire to be a member of the Red Cross organization.

Red Cross Nursing and Health Services provides an excellent opportunity for students in schools of nursing to participate in community health activities. Directors of schools of professional nursing frequently include Red Cross experience as part of the curriculum or encourage their students to participate in Red Cross activities. The student participating can become an enrolled Red Cross nurse following registration as a professional nurse by presenting the credentials received as a student to the local chapter. The nurse will receive the Red Cross nurse's badge when the request has been processed.

Volunteer and paid Red Cross nurses follow the same procedure for requesting enrollment. Nurses who join the paid staff almost invariably have formerly served as volunteers. To enroll in the Red Cross, nurses should write or phone the local chapter office for further information. If there is no local chapter in a nurse's area, nurses can obtain information by writing to the National Director, Program Operations, Nursing and Health Services, American Red Cross, 17th and D Streets, N.W., Washington, D.C. 20006.

A professional nurse officially accepted for Red Cross service receives an appointment card certifying enrollment and a Red Cross badge bearing an individual identification number.

COMMISSION ON GRADUATES OF FOREIGN NURSING SCHOOLS

The Commission on Graduates of Foreign Nursing Schools (CGFNS) was established in January 1977 as a nonprofit, independent organization sponsored by the American Nurses' Association and the National League for Nursing. CGFNS supports the United Nations Declaration of Human Rights which affirms the individual's freedom to migrate; however, CGFNS neither encourages nor discourages immigration. The purpose of CGFNS is to prevent the exploitation of graduates of foreign nursing schools who come to the United States to practice nursing, but are prevented from doing so as a result of failure to pass state licensing examinations. (Only about twenty percent pass on the first try.) Another purpose is to help assure safe patient care for the American public. To attain these purposes, CGFNS screens and examines foreign nursing school graduates while they are still in their own countries to determine their probable eligibility for professional nursing practice in the United States. The first preimmigration screening examination was conducted in October 1978; about 10 percent of the candidates passed. The Commission received a grant from the W. K. Kellogg Foundation to provide four worldwide screening examinations testing both English comprehension and nursing proficiency, in 1979-80. The Commission's governing body is a board of trustees of six nurses and up to five trustees-at-large who specifically represent the interest of the general public. An executive director assumes the administrative responsibilities of the organization. CGFNS is located at 3624 Market Street, Philadelphia, Pa. 19104.

MIDWEST ALLIANCE IN NURSING

The Midwest Alliance in Nursing (MAIN) was established in 1978 and aims to advance and protect the health of persons in the Midwest by promoting an improved system of higher education in nursing, improving nursing practice, and advancing nursing research. One of the organization's prime functions is to foster productive relationships and better communications between personnel in nursing education, nursing service institutions, and liaison agencies and organizations. MAIN will be concerned with nursing activities in Indiana, Illinois, Iowa, Kansas, Michigan, Minnesota, Missouri, Nebraska, North Dakota, Ohio, Oklahoma, South Dakota, and Wisconsin.

In addition to providing continuing education MAIN also aims to promote regional planning for nursing education and service. It will work toward resolution of nursing issues, such as the separation of education and service, and encourage a multidisciplinary approach to health care. All educational institutions preparing nurses for licensure from diploma through graduate level and health care agencies offering acute, long-term and ambulatory services will be invited to join the organization as well as special organizations, such as state and regional planning agencies. MAIN headquarters is at the Indiana University School of Nursing, Indianapolis, Indiana 46223.

NATIONAL ASSOCIATION FOR PRACTICAL NURSE EDUCATION AND SERVICE

The National Association for Practical Nurse Education and Service, Inc. (NAPNES) is the oldest organization for practical nurses in the United States. It was founded in 1941 by a group of nurse educators for the purpose of improving and extending the education of the practical nurse to meet the critical need for more nursing personnel. Founded as the Association of Practical Nurse Schools, the name was changed to the National Association for Practical Nurse Education in 1942; *and Service* was added to the title in 1959.

Within a few years, after professionally planned curricula has been set up and duties of the practical nurse defined, NAPNES expanded its activities to include a broad program of service to schools of practical nursing and the licensed practical vocational nurse (LP/VN). Important among these were the establishment in 1945 of the first accrediting service for programs of practical nursing education now recognized by the United States Office of Education (USOE) and the Council on Postsecondary Accredidation (COPA) as one of the accrediting bodies for practical nurse education.

NAPNES activities include working closely with its constituent state associations to provide guidance and assistance in initiating and carrying out a wide range of programs; conducting workshops and seminars to keep licensed practical/vocational nurses (LP/VNs) abreast of new nursing and medical techniques; providing guidelines for courses to upgrade and expand the capabilities of the LP/VN; sponsorship of continuing education programs; evaluation of such programs sponsored by other agencies for continuing education credit; a computerized record-keeping system for maintaining an accurate record of an individual's continuing education activities; awarding of scholarships to deserving students; dissemination of recruitment materials; conducting an annual survey of state boards of nursing to gather data on LP/VN licensure; and information on and interpretation of practical nursing education and practice to the public. NAPNES serves as one of the spokesmen of the licensed practical nurse on federal and state levels on such matters as licensing, laws governing LP/VN practice, educational opportunities for the licensed practical/vocational nurse, and matters of general welfare. NAPNES publishes the *Journal of Practical Nursing* monthly, which is geared exclusively to meeting the needs of LP/VNs, students, and practical/vocational nurse educators.

Membership is open to all licensed practical/vocational nurses, professional nurses, nurse educators, physicians, hospital and nursing home administrators, and lay citizens interested in practical nursing's role in the health field. Agency membership is open to hospitals, nursing homes, schools of practical nursing, alumni groups, civic organizations, and others interested in the objectives of NAPNES. Students in schools of practical nursing are welcomed as student members. NAPNES headquarters office is at 122 East 42nd Street, New York, N.Y. 10017.

NATIONAL FEDERATION OF LICENSED PRACTICAL NURSES

The membership of the National Federation of Licensed Practical Nurses (NFLPN), a federation of state associations organized in 1949, is made up entirely of licensed practical or vocational nurses. In states with a practical nurses' association affiliated with the federation, members enroll through the state association. In other states, individual practical or vocational nurses may join NFLPN as members-at-large. Each member participates in formulating policies and programs through election of a House of Delegates, which meets during the annual convention. In 1980 there were 16,000 members and more than 3,000 student affiliates. The latter may attend meetings with voice but no vote.

Some of the major purposes of the NFLPN are to preserve and foster the ideal of comprehensive care for the ill and the aged, to associate together all licensed practical nurses or persons with equivalent titles; to secure recognition and effective utilization of the skills of licensed practical nurses; to promote the welfare and interests of licensed practical nurses; to improve standards of practice in practical nursing; to speak for licensed practical nurses and interpret their aims and objectives to other groups and the public; to cooperate with other groups and the public; to cooperate with groups concerned with better patient care; to serve as a clearinghouse for information on practical nursing; and to continue improvement in the education of licensed practical nurses. A code of ethics for licensed practical nurses that stresses many of the same points as the ANA code has been developed by the NFLPN as a "motivation for establishing and elevating professional standards."

To help carry out its objectives, NFLPN maintains a government relations consultant in Washington, D.C., and other consultants on labor relations. In 1962 NFLPN established the National Licensed Practical Nurses' Educational Foundation "for scientific, educational, and charitable purposes." The foundation grants scholarships to qualified students entering approved schools of practical nursing.

Seminars, workshops, and conferences are financed by the federation, as well as leadership training conferences for persons engaged in practical nurse association activities at the national, state, or local level. NFLPN encourages continuing education through sponsorship of the Continuing Education Unit (CEU) system for measuring and permanently recording the participation of individual LPNs in continuing education activities. Adopted by the NFLPN House of Delegates in 1974, the CEU system involves program assessment and approval processes, and provides yearly uniform data to support specifics of continuing education program types, provider agency types, and program lengths in regional and national configura-

tions. An individual CEU Data Bank Account is an automatic benefit of membership in NFLPN, and nonmember LPNs may also arrange for an account and service. Official transcript service is also available.

Both the American Nurses' Association and the National League for Nursing work with NFLPN in matters of mutual concern, principally through liaison committees. The NFLPN supports the National League for Nursing as the recognized agency for accreditation. NFLPN also supports NLN efforts in the development and improvement of practical nurse programs. Members of NFLPN staff or appointed representatives serve on committees with other health personnel and organizations.

NFLPN's official publication is *The Journal of Nursing Care*, a monthly. Other materials on practical nursing, such as the statement on Standards of Practice, are also available. NFLPN headquarters is at 888 Seventh Avenue, New York, N.Y. 10019.

NATIONAL JOINT PRACTICE COMMISSION

In the 1960s there were a number of efforts between the American Nurses' Association and the American Medical Association to encourage increased collaboration between the professions, including three joint conferences on patient care. However, a major impetus for the formation of the commission came from the National Commission for the Study of Nursing and Nursing Education (NCSNNE). One of the major recommendations was that "a National Joint Practice Commission, with state counterpart committees, be established between medicine and nursing to discuss and make recommendations concerning the congruent roles of the physician and the nurse in providing quality health care."[9] NCSNNE asked the AMA and ANA to jointly sponsor the Commission. By the concurrent action of the AMA Board of Trustees and the ANA Board of

Directors, the National Joint Practice Commission (NJPC) was created in September 1971.* The sixteen Commissioners, eight physicians named by the AMA and eight nurses named by the ANA, first met in January 1972, and established these guidelines:

- The Commission should initially concern itself with generating, rather than implementing, concepts.
- The Commission should represent the interests of the public rather than of medicine and nursing *per se.*
- Commission members should regard themselves as consultants on the problems of medicine and nursing, not as advocates for positions within their professions.

The Commission agreed that its primary aim should be "to discuss, study, and make recommendations concerning the roles of the physician and nurse in providing quality health care to our nation's people." It was further agreed that

> Nursing has recognized its need to expand its role, using the capabilities of nurses to the fullest; and medicine has recognized that physicians need to concentrate on their best areas of expertise, in part relinquishing some of what they do to other professions, especially to nursing. Out of these parallel desires, we should be able to develop better role relationships that can result in better health care systems.[10]

Both the ANA and AMA provided the initial funds for the NJPC. A series of grants by the W. K. Kellogg Foundation and continued ANA/AMA funding enabled NJPC to implement important new programs.

The aims of the NJPC were to examine the roles and functions of both professions and to define new roles and relationships, recommend changes in professional education to support new roles, remove sources of professional differences, and assist in the development and support of state joint practice committees.

---

*The NJPC ceased operation when the AMA decided in June, 1980, to discontinue funding and participation as of January, 1981.

These intents are demonstrated by a number of statements made by NJPC: "Medical and Nurse Practice Acts" (1974) encourages flexibility and breadth; "Certification of Nurses and Physicians" (1974), supports certification by each profession of its own practitioners; "Nursing Staffs in Hospitals" (1977), recommends that organized professional nursing staffs at hospitals exercise the responsibility for quality of nursing care; "Definition of Joint or Collaborative Practice in Hospitals" (1977), lists elements of joint practice; and "Joint Practice in Primary Care: Definition and Guidelines" (1977), describes characteristics of joint practice.

In addition, the NJPC has produced several publications: a *Selected Bibliography with Abstracts on Joint Practice* (now out of print); *The Statutory Regulation of the Scope of Nursing Practice—A Critical Survey,* by Virginia C. Hall (1975), intended as an aid to those planning to amend state nurse and medical practice acts; and a casebook of joint practices, published in April 1977, under the title *Together,* and aided by a grant from the Robert Wood Johnson Foundation.

In 1977, the NJPC also initiated a special project to develop joint practice in hospitals through the demonstration of joint practice in four selected hospitals. Five basic elements constitute the activities included in the project. These are to introduce primary nursing, encourage nurses' clinical decision making, integrate the patient record, conduct joint patient care record review, and establish a joint practice committee. In addition, the committee continued to examine the issues in medicine and nursing in primary care settings whose clarification will encourage closer collaboration with joint practice.[11]

Programs have been held at both ANA and AMA meetings, and several National Conferences on Joint Practice have been held. Publication of a quarterly *NJPC Bulletin,* beginning in June 1975, was intended to maintain communication between NJPC and state joint practice committees. Almost all states have such committees, but they function with a varying amount of success. The rather unexpected dissolution of the NJPC presumably should not affect such committees or those at practice sites.

NEW ENGLAND BOARD OF HIGHER EDUCATION (NEW ENGLAND COUNCIL ON HIGHER EDUCATION FOR NURSING)

The New England Board of Higher Education (NEBHE), composed of representatives appointed by the governors of the six states comprising New England, exists to promote and develop activities that will expand educational opportunities for the people of the region and that will most efficiently utilize all of the region's higher education facilities. The board attempts to develop areas of cooperation and mutual interest among more than 250 private and public universities, colleges, and institutes in New England.

In 1964 NEBHE formed the New England Council on Higher Education for Nursing (NECHEN). This action indicates both the recognition of the need for a broad regional approach to improvement of nursing care and education, and also the commitment of the board to assist institutions of higher education in their responsibilities for nursing education.

In 1978, NECHEN was composed of 137 nurse representatives appointed from fifty-eight colleges and universities in New England that offer nursing programs leading to associate, baccalaureate, and graduate degrees in nursing.

The purpose of NECHEN is to promote, improve, and coordinate educational opportunities for the preparation of professional and technical nurses through cooperative planning and consultation among New England institutions of higher education. To carry out these purposes, the council supports, promotes, and undertakes cooperative planning for educational programs with New England institutions of higher learning, provides opportunities for exchanges of ideas and information among nursing and other faculty members in these institutions, promotes and cooperatively plans continuing

education programs, and supports, promotes and undertakes studies and research related to nursing education. NECHEN has had a significant impact on college-based schools of nursing in New England for nearly fifteen years, particularly through continuing education of faculty members.

Representatives of member colleges and universities include the chief nurse administrative officer and a faculty member from each nursing program offered by the institution. An executive committee is elected by the council to help carry out the purposes and functions of the council between meetings. NEBHE employs a full-time program director for nursing education who provides staff assistance to NECHEN and acts as liaison between NECHEN and NEBHE. The board provides general administrative support for those NECHEN activities not funded from other sources.

NECHEN sponsors at least three major conferences each year on issues of importance to nursing education and topics that will contribute to the development of faculty members in NECHEN schools. Communication between NEBHE and NECHEN representatives is facilitated by a newsletter, *NECHEN News*, which includes information about regional nursing activities, data about nursing education in New England, and developments in the health manpower field of particular relevance to nursing education in New England. Since 1973, NEBHE has sponsored nursing projects funded by federal grants and contracts in several areas.

The address of NECHEN is c/o New England Board of Higher Education, 40 Grove Street, Wellesley, Massachusetts 02181.

PUBLIC HEALTH SERVICE, DEPARTMENT OF HEALTH AND HUMAN SERVICES

As its name implies, the Public Health Service (PHS) is not an organization but a federal government agency, and an exceedingly important one as far as health and nursing are concerned. Established in 1798 as a hospital service for sick and disabled seamen, the PHS has steadily expanded its scope and activities over the years and is now the federal agency charged with overall responsibility for promotion and protection of the nation's health. Since the Department of Health, Education, and Welfare (HEW)* was created in 1953, the PHS has been a component of that department.

Among the many subdivisions of the PHS is the Division of Nursing, which is the one unit in the federal government concerned exclusively with nursing. It is within the Division of Nursing that the PHS focuses on the nation's nursing situation.[12] Its roots go far back into the history of nursing in the Public Health Service, however. In 1933, the first public health nursing unit was created within the PHS, primarily to implement the health provisions of the Social Security Act and to conduct the first national census of nurses in public health work. In 1941, PHS established a unit on nursing education to administer federal programs, among them the United States Cadet Nurse Corps, which produced nurses during the emergency caused by World War II. In 1946, the Division of Nursing had been established within the Office of the Surgeon General. Formally, the Division of Nursing was known as the Division of Nurse Education. During 1949, the Public Health Service was reorganized to better coordinate its activities. The Division of Nursing in the Surgeon General's Office was abolished and its functions were taken over by the Division of Nursing Resources of the Bureau of Medical Services. In 1960, a restructuring of the Public Health Service again occurred uniting the Division of Nursing Resources and the Division of Public Health Nursing into the present day Division of Nursing.

The division's overall purpose is to work toward the achievement of high-quality nursing care for the nation's growing population and to approach this goal through aid to nursing education, consultation, support of research in nursing, and preparation of nurses for expanded roles in the primary care and teaching of patients.* The division "seeks to find out what exists in nursing care, what is needed, and how improvements can be made. . . ."[13] The Division of Nursing is a "catalyst for the . . . process . . . that begins with producing nurses (and) further entails keeping them in nursing and heightening their contribution to patients through nursing practice of a high new order."[14]

The division consists of three branches, each primarily responsible for one of the following areas of program activity: the Nursing Education Branch supports programs related to the development, financing, and use of educational resources for the improvement of nurse training; the Nursing Practice Branch designs, conducts, and supports a national program to improve the quality of nursing practice and health care; and the Nursing Research Branch conducts and supports a nurse fellowship program and research projects to expand the scientific base of nursing practice. There is also an Advanced Nurse Training Program Staff that provides support to develop or maintain graduate nursing education programs and a Nurse Practitioner Program Staff that supports programs to prepare RNs for expanded roles in primary health care in various health care settings. The latter report directly to the director.

Through research, the division (and its predecessor units) has exerted significant influence and leadership within the nursing profession. Not only does the division conduct research, but it contracts out special research projects in which it is interested and has also encouraged, promoted, and sup-

---

*When a separate Department of Education was created in 1980, HEW became the Department of Health and Human Services (HHS).

*Until 1979, the Division was also concerned with nurse manpower, but at that time the manpower analysis and research branch was moved into another HEW section.

ported many research projects in nursing carried on by others. It is responsible for grant programs that assist nurses to acquire additional education to prepare themselves for research to increase the nursing controbution to health care. Still another grant program has helped to prepare nurses for teaching, supervision, administration, and clinical specialization.

Through the research program, the Division of Nursing personnel have placed considerable emphasis on the development of methodology—study and research procedures—that could be used by others in studying nursing problems. Over the years, the division has developed many significant publications to that end. Other publications have been based on the various research projects done by external groups, as well as significant reports of special committees, such as that on the extended role of the nurse (discussed in Chapter 5) that helped launch federal financing for nurse practitioners.* Consultation services in many nursing areas are available through the division. For example, groups who wish to experiment with new teaching methods in a school of nursing or study the way nursing services are provided in a public health agency may receive help from the division.

HHS has ten regional offices throughout the United States, each headed by a Regional Health Administrator. PHS has always recognized the importance of nursing in the total scheme of providing health services, and there is scarcely a PHS program that does not have a nurse involved in some way. At one time, there was a regional nursing program director in each region, but in the cutback of the 1970s, that was discontinued and now the assigned nurse acts as a general consultant. A look through the PHS listings in a directory issue of the *American Journal of Nursing* gives added insight into the pro-

grams of PHS and also demonstrates the extent to which nursing is an integral part of them.

Further information may be obtained by writing the Division of Nursing, Bureau of Health Manpower, Health Resources Administration, U.S. Department of Health and Human Services, Public Health Service, 3700 East-West Highway, Hyattsville, Maryland 20782.

SOUTHERN REGIONAL EDUCATION BOARD (COUNCIL ON COLLEGIATE EDUCATION FOR NURSING)

The Southern Regional Education Board (SREB), operating agency of the nation's first interstate compact for higher education, is a coalition of educators, government officials, and civic leaders working to advance knowledge and improve the social and economic life of the South. Created in 1948 at the direction of the Southern Governors' Conference, the board's member states are Alabama, Arkansas, Florida, Georgia, Kentucky, Louisiana, Maryland, Mississippi, North Carolina, South Carolina, Tennessee, Texas, Virginia, and West Virginia.

The board conducts studies and reports on needs, problems, and developments in higher education; directs cooperative programs to improve education at undergraduate, graduate, professional, and technical levels; serves as the fiscal agency for interstate arrangements for regional educational services and institutions; and offers consultation to the states, their planning and coordinating agencies for higher education, and their institutions.

Membership on the board consists of the governor of each state and four other persons, one of whom must be a state legislator and another of whom must be an educator. All appointments are made by the governor for four-year staggered terms. SREB's basic operating support comes from the fourteen participating states. Federal agencies and

---

*A complete list of publications and reports is available from the Division of Nursing.

foundations provide the bulk of funds for program activity.

In 1954 SREB sponsored the first regional project in nursing education, a five-year project in graduate education and research. The region that had offered no graduate degrees in nursing at all then developing six. Three other projects in nursing education followed, funded first by Kellogg and then by the HEW Division of Nursing. These projects resulted in improvement and expansion of nursing education programs and faculty and the gathering of vital data.

The Council on Collegiate Education for Nursing was formed by SREB in 1962 to facilitate relationships between the regional nursing programs in higher education and SREB in implementation of the second nursing project.

Participation in the council is open to regionally accredited colleges and universities in SREB states that offer nursing programs leading to associate, baccalaureate, and master's degrees. There are now approximately 223 participating institutions. The council functions as a forum where heads of programs can obtain information and discuss developments at national, state, and local levels. It also advises on the development of regional activities and assists in implementing them. The council members, who feel the necessity for ongoing regional planning and continued existence of the council, are making long-range plans in this direction. SREB does not sponsor the council per se but, rather, the project under which the council exists.

A number of seminars, workshops, and conferences are held in relation to funded projects, chiefly involving faculty of the member schools. Other activities provide contact with nursing service personnel in hospitals and other agencies and staff in state organizations and agencies. Publications are generally related to the projects, including papers given at the council meetings. SREB headquarters is 130 Sixth Street, N.W., Atlanta, Ga. 30313.

WESTERN INTERSTATE COMMISSION FOR HIGHER EDUCATION (WESTERN COUNCIL ON HIGHER EDUCATION FOR NURSING)

The Western Council on Higher Education for Nursing (WCHEN) is a part of the Western Interstate Commission for Higher Education (WICHE). WICHE was founded in 1952 as a public agency with thirteen member states: Alaska, Arizona, California, Colorado, Hawaii, Idaho, Montana, Nevada, New Mexico, Oregon, Utah, Washington, and Wyoming. Its major purposes involve increasing educational opportunity, improving educational programs in higher education, expanding the supply of specialized manpower, and informing the public of higher education needs.

One of its forty-five programs in higher education is WCHEN, which was founded in 1957. The major functions of the council are to undertake cooperative planning for nursing education; identify and study problems; stimulate research; provide information and a medium for exchange of ideas and experiences among nursing education programs in higher education, their cooperating clinical agencies, and certain governmental agencies; encourage interdisciplinary discussion on health issues; encourage participation of men and ethnic minorities in nursing, recommend to the commission policies relating to education and research in nursing.

Membership in the council, which numbers more than 160, is open to accredited colleges and universities of the thirteen member states. Representatives are the dean plus one seat each for associate degree, baccalaureate, graduate, and continuing education programs, and one nurse representative from a clinical agency designated by each member school. Others are also invited to attend the yearly council meetings. An elected executive committee develops broad priorities and charts directions for the council. Elected members of steering committees in research, curriculum and teaching, nursing roles and practice, minority issues, and sociopolitical issues delineate issues, develop plans, and make recommendations to the executive board with the help of appointed subcommittees and ad hoc groups. A professional staff is maintained to assist the council.

WCHEN has carried out a number of projects in curriculum, research, and continuing education. Reports on the projects are part of the publications available from WCHEN. Recent projects are related to minority group needs, utilization of nursing research, and the three-and-one-half-year contract with the Division of Nursing: "Analysis and Planning for Improved Distribution of Nursing Personnel and Services." (The contract was completed in 1978 and copies of many of the reports are available.) Conferences and workshops are frequently held for the schools participating in these projects. WICHE maintains a large library and has numerous publications. The address of WICHE and WCHEN is P.O. Drawer P, Boulder, Colorado 80302.

REFERENCES

1. "Nursing Organizations Meet at ANA Headquarters to Plan Greater Coordination of Activities," *Am. J. Nurs.*, **73**:7 (Jan. 1973).
2. "Nursing Groups Reject Umbrella Congress, Agree on Need for Talks, Support on Issues," *Am. J. Nurs.*, **73**:420 (Mar. 1973).
3. "Nursing Organizations Adopt Group Name," *Am. J. Nurs.*, **73**:1306 (Aug. 1973).
4. "Groups Call for Better Use of RN," *Am. Nurse*, **5**:8 (July 1973).
5. "ANA, Collegiate Schools Form Alliance," *Am. J. Nurs.*, **74**:215 (Feb. 1974).
6. "Indian Nurses Hold National Conference," *Am. Nurse*, **7**:8 (June 1975).
7. Gloria Smith, "From Invisibility to Blackness: The Story of the National Black Nurses' Association," *Nurs. Outlook*, **23**:225–229 (Apr. 1975).
8. Carolyn Widmer, "Sigma Theta Tau:

9. Golden Anniversary," *Nurs. Outlook*, **20**:786–788 (Dec. 1972).
9. Jerome Lysaught, *An Abstract for Action* (New York: McGraw Hill Book Company, 1970), p. 159.
10. *NJPC, A Brief Background Statement* (Chicago, Ill.: The Commission, 1979), pp. 3–4.
11. Alan Appelbaum, "Commission Leads Way to Joint Practice for Nurses and Physicians," *Hospitals*, **52**:78–81 (July 16, 1978).
12. Philip Kalisch and Beatrice Kalisch, "Nurturer of Nurses: A History of the Division of Nursing of the U.S. Public Health Service and Its Antecedents 1798–1977—Summary Review," report to the Division of Nursing, March 1977.
13. Gladys Uhl, "The Division of Nursing, USPHS," *Am. J. Nurs.*, **65**:82–85 (July 1965).
14. Jessie M. Scott, "Federal Support for Nursing Education 1964 to 1972," *Am. J. Nurs.*, **72**:1855–1861 (Oct. 1972).

BIBLIOGRAPHY

"Federation Becomes Stronger Voice for Nursing Groups." Editorial, *AORN J.*, **27** (Apr. 1978), 809. Reviews organization of Federation and expresses hope for the future.

"Special Interest Groups or the ANA: An Analysis." In *Current Perspectives in Nursing: Social Issues and Trends*. Ed. by Michael Miller and Beverly Flynn. St. Louis, Mo.: C. V. Mosby Company, 1977, pp. 111–119. Analysis of formation of specialty organizations ties them to ANA's new emphasis on economic security in 1968.

Gortner, Susan. "Research in Nursing—The Federal Interest and Grant Program." *Am. J. Nurs.*, **73** (June 1973) 1052–1055. Reviews the program of the Division of Nursing, NIH, which administers federal funds for nursing research, pointing out key activities and studies funded since the 1950s.

Kalisch, Beatrice, and Philip Kalisch. *Nurturer of Nurses: A History of the Division of Nursing of the U.S. Public Health Service and Its Antecedents, 1798–1977*. Summary report of a study for Division of Nursing (Mar. 1977). Presents overview of impact of federal influence on nursing.

McNeil, Ella. *A History of the Public Health Nursing Section, 1922–1972.* Washington, D.C.: Public Health Association. Excellent but brief reference on public health nursing cites many original sources.

Scott, Jessie. "Federal Support for Nursing Education to Improve Quality of Practice." *Pub. Health Rep.,* **94** (Jan./Feb. 1979), 31–35. Reviews Division of Nursing report on nursing education and practice.

See also references for Chapter 27, the journals, newsletters, and other published material of the various organizations for further information or updating on each. *AJN* usually reports meetings and/or statements of the Federation and often of other groups.

International Organizations

The organizations discussed in the preceding chapters have all been national ones, although some have international affiliations. Included in this chapter are the major international organizations related to nursing and health.

INTERNATIONAL COUNCIL OF NURSES

Nursing claims the distinction of the oldest international association of professional women, the International Council of Nurses (ICN).[1] Antedating by many years the international hospital and medical associations, ICN is the largest international organization primarily made up of professional women in the world. (There are, of course, men in ICN.)

The originator and prime mover of the International Council of Nurses was a distinguished and energetic English nurse, Ethel Gordon Fenwick (Mrs. Bedford Fenwick), who first proposed the idea of an international nursing organization in July 1899.[2] Among the American nurses present in London at that time, attending a meeting of the International Council of Women, was one whose name figures prominently in the nursing history of our own country, Lavinia Dock. She was quick to support Mrs. Fenwick's idea and, shortly thereafter, a committee of nurses from nine different countries began laying the groundwork and drawing up a constitution for the proposed new organization. When ICN was officially established in 1900, Mrs. Fenwick became its first president. Miss Dock became its first secretary, a position she held for the next twenty-two years. Annie Goodrich became the first president from the United States.

The essential idea for which the ICN stands is, in Miss Dock's words,

. . . self government of nurses in their associations, with the aim of raising ever higher the standards of education and professional ethics, public usefulness, and civic spirit of their members. The International Council of Nurses does not stand for a narrow professionalism, but for that full development of the human being and citizen in every nurse, which shall best enable her to bring her professional knowledge and skill to the many-sided service that modern society demands of her.[3]

Today the ICN is sometimes referred to informally as the "United Nations of Nurses," an appropriate enough title. Although nonpolitical, and certainly less affluent than the UN, ICN does bring together persons from many countries who have a common interest in nursing and a common purpose, the development of nursing throughout the world.

Membership

From the beginning, the ICN was intended to be a federation of national nursing organizations. The association was a little ahead of its time, however, because, in 1900, very few countries had organized nursing associations. Until 1904, therefore, ICN had individual members. (These included men nurses, although the first time men were specifically mentioned as attending an ICN Congress was in 1912 in Cologne, where greetings were given from the president of the association of men nurses in Berlin.) In 1904 three countries reported that their national nursing organizations were "ready and eager to affiliate with the International Council of Nurses," and thus Great Britain, the United States, and Germany became the three charter members of the ICN.[4]

The ICN today is a federation of national nurses' associations in ninety-three countries. The requirements for membership have been, essentially, that the national association be an autonomous, self-directing, and self-governing body, nonpolitical, nonsectarian, with no form of racial discrimination, whose voting membership is composed exclusively of nurses and is broadly representative of the nurses in that country. Its objectives must be in harmony with ICN's stated objective: to provide a medium through which national nurses' associations may share their common interests, working together to develop the contribution of nursing to the promotion of the health of people and the care of the sick.[5] A majority vote by the ICN's governing body determines the admission of national associations into membership.

At the 1973 meeting of the ICN a constitutional change was made to broaden criteria for membership to include nurses who are a section or chapter of a national organization composed of other health workers as well as nurses. The ICN definition of *nurse* (the basis for national membership eligibility) was also broadened.[6]

A reiteration of the principle of nondiscrimination was also reinforced at this meeting through a resolution requiring the South African Nursing Association to take action to enable nonwhite nurses to serve on SANA's board of directors or face the possibility of expulsion from ICN. (This discrimination apparently exists because of certain clauses in that country's nursing practice act, which must therefore be changed.) Later that year, SANA withdrew from ICN because of stated inability to comply with the mandate.

Each country may be represented in ICN by only one national nursing organization. For the United States, the ICN member is the American Nurses' Association, which allocates a small percentage of each individual member's dues to the support of ICN. Thus, even though individual nurses are not ICN members, those who are ANA members can consider themselves part of this great international fellowship.

Organization

The governing body of ICN, according to a new constitution adopted in 1965, is the Council of National Representatives, consisting of the presidents of the member associations. This group meets at least every two years to establish ICN policies. It also has the responsibility of electing the members and appointing the chairmen of standing committees.

ICN's Board of Directors consists of its four officers (president and three vice presidents) plus eleven additional members, all elected by the Council of National Representatives. As of 1973, nearly half the board is elected by geographic area.[7] The board, which meets at least once a year, carries on the general business of ICN, reporting to the council. The ICN president and vice presidents constitute its Administrative and Finance Committee, responsible for general

ICN Member Countries (1980)

Argentina	Ethiopia	Israel	Norway	Sweden
Australia	Fiji	Italy	Pakistan	Switzerland
Austria	Finland	Jamaica	Panama	Swaziland
Bahamas	France	Japan	Paraguay	Taiwan
Barbados	Gambia	Jordan	Peru	Tanzania
Belgium	**Guatemala**	Kenya	Philippines	Thailand
Bermuda	German Federal	Korea	Poland	**Tonga**
Bolivia	Republic	Lebanon	Portugal	Trinidad/Tobago
Botswana	Ghana	Liberia	Puerto Rico	Turkey
Brazil	Greece	Luxembourg	Rhodesia	Uganda
Burma	Guyana	Malaysia	Salvador (El)	United Kingdom
Canada	Haiti	Mauritius	Senegal	United States
Chile	Honduras	Mexico	**Seychelles**	Uruguay
Colombia	Hong Kong	Morocco	Sierre Leone	Venezuela
Costa Rica	**Hungary**	Nepal	Singapore	Western Samoa
Cyprus	Iceland	Netherlands	Spain	Yugoslavia
Denmark	India	New Zealand	Sri Lanka	Zaire
Ecuador	Iran	Nicaragua	St. Lucia	Zambia
Egypt (UAR)	Ireland	Nigeria	Sudan	

administration of ICN affairs and advice in relation to investments.

Finally, the ICN constitution calls for one standing committee on professional services. This committee studies and makes recommendations in relation to the three broad areas with which ICN is concerned—nursing education, nursing practice, and the social and economic welfare of nurses. Interestingly enough, these are the same three areas represented by the American Nurses' Association's commissions. The membership committee, which investigated the eligibility of national associations applying for membership, made appropriate recommendations to the Council of National Representatives and reviewed the current status of member associations to ensure their continued eligibility, was discontinued after the 1973 ICN meeting. Its functions are now handled administratively.[8]

Assisting the ICN executive staff, standing committees, and board in their work is an Expert Advisory Panel, consisting of nurses expert in various fields of nursing as well as persons expert in other appropriate fields. Members of this panel, appointed by the Board of Directors for four-year periods of service, provide information, advice, and

consultant services and, through their specialized knowledge and experience, serve to facilitate the work of ICN.

Carrying out ICN's day-to-day activities is its headquarters staff—a group of seven professional nurses, including ICN's executive director. These nurses represent ICN's executive staff, but in their relationships with and services to the member associations, they serve in an advisory and consultative capacity. Staff members are selected from various member countries. Usually all of them speak more than one language and have special qualifications in one or more of ICN's areas of activity and service.

Since mid-1966, ICN headquarters has been located at 37 Rue de Vermont, 1202 Geneva, Switzerland (mailing address: P.O. Box 42, 1211 Geneva 20, Switzerland). For many of the preceding years, its headquarters was in London. The move to Geneva, however, locates ICN close to the many other international bodies in that city.

ICN Congresses

Once every four years the ICN holds what is always referred to as its Quadrennial Congress: a meeting of the members of the national nurses' associations in membership with ICN. Nursing students are usually eligible to attend ICN congresses, too, if they are sponsored, and their applications processed, by their national nurses' association. In the new quadrennial, an interest session for students is planned. The most recent congress, in Japan in 1977, was the sixteenth such international meeting. (The ICN did not meet quite so regularly in its early years, and the two world wars in the course of its history have also caused the canceling of meetings during these periods. The first, which was to have been held in the United States in 1915, was disrupted by World War I. Instead, the business of ICN was carried on during the ANA convention in San Francisco that year, attended by American nurses and a few intrepid English nurses who braved the submarine-infested Atlantic Ocean.) The Seventeenth Quadrennial Congress is scheduled for 1981 in Los Angeles.

Those who have attended any of the congresses will testify to the fact that they fully live up to the pomp and ceremony of their name. Held in various countries, upon invitation of the national nurses' association of that country, the congresses are inspiring demonstrations of international communication and fellowship in nursing. In conjunction with each congress, the Council of National Representatives (CNR) holds its meeting, with all those in attendance at the congress free to observe the council's deliberations. The official language of the congress is English, but facilitating communication is a system of simultaneous translation into the official congress languages, English, French, and Spanish. Each seat in the conference hall is usually provided with earphones tuned into this system, and the individual nurse has only to select the language of her/his choice. There is also a daily convention paper in all three languages distributed during the congress.

One of the interesting traditions of the congress is that each outgoing president leaves a watchword for the next four years. The first, left by Mrs. Fenwick in 1901, was *courage.* That left by an American, Dorothy

Cornelius, in 1977 was *accountability.* Each watchword is engraved on a link of the silver chain of office of the ICN president and becomes a permanent part of ICN history.

At the congress special program sessions are held, usually linked to one unifying theme. Among the most outstanding achievements of the CNR meetings at the 1973 congress was the acceptance of a new code of ethics (see Chapter 10), which makes explicit the nurse's responsibility and accountability for nursing care. Eliminated, for instance, were statements that abrogated the nurse's judgment and personal responsibility and stressed a dependency on physicians, which nurses throughout the world no longer saw as appropriate. There was also a major statement on the developing role of the nurse, which read

> In the light of scientific and social change and the goals of social and health policy to extend health services to the total population, nursing and other health professions are faced with the need to adapt and expand their roles.
>
> In planning to meet health needs it is imperative that nurses and physicians collaborate to promote the development and optimum utilization of both professions. A variety of practices may evolve in different settings, including the creation of new categories of health workers.
>
> Although this may require nurses to delegate some of their traditional activities and undertake new responsibilities, the core of their practice and their title should remain distinctly nursing, and education programs should be available to prepare them for their expanding role in the various areas of nursing practice.[9]

Other major areas of discussion, either in the plenary and special interest sessions or in the CNR meetings, included continuing education for nurses, the career ladder, economic security, health care for the aged, health care innovations, and disease prevention.

The Sixteenth Quadrennial Congress of the International Council of Nurses in Tokyo, Japan, was the largest international conference of nurses ever convened. Program sessions focused on changes in nursing practice around the world, how to educate nurses for such changes in practice, and what the changes mean in terms of nursing responsibility. At the first major program, seven speakers presented trends in nursing practice. Despite differences in methods and cultural influences, it was noted that all nurses are moving in the direction of primary health care. Other sessions discussed the rights of nurses, self-regulation for nursing, and directions in education, in which lengthy debates centered on traditional versus modern technological methods of teaching. New dimensions of professional responsibility of nurses in view of expanding roles and primary care were emphasized at the final program session. Major actions adopted at CNR in 1977 were statements on the economic and general welfare of nurses, including a resolution endorsing collective bargaining, the international migration of nurses, the development and utilization of nursing research, continuing education, and career mobility in nursing.[10] A commemorative stamp was also issued for the occasion.

Functions and Activities

In the foreword to its 1965 constitution, the ICN points out that the primary purpose of nurses the world over is "to provide and develop a service for the public" and that ICN, as a federation of national nursing associations, provides for sharing of knowledge so that "nursing practice throughout the world is strengthened and improved." In pursuit of this objective, ICN promotes the organization of national nurses' associations and advises them in developing and improving health service for the public, the practice of nursing, and the social and economic welfare of nurses; provides a means of communication, understanding, and cooperation among nurses throughout the world; establishes and maintains liaison and cooperation with other international organizations; and serves as representative and spokesman for nurses at an international level.

An attempt to broaden the goals and activities of the ICN by changing the constitution and regulations was defeated at the 1973 meeting, perhaps in part because of the previous defeat of increased dues. The CNR voted to maintain ICN's functions as outlined in the 1965 constitution.

From the very beginning ICN has always been concerned with three main areas— nursing education, nursing service, and nurses' social and economic welfare. Two of its first objectives were to provide for the registration of trained nurses in order to protect the public from practice by unqualified practitioners, and to promote a standardized and upgraded system of nursing education. At the 1969 congress, for instance, statements on basic belief about and principles of nursing education, practice, and service and social and economic welfare were agreed upon. The nursing education statement indicated that nursing education should be in institutions where education is the primary concern and that supervised experience related to theory should be in preventive and curative facilities. The nursing practice statement stressed health care and security as a basic human right, and the economic welfare statement called for joint consultation in determining conditions of employment, and nurses' rights to participate in their national organization.

Whenever possible, ICN has sought common denominators in education and practice throughout the world. One such common denominator, for instance, is the international Code of Ethics adopted by ICN and equally applicable by nurses in every country from Australia to Zambia. Another example is the ICN publication *ICN Basic Principles of Nursing Care*, now available in fifteen languages and useful to nurses throughout the world.[11] At the same time, ICN has always recognized the autonomy of its member associations and the principle that each country will develop the systems of education and practice best suited to its individual culture and needs.

Throughout the years ICN has both collected and disseminated data on patterns of nursing education and service throughout the world, and provided information and advisory and consultative services in both areas to member associations requesting such service. Some of its activities in the educational field are financed, in whole or in part, by the Florence Nightingale International Foundation (FNIF), which is associated with ICN. The FNIF was established in 1934 as an educational trust in honor of Miss Nightingale. FNIF trust funds have also been used by ICN to encourage and stimulate research activities in nursing. A new document developed by FNIF is "The Nurse's Dilemma, Ethical Considerations in Nursing Practice," published in 1977.

ICN administers two annual scholarships of $6,000 each plus $200 to each national winner submitted by national nurses' associations.

Within recent years, ICN has been particularly active in the area of nurses' social and economic welfare, and its staff has carried on field work to assist national associations in this area. Published in 1977 was "An Underestimated Problem in Nursing: The Effect of the Economic and Social Welfare of Nurses on Patient Care," by Ada Jacox, and in the 1979 CNR meeting, the economic and general welfare of nurses was considered a concern of top priority.

ICN is ready to supply general information relative to new developments in this area as well as guidance to national associations wishing to develop or strengthen their social and economic welfare programs. ICN has already collected data on employment conditions of nurses in selected European countries and will undoubtedly extend this data gathering in the future.

At one time, facilitating arrangements whereby nurses from one country could observe, study, or work in another was an ICN activity. As of 1969, direct participation in such arrangements was discontinued and arrangements are now made through the individual countries. Each member association provides guidance and assistance for nurses planning to come in or go out of its particular

country. Providing liaison for nurses with other international groups is one of the ICN's most significant contributions to world nursing. Among the organizations, governmental and nongovernmental, with which ICN is associated in one way or another are the World Health Organization, the World Federation of Mental Health, the International Labor Organization, the World Medical Association, the International Hospital Federation, the League of Red Cross Societies, the International Committee of the Red Cross, United Nations Educational, Scientific and Cultural Organization (UNESCO), and the Union of International Associations.

Publications

Since 1929 ICN's official organ has been the *International Nursing Review*, published six times a year from ICN headquarters in Geneva. In addition to reports of ICN activities, the *Review* also carries nursing articles of international interest, usually written by nurses from the ICN member countries. Occasionally it reprints articles from the official publications of member countries. Its primary language is English but some articles are published in other languages; sometimes, an article may appear in several languages. Subscription requests to the *Review* should be addressed to ICN headquarters. The journals of member associations—the *American Journal of Nursing*, for instance—also carry reports of ICN activities and actions.

Issued every four years is the book *Reports of ICN Members Associations*. The 1977 edition contains up-to-date and detailed data on sixty of the national nurses' associations affiliated with ICN.

The ICN also publishes documents from time to time on various aspects of nursing. These publications, as well as a list of those available, can be obtained from ICN headquarters. Some are free; for others there is a charge.

The Past and the Future

The preamble to ICN's original constitution stated, "We, nurses of all nations, sincerely believing that the best good of our Profession will be advanced by greater unity of thought, sympathy and purpose, do hereby band outselves in a confederation of workers to further the efficient care of the sick, and to secure the honour and interests of the Nursing Profession."[12] From the beginning, the ICN and its officers were farsighted and pioneering. Included were members of every race and creed. The courageous Mrs. Fenwick stood firmly for her beliefs in woman's suffrage and often spoke of the organization as a federation of women's organizations (for all its men members) with woman's suffrage as one of its objectives. In 1901 she was firmly stating a need for nursing education to be in colleges and universities and for nurses to be licensed. (Lavinia Dock missed one major ICN meeting because she was too busy lobbying for women's suffrage.)

In conservative 1900, at the ICN program meeting in London, one subject discussed was venereal disease. Nurses stood up and demanded early sex education for children and accessible treatment with no moral stigma attached. The members greeted this with a storm of applause. At other meetings they tackled such subjects as criminal assault on young girls, the role of nurses in prisons, and many other taboo topics. They reached out to effect change and for more than seventy years have been carrying on activities to meet their broadening objectives. It is impressive to see how an international group of nurses with such diverse membership can agree on common goals on education, practice, and economic security when often nurses within an individual country, including the United States, cannot agree. There are clearly financial problems with which the ICN must cope, reflecting perhaps the financial problems of each country's own association. Currently, ICN's four new objectives are "to assist national associations to (1) improve standards of nursing and the competence of nurses, (2) to promote the development of strong national nurses' associations, (3) to serve as the authoritative voice for nurses and nursing internationally

and (4) to improve the status of nursing."[13] To fulfill these objectives will require the same kind of innovative and challenging spirit that the founders of ICN had so abundantly. At times, it may be questionable whether the nations of the world are coming closer together for the betterment of mankind, but it might well be that the International Council of Nursing can play a significant role in improving the health of mankind.

INTERNATIONAL ASSOCIATION FOR ENTEROSTOMAL THERAPY, INC.

The International Association for Enterostomal Therapy, Inc. (IAET) is the professional association for enterostomal therapy. Currently one must be an enterostomal therapist to be a member of IAET. As of September 1976, only registered nurses are permitted to pursue Enterostomal Therapy (ET) education. In addition, candidates must have two recent years of full-time clinical experience prior to admission.

Membership in the IAET totals approximately 950. Current activities include involvement in advancing continuing education, studying cost-effectiveness of ET services, securing reimbursement for care of their clients, and certification.

The scientific publication, *E.T. Journal*, is published quarterly. In an effort to advance education and research activities, the Enterostomal Therapy Foundation was established. Headquarters is located at 1701 Lake Avenue, Glenview, Illinois 60025.

WORLD FEDERATION OF NEUROSURGICAL NURSES

The World Federation of Neurosurgical Nurses (WFNN) was formed during the 1969 World Congress of Neurological Services in New York at the suggestion of the president of the International Congress of Neurological Surgery. It is affiliated with the World Federation of Neurosurgical Societies and its first international meeting was in conjunction with the surgeons at the Fifth International Congress of Neurosurgical Surgery in Japan in 1973.

The organization devotes itself to the improvement of neurosurgical patient care, the exchange and dissemination of knowledge and ideas among neurosurgical nurses around the world, and the fostering of research in clinical nursing. Membership in the federation is generally limited to neurosurgical nurses through member societies throughout the world.

Because the address for communication with WFNN changes in relation to the officers elected, the best contact is probably made through the national constituent member or the AJN directory of organizations.

WORLD HEALTH ORGANIZATION

The World Health Organization (WHO), one of the largest of the specialized agencies set up by the United Nations, has its headquarters at 1211 Geneva, 27, Switzerland. Established in 1948, WHO's constitution gives as one of its beliefs: "The enjoyment of the highest attainable standard of health is one of the fundamental rights of every human being without the distinction of race, religion, political, economic or social condition" and defines *health* as "a state of complete physical, mental, and social well-being and not merely the absence of disease. . . ."

Membership in WHO is open to all countries, including those that do not belong to the United Nations. WHO is organized on a regional basis, the regions subdivided into zones, so that WHO and the nations within each region or zone can work together on matters of mutual concern. The six regions are Southeast Asia, Eastern Mediterranean, Western Pacific, Africa, Europe, and the Americas. The American region is served by the Pan American Health Organization, (PAHO) which also acts as the WHO regional organization.

An executive board directs the work of WHO, which is administered by a director general. Among its working force, known as the secretariat, are members of the health professions, including nurses. WHO's activities are largely financed by assessments on the member countries, on the basis of a scale authorized by the World Health Assembly.

World Health Assembly

WHO's governing body is the World Health Assembly. It is made up of delegates from all member countries and meets once a year. The United States was the only country to include a nurse (Lucile Petry Leone) in its delegation to the first World Health Assembly and has followed this practice ever since. Some other countries now include nurses in their delegations, too.

In her report on the first World Health Assembly, Mrs. Leone commented:

> *Nursing was mentioned in many ways by a large number of the delegates. Everywhere there seemed recognition of the importance of nurses in the health activities which are recommended by the WHO. I was frequently consulted by delegates of many countries when they found that a nurse was present in the assembly. . . . The delegations of Ireland and the United States presented [a] resolution on nursing which formed the basis for the inclusion of nursing in WHO.*[14]

The first World Health Assembly planned to include nurses only on specialized teams concerned with such health problems as malaria, tuberculosis, venereal diseases, and maternal and child health. Within a year, however, the importance of having nurses help with all phases of world nursing was recognized, and in 1949 a nurse consultant was appointed to WHO's headquarters staff, and an Expert Committee on Nursing was appointed to consider nursing education and nursing service on a worldwide basis. Since then, nursing has been an integral part of a great many WHO programs, with WHO's nursing staff including not only those nurses assigned to the headquarters and regional offices but also those providing direct assistance with health and nursing projects in many countries throughout the world.

National and International Services

WHO's services are divided into three broad areas: (1) assisting governments, on request, with their health problems, (2) providing a number of worldwide health services, and (3) encouraging and coordinating international research on health problems. The trained staff of technical advisors, doctors, dentists, sanitary engineers, nurses, and others who are dispatched to help and advise any nation requesting aid works with the national ministry of health, the main emphasis being on making health care available to all persons.

Personnel are trained to initiate problem-solving programs and, when progress toward solution is assured, to teach people in the locality or country to carry on by themselves. WHO personnel recognize the influence of a people's social and economic status on health practices and attempt to effect improvement in those areas also. In 1978, WHO's Programme on Appropriate Technology for Health (ATH) published its first directory of those involved or interested in working in the ATH field. The directory is a product of activities concerned with the collaboration of ATH with member states and organizations, institutions, groups and individuals in the collection, assessment, compilation, and dissemination of information.[15] It is expected to be updated yearly. WHO encourages the creation of schools for the health professions, provides consultation, and advises on education and training guidelines where needed.

Among WHO's major programs in individual countries are aid to strengthen local health services through better administration; eradication or control of such communicable diseases as smallpox, malaria, typhoid fever, tuberculosis, syphilis, trachoma, and yaws; provision of better care for mothers and babies; development of better sanitation facilities; and improvement of mental health. WHO also provides fellowships, usually short-term, to enable health workers to observe or study in other countries, with the goal of improving practice or services in their own country. United States nurses are among those eligible for these fellowships.

On the international plane, WHO, in cooperation with member nations, collects and disseminates epidemiological information, develops and administers international quarantine regulations, establishes a uniform system of health statistics, promotes standards of strength and purity for drugs and recommends names for pharmaceutical products, keeps countries advised of the possible dangers in the use of radioisotopes and helps train personnel in protection measures, and institutes international vaccination programs as, for example, those against poliomyelitis. Within the last several years, WHO has emphasized primary care and is also intensifying its promotion of the medical systems used by the majority of people. In the Third World countries, most people depend on traditional healers, who have often been quite effective in caring for people. Their integration into the general health system is considered essential at this point of development and health care delivery.[16]

Nursing Within WHO

As was mentioned earlier, delegates at the first World Health Assembly realized that nursing was of worldwide interest and concern. More and better nurses were needed in every section of the globe.[17] In some countries—in 1948—there was not a single fully qualified nurse. Health care was given entirely by aides who often had little or no training. In other countries, as in the United States, there were adequate nursing services that could have been even better if more nurses were available. In between these two extremes were countries with widely varying numbers of nurses and vastly different educational patterns for preparing them. The largest part of WHO's nursing assistance has naturally been directed toward the relatively less developed, underprivileged countries with the most urgent health and nursing needs.

WHO nurses work primarily in an advisory capacity, helping the nurses in a country with their specific problems. Sometimes, however, WHO nurses must temporarily assume operational responsibilities until one of the country's own nurses has been prepared for the job. Thus, in establishing a postgraduate nursing program in a university, the WHO nurse may have to serve as director of the program in its early stages.

The areas in which WHO is called upon to provide assistance cover practically all of nursing—nursing education, organization and administration of hospital and public health nursing services, mental health, maternal and child health, clinical nursing specialties, and community health care planning. Improved midwifery services and education are vitally needed in many countries; so are programs to increase the numbers and upgrade the training of auxiliary nursing personnel. WHO helps in these areas by cooperating with manpower planning. Assistance from WHO is also available to governments and their nursing divisions (if they have any) to plan for the development of nursing in those countries and to promote nursing legislation in the interests of both nurses and the public.

Another WHO nursing activity is the sponsoring, sometimes in cooperation with other agencies, of regional conferences and seminars that focus on the changing role of the nurse in relation to current health policies. These enable nurses with similar backgrounds and problems to exchange information and work toward solutions, under the guidance of expert nurses from WHO or other international health agencies. Many of these nurses have never before had an opportunity to meet with members of their profession from other countries, and they derive not only knowledge but encouragement and moral support from such conferences.

It is obvious that WHO's nursing activities call for highly qualified nurses, expert in at least one of the fields in which WHO offers advisory services.* Language requirements depend upon the country of assignment, but it is desirable for a nurse to be proficient in at least one language other than her own. The official languages of WHO are Spanish, English, French, Russian, Chinese, and Arabic. In addition to its more or less regularly employed nursing staff, WHO also engages nurses for limited periods of time to carry out special projects in various countries. WHO nurses often work in collaboration with nurses from other agencies—the United States Agency for International Development, for instance—who are also helping with nursing development in a given country.

In addition to its advisory services, WHO has published a variety of documents in relation to nursing, most of them of a basic nature and intended to be widely applicable in many countries. Two examples are *Basic Nursing Education Programmes: A Guide to Their Planning*, and *The Staffing of Public Health and Outpatient Nursing Services: Methods of Study*. WHO also publishes *World Health*, a monthly magazine on world health intended for the lay public. *International Digest of Health Legislation*, *World Health Statistics Annual*, directories of schools of the health professions, and a variety of technical papers, journals, and reports.*

After twenty-five years of existence, WHO has had a part in many of the major developments in the international health field such as increase in the average life-span; decrease in infant mortality; almost total eradication of smallpox; major reduction in poliomyelitis and malaria; and increase in medical and other health profession schools.

OTHER UN AGENCIES

WHO works closely with other intergovernmental agencies of the United Nations that are concerned with the health of world citizens: the United Nations International

---

*See Chapter 15.

*A complete catalog of World Health Organization publications is available on request from the Public Information Office, United Nations, New York, N.Y.

Children's Emergency Fund (UNICEF), the United Nations Educational, Scientific and Cultural Organization (UNESCO), the Food and Agriculture Organization (FAO), and United Nations Development Program (UNDP). News items and articles about these organizations appear frequently in the popular press.

The United Nations International Children's Emergency Fund is an outgrowth of another organization, the United Nations Relief and Rehabilitation Administration (UNRRA), which was established in 1943 during World War II to help care for the millions of refugees and displaced persons in liberated countries. UNRRA went out of existence in 1947, two years after the end of the war.

For the next two years, the United Nations asked for aid in easing the plight of children all over the world and, in 1950, organized UNICEF, which has earned the support and esteem of governments, individuals, and organizations. The American Nurses' Association promptly pledged its support, and nursing publications have carried articles urging individual nurses to contribute as much as they can.

UNICEF provides food, clothing, and vaccines and other medical supplies for children and helps to fight children's diseases. It supports positive health programs and is vitally interested in the care of mothers and infants. Although it does not employ a staff of nurses, it provides equipment to help with nursing and midwifery services and training programs. It has also provided grants for the training of doctors, nurses, midwives, and other health workers. Family planning information is provided in those countries wishing help in their population control programs. Other major efforts are directed toward fighting malnutrition.

The work of the United Nations Educational, Scientific and Cultural Organization, as its title implies, is not directly concerned with health problems, but has an extremely important bearing on them. For example, more and better elementary and secondary

schools for youngsters means more and better potential nurses and other health workers. It also means that larger segments of the world population are able to comprehend the health-related literature that is distributed to them and to take an active part in health programs in their own and other countries.

The Food and Agriculture Organization's objective is to help countries produce the food their citizens need for adequate nutrition. This naturally influences the health of individuals. WHO programs to control and eradicate disease assist in the FAO's work by providing healthier personnel and workers to carry on agricultural activities.

Specific details of the activities of these agencies are found in their individual annual reports and in papers published about specific programs. They provide a fascinating picture of the problems and progress of the world's health.

The WHO address is Avenue Appia, 1211 Geneva 27, Switzerland. The Pan American Health Organization address is Pan American Sanitary Bureau, WHO Regional Office for the Americas, 525 23rd St. N.W., Washington, D.C. 20037.

AGENCY FOR INTERNATIONAL DEVELOPMENT

The Agency for International Development (AID), administered by the U.S. Department of State, is one of a succession of agencies through which the United States has assisted other countries in their social and economic development, with nursing one of the areas in which assistance has been provided. AID is a national, rather than an international, agency, but is included in this section because of the worldwide nature of its activities.

The distinguishing feature of the health and other technical assistance programs that have been carried out by AID and its predecessor agencies is that they have been bilateral in nature—that is, undertaken cooperatively with the government of the country being assisted, upon the request of that country and with both nations sharing in the determination of the programs to be carried out and the goals to be achieved. These bilateral health programs had their beginnings in 1942 with the establishment of the Institute of Inter-American Affairs to work cooperatively with Latin American countries in improving their health and welfare services. Since that time, U.S. technical assistance in nursing has been provided under a variety of administrative auspices (Economic Security Administration, Foreign Operations Administration, International Cooperation Administration, and others), culminating with the establishment of AID in 1961.

The early nursing assistance projects were highly concerned with the development and improvement of public health nursing services; this was the most pressing health need in Central and South America in the 1940s. The United States nurses working in these programs, however, soon discovered that public health nursing services could not be permanently strengthened without a continuing supply of well-prepared nurses, which would, of course, require improved nursing school systems and facilities. In turn, if nursing students were to have their clinical experience in a true learning environment, hospital nursing services also needed improvement.

These three areas—public health nursing, nursing education, and hospital nursing services—have represented the target of most nursing assistance projects carried out under AID's auspices. Like WHO, however, AID has also provided assistance in other nursing areas, such as midwifery services, the preparation of auxiliary personnel, and the establishment of postgraduate programs to prepare nurses for teaching and administrative responsibilities, among others. AID also operates a "participant training" program whereby qualified individuals—nurses among them—in the assisted countries are given an opportunity to get the basic or advanced education they need in educational institutions in this country or elsewhere.

AID employs nurses on a short- or long-term basis to carry out its nursing assistance projects. Some AID nurses have been with the agency or one of its predecessors for many years, assisting with projects in various countries. Others are recruited on a more limited basis.

Summary

The purpose of this chapter was to provide only an overview of international health and nursing activities. Therefore, only the largest and most significant of the organizations and agencies operating in this area have been included. There are many other organized groups—religious and lay, private and governmental, societies and foundations—carrying on similar or related functions. For additional information, the heading *international* in any nursing, hospital, or medical literature index will provide additional information about the activities being carried on around the world in behalf of the health and nursing needs of its people.

REFERENCES

1. Daisy C. Bridges, "Events in the History of the International Council of Nurses," *Am. J. Nurs.,* **49**:594–595 (Sept. 1949).
2. Margaret Breay and Ethel Bedford Fenwick, *The History of the International Council of Nurses, 1899–1925* (Geneva: The International Council of Nurses, 1931). This is a detailed, fascinating, and informative account of the ICN's founding and first twenty-five years, throwing considerable light on the nursing problems and personalities of this period.
3. According to ICN records, Miss Dock wrote these words as part of a foreword to the program of the ICN's Second Quinquennial Meeting, held in London in 1909.
4. Mary M. Roberts, *American Nursing: History and Interpretation* (New York: Macmillan Publishing Co., Inc., 1954), pp. 80–81.
5. International Council of Nurses, *Basic Documents: Constitution and Regula-*

tions. Rules. Procedure at Meetings (Geneva: The Council. 1966). p. 8.

6. "ICN." *Am. J. Nurs..* **73**: 1388. 1352 (Aug. 1973).
7. Ibid.. p. 1352.
8. Ibid.
9. Ibid.
10. "ICN '77." *Am. J. Nurs..* **77**:1303–1310 (Aug. 1977).
11. Virginia Henderson. *ICN Basic Principles of Nursing Care* (London: International Council of Nurses. 1958).
12. Breay and Fenwick. op. cit.. p. 12.
13. "ICN–1973." op. cit.. p. 509.
14. Lucile Petry. "World Health Organization and Nursing." *Am. J. Nurs..* **48**:611 (Oct. 1948).
15. *Appropriate Technology for Health Directory* (Geneva: WHO. April 1978).
16. "WHO Pushes Traditional Healing." *The Nation's Health.* **9**:3 (May 1979).
17. World Health Organization. *The First*

Ten Years of WHO (Geneva: WHO. 1958). pp. 391 ff.

BIBLIOGRAPHY

Bridges, Daisy Caroline. *A History of the International Council of Nurses. 1899–1964.* Philadelphia: J. B. Lippincott Company. 1967. A detailed and authoritative history of the ICN's first 65 years. written by its former executive director.

"The ICN in the New World." *Am. J. Nurs..* **74**:1286–1287 (July 1974). As ICN celebrates its 75th anniversary, pictures and text show the involvement of American nurses through the years.

See also reports of ICN congresses in *Am. J. Nurs.. Nurs. Outlook.* and other nursing journals that usually carry news items about ICN activities. Other news is carried in the *International Nursing Review.*

The Professional Literature

Nursing is no exception to the publication explosion that is affecting all professions today. New nursing knowledge is accumulating rapidly, partly as a result of the extensive research now being carried on. Rapid advances in scientific knowledge and in medical therapies call for the development of corresponding nursing care techniques. New fields of nursing practice and new ways of delivering nursing services continue to emerge. More and more, as the nursing profession becomes more mature and sophisticated, nurses recognize the need to share their concepts, research findings, and nursing care knowledge with their colleagues.

The result is a proliferation of nursing literature—books, periodicals, and pamphlets, as well as many specialized publications. Not too long ago, text or reference books in nursing were generally limited to the major clinical fields. Now there is scarcely any area relating to nursing that does not have books on the subject. New titles show the extremely diverse nature of the subjects that nurses must read and write about today. Many of these books (this one, for instance) must be frequently revised and brought out in new, updated editions to keep up with new knowledge and expanding concepts.

Reading the book advertisements in the nursing magazines is almost an education in itself; by doing this the nurse is reminded of the pressing topics of the day—or of tomorrow. Even more important is reading the reviews of these books, also published in the nursing journals. That way, the reader will gain a better knowledge of their content and the reviewer's estimate (and he or she is usually an expert in the field) of their value. Then it is easier to decide whether to buy it, borrow it from the library, glance through it there, or forget all about it. Certainly it is impossible to read all the books published in the nursing field today, so nurses will want to select those that promise to hold the most value for them and their individual interests.

It is the nursing journals, however, that will keep the nurse up-to-date and well-informed. Usually at least six months passes between the writing of a book and its appearance in print, and it may be still a few more months before it is reviewed. But the nursing journals, especially those that come out monthly, make available news, reviews, and information promptly. Just within the past ten years, there has been a remarkable increase in the numbers and kinds of nursing magazines. Some the nurse will undoubtedly want to subscribe to and keep for reference, others to look at each month in the library. It is helpful to have at least an idea of the content, purpose, and approach of all of them.[1]

In academia, there is some tendency to consider as more scholarly and prestigious those journals that are "refereed," that is, have peer review. This means, in general, that the article (paper) written has been reviewed by other experts in the field before being published. These reviewers may be called an editorial board, advisory board, editorial advisors, associate editors, co-editors, or assistant editors. They are usually volunteers, not paid, and generally are not involved in the production of the journal. There are mixed opinions as to whether these journals are really of better quality.[2,3] At times there is also a problem determining just how much involvement these expert volunteers have; some never see a manuscript, but their names are on the mastheads.

It is not feasible to review the content of all these periodicals, so attention is directed primarily to the periodicals and services presented by the American Journal of Nursing Company. However, the names and addresses of the major nursing journals and serials published in the United States, Canada, and England and some international journals are listed in this chapter. Not included are the national journals of other countries and the journals of the state nurses' associations. However, it is well worthwhile to review these journals, if possible (they are not subscribed to in many libraries), because they also contain useful information. A full listing of all nursing journals and serials is published in the *International Nursing Index*.

AMERICAN JOURNAL OF NURSING

Oldest of the nursing periodicals now in existence, the *American Journal of Nursing*

first appeared in October 1900, and has been published monthly ever since.* The *Journal* is the professional journal of the American Nurses' Association and is published by the American Journal of Nursing Company, a nonprofit corporation owned by ANA, which also publishes *Nursing Research, Nursing Outlook, MCN, Geriatric Nursing*, and *International Nursing Index*.

The *Journal*, intended for all nurses, cuts across all fields and levels of nursing practice and education, with special emphasis on the clinical practice of nursing. Almost as fast as new nursing care principles or techniques evolve, they are reported in the *Journal* in articles written by nurse experts in each area.

New ideas about nursing in general—its scope, its definition, and its problems—will be found in the *AJN* pages. And, not least important, the *Journal*, as an official publication of nursing's professional organization, the ANA, carries full and up-to-date information about ANA's programs and activities.

Journal coverage, in news content, ranges from local (the appointment of new faculty members in various schools of nursing, and legislative efforts of individual states, for instance) to international (reports of ICN congresses and interim activities). In recent years there have been special supplements on clinical problems, such as pain (March 1974), and issues such as ethics (May 1977) and programmed instruction, such as the series on assessment technique, which began in the February 1974, issue and a series on crutchwalking (June 1979). It also provides other professional services, such as a yearly listing of the addresses of nursing and health organizations; both annual and five-year cumulative indexes; lists of major meetings and continuing education programs; classified and other advertisements of job opportunities.

The Trained Nurse and Hospital Review (later *Nursing World*) antedated the *Journal* by twelve years. It ceased publication in 1960.

Through the years *AJN* has done more than reflect changes and trends in nursing as a clinical practice and as a profession. It frequently has helped shape those changes. The most recent example of this is the publication, in *AJN*, of material through which nurses can earn continuing education contact hours by home study. As the trend toward mandatory continuing education for relicensure gains momentum, a major problem facing the profession is availability of offerings through which nurses can obtain the credits they need. *AJN* was the first nursing publication to offer such material. Continuing education units, approved for contact hours under the ANA Mechanism for Approval of Continuing Education in Nursing, have been published in four issues each year since March 1977. Nurses wishing to acquire CE contact hours through these home-study units, which are usually on clinical topics, can do so by passing an examination on the material. *AJN*'s CE program includes the preparation, scoring, and handling of these exams. For this service to its readers, *AJN* won the 1979 National Magazine Award, in competition with consumer, business, and professional publications. The National Magazine Awards are regarded as the most prestigious in the magazine field.

The *AJN*'s editorial staff is largely, but not exclusively, made up of nurses chosen because of their expertise in a given nursing area plus journalistic ability. And, as nursing expands, so does the *Journal*. Averaging about 175 pages an issue (this includes advertising and educational reading), the *AJN* in 1980 had about 345,000 subscribers. The *Journal*, unlike most official magazines of a professional association, does not come automatically with membership in the association; it must be subscribed to and paid for independently. It is, however, available at a reduced rate to ANA members.

The history of the *Journal*'s founding and subsequent development as a publication "managed, edited, and owned by the profession" is one of which nurses can be proud. This is related in *The American Journal of Nursing and its Company: A Chronicle, 1900 –1975*, and various histories of nursing.

NURSING OUTLOOK

Nursing Outlook, also published by the American Journal of Nursing Company, was, until 1979, the official publication of the National League for Nursing and has about 27,000 subscribers. It is much younger than the *Journal*, its first issue having appeared in January 1953, less than a year after the League was organized. It is the successor to *Public Health Nursing*, which had been the official journal of the National Organization of Public Health Nursing, one of the associations that disbanded and became an integral part of the NLN.

Outlook's content was originally directed toward the concerns of the NLN—nursing service and education, especially their administrative and community aspects. However, the journal is now broadly based, frequently focusing on controversial or new issues in nursing and health, such as institutional licensure, independent nursing practice, HMOs, national health insurance, physician's assistants, and mandatory continuing education. For those interested in current trends in education, there are articles on curriculum development, theoretical models, approaches to teaching, and development of new nursing programs. There is also information on current community, hospital, nursing home, clinic, and independent nursing practice. Each issue contains some sixty pages and features articles on these subjects. Certain issues every year have listed NLN-accredited nursing education programs, as well as an annual NLN report on admissions, enrollments, and graduations in all nursing education programs. Information of this kind is now published by NLN's official journal.

Like *AJN*, news, book reviews, educational programs, and notices of major meetings are published in addition to teaching aids and classified and other advertisements.

The July issues carry an official directory of nursing and health organizations.

The *Nursing Outlook* editorial staff, although considerably smaller than that of *AJN*, is also of outstanding caliber.

NURSING RESEARCH

Still another publication of the American Journal of Nursing Company is *Nursing Research*, a bimonthly journal established in 1952 for the purposes of stimulating and reporting research and scientific studies in nursing. Jointly sponsored by the ANA and NLN, *Nursing Research* has an editorial advisory committee and nurse editors who are qualified nurse researchers. *Nursing Research* carries reports of research projects, articles on research methods, and news about research activities.*

MCN, THE AMERICAN JOURNAL OF MATERNAL CHILD NURSING

MCN, The American Journal of Maternal Child Nursing first appeared in January 1976 and the journal quickly acquired approximately 26,500 subscribers. It is a bimonthly publication established to help the practicing nurse so that care given to individuals and families during the childbearing and child-rearing phases of the life cycle can be of high quality. *MCN* is a refereed journal whose review panel is made up of practicing nurses and nurse researchers who are active in the field of maternal child nursing. The editor is a clinical specialist in maternal child nursing.

MCN primarily focuses on clinical practice, with particular emphasis on nursing intervention. The scope of topics range from preconception through adolescence. Most issues have a special section that highlights

*The idea for a magazine such as *Nursing Research* came initially from the Association of Collegiate Schools of Nursing, an organization that was merged into the NLN in 1952.

such areas as human sexuality, maternal child relationships, or the school-aged child. Occasionally, when merited, an entire issue of the journal is devoted to one subject, such as nutrition or the family. A recent addition is the development of a format to present pertinent research that focuses on those areas. Space is also devoted to the discussion of other issues about which practicing nurses must be knowledgeable. A section, "Professionally Speaking," includes such areas as how to write to a legislator, how to bring about change, and how to testify as an expert witness. Each issue also carries book reviews, occasional film reviews, and notices of major meetings in the field of maternal child care.

GERIATRIC NURSING

The newest of the AJN company journals is *Geriatric Nursing*, which began publication with the May/June 1980 issue. Emphasis is on clinical articles on common diseases, disabilities and living problems of the aged, including ways to meet their visual, hearing, mental-emotional, and other needs, and nutritional information. News, current events, and other items of interest to nurses concerned with the care of the elderly are also included.

OTHER AMERICAN JOURNAL OF NURSING COMPANY SERVICES

The *American Journal of Nursing, Nursing Outlook, MCN, Geriatric Nursing*, and *Nursing Research* might be considered the "official" publications of the nursing profession. Their official status derives from the fact that they are all published by the American Journal of Nursing Company, a non-profit corporation owned by ANA. The magazines are not published as commercial ventures, but as a service to the nursing profession. In addition to the magazines, the Journal Company also provides a variety of other services related to the publications and communications fields.

For example, in 1973, the AJN Company assumed administrative responsibility for the Nurses' Educational Funds, Inc. However, NEF remains a separate entity, its functioning enhanced by these services.

As a nonprofit entity, the Journal Company also gives some support to various nursing activities, including contributions to the American Nurses' Foundation; NEF Scholarships; the Nursing Archive of Mugar Library at Boston University; and provides for speakers, moderators, and programs for the National Student Nurses' Association.

Microfilm or Microfiche Issues

To meet the demand for unavailable back issues of its publications, the Journal Company has given University Microfilms permission to reproduce on microfilm or microfiche out-of-print volumes of the magazines. Some organizations, individuals, and libraries also like microfilm/microfiche volumes because they require less storage space than original magazines.

University Microfilms also reproduces current out-of-stock issues of the magazines, on order, by photocopy, producing a very readable facsimile of the original publications, but with some limitations. Inquiries about prices and other details of this service should be sent directly to University Microfilms, 300 North Zeeb Road, Ann Arbor, Mich. 48106.

The Journal Company has a policy governing the reproduction of material on which it holds copyright. Generally, permission is granted except when the material is available from the Educational Services Division. Material may not be reproduced without *written* permission. Requests should be directed to the permissions editor at the company address, 555 West 57th Street, New York, N.Y. 10019. A charge may be made to commercial organizations.

The company has a special policy covering the reproducing of its material for library re-

serve collections. Interested organizations should write for this policy.

Sophia F. Palmer Memorial Library

For many years the American Journal of Nursing Company has maintained a library at its headquarters. Intended originally for the use of the magazines' editors and the staffs of the ANA and NLN, the library's facilities have for some years now been available to a limited number of nurses and other individuals seeking information about nursing. They must come to the library, however; there is no mail or loan service and no material may be taken out of the library.

In 1953 the library was named the Sophia F. Palmer Memorial Library in honor of the *Journal's* first editor. Under the administration of a professional librarian, the library contains a wealth of nursing literature, including textbooks, periodicals, numerous bulletins, reports, and official publications of all kinds, as well as some rare and old material about nursing not available elsewhere. A Reader Service answers letters and other requests for information in all areas of nursing. Most queries are handled by the librarians, a few are referred to other organizations or to editorial staff members for reply.

The Educational Services Division

The Educational Services Division was established in 1970, when the AJN Company absorbed the ANA–NLN Film Service and combined this with the existing service of providing reprints of articles from the company periodicals. In the same year, the Contemporary Nursing Series was initiated with the publication of *The Clinical Nurse Specialist*, a compilation of articles from the three AJN Company periodicals. In addition, three special publications were produced: *Closed Urinary Drainage System*, the first original clinical publication from the division; the *National Survey of Audiovisual Materials*, supported by a PHS grant; and the *Editor's Manual*, a source book for the production of any kind of publication. Other services given by the division in its first year were the provision of closed circuit television reports at the ANA convention, in conjunction with Televised Medicine, Inc.; assumption of the responsibility for the convention newspaper; and selection of films and commentators for the film program at the ANA convention. Thus from its inception the division has had three components: publications, audiovisuals, and general services. As the services of the division have increased, effort has been made to maintain a reasonable balance between these three components.

Since 1970 the Film Library has been pruned of some of the outdated material and newer films have been added. Several slide sets and filmstrips were included in 1972. Early in 1973 the division produced for sale the first of its Audio Learning Series, an eight-unit audio cassette, programmed-instruction module, which has proved very successful. Also in 1973 final arrangements were made for the company to acquire Video Nursing, Inc. This non-profit corporation was started in 1966 through a five-year PHS grant, to provide audiovisual educational tools. In 1971, when its grant terminated, the company had demonstrated its ability to produce audiovisuals of high quality, and it continued its work, depending on income from sales, rentals, and consultation services to finance its operation. By 1972 it was clear that a small company of this nature could not maintain a sound fiscal position, and ultimately, arrangements for acquisition by the AJN Company were completed. As a result, the company more than doubled its audiovisual holdings, and has added to its services different types of multimedia, coordinated educational courses.

Today, the Educational Services Division produces and distributes a wide range of multimedia programs for generic and in-service nursing education. The Contemporary Nursing Series continually adds new titles. These compilations are very popular with individual nurses and are also used by numerous schools of nursing as source material. A number of these programs have been approved for continuing education contact hours under the ANA Mechanism for Approval of Continuing Education in Nursing. In addition, the division publishes books, compilations, and reprints of special features appearing in its journals. Consultation service is offered to help faculties of schools of nursing and in-service departments integrate media into their curricula. The division publishes an annual catalog of its materials and services, available on request.

In 1979, the division established Nursing Boards Review (NBR) in answer to a growing demand from new graduates for an organized study program to assist them in preparing for the State Board Examination. This comprehensive, five-day program reviews the clinical nursing subjects covered in the State Board Exams: medical, surgical, pediatric, obstetric, and psychiatric nursing. The program is offered each January and June in various cities throughout the United States. Finally, the division publishes the news concerning convention activities and business for the ANA and NLN and organizes film programs for both conventions. These services were extended to the ICN Congress in 1973. The staff of whichever organization is meeting prepares the material, with the Journal Company staff assuming publication responsibilities. The newspaper is called *Convention Journal* or *Convention Outlook* at the ANA or NLN conventions, respectively.*

Writing Awards

In 1950, when the *American Journal of Nursing* celebrated its fiftieth anniversary, the company established the Mary M. Roberts Fellowship (later, the Mary M. Roberts Writing Awards) in honor of Miss Roberts, who had retired as editor of the *Journal* the

---

*NLN will probably be making its own arrangements for convention coverage after 1980.

previous year after twenty-eight years (1921–1949). The purpose of these awards, as originally described, was to "afford specialized training in writing and other journalistic skills to a nurse [now, nurses] who has demonstrated talent for writing about subjects significant to nursing, addressed to nurses and other professional groups, and the general public."

The nature of these awards has varied over the years since this special fund was first established. For some ten years, six nurses or more annually attended, with all expenses paid, a writers' conference workshop or program for two-week to one-month periods. Currently, the annual nurse writing awards, co-sponsored by participating constituent nursing organizations, are intended primarily to encourage nurses to sharpen their writing skills to promote better communication within the profession and with the general public. An award certificate and a monetary prize are given.

State Publications Awards

To recognize excellence in the official publications of all professional state nurses' associations, the Journal Company makes awards every two years to state bulletins or journals in various areas of excellence such as total editorial content, best feature or news article, and production excellence. To achieve fairness in making the awards, the association publications are grouped according to association membership.

An awards committee of outstanding non-nurse editors and publishers and professional nurses selects the winners of the awards, which are presented at each ANA biennial convention. They are not financial awards but, rather, certificates of merit.

INTERNATIONAL NURSING INDEX

One of the Journal Company's most significant services to the profession is the *International Nursing Index*, which it publishes in cooperation with the National Library of Medicine. This quarterly publication, whose first issue appeared in the spring of 1966, provides a categorized listing of the articles published in some 200 nursing journals throughout the world, many of them in languages other than English, plus articles relevant to nursing that appear in journals listed in *Index Medicus*. The first three issues of the *INI* each year are paperbound and noncumulated; the fourth issue is a cloth-bound cumulation of the three previous issues plus new material to the end of the year.

Representing a comprehensive and continuing index of the world literature pertaining to nursing, the *International Nursing Index* is important to nursing and nurses. In the words of the Journal Company's publishing director, in announcing the inauguration of the *INI*:

> On the practical level, it means that the nurse looking for material on, say, the supervision of nursing services in a psychiatric hospital will no longer have to search through a whole battery of separate indexes; instead, she will find all the relevant references brought together in a single place: the International Nursing Index. And, on the professional level initiation of INI means that nursing, like other professions, has a bibliographic instrument for the control of its scholarly record.[4]

The Index has a circulation of about 1,700; copies are found in most every nursing school, health profession (and probably, hospital) library, and nurses will want to become familiar with it. It gives an idea of the scope, quantity, and variety of material about nursing being published today.

OTHER REFERENCE SOURCES

Most schools of nursing today do not have a collection adequate enough to meet the needs of a serious scholar, or even someone who wants to go beyond the major nursing journals and books. Because of limitations of space and money, a decision is usually made by faculty and library staff about what is most essential for that particular nursing program. Interprofessional health sciences libraries in medical centers and professional schools have collections that cover the various health professions, including international journals and other publications. Other disciplines also have their specialized libraries. What about access? A nurse enrolled in an educational program has access to all of that institution's learning resources, including libraries, audio-visual centers, faculty, and staff. Those same resources may be completely off limits for one not enrolled; at times, even those in university continuing education programs have only limited access. If the nurse is permitted admission to read and browse, chances are that nothing can be taken out.

Hospitals usually have some kind of medical library. Even should the acquisitions be useful to the nurse (and often they are), this librarian, too, has a primary responsibility to others—physicians, medical students (rarely other students), and perhaps administrative personnel and clinical specialists. Nevertheless, nurses who learn how to use the library, the interlibrary loan service, and the various computer information retrieval services will find a new world of reference sources.

There are a number of ways to become knowledgeable about these sources. One that is readily available is "Reference Sources for Nursing," published periodically in *Nursing Outlook*, which provides necessary or helpful sources that all libraries serving nurses should have, and informs nurses and others of what is potentially available. Included are listings of abstract journals, audio-visual catalogs, bibliographies and book lists, dictionaries and workbooks, directories, drug lists and pharmacologies, educational programs in nursing, histories, indexes, legal guides, library administration and organization, research and statistical sources, research grants, on-line resources, and writer's manuals. Both United States and Canadian listings are given.

These are prepared by the Interagency Council on Library Resources, organized in 1960. Seven national nursing organizations in the United States are represented on the Council, as well as the American Journal of Nursing Company, the Canadian Nurses' Association, the Nursing Archive Collection of the Mugar Memorial Library of Boston University (which houses the ANA's Archives), three national hospital associations, three national library associations, the Nursing Division of the United States Public Health Service, and the National Library of Medicine. This Interagency Council has no budget and no executive function, but its recommendations to the agencies represented on it carry weight.[5]

Interlibrary loans extend not only to other on-campus or intracity libraries, but include the vast resources of the National Library of Medicine and designated regional medical libraries.

> *The National Library of Medicine now contains over 1,500,000 items. Since 1967, the National Medical Audiovisual Center in Atlanta, Georgia, has been a component of the National Library of Medicine. Eventually, it will be moved to Bethesda where it will be housed in the Library's Lister Hill Center Building. Under the Medical Library Assistance Act of 1965 (Public Law 89–291), eleven medical libraries in the United States were established as Regional Medical Libraries.*
>
> *. . . Through photoduplication for interlibrary loans and computerized storage and retrieval systems, and approximately 30 indexes or "recurring bibliographies" (among them the Index Medicus and the International Nursing Index), the population of the United States and other nations can benefit from what is said to be the world's largest research library in a single scientific and professional field.[6]*

A more recent source of information is the Nursing Information Center (NIC), made operational through the efforts of the Division of Nursing, HHS. This center "employs complex computer system designs and operations and utilizes modern, on-line, full-text storage and computer retrieval and microfilm technology."

It has three major features: (1) a computer-ized, on-line searchable information file of abstracts of the literature on nursing ser-vices, nursing resources, and nurse planning, and resources development, practice, and methodology; (2) a reference service that pro-vides informative responses to specific inquir-ies, including an annotated bibliography; (3) access to reprints of the referenced literature in paper copy and microfiche.

Unique to the Nursing Information Center (NIC) is its collection of "fugitive" docu-ments. These documents include doctoral dissertations, reports from federally funded projects and studies, state and local govern-ment and nursing association studies and plans, and so forth. These "fugitive" docu-ments were originally unpublished or were published in limited numbers and are rarely identified as part of the formal nursing literature.[7]

Although particularly useful for nurse manpower planners, NIC's subject scope in-cludes all aspects of planning health care needs and delivery of health services and health costs. Services include literature searches, access to copies of documents (which may also be purchased), annotated bibliographies, and referral to other appro-priate sources. To utilize the services, an in-dividual may call or write National Health Planning Information Center, P.O. Box 1600, Prince Georges Plaza Branch, Hyatts-ville, Maryland 20788.

For practicing nurses, it is useful to know which of the many new procedure reference manuals might serve their particular pur-pose. Sending for review copies or checking them in the exhibit areas of major conven-tions is probably the best way to review them. One journal has also provided a com-parison guide.[8]

Of course, all the reference sources in the world are of little value if an individual can-not utilize them properly. Taylor provides some good guidelines,[9] and Henderson delin-eates specific skills.[10]

1. Searching a card catalogue to find books and pamphlets.

2. Using indexes to find journal and serial publications.

3. Finding and using abstracting and ex-cerpting journals, or serials that shortcut finding, scanning, or reading books, pam-phlets, or journals on a given subject.

4. Finding and using lists and bibliographies that enable each worker to build on the searches of others. (Such lists or bibliog-raphies may cite exclusively books and pamphlets, journal articles, or audio-vis-ual materials, or any combination of these.)

5. Finding and using dictionaries, ency-clopedias, directories, statistical and legal guides, fact books, and yearbooks.

6. Making correct citations for each item of information sought or found and prepar-ing a file of these items organized in such a way that the maker of the file and any trained filing clerk can find (or retrieve) the item.

7. Finding nonprint learning media in cata-logues, indexes, and lists.

8. Using viewers, projectors, and other me-chanical devices for reading or looking at both print and nonprint media.

9. Making full (but considerate) use of the services of librarians and other members of the learning center staff in:
   a. Seeking general information in the use of the resources.
   b. Asking for bibliographical help.
   c. Getting an interlibrary loan.
   d. Using retrieval systems such as AV-LINE, CANCER LINE, MED-LINE or TOXLINE.[11,12,13,14,15,16,17]

Well-informed nurses will not want to con-fine themselves to the limits of their own pro-fession's literature. The publications of med-ical and hospital groups, allied professions, education, administration, the social ser-vices, and other related fields frequently contain material of interest to the nurse as a member of the total health team. Under-standing of social, economic, educational, and other issues is as important to under-standing current and future changes in nurs-ing as knowledge of medical and scientific progress. Professional nurses never limit their interests and activities to their own field only, but maintain active participation in broader areas as well.

WRITING FOR PUBLICATION

The nursing profession needs nurse writers to write articles about nursing for publication in professional journals and in magazines read by the general public; to write books on nursing and allied subjects; and to prepare pamphlets, releases, and other written communications for publication and distribution as indicated. Nurses who have any inclination at all toward writing should begin to develop this ability early in their career.

Why write? There are, of course personal/professional reasons, and the most obvious is that a person has something to say, something to share with others. Sometimes it is to react to an issue, a concern, an event, or situation in nursing or elsewhere that affects nursing. It may be in response to an article read that could result in a letter to the editor, a reaction paper, or a follow-up article. A logical reason is that there hasn't been anything, or not much, in the literature on that particular topic, especially if this is in the area of clinical practice. Or a nurse may be involved in development of new techniques, use of new equipment or an innovative approach to caring for a particular kind of patient. Sharing such information is satisfying in itself, but it is also a contribution to the profession. The most important reason for nurses to write (always assuming of course that what is written has substance) is the survival of the profession.

A profession must have an adequate body of literature documenting the theoretical and philosophical base of its practice and how its practitioners operate to provide the service that is the essence of professionalism. Informational voids encourage the multiple misconceptions and stereotypes of nursing already existing and also tempt others to fill the void on the basis of their own prejudices and their own interests.

It is true, of course, that both the quantity and quality of the nursing literature have grown in all its dimensions. In journals alone, the increase in clinical articles attest to nurses' interest in improving their clinical practice. More journals concentrating on a clinical specialty have sprung up. Functional specialties such as administration and education or the broad specialties of school and occupational nursing also have their journals and their interest groups. New authors are emerging. Many nurses, who were traditionally not seen as writers, through a broader formal educational base or writing workshops, have discovered that they have something to say and are learning to express it in writing. They do not yet have a long wait from the time of submission of an article to publication, as is true of many other disciplines.

Nevertheless, there are still a number of informational gaps in the nursing literature in the clinical area, because research and practice follow-through are just beginning to hit their stride. But some other deficiencies may not be as easily detected. For instance, just a few years ago, a noted lay commentator on the health scene did not know that nurses had developed a patient's bill of rights long before the AHA statement. More recently, a computer search on "professional discipline in nursing" brought a horrified non-nurse doctoral student to a professor saying, "Do you mean to say that all professional discipline means to nurses is how cooperative and obedient a nurse employee is, according to her evaluation form?" Finally, consider the legislator who remarked coldly to a group of nurses, "Don't tell me about the need for baccalaureate education; there's nothing much in your own literature that gives *objective* evidence of the benefits to the public." Doubtless, other instances come to mind. Yet, in meetings, workplaces, and schools, some nurse is talking about a concept, or an experiment, or a practice that excites a whole group.[18]

So why don't nurses write? Or at least as

much as other professionals do? Perhaps the first reason is that too many nurses think that writing is for the academician, who must function in a "publish or perish" environment; or the researcher who, in somewhat obscure language, adds to the theory of nursing. The "average" nurse has a string of excuses, "I don't have anything to say; I don't have a degree; I don't have time; I don't know how." All those don'ts can be overcome. A person has to start somewhere, and except for that handful who have an innate talent and inclination for writing, it takes a little self-discipline and maybe some tutoring. There are great satisfactions. As Styles says,

> the thrill of expressing oneself (and perhaps even gaining nursing immortality); of seeing one's ideas applied; of learning that one's published work is the basis of teaching, of seeing that it has stimulated or contributed to the work of others; of finding one's circle of professional friends and scope of influence extending, of being invited to speak, of being recognized by awards, not to mention possibly receiving promotions, better jobs and increased income.[19]

No doubt the writing novice will not find all these rewards immediately, but for the professional career nurse, writing is an essential step in the ladder of success.

It's not all easy as shown by this litany of "pains"—the need for discipline, finding the time, searching out and documenting sources, having one's cherished ideas (or pet phrases) criticized, finding the right editors, even being rejected.[20] For those who want to write, but feel that they don't know how, there are various practical steps. Anyone who has graduated from a nursing program should have the basic tools of writing; a firm grasp of grammar, punctuation, spelling, and word usage. If not, that is an embarrassment for the individual and the profession, and there is little excuse for not remedying the situation. However, to go a step further, for the purpose of writing, there are three indispensable tools: a good dictionary; *Roget's Thesaurus* (a dictionary of syn-

onyms and antonyms, something to turn to when one knows the meaning but can't think of the word); and William Strunk Jr. and E.B. White, *The Elements of Style*, second edition (New York: Macmillan Publishing Co., Inc., 1972), which is easily read and includes basic rules of composition, grammar, punctuation, and word usage. In addition, there is a new surge of "how to" articles and books that can be extremely helpful, some of which, directed specifically to nurses, are cited in the references and bibliography of this chapter. However, a word about style is appropriate: the best writers write so that they are understood; there is little that cannot be said without the use of long words, and there is absolutely no excuse for pretentious prose. This does not mean that the technical words that may be essential to a clinical article should be omitted. It does mean that a simple collection of noun, verb, participle, clause, or whatever makes sense serves as well, if not better, than a convoluted sentence that says nothing more.* The most common writing weaknesses cited by a group of editors were overly formal and pedagogic writing; poor organization, absence of introduction and summary; poor sentence structure (too long and "doesn't flow"), poor or fabricated documentation and use of jargon.[21] Today, use of nonsexist gender is also desirable, whenever possible.

Most nurses start their writing ventures with letters to the editor or articles in state or national journals, although there are some who, with or without a co-author, may publish a book first. One editor suggests certain basic guidelines as a beginning:

> 1. Know as much as possible about your subject. Research those areas you're not sure about (library, interviewing people involved or who have an opinion to offer). Make careful notes as you do this.

---

*For some amusing examples, check the *Nursing Outlook* editorials and cartoons on the subject, some of which are collected in *Toward Getting Published: Guidelines for Nurses Who Want to Write* (New York: A.J.N. Co., 1979).

2. *List all the ideas. arguments. facts. and illustrations you can think of.*
3. *Establish the what. where. when. why. how. and who for your beginning paragraphs.*
4. *Sort out your ideas. putting them in order so you provide continuity as you write.*
5. *Come to a logical conclusion—and make a note of that too.*[22]

The article can be written first in draft form. then polished (a second look brings amazing insight). Sometimes a friend who writes or who is an editor can be helpful in making suggestions. However, it is the writer's responsibility to see that content is accurate and that references and bibliography are properly cited.

Selecting the appropriate journal for submission of an article is crucial. Some editors will return an article with a suggestion that another specific journal might be better for that type of paper,* but most do not. (Nor do most bother to critique it, in part because of the volume of mail they must deal with.) One way to determine which is the "right" journal is to check them all for content and style, but in the last few years, there have also been some helpful publications that compare the various journals in which nurses might want to publish.[23,24] The *Directory of Publishing Opportunities* provides an even more complete listing of non-nursing journals.

At times, authors, especially if they have no track record, may choose to approach an editor first to see whether there is any interest in a particular type of article. In that case, the usual procedure is as follows:

1. Write to the editor. If you know a particular editor of that journal, address it to him/her. Explain what you would like to write about; send an outline of major points; give brief autobiographical information to indicate that you are qualified to write on the subject; list previous writings, if any, and enclose reprints if available; state whether or not you expect re-

---

*Before publication. an article is properly called a paper or manuscript.

muneration other than what the journal usually pays. (Only if you feel strongly about the latter—nursing journals are not noted for extravagant fees.)

2. Wait for the editor's reply. If your idea is appealing, a letter or telephone call will follow with instructions regarding length and due date; information about payment; and possibly suggestions about content, development, and style.

3. Acknowledge the editor's letter promptly, either indicating that all instructions are clear or asking for further information as the case may be.

4. Prepare an outline first; then start to write the manuscript, keeping both the reader and the journal in mind as you write.

5. Type, double spaced, leaving 1-inch margins at top, bottom and right-hand side, $1\frac{1}{2}$-inch margin at left. Include references or bibliography and your autobiography as you would like to have it published with your article.

6. Send the article to the editor first-class mail, together with pictures, or other illustrations (protected with cardboard), and a covering letter. Keep a copy.

7. You should receive an acknowledgement of receipt of the manuscript and, usually a little later, a letter stating whether or not your article has been accepted for publication. Occasionally the editor will ask you to send more information or possibly to revise part or all of your article.

8. The magazine's editorial staff will edit your manuscript and prepare it for the printer. They may send the edited copy for you to check and approve or they may send you the galley proof after the article is set in type. Sometimes both edited copy and proof are sent. Read the copy promptly, request only such changes as you feel are necessary for clarity and accuracy, and return it to the editor's office right away. Delay may mean that your article will not appear in the issue it was planned for and may disrupt the magazine's production schedule.

9. One or more complimentary copies of the

issue in which your article is published will be mailed to you. If you wish extra copies, you will usually find the cost per copy on the magazine's table of contents page. If you want reprints, write at once to the magazine's business office for information regarding the policy for ordering and the price.

Much of the same process occurs when submitting an unsolicited manuscript. It is not ethical to submit copies of the same manuscript to more than one journal at a time. An editor should return a paper promptly if it cannot be used, and then it can be sent to another editor.

An article or lesser item, such as a letter to the editor, a news item, or book review also requires careful planning, organizing, and writing. It, too, must be acceptable to the editors of a publication, or it will never appear in print.

The procedure for writing a book is similar to that for a magazine article, but it is often more exacting and usually much more time consuming.[25] There is more of everything, including satisfactions and remuneration. In addition to the manuscript for the main portion or body of the book, the author is usually responsible for writing the foreword or preface, preparing the index, and reading the galley proof. She/he must obtain written permission to use material quoted or adapted from other sources, being sure that credits are included in the book as indicated in order to avoid any embarrassment or difficulty for all concerned.

The editorial staff of a book publishing company is willing to help the author in every way possible. But only in unusual instances does the staff relieve the author of the responsibility of checking data and presenting it in proper form.

It is customary for a book publisher and an author to negotiate a contract covering the main considerations in the preparation of the manuscript, responsibilities for illustrative materials, revisions, and royalty rates.

Because royalties, support or advances, and marketing vary among publishers, it is wise to "shop around" to find the one most suitable. Sometimes a lawyer or someone who has had considerable experience with publishers can be extremely helpful.

Not all nurses have writing skills, but many do have ideas that are worth sharing.[26] There are two solutions—developing those skills through practice, study, and workshops, or joining forces with someone who does write well, with one taking primary responsibility for the research or background and the other writing the article. This is a perfectly acceptable way to function. Many research publications have multiple authors, only one of whom may do the actual writing; the others have contributed various aspects of the research. The important point is that the person who has something worthwhile to say finds a way to say it; this is a professional responsibility and a satisfying one.

MAJOR NURSING JOURNALS

AANA Journal
American Association of Nurse Anesthetists
111 East Wacker Drive, Suite 929
Chicago, Ill. 60601

AANNT
6352 W. Oakton Street
Morton Grove, Ill. 60053

American Journal of Nursing
The American Journal of Nursing Company
555 W. 57th Street
New York, N.Y. 10019

A.N.S. Advances in Nursing Sciences
Aspen Systems Corp.
20010 Century Blvd.
Germantown, Md. 20767

AORN Journal
Association of Operating Room Nurses
10170 E. Mississippi Ave.
Denver, Colo. 80231

Canadian Journal of Psychiatric Nursing
Psychiatric Nurses' Association of Canada
871 Notre Dame Ave.

Winnipeg, Manitoba, R3E 0M8
Canada

Canadian Nurse
50, The Driveway
Ottawa, Ont., K2P 1E2
Canada

Cardiovascular Nursing
American Heart Association
44 E. 23rd Street
New York, N.Y. 10010

Geriatric Nursing
The American Journal of Nursing Company
555 W. 57th St.
New York, N.Y. 10019

Image
Sigma Theta Tau
National Honor Society of Nursing
1232 West Michigan
Room 347
Indianapolis, Ind. 46202

Imprint
National Student Nurses' Association
10 Columbus Circle
New York, N.Y. 10019

In-Service Training and Education
Health Care Publications, Inc.
125 Elm Street
P.O. Box 696
New Canaan, Conn. 06840

International Journal of Nursing Studies
Pergamon Press
Maxwell House, Fairview Park
Elmsford, N.Y. 10523

International Nursing Review
International Council of Nursing
Box 42
1211 Geneva 20, Switzerland

Journal of Continuing Education in Nursing
Charles B. Slack, Inc.
6900 Grove Road
Thorofare, N.J. 08086

Journal of Emergency Nursing
Emergency Department Nurses Association

241 East Saginaw
East Lansing, Mich. 48823

Journal of Gerontological Nursing
Charles B. Slack, Inc.
6900 Grove Road
Thorofare, New Jersey 08086

Journal of Neurosurgical Nursing
American Association of Neurosurgical
  Nurses
428 E. Preston Street
Baltimore, Md. 21202

Journal of Nursing Administration
'Concept Development, Inc.
12 Lakeside Park
607 North Avenue
Wakefield, Mass. 01880

Journal of Nursing Education
Charles B. Slack, Inc.
6900 Grove Road
Thorofare, New Jersey 08086

Journal of Nurse-Midwifery
American College of Nurse-Midwives
100 Vermont Avenue, N.W.
Washington, D.C. 20005

Journal of Obstetric Gynecologic and Neonatal Nursing
Harper & Row, Publishers
235C Virginia Avenue
Hagerstown, Md. 21704

Journal of Practical Nursing
National Association for Practical Nurse Education and Service, Inc.
122 E. 42nd Street
New York, N.Y. 10017

Journal of Psychiatric Nursing and Mental
  Health Services
Charles B. Slack, Inc.
6900 Grove Road
Thorofare, N.J. 08086

Journal of School Health
American School Health Association
7263 State Road, No. 43
Kent, Ohio 44240

MCN
American Journal of Maternal Child Nursing
The American Journal of Nursing Company
555 W. 57th Street
New York, N.Y. 10019

Nursing Educator
Concept Development, Inc.
12 Lakeside Park
607 North Avenue
Wakefield, Mass. 01880

Nursing 80 (Year changes)
Intermed Communications, Inc.
14 Benjamin Fox Pavilion
Jenkintown, Pa. 19046

Nursing Administration Quarterly
Aspen Systems Corp.
20010 Century Blvd.
Germantown, Md. 20767

Nursing Care
Dual Publishing Corp.
75 E. 55th Street
New York, N.Y. 10022

Nursing Clinics of North America
W. B. Saunders Company
West Washington Square
Philadelphia, Pa. 19105

The Nurse Practitioner
Health Sciences Media and Research Services, Inc.
3845 – 42nd Ave., N.E.
Seattle, Wash. 98105

Nursing Dimensions
Concept Development, Inc.
12 Lakeside Park
607 North Ave.
Wakefield, Mass. 01880

Nursing Forum
Nursing Publications
P.O. Box 218
Hillsdale, N.J. 07642

Nursing Leadership
Charles B. Slack, Inc.
6900 Grove Road
Thorofare, N.J. 08086

Nursing Outlook
American Journal of Nursing Company
555 W. 57th Street
New York, N.Y. 10019

Nursing Research
American Journal of Nursing Company
555 W. 57th Street
New York, N.Y. 10019

Nursing Research Report
American Nurses' Foundation
2420 Pershing Road
Kansas City, Mo. 64108

Nursing Times
Macmillan Limited
Houndsmill
Basingstake
RG21 2X5 England

Occupational Health Nursing
Charles B. Slack, Inc.
6900 Grove Road
Thorofare, N.J. 08086

The ONA Journal
Charles B. Slack, Inc.
6900 Grove Road
Thorofare, N.J. 08086

Pediatric Nursing
Anthony J. Jannetti and Associates
North Woodbury Road
Box 56
Pitman, N.J. 08071

Perspectives in Psychiatric Care
Nursing Publications, Inc.
Box 218
Hillsdale, N.J. 07642

Research in Nursing and Health
John Wiley & Sons, Inc.
605 – 3rd Ave.
New York, N.Y. 10016

RN Magazine
Litton Publications
550 Kinderkamack Road
Oradell, N.J. 07649

Supervisor Nurse
S-N Publications, Inc.
18 South Michigan Ave.
Chicago, Ill. 60603

REFERENCES

1. Joanne McClosky, "Publishing Opportunities for Nurses: A Comparison of 65 Journals," *Nurse Educator.* 1:2:4–13 (July-August 1977).
2. Franz Ingelfinger, "Peer Review in Biomedical Publication," *Am. J. Med.,* 56:686–692 (May 1974).
3. "A Peerless Publication" Editorial, *Nurs. Outlook* 28:225–226 (Apr. 1980).
4. Philip E. Day, "The International Nursing Index," *Am. J. Nurs.* 66:783–786 (Apr. 1966).
5. Virginia Henderson, "Awareness of Library Resources: A Characteristic of Professional Workers, An Essential in Research and Continuing Education," in *Reference Sources for Research and Continuing Education in Nursing* (Kansas City, Mo.: ANA, 1977), p. 3.
6. Ibid. p. 8.
7. Virginia Saba and Kathleen Shapiro, "Nursing Information Center," *Am. J. Nurs.* 79:86–87 (Jan. 1979).
8. Estelle Beaumont and Judy Warmuth, "The New Procedure Reference Manuals," *Nurs '79* 9:72–77 (Apr. 1979).
9. Susan Taylor, "How to Search the Literature," *Am. J. Nurs.* 74:1457–1459 (Aug. 1974).
10. Henderson, op. cit., pp. 11–12.
11. U.S. National Library of Medicine. *Fact Sheet NLM Policies for Reference Service* (Bethesda, Md.: The National Library of Medicine, 1974).
12. ———. Cancer Project, National Cancer Institute's On-Line–Data Base of Ongoing Cancer Research Projects. (Bethesda, Md.: The National Library of Medicine, 1976. Revised every four months).
13. ———. CANCERLINE [Cancer On-Line] (Bethesda, Md.: The National Library of Medicine, 1976).
14. ———. TOXLINE [Toxicology Information On-Line] (Bethesda, Md.: The National Library of Medicine, 1976).
15. ———. Fact Sheet-CATLINE [Catalog On-Line] (Bethesda, Md.: The National Library of Medicine, 1975).
16. ———. Fact Sheet-Interlibrary Loan Policy, Rev. (Bethesda, Md.: The National Library of Medicine, 1975).
17. ———. Fact Sheet-MEDLINE [Medical Literature Analysis and Retrieval System On-Line] (Bethesda, Md.: The National Library of Medicine, 1976).
18. Lucie Young Kelly, "Voices for Nurses," *Image.* 10:4 (Feb. 1978).
19. Margretta Styles, "Why Publish?" *Image,* 10:30–31 (June 1978).
20. Ibid. p. 31.
21. Jane Berger, "Writing for Publication: A Survey of Nursing Journal Editors," *J. Nurs. Admin.* 9:50–52 (Jan. 1979).
22. Alice Robinson, "Want To Get Your Message Across? Write About It." *Imprint.* 23:45 (Oct. 1976).
23. Joanne McCloskey, "Publishing Opportunities for Nurses: A Comparison of 65 Journals," *Nurse Educator.* 2:4–13 (July-August 1977).
24. Ida Martinson, ed. *A Guide to Publishing Opportunities* (Minneapolis: University of Minnesota, 1977).
25. Gail Stuart, et al. "Getting a Book Published," *Nurs. Outlook.* 25:316–318 (May 1977).
26. Elida Murat. "Why Don't Nurses Write?" *Nurse Educator.* 2:6 (Mar.-Apr. 1977).

BIBLIOGRAPHY

Berger, Jane, and Ann Huntsman. "Keeping Up: The Staff Development Educator and the Professional Literature." *Nurse Educator,* 4 (May-June 1979), 19–22. Survey identifies the periodical indexes and journals most used by staff development educators.

Brandon, Alfred, and Dorothy Hill. "Selected List of Nursing Books and Journals," *Nurs. Outlook* 27 (Oct. 1979), 672–680. Lists key books, journals, and reference sources for nurses.

Bunge, Helen L. "The First Decade of Nursing Research," *Nurs. Res.,* 2 (Summer 1962), 132–137. The words *Nursing Research* in the title refer to the magazine of that name published by the American Journal of Nursing Company. A review of the people and events instrumental in the development of this journal.

Hodgman, Eileen. "On Writing and Writing Workshops," *Nurs. Outlook,* 28 (June 1980), 366–371. Author describes content of writing workshops, analyzing what can and can't be done. Factors that facilitate or inhibit would-be writers' motivation and persistence are cited.

King, Lester. *Why Not Say It Clearly: A Guide to Scientific Writing.* (Boston: Little, Brown, and Co.) 1978. Suggests modes of writing that hinder clear expression and offers suggestions for improvement.

Kientz, Carol. "How to Make Your Own Reference File," *Nurs. Outlook*, 15 (Jan. 1967), 57–58. Describes the construction and use of keysort punch cards in constructing a card file index of professional readings.

Miller, Lois, and Edith Rathburn. "Growth and Development of Nursing Literature," *Bull. Med. Lib. Assoc.*, 52 (Apr. 1964), 420–426. A former AJN Company librarian presents interesting background on subject, including development of nursing research and bibliographies. Pertinent references cited.

Montag, Mildred. "Nurses' Educational Funds, Inc." *Nurs. Outlook*, 22 (July 1974), 444–447. Background, current status, and current activities of NEF are described by one of the board of directors.

O'Connor, Andrea. *Writing for Nursing Publications.* (Thorofare, N.J.: Charles B. Slack, Inc.,) 1976. A clear and simple guide to writing, including an index to nursing and related journals.

O'Farrell, Elizabeth. "Write for the Reader, He May Need to Know What You Have to Say." *J. Nurs. Admin.* 4 (Sept.-Oct. 1974), 49–53. Good presentation on planning, organizing, and preparing a manuscript and the publication and production process.

Pings, Vern M. "Nursing Libraries in Historical Perspective," *Am. J. Nurs.*, 65 (Nov. 1965), 115–120. The author reviews pertinent literature to illustrate serious shortcomings of our present nursing libraries. Still has some pertinence.

Raisig, L. Miles. "The Index to Current Nursing Periodical Literature in the United States," *Nurs. Forum*, 3 No. 3 (1964), 96–109. Historical overview of the development of a need for this type of index, and description of past and present efforts to meet this need.

Rajecki, Aldona, and Margaret Muntz. "An Introduction to Medical/Nursing Libraries and Available Resource Tools," *Nurs. Forum* 7-1 (1978), 103–112. How and where to locate information.

"Reference Sources for Nursing," *Nurs. Outlook*, 26 (May 1978), 325–338. The tenth revision, including a Canadian supplement of a list of reference works designed for nurses, developed by the Interagency Council on Library Resources for Nursing.

Styles, Margretta. "Why Publish?" *Image*, 10 (June 1978), 28–32. Excellent article on pains and pleasure of writing, selection of journal. Extensive bibliography worth checking.

See also references and bibliography, chapters 14 and 29 for research resources, and the various non-nursing manuals, articles, and books published on "how to write."

Transition
Into
Practice

30

Employment Guidelines

Long before graduation, even before entering nursing school, many students will have considered seriously what they would like to do after they graduate, or at least have found out about some of the career opportunities in nursing. Often their minds are not completely made up, however, and it is usually helpful to talk over career plans with the school's director, faculty, or someone else prepared to assist students in this way at some time in the educational program. Once a career is selected, the student, in some schools, may choose electives, clinical experiences, or individual projects that give additional pertinent background and aid in attaining the career objectives, although, of course, the basic student's major responsibility is to meet the requirements of the general basic program. At any rate, if such experiences are possible, they will broaden a student's nursing views.

Career goals in nursing undoubtedly can change, and they often do. It may take practical experience to confirm, or disaffirm, one's early convictions about what one wants to do in life. Values may change. Sometimes individuals must face the fact that they do not have the ability or resources to attain the goal they had in mind. And sometimes they find that once they have reached it, it no longer holds a challenge and they set their sights higher.

The new graduates with a planned future in nursing will want to keep that plan in mind as they consider their first job following graduation from nursing school. Very often they will be able to find a position that will definitely advance them toward their career goals.

There are many employment opportunities for nurses today although the place of employment preferred may not offer the exact hours, specialty, opportunities, or assistance a new graduate might want. The pockets of unemployment most often result from budgeting factors and a tightening of the economy. Although nurses may be *needed*, sometimes seriously needed, the tendency of hospitals and other health agencies in a budget squeeze is to reduce numbers of personnel, sometimes retaining those on lower salaries, although less qualified, and eliminating patient care services. Another problem is maldistribution, with not enough nurses opting to work in ghetto areas or poor rural areas, although the need there is serious. Conversely, small communities may be flooded by nursing graduates of a community college who wish to stay in that community.*

Even with these social and economic factors, new nursing opportunities are constantly emerging. And certainly there is no overabundance of nurses with graduate degrees (or baccalaureate degrees for that matter), because the 1963 surgeon general's recommendations for educational requirements for nursing have not yet been met, after more than fifteen years.

There are still pages of advertisements for nurses in the nursing journals and advertisements in local newspapers. A quick survey shows that there are positions offered in just about any type of position a nurse could fill. How, then, can a nurse, particularly a new graduate decide what the best job would be for him or her? How can that job be found?

SOME BASIC CONSIDERATIONS

Although it is true that most new graduates are eager to start earning money at the earliest possible date, it is well to take time to survey the opportunities for employment and to apply for the job that seems best suited to one's present need and wish. It is possible that some help will be received from the director or faculty of one's school, who are generally aware of each student's ability. There also are several basic considerations that should be given serious thought.

Licensure

The first major step in the career of graduate professional nurses is to become licensed in the state in which they intend to practice. Information about how to apply to take the state board examination leading to licensure and other significant information is found in Chapter 20. The procedure for becoming licensed, either initially or later, may take from four to six months. State boards of

---

*See Chapter 15 for career opportunities and a discussion of issues and concerns about nurse employment.

nursing in most states permit nurses to practice temporarily while the application for licensure is being processed.

Marital Status and Plans

Statistics show that most nurses are married; in fact it is becoming more common for nursing students to be married and also to have children. A mature married woman entering nursing probably has made plans to continue working in the profession. Many younger women also plan to continue in their careers with or without interruption for children. Almost inevitably men entering the field plan their careers on a long-term basis.

Nevertheless, there are always some nurses, newly graduated, who prefer to devote time to family and home, with the thought of returning to nursing at some later date. This is, of course, an individual choice. Although there are beginning to be changes in women's views of themselves (see Chapters 6 and 11), many married women still consider their first responsibility to be their family and home. If the nurse's husband's work requires her to assist him in any way or to move from place to place, she may adjust her life accordingly. As a mother, she may believe that her children need her personal attention through the formative years, and that therefore she cannot work at all. During this time, however, she can keep in touch with nurses and nursing by maintaining membership in her alumni association (if any) and her professional nursing organization, and by reading the professional literature. Then when she is ready she can return to active nursing with continued interest and self-confidence.

Often the married nurse with family responsibilities is able to work part time, although not always at the most desirable hours. Even so, the nurse can make a needed contribution to patient care, for part-time nurses are usually employed only if it is not possible to staff adequately with full-time nurses. She also is contributing to the security of herself and her family. She does this in several ways besides the obvious one of increasing the family's income, which may be necessary in times of economic crisis. For example, while working she can keep abreast of theories and techniques in nursing and medical knowledge. She can help advance nursing knowledge and practice while on the job in ways that would be impossible if she stayed at home. She keeps in touch with other nurses and health personnel and, if in a clinical situation, with patients and the many facets of their care. She keeps herself prepared as a competent practitioner and earns a substantial income as well. This offers much more personal security than letting herself get so out of date that the tought of returning to nursing later may be almost frightening.

If the young married nurse decides that she does not want to work immediately she should at least take her state board examinations, become licensed to practice nursing, and continue learning. Unused knowledge has a way of disappearing completely from the mind or becoming so encapsulated that even the nurse who was an excellent student may be unable to pass the examination later without retaking courses. It should be remembered, however, that merely being *licensed* to practice does not mean that the nurse is a competent practitioner unless she has continued to learn. Most nurses who have been out of nursing for as little as three years find that they need a refresher course or comprehensive orientation before assuming full nursing responsibility. It is quite possible that a married nurse will want to return to nursing later, although, at the moment, it may seem an unlikely possibility to her. A great many women in all occupational groups have found it necessary to go back to work because of unexpected developments in their personal lives, but increasingly they choose to return to (or never completely leave) a professional career because of its stimulation. Among the latter is the professionally oriented nurse who maintains a commitment to nursing.

Many positions in nursing require a college degree. The married professional nurse without one often can work toward obtaining it while maintaining a home and fulfilling her responsibilities in the community, by part- or full-time study at a college in the vicinity. The nurse with a bachelor's degree can work toward her master's on a similar basis, although some colleges and universities require that the student attend classes full time for at least one semester of the program, and the entire program usually must be completed within a specified period. Some graduate programs also require some nursing experience before admission.

It is probably wise for any nurse with the intellectual ability and the interest to begin advanced studies as soon after graduation as possible, perhaps on a part-time basis. There is a practical point in this connection that is worth mentioning. It is more economical to obtain a college degree promptly than it is to wait, unless, of course, the cost of living—and education—goes down instead of following its current trend upward.

Personal and Occupational Assessment

New graduates too often neglect to think through their career goals before accepting a first position.

Hospitals affiliated with schools of nursing may offer new graduates positions on the general duty nursing staff. That has several advantages for the hospital and usually for the student. The hospital welcomes nurses who are familiar with the personnel policies, procedures, and physical facilities of the hospital. It gives an often pressed nursing staff the additional assistance so badly needed in most hospitals today.

There are also benefits for the new graduates. During these first months after graduation, she/he can gain valuable experience in familiar surroundings, practicing nursing with less supervision than as a student, and gaining poise and skill with the responsibilities of a graduate nurse.

There are opportunities to develop leadership and teaching skills and practice clinical and other skills under less pressure because people, places, and routines will not be totally unknown. The potential trauma of relocating and readjusting one's personal life is not combined with the tension of being both a new, untried graduate and a new employee. And it may be a wonderful place to work.

However, if the experiences offered do not help the nurse to develop and advance, if the milieu is one that makes the nurse resistant, resentful, indifferent, unhappy, or disinterested, the tone may be set for a lifetime of nursing jobs, not a professional career. The nurse may be competent, but undecided. What the nurse is and wants is of primary importance. Self-assessment of manual skills, temperament, communication skills, stamina, spiritual values, role position preference, and cognitive skills will help the nurse gain realistic self-knowledge. Reres delineates specifically the kinds of questions that can be asked of oneself to help the individual pinpoint a practice area that will, at least potentially, bring mutual satisfaction to employee and employer.[1]

Except in times of great shortage, employers of nurses prefer to hire nurses who have the potential for success in the area of nursing for which they are being employed. For a career-oriented nurse, looking at the potential of various fields or specialties is equally important, assuming that a person does not have a firm commitment for or antithesis to a particular field. Several areas of interest might be compared in relation to current and future demand, stability, educational, professional, and personal qualifications needed, degree of autonomy, opportunities, types of patients/clients and co-workers likely, conditions of employment, earnings, and other benefits. Chapter 15 should be helpful as an overview of the opportunities available, but reading the literature, talking to practitioners in the field and, if possible, getting exposure to the actual practice at some time during one's educational program will help answer some specific questions.

There are undoubtedly other strictly personal considerations related to the first position in nursing, such as the off-duty activities

particularly enjoyed, desire for a change of environment or satisfaction with one's present location, home ties, and interest in meeting new people, possibly a prospective husband or wife. All of these factors should be considered seriously. The major steps taken can rarely be retraced. At best, time is wasted. It is much better to move carefully when selecting the first "permanent" job in nursing and to make sure one is progressing in the direction desired.

SOURCES OF INFORMATION ABOUT POSITIONS

Four principal sources of information are available to graduate professional nurses who are looking for a position: (1) personal contacts and inquiries; (2) advertisements and recruiters; (3) nurses' registries approved by district or state nurses' associations; and (4) commercial placement agencies. At some time, every nurse may have occasion to use the services of each of these. It is well, therefore, to know how to go about using them intelligently and to the best advantage.

Personal Contacts and Inquiries

The nursing service director or a member of the nursing staff of a student affiliated agency, instructors, other nurses, friends, and family may suggest available positions in health agencies or make other job suggestions. Hospitals not affiliated with schools of nursing may ask the heads of nursing schools to refer graduates to them for possible placement on their staffs. Often, letters or announcements of such positions are posted on the school bulletin board or are available in a file. The nurse's own inquiries are likely to be equally productive in turning up just the sort of position desired. A nurse interested in a position in a particular agency in a particular city should write a letter of inquiry, expressing interest in a position there and outlining his or her qualifications and interests. Employers expect this type of communication and usually respond reasonably promptly with information as to whether positions are available and when an appointment for an interview can be made.

Advertisements

Local newspapers, journals of local health organizations, and official organs of district and state nurses' associations often carry advertisements of positions for professional nurses. National nursing magazines list positions for nurses in all categories of employment, usually classified into the various geographic areas of the country. National medical, public health, and hospital magazines carry advertisements for nurses, but they usually are for head nurse positions or higher, or for special personnel such as nurse anesthetists or nurse consultants.

All publications carry classified advertisements for information only, and of course, as a source of revenue. Rarely, if ever, does the publisher assume responsibility for the information in the advertisement beyond conformance to such legal requirements as may apply and to the laws of decency and good taste. The nurse who accepts an advertised position that does not turn out to be what was expected cannot hold the publication responsible.

In seeking employment by this means, therefore, it is important to read very carefully every advertisement of interest. Is the hospital or health agency well known and of good reputation? Is the information clear and inclusive? Does it sound effusive and over-stress the advantages and delights of joining the staff? What can be read between the lines? How much more information is needed before deciding whether the job, if available, is suitable? Some of these questions can be resolved through correspondence or telephone contact.

At some time a nurse may want to place an advertisement in the "Positions Wanted" column of a professional nursing publication. In that event, the individual should obtain a copy of the magazine and read the directions for submitting a classified adver-

tisement. They will be very explicit, and should be followed to the letter; otherwise publication of the advertisement may be delayed. The editor will arrange the information to conform to the publication's style, but will not change the material sent, unless asked to. Therefore all the information needed to attract a prospective employer *within the limits of professional ethics* should be included in a clear and concise manner.

A recent innovation is the "Career Directory," published periodically by some nursing journals or other commercial sources. They are free to the job seeker and are supported by the prospective employer by placement of relatively extensive advertisements with much more detailed information than is in the usual ad. The other added advantage is instant comparison and geographic separation, with preprinted, prepaid postcards that will be sent to the health agency of interest. (Most are generally geared toward hospital recruitment.) They are frequently made available in the exhibit section of student and other nursing conventions. At least one carries reprints of its articles on careers, licensure, job seeking, and other pertinent information.[2] Some journals also do periodic surveys on job salaries and fringe benefits that can be useful when considering various geographic areas.[3]

Recruiters for hospitals and other agencies are usually present at booths representing that hospital in the exhibit areas of conventions; some also have suites where they have an open house. Recruiters who may or may not be nurses also visit nursing schools or set up in a hotel for preliminary interviews. Notices may be placed in newspapers or sent to schools. There are advantages to the personalized recruiter approach because it is possible to have questions answered directly, as well as to get a "feel" for attitude, especially if nurses accompany the recruiter. However, it is necessary to remember that recruiters are selected for their recruiting ability.

Registries and Temporary Nurse Services

A nurses' registry, as the name implies, is

a list of nurses who are available for nursing work. A registry usually is concerned chiefly with private duty nurses, but its services may be offered to all nurses.

There are two general classifications of registries for nurses. Professional registries are operated on a nonprofit basis, usually under the auspices of a district or state nurses' association. Commercial registries are run by private individuals for the purpose of making a profit. Both types usually provide twenty-four-hour service to patients, doctors, hospitals, and other health agencies in need of a nurse or nurses.

When private duty was a larger field, ANA-associated professional registries were a popular source of employment. Today, there are still some functioning, although many hospitals seem to have their own "private duty registry."

The objectives of a professional registry are threefold: (1) to provide the public with safe nursing care; (2) to serve as a center from which the community can obtain nurses; and (3) to administer a call service for private duty nurses and others seeking positions.

It follows, therefore, that the registry must be careful in the selection of nurses for enrollment. Registrants must be qualified by education and experience for the assignments they will be asked to fill. All nurses must be licensed and currently registered to practice in the state in which the registry is located.

Nurses who wish to register with a professional registry should (1) find out whether there is one in the locality in which they want to work; (2) write or telephone the registrar expressing their intention; and (3) follow the registrar's instructions thereafter, which very likely will include a personal interview, completion of an application form, and submission of credentials and references.

Nurses accepted for registration will be so notified, and their names will be placed on the list in the employment category that they designate. Nurses are assigned in rotation when their qualifications are adequate for the assignment.

To defray the cost of operation, a professional registry charges registrants a registration fee, which varies in amount from place to place. It is usually a stated sum paid annually or semiannually. Hospitals usually do not make a charge for the service because it is done to serve their own patients. A nurse is employed and paid by the individual patient. Many commercial registries are reputable and reliable in every way; others are careless in their selection of registrants and fail to make sure that they are licensed to practice nursing. Some are not conscientious about making assignments and thus may subject the public to unsafe and unskilled care.

The law in every state requires a commercial registry to be licensed. These registries are not subject to inspection by any approving body of a state nurses' association. Many advertise in newspapers.

The registrant's fee is considerable in a commercial agency and unless controlled by state law, may be as high as 10 per cent of the nurse's earnings from every assignment. Some registries charge the employer a fee also, especially if he is the patient or the person responsible for paying the patient's bills.

Nurses considering registration with a commercial agency should determine its reputation and mode of operation in advance and make sure that the benefits to them will be worth the cost in every way.

The relatively new temporary nurse service functions quite differently (see Chapter 15), but is an employment source.[4] Nurses are usually placed in short-term situations in hospitals, but some services advertise home care. The single most important factor that seems to attract nurses to TNS' is control over working conditions including time, place, type of assignment, and so on. New graduates may find this type of employment attractive as a temporary measure since the nonavailability of fringe benefits may not be important to them. There is also an opportunity to try out different types of nursing, but for the new nurse, the lack of individual support and supervision is a disadvantage.

BUSINESS CORRESPONDENCE

New nursing graduates today present a wider variety of personal and educational backgrounds than a few years ago. Many have held responsible positions in other fields and even more have worked part- or full-time in some kind of position before or during their educational programs.

Therefore the *suggested* procedures for application and resignation presented are just that. They review generally accepted ways to go about certain inevitable professional matters in a sophisticated and businesslike way, and may serve as a refresher for those already familiar with these or other equally acceptable ways of relating and communicating in professional business relationships. For the younger, less-experienced nurse, this provides a convenient reference and guide.

Inherent in all these relationships is the desirability—indeed the necessity—of doing one's share to maintain courteous, professional, and businesslike relationships with a prospective or present employer and all others who are connected in any official capacity with one's position. Emotional maturity is particularly important. This is revealed in the ability to help create a favorable climate for productive discussion of all aspects of the employment situation.

Courtesy in business arrangements involves consideration as revealed in a thorough preparation for an interview, the careful construction of letters, the timing and brevity of telephone conversations, the appropriateness of personal appearance for interviews, and promptness in every respect. In return for such courtesy, one has a right to expect comparable consideration from others. But, whether this is received or not, there is no reason to relax one's standards of personal deportment in business relationships. This principle can be extended to other business matters as well as those directly connected with a nursing position.

The first contact with a prospective employer is usually made by letter, followed by a personal interview, telephone conversa-

tions, and, occasionally, telegrams. Every business letter makes some kind of an impression on its reader, an impression that may be favorable, unfavorable, or indifferent. For the best effect, the stationery on which it is written should be in good taste; the message accurate and complete, yet concise; the tone appropriate; the form, grammar, and spelling correct.

Stationery

Business letters should be neatly and legibly typed or handwritten in black or blue ink on unlined white stationery. Single sheets no smaller than 7- by 9-in. or larger than $8^1/_2$- by 11-in. are more suitable than folded sheets. Personal stationery is acceptable if it is of the right size; white, light grey, or off-white; and the envelopes are unlined. Notebook paper should never be used for business correspondence; neither should someone else's personal stationery or the stationery of a hospital, hotel, or place of business. Good quality typing paper is always in good taste, if a suitable envelope is used with it.

It is usually best to type a business letter because it is easier for the receiver to read it. The fact that a letter is typed, however, does not ensure that it will make a good impression. Margin and spacing should be uniform with no incorrectly merged letters or extra spaces left between letters or words. This often requires painstaking typing, particularly if the typewriter tends to skip spaces or is very sensitive to touch. The typewriter ribbon should be fresh, the color black or dark blue. There should be no typed-over letters and no erasures. It is better to retype a letter several times if necessary than to send one that does not do credit to one's knowledge of what constitutes a proper business communication.

The signature for a typewritten letter should always be handwritten above a typed signature as shown in the sample letter in this chapter.

One advantage of a typewritten letter is that it is easy to make a carbon copy to retain for one's files, an important consideration in all business correspondence. A copied letter has little or no business or legal value; a carbon copy of a letter often does. (Photocopies are also popular now and equally suitable for one's records.)

An attractive handwritten letter may have certain advantages over a typed one. For example, it can show one's ability to prepare neat and legible records and reports and can indicate preciseness and careful attention to details. A nicely handprinted letter may also make a good impression on the recipient, perhaps because so few individuals have the patience and skill to do it.

Message

The information included in a business letter should be presented with great care, giving all pertinent data but avoiding unnecessary details and divulging nothing that would be better withheld, at least until a later date. Even for experienced business executives, this requires attention to every letter that goes out over their signatures, whether they see to it personally or leave it to a competent assistant or secretary. The young nurse applying for a position or carrying on continued correspondence about it must exercise comparable care. Furthermore, composing correct and commendable business correspondence is excellent experience for a person's nursing career and for general business letters as well.

Beginning career letters will be quite different from the letters written to meet class requirements in high school or when corresponding with the director of a school of nursing prior to admission. They will reflect the level of growth attained during one's educational program just as later letters will reflect added years of experience and advanced education.

It is often helpful to outline, draft, and edit a business letter just as one would a term paper. This requires an individual to think it through from beginning to end to ensure completeness and accuracy, and helps to tailor it to fit a well-spaced single page, if possible, or two at the most.

An outline for a letter applying for a position might contain the following information.

A. Reason for writing
  1. To apply for position for staff nurse advertised in June issue of *American Journal of Nursing.*
  2. Position interests me because of location of hospital, salary scale, insurance and retirement benefits, and opportunities for advancement and continued education mentioned in ad.
B. Qualifications: single, twenty-one years old, graduate Northfield College School of Nursing, Chelsea, Ill., June, 1980; will take state boards in July; worked two summers as ward clerk.
C. References: director of my school of nursing; will supply others if desired.
D. Can arrange to go to Chicago for personal interview, preferably in late afternoon because no conflicting classes at that time.
E. Look forward to reply. Thanks for consideration.

A letter written according to this outline should contain all of the information that the prospective employer will need at this point. If she/he is interested in having the nurse join the staff, an application form will be sent. In this event, it should be completed promptly and fully with careful attention to spelling, neatness, and accuracy of all information, and returned with a very brief covering letter. A copy may be kept for the nurse's files.

It is quite possible that a nurse does not want actually to apply for a position but will only want to express interest in it and ask for more information. In that instance, the outline might follow this pattern.

A. Reason for writing
  1. Saw advertisement for general duty nurses in December issue of *Nursing Outlook.*
  2. Position on staff interests me because of location and known good reputation of hospital but would like to know whether general duty nurses have a staff organization and whether I could be assigned to pediatric division, my major interest in nursing.

B. Qualifications: single, twenty-four years old, no dependents; graduated Jackson Hospital School of Nursing, Mineola, Md., Sept., 1979; registered in Maryland. Now working as general duty nurse in recovery room in Jackson Hospital.

C. Will appreciate consideration given letter. If answers to queries are in the affirmative, would like to make formal application for position. Eager to get started on career in pediatric nursing.

This type of exploring letter should bring the information needed plus a reply that may help the nurse decide whether she/he really wants to join the staff of that institution. Communications are two-way streets on which the prospective employer should be just as prompt, informative, and courteous as the prospective employee. The nurse graduate will be wise to ascertain that the prospective new position is really what is desired, and the attitude conveyed in the employer's letter may be as much of an indication of whether the position is desirable as the stated information.

Should the reply received be favorable, the nurse should send the additional information or return the application blank promptly and continue to follow through until final arrangements have been made.

If the nurse decides not to apply for the position after all, it is courteous to inform the person with whom there has been correspondence. Specific reasons need only be given (briefly) if such a decision is made *after* first accepting the position. This is not only courteous, but advisable, because the nurse may wish to join that staff at another time or may have other contacts with the nurse administrator.

Tone

The tone of a business letter has considerable influence on the impression it makes and the attention it receives. It is probably better to lean toward formality than informality, although a happy medium is most desirable. Friendliness without undue familiarity, cordiality without overenthusiasm, sincerity, frankness, and obvious respect for the person to whom the letter is addressed set the most appropriate tone for correspondence about a position in nursing.

Form

Books on English composition and secretary's handbooks include correct forms for writing business letters. Two or more variations may be given and the choice is the individual's to make. It usually is advisable to select one correct form and use it for all business letters, thus avoiding inconsistencies in later correspondence.

The block form is employed most widely in business correspondence and, therefore, is selected for illustration here. This means that the left-hand words or margins are aligned throughout the letter, with extra space between paragraphs.

Commas are used sparsely in this form and a colon is used following the salutation. No abbreviations are used. If any abbreviations, such as Ave. or Aug., are used, the names of the states should also be abbreviated. The addressee's title should never be abbreviated. If it is too long to carry on the line with the person's name, it may be placed on the line immediately below. If personal stationery on which name and address are engraved or printed is used, these should be omitted from the heading of the letter and only the date given. Zip codes should be used.

17 Eastern Avenue
Belmont, Montana 00000

August 16, 1979

Miss Sarah Pierce, R.N., Director of Nursing
Columbia Memorial Hospital
Hastings, Alabama 00000

Dear Miss Pierce:

I should like to apply for the general duty nursing position at your hospital which was advertised in the June issue of the American Journal of Nursing.

Alice Hagar

....

Sincerely yours,

(Miss) Alice Hagar

The inside address and the envelope address should be identical. People are sensitive about their names and titles; care should be taken to be accurate. It is easy to write Macdonald as MacDonald, Larsen as Larson, or Peake as Peak, but it usually is inexcusable.

It is correct to give a title before the name in an address in the heading and on the envelope—not in the form of initials after the name. For example: Dr. Constance E. Wright rather than Constance E. Wright, Ed.D. In a signature, however, it is preferable to reverse this and place the degree initials after the name of the signer of the letter. Never use both the title and the initials in an address: Dr. Constance E. Wright, Ed.D.

It is quite suitable, and even desirable, to use RN after the name of a nurse, particularly in professional correspondence. Many nurses with doctorates sign their names with an RN, Ph.D., or RN, Ed.D., added to clarify that they are nurses as well as "doctors."

Mrs. John, Mrs. Mary, or Ms.? Books of social etiquette almost invariably have insisted that a woman who has ever been married is committing a social error whenever she uses the title *Mrs.* with her given name: Mrs. Mary Holmes. The only correct form, they contend, is Mrs. John Holmes, because the title *Mrs.*, translated loosely, means "I am (or have been) married to a man named John Holmes." Following this reasoning, it obviously is incorrect to use *Mrs.* with a feminine name.

This rule of etiquette may be followed in social correspondence, but a professional or business woman usually does not use her husband's name at all in connection with her work. However, she can use the title *Mrs.* to identify her as a person who is, or has been, married if she desires. Because the purpose of a letter is to communicate, this seems logical and practical. Although it is generally assumed that a woman is single if no title appears before her name, this is not always true. Many times a person makes this assumption and addresses the other as *Miss* only to learn at some later date, possibly un-

der embarrassing circumstances, that she should have been addressed as *Mrs.*

When so many business and professional women are married, it has seemed reasonable to adopt a consistent address style and always use either *Miss* or *Mrs.* before an adult female's name unless she should be addressed as *Dr., Dean,* or by some other academic or occupational title. Thus a letter would be addressed to Miss Mary Holmes or Mrs. Mary Holmes and the typed signature would be (Miss) Elizabeth Kellogg or (Mrs.) Elizabeth Kellogg, as the case might be. The written signature would omit the title. In a letter that is completely handwritten, however, *Miss* or *Mrs.* would be written and enclosed in parentheses. This is still an acceptable approach. However, with new attention being given to women's rights, women's liberation, and women's professional freedom, these standard rules of etiquette are no longer acceptable to all. Some professional (or nonprofessional) women combine their maiden names and married names in hyphenated form or retain their maiden names with either a Miss or the newer Ms. title. Others use Ms. with their married names. Currently, some journals and many individuals use the Ms. title with a surname for *any* woman addressed. As might be expected, this is highly acceptable to some women and equally unacceptable to others. On this point it is probably more a matter of good sense and one's own philosophy rather than of etiquette.

If a woman uses her husband's name in the signature of a letter she has written, she should enclose it in parentheses and write her name above:

Mary Holmes

(Mrs. John Holmes)

Other Important Points. It is always advisable to address a person in business correspondence exactly as his name appears on his own letters. The full title and position should be used no matter how long it may be or how tedious it is to write or type. It is better to place the lengthy name of a position on the line below the addressee's name, and break up a long address also in the interest of neat appearance, remembering to indent continuation lines as follows:

Miss Selma T. Henderson, RN
Director, School of Nursing and Inservice
    Education Program for Nurses
The Reddington J. Mason Memorial Hospital
    School of Nursing
1763 Avenue of the Nineteenth Century
Chesapeake-on-Hudson, Ohio 00000

If the name of the person to whom one is writing to inquire about a position is not known, the letter may be addressed to the director or supervisor of the appropriate division, e.g., Director of the Department of Nursing, or Operating Room Supervisor. The salutation would then be Dear Madam or Dear Sir. Using the person's name, if it is at all possible, is by far the most preferable choice.

Reference may be made to a secretary's handbook for other variations in addresses, signatures, and titles. The best complimentary close for almost any business letter is Sincerely yours or Sincerely. Others are acceptable, such as Yours truly and Very truly yours, but are used less frequently today.

PROFESSIONAL BIOGRAPHIES AND RÉSUMÉS

No matter how the nurse obtains a position in nursing she/he probably will be asked to submit a résumé or summary of qualifications for the job. This might include a personal history, education and experience, character and performance references, professional credentials, such as license registration number and a transcript of education records.

It is possible, of course, to prepare this professional biography oneself, updating it every time there is a change of position, adding new references, and subjecting former educators and employers to repeated requests for information and references. A better idea, however, is to have one's professional biography compiled and kept on file, if possible. The ANA no longer maintains this service, but some universities and colleges do, for a fee. The advantages are that the prospective employer receives an organized summary of all relevant information without the necessity of the nurse listing educational qualifications, nursing experience, or names and addresses of references each time he or she changes positions. Moreover, former teachers and employers do not have to refresh their memories constantly and consult their files to write a reference about someone they may scarcely remember. It is also much quicker than waiting for an assortment of records to be sent from many places.

However, the reality is that not only is such a compilation of records less likely to be available than before, but many employers now prefer that the applicant send a résumé. A résumé is a relatively short biography. (In academia, a curriculum vitae, or CV, which is somewhat lengthier and contains different and more detailed information, is the appropriate form of professional biography.)[5] Résumés are seen as being shorter than CVs.

The résumé, like the letter of application, should be businesslike, typed neatly on one side of good-quality plain white paper, 8½ by 11 inches, with a good margin all around. Two or three pages are usually recommended.

There are a number of sources on writing a résumé,[6,7] and some colleges and universities offer a placement or career guidance service that helps the individual to develop the type of résumé that is best for that person's career goals and shows her/his background to the best advantage.

The usual form is as follows:

1. Name, address, telephone number at top (home and work number, if necessary). Marital status and number of dependents may be included, but are not required.
2. License registration number(s) and state certification, if appropriate.
3. Education: name and location of school(s) attended, date of graduation

and/or year attended, and any advanced or nonmatriculated credits taken.

4. Experience: title of position held, name and address of employer, dates of employment listed in *reverse* chronological order. Description of principal duties and responsibility for each position (military duty may be included here).

5. Memberships, activities, accomplishments, major honors. Professional membership (office and committee positions, if any). Any special recognition received at work or school. Relevant voluntary or community contributions.

6. References: full names, titles, and business addresses of about three people who are qualified to evaluate the applicant's professional ability, scholarship, character, and personality. Most suitable are teachers and former employers. Permission to use these names as references should have been requested.

Some variations include listing first the job objectives; placing the work history before the education; including a brief summary of personal characteristics, appearance, and abilities; including special skills (speaking and writing ability, languages); listing publications and research. Usually salaries of the last job are not listed. Multiple clear copies should be made (photocopy or other method) and sent with letter of inquiry. It should be considered the applicant's personal advertisement.

Applications

Applications are not just routine red tape. Whether or not a résumé is requested or submitted, the formal application, which is developed to give the employing agency the information it wants, can be critical in who is finally hired. Even if the information is repetitious of information offered in the résumé, it should be entered. It is usually acceptable to attach the résumé or a separate sheet if there is not adequate space to give complete information. It is a good idea to read through the application first so that information is put in the correct place. Neatness is essential.

Erasures, misspellings, and wrinkled forms leave a poor impression. Abbreviations, except for state names and dates, should not be used.

If the form must be completed away from home, it is wise to think ahead and bring anticipated data—social security and registration number, places, dates and names. Although occupational counselors say that it is not necessary to give all the information requested (such as arrests, health, color, some of which are illegal to request),* it is probably not wise to leave big gaps in one's work history without explanation.

Personal Interview

An interview may be the deciding factor in getting a job. Anyone who has an appointment for a personal interview should be prepared for it physically, mentally, emotionally, and psychologically.[8,9] The degree of preparation will depend on the purpose of the interview and what has preceded it. Assuming that the nurse has written to a prospective employer about a position and an interview has been arranged, preparation might include the following:

Physical Preparation. Be rested, alert, and in good health. Dress suitably for that job, but wear something in which you feel at ease. It is important for a man or woman to be well groomed and as attractive as possible. First appearances are important, and given a choice, no one selects a sloppy or overdressed person over someone who is neat and appropriately dressed. Have enough money with you to meet all anticipated expenses. If you are to be reimbursed by the employing agency, keep an itemized record of expenses for submission later. Arrive at your destination well ahead of time, but do not go to your prospective employer's office earlier than five minutes before the designated time.

Mental Preparation. Review all informa-

---

*See Chapter 19 regarding federal legislation on employment rights.

tion and previous communications about the position. Showing that you know about the hospital or agency is desirable and impressive. Make certain that you know the exact name or names of persons whom you expect to meet and can pronounce them properly. Decide what additional information you want to obtain during the interview. Consider how you will phrase your leading questions. Carry a small notebook or card on which you have listed names of references and other data that you may need during the interview. If you bring an application form with you, make sure it is complete, accurate, and neatly filled out. Fold it carefully, place it in a fresh envelope which you leave unsealed, and have it ready to hand to the interviewer when she/he asks for it or, if it seems indicated, offer it at the appropriate time.

Emotional and Psychological Preparation. If you have any worries or fears in connection with the interview, try to overcome them by thinking calmly and objectively about what is likely to take place. Thorough physical and mental preparation is the best stabilizer of emotions at such a time. Be ready to adjust to whatever may develop during the interview. For example, you may expect to have an extended conversation with the director of nurses and find when you arrive that a personnel officer who is not a nurse will interview you. She/he may interview you in a very few minutes and in what seems to be an impersonal way. Or you may have visualized the job setting as quite different.

Acceptance of things as you find them, while reserving the privilege of making a decision after thoughtful consideration of the total job situation, is the most desirable attitude. If a stimulating challenge is inherent in the position, you will sense it during the interview or you may have reason to believe that it will develop after you assume your duties. However, you cannot demand a challenge, and if one is "created" for you spontaneously by the interviewer, take the prom-

ise with the proverbial grain of salt, knowing that rarely does an employment situation adjust to the new employee. Psychological sensitivity can be very helpful in selecting a position at any stage in your career.

During the Interview

Usually, the interviewer will take the initiative in starting the conference and closing it. You should follow that lead courteously and attentively. Shake hands. Be prepared to give a brief overview of your experiences and interests, if asked. At some point you will be asked if you have any questions, and you should be prepared to ask for additional information if you would like to have it. Should the interviewer appear to be about to close the conference without giving you this opportunity, you may say, "May I ask a question, please?" It is perfectly acceptable to ask, before the interview is over, about salary, fringe benefits, and other conditions of employment, if a contract or explanatory paper has not been given you. In fact, it would be foolish to appear indifferent. A contract is desirable (see Chapter 22), but if that is not the accepted procedure, it is important to understand what is involved in the job. The job description should be accessible in writing and it is best that you have a copy. If not asked, say what you want and expect as salary, benefits, work conditions, but it is better to wait for a lead.

Most interviewers agree that an outgoing candidate who volunteers appropriate information is likeable. On the other hand, many use the technique of selective silence, which is anxiety-provoking to most people, to see what the interviewee will say or do. A good interviewer will try to make the applicant comfortable, in part to relax him/her into self-revelation; most do not favor aggressive methods. Good eye contact is fine, but don't stare. Be sensitive to the interviewer's being disinterested in a certain response; maybe it's too lengthy.

When the interview is completed, thank the interviewer, shake hands, and leave promptly. You may or may not have been offered the position, or you may not have accepted it if it was offered. If it was offered to you, it is usually well to delay your decision for at least a day or two until you have had time to think the matter over carefully from every practical point of view. Perhaps you will want more information, in which case you may write a letter, send a telegram, or make a phone call to your prospective employer. It is always courteous and sometimes acts as a reminder to send a thank-you letter.

Telephone Conversations and Telegrams

During the procedure of acquiring a position, a nurse may have occasion to discuss some aspect of it over the telephone with the prospective employer. If the nurse makes the call, she/he should be brief, courteous, and to the point, with notes handy, if needed. It may be helpful to make notations of the conversation. It is sensible to listen carefully and not interrupt.

If the nurse receives a call and is unprepared for it, he or she can be courteous but cautious and, perhaps, ask for time to think over the proposal—or whatever may have been the purpose of the call.

Agreements about a position made over the phone should be confirmed promptly in writing. If it is the nurse's place to do so, she/he might say, while speaking with the person, "I will send you a confirming letter tomorrow." If it is the responsibility of the other party to confirm an agreement, but she/he does not mention it, the nurse may ask, "May I have a letter of confirmation, please?"

If any business arrangements are made by telegram, the telegram or copy should be filed with other related correspondence.

For positions sought through a nurses' registry or employment agency, the same courteous, thorough, and businesslike procedures used when dealing directly with a prospective employer are appropriate. A brief thank-you note for help received shows consideration of the agency's efforts in the nurse's behalf. After any interview or conversation, it is useful to make notes about what happened, both for future use and reference.

CHANGING POSITIONS

There seems to be an unwritten rule that nurses should remain in any permanent position they accept for at least a year. Certainly this is not too long—except in the most unusual circumstances—for a nurse to adjust to the employment situation and find a place on the staff in which to use one's ability and talents to the fullest potential. Furthermore, a person who changes jobs frequently in any profession or occupation soon gains a reputation for being a "flitter," and some employers are reluctant to hire him or her. However, should it be desirable or necessary to change positions, a number of points might be observed. Consider your employer and co-workers as well as yourself and leave under amicable and constructive circumstances. Try to finish any major projects you have started, such as the revision of written directives; arrange in good order the books, equipment, and materials your successor will "inherit"; prepare memos and helpful guides to assist the nurse who will assume your duties. Tell your immediate superiors about aspects of your work that may be helpful to them. If requested by the administration, help select the person who will succeed you, being extremely careful to be objective. If this is impossible because of personal considerations, ask to be excused from this obligation.

Terminal interviews are considered good administrative practice, and are sometimes used for a final performance evaluation and/or a means to determine reasons for resignation. There is some question of how open the employee is about resignation (unless the reason is illness, necessary relocation, and so on), perhaps because of fear of reprisal in references or even a simple desire to avoid unpleasantness. This is a decision the nurse must make in each individual situation.

A nurse who plans to continue to work should be reasonably sure that she/he has acquired a new position before resigning from the current job. Depending on the reasons for leaving and how eager one is to make a change, some writers suggest that before definitely accepting the new position, the present employer might be informed about the nurse's desire to leave and why. It may be that, depending on the employer's concept of the nurse's value to the institution, a new, more desirable position might be offered.

It is important to give reasonable notice of intention to resign. If there is a contract, the length of the notice will very likely be stipulated. Two weeks to a month is the usual period, depending principally upon the position held and the anticipated difficulty in hiring a replacement.

A letter of resignation is always indicated when leaving a position, unless one is asked to leave or dismissed. In that case, it is vital to know why. If a problem situation has existed and the nurse is at fault, this should be known, with some understanding acquired for avoiding similar situations. If the nurse is not at fault, full efforts should be made to remedy the situation, particularly in light of probable unfair negative references. If the situation is serious, the nurse who is a member of ANA may choose to seek the help of the state organization's economic security division. If the dismissal is a "lay-off" because of economic reasons, it would be well for the nurse to have a letter to this effect, both in terms of professional security and in order to obtain unemployment benefits, if necessary (see Chapter 19). A letter of resignation should state simply and briefly, but in a professional manner, intention of leaving, the date on which the resignation will become effective, and the reasons for making the change. A sincere comment or two about the satisfactions experienced in the position and regrets at leaving will close the letter graciously.

There should be no hint of animosity nor harbored resentment because this will serve no constructive purpose and may boomerang to the nurse's disadvantage later.

One nurse author comments, appropriately:

> When the nurse leaves a position, she does not burn her bridges or close a chapter. The reputation she made will go with her. Her old employer will be asked many times for comments on her performance, on her professional and social conduct, on her character and integrity. Her contribution in the nursing group and in the community will be scrutinized and evaluated and her readiness and ability to take over a new appointment will be judged largely in terms of what she did in the old one. Did she leave in a huff? Was she difficult to get along with? Or did she fill a difficult spot capably and is she missed? No greater compliment can be paid a person than to say that the agency concerned not only regrets her leaving, but would be glad of an opportunity to reemploy her. [11]

REFERENCES

1. Mary Reres, "Assessing Growth Potential," *Am. J. Nurs.*, 74:670–676 (Apr. 1974).
2. *Nursing '79 Career Directory.*
3. Marjorie Godfrey, "Nursing Salaries Today: Where You Can Earn the Most and the Least," *Nurs. 77*, **81**:97 (June 1977).
4. Patricia Prescott and Teddy Longford, "Supplemental Nursing Service: Boon or Bane?" *Am. J. Nurs.*, 79:2140–2144 (Dec. 1979).
5. Joan Newcomb and Patricia Murphy, "The Curriculum Vitae—What It Is and What It Is Not," *Nurs. Outlook*, **27**:580–583 (Sept. 1979).
6. William Walsh, "Preparing a Résumé," *Am. J. Nurs.*, 74:677–679 (Apr. 1974).
7. Mary Parker, "How to Write Your Résumé," *Am. J. Nurs.*, 79:1739–1741 (Oct. 1979).
8. Reres, op. cit.
9. Dick Irish, "17 Ways to Shine at a Job Interview," *Glamour* (Sept. 1978), pp. 38–42.
10. "Make That First Impression Count," *Nurs. 79 Career Directory*, pp. 30–31.

11. Frances M. McKenna, *Thresholds to Professional Nursing Practice*, 2nd ed. (Philadelphia: W. B. Saunders Company, 1960), p. 78.

BIBLIOGRAPHY

Hamburg, Alvin A. "Evaluate Before Employment," *Nurs. Outlook*, **13** (Mar. 1965), 45–47. A very helpful guide for the nurse seeking a position. Includes an evaluation checklist for assessing important characteristics of the prospective employing agency.

Heneman, Herbert G., and Mary Sue Kern. "Exit Interviews," *Nurs. Outlook*, **4** (Aug. 1956), 436–438. To retain the employee's goodwill and help identify trouble spots in the organization, a well-trained interviewer has a personal talk with everyone who is about to leave. Still useful.

Rotkovich, Rachel. "Hiring a Nurse," *Am. J. Nurs.*, **74** (Apr. 1974), 680–681. A director of nursing tells what she looks for in an applicant.

Walsh, William. "Preparing a Résumé," *Am. J. Nurs.*, **74** (Apr. 1974), 677–679. How to prepare a résumé that will clearly identify the applicant's preparation and abilities to a prospective employer.

See also references at end of Chapter 30, references and bibliography in Chapters 6, 11, 15, 16, 19, and 22. The popular literature and business journals have numerous articles on getting a job; women's magazines are giving this a great deal of attention. Among the career resource books that have been recommended are: *The Ambitious Woman's Guide to a Successful Career*, Margaret V. Higginson and Thomas L. Quick, New York: Amacom, 1975; *The Career Game*, Charles G. Moore, PhD. New York: National Institute of Career Planning, 1976; *Career Satisfaction and Success: A Guide to Job Freedom*, Bernard Haldane. New York: Amacom, 1974; *How To Be Successful in the Employment Interview: A Step by Step Approach for the Candidate*, Forest M. Amsden and Noel D. White. Cheney, Wash.: Interviewing Dynamics, P.O. Box 223, 1975; *The Professional Job Changing System. World's Fastest Way To Get a Better Job*, 1978 Edition, Robert Jameson and the Staff of Performance Dynamics, Parsippany, N.J., December 1977; *Get the Best of Yourself: How To Find Your Success Pattern and Make It Work for You*, Katherine Nash, New York: Grosset and Dunlap, 1976; *"Résumé Preparation Manual: A Step-by-Step Guide for Women."* May be obtained from Catalyst, 14 East 60th Street, New York, N.Y. 10022.

Surviving Reality Shock:
The Challenge of Professionalism

SOCIALIZATION AND RESOCIALIZATION

The transition from student to RN is a psychological, sociological, and legal phenomenon. The student has spent two to four years being socialized into nursing in the education setting; now resocialization into the work world is necessary. Socialization into a new role is not usually a conscious process, although both the individual being socialized and those doing the socializing consciously make certain efforts. Hinshaw describes socialization as a sequential set of phases, a "chain of events." In an adaptation from Simpson,[1] she identifies the phases as:

1. *Transition from anticipatory expectation of role to specific expectations of role as defined by the societal group.*
2. *Attachment to significant others in the social system milieu; labeling incongruencies in role expectations.*
3. *Internalization, adaptation, or integration of role values and standards.*[2]

A further delineation of this process and the resocialization is described by Hinshaw,[3] using Davis' classical description of the doctrinal conversion process among student nurses.

Stage One. Initial innocence: students enter profession with image of what they expect to become and how they should behave, often based on public stereotypes. Most have had some degree of a "serving humanity" mentality, with emphasis on touching and doing. In the educational system, they are praised for presenting an analysis of the action more than the action itself.

Stage Two. Labeled recognition of incongruity: students sharing their concern can begin to recognize what is different from their expectations.

Stages Three and Four. "Psyching out" and role simulation: those individuals who want to continue in nursing must identify appropriate behaviors and role model them. Soon those behaviors become part of that person's own repertoire of how to act.

Stages Five and Six. Provisional and stable internalization: First the nurse vacillates between behaviors now attached to the new professional imagery and those reflecting previous lay imagery. But as they become more comfortable in practicing those behaviors and have increasing identification with nurse-teacher role models, they move to stage six, in which the imagery and behavior of the newly socialized nurse-student reflect the professionally, educationally approved model.

However, for all but a few new graduates, the first job is as an employee in some bureaucratic setting, the antithesis of professionalism. A comparison of characteristics of a profession and a bureaucracy clearly shows the differences.

Characteristics of a Bureaucracy

Specialization of roles and tasks.
Autonomous rational rules.
Overall orientation to rational, efficient implementation of specific goals.
Organization of positions into a hierarchical authority structure.
The impersonal orientation of contacts between officials and clients.

Characteristics of a Profession

Specialization competence having an intellectual component.
Extensive autonomy in exercising this special competence.
Strong commitment to a career based on a special competence.
Influence and responsibility in the use of special competence.
Development of training facilities that are controlled by the professional group.
Decision making governed by internalized standards.[4]

Kramer, in an extensive longitudinal study, has identified the problems of new graduates in resolving their role in a bureaucratic-professional conflict and has termed it *reality shock,* "the specific shocklike reactions of new workers when they find themselves in a work situation for which they have spent several years preparing and for which they thought they were going to be prepared, and then suddenly find that they are not."[5] The phenomenon is seen as different from, but related to, both culture shock and future shock.[6]

Thus, when the new nurse, who has been in the work setting, but not of it, embarks on what is thought to be the first professional work experience, there is not an easy adapta-

tion of previously learned attitudes and behaviors, but the necessity for an entirely new socialization. Kramer has categorized and described these as follows:

1. *Skill and routine mastery: The expectations are those of the employment setting. A major value is competent, efficient delivery of procedures and techniques to clients, not necessarily including psychological support. The new graduate immediately concentrates on skill and routine mastery.*
2. *Social integration: getting along with the group; being taught by them how to work and behave; the "backstage" reality behaviors. If the individual stays at stage one, she/he may not be perceived as a competent peer; if she/he tries to incorporate some of the professional concepts brought over from the educational setting and adheres to those values, the group may be alienated.*
3. *Moral outrage: With the incongruencies identified and labeled, new graduates feel angry and betrayed by both their teachers and their employers. They weren't told how it would be and they aren't allowed to practice as they were taught.*
4. *Conflict resolution: The graduates may and do change their behavior, but maintain their values; change both values and behaviors to match the work setting; change neither values nor behavior; or work out a relationship that allows them to keep their values, but begin to integrate them into the new setting.*[7]

The individuals who make the first choice have selected what is called *behavioral capitulation.* They may be the group with potential for making change; they may simply slide into the bureaucratic mold, but more likely they withdraw from nursing practice altogether. Those who choose bureaucracy *(value capitulation),* may either become "rutters," with an "it's a job" attitude, or they may eventually reject the values of both. Others become organization men and women, who move rapidly into the administrative ranks and have totally absorbed the bureaucratic values. Those who will change neither values nor behavior, what might be called "going it alone", either seek to practice where professional values are accepted or try the "academic lateral arabesque" (also used by the first group), going on to advanced education with the hope of new horizons or escape. The most desirable choice, says Kramer, is *biculturalism*.

In this approach the nurse has learned that she possesses a value orientation that is perhaps different from the dominant one in the work organization, but that she has the responsibility to listen to and seek out the ideas of others as resource material in effecting a viable integration of both value systems. She has learned that she is not just a target of influence and pressure from others, but that she is in a reciprocal relationship with others and has the right and responsibility to attempt to influence them and to direct their influence attempts on her. She has learned a basic posture of interdependence with respect to the conflicting value systems.[8]

THE REALITY OF REALITY SHOCK

Kramer, both in her book and in other articles, has documented that new graduates do indeed go through variations of the socialization process described.[9,10,11,12] One graduate linked the reality shock to physiological shock and drew up a list of "treatments," such as keeping communications open, arresting feelings of inadequacy, getting information and feedback, and watching for openings to inject your own ideas.[13] Others have cited the trauma of adjustment, the insecurities, the tensions with co-workers, the doctor-nurse games.[14,15,16,17] That there has really been little change in the adjustment process for decades can be seen by reviewing journals in the interim and by the nomadic patterns of nursing that must reflect deep-seated job dissatisfaction. In some places nurse turnover is as high as 200 per cent; it is said that 70 per cent is not unusual, a higher rate than that of waitresses. Turnover and absenteeism are signs of boredom, lack of involvement, and apathy. New graduates are responsible for a large part of these statistics, but it may be even more shocking

to know that an unusually large percentage leave nursing altogether. Kramer reports 29 per cent of the baccalaureate graduates she studied left nursing within two years. Even if they do not, their disillusionment, if unchecked, does not bode well for the profession. Statements made by some of Kramer's subjects more than ten years ago can be echoed today:

'I think, in general, most of the nurses in the hospital are not really very happy as nurses; I think it's just more or less a job that they come to every day. They just don't seem to care. . . .'

'A nurse I was talking with one night said, "Don't stay in hospitals. Get out as fast as you can because you're going to become bitter." I can see her point; you do relax; you lower your standards a little bit when you get busy.'

'If I stay in the hospital much longer, I'll get into the same rut as the other nurses. You can't help yourself. I hope that I won't get like the rest of them, but I'm afraid I might.'[18]

Some of these issues seem to focus on the hospital, which certainly is a bureaucracy, but that is also where most new graduates choose to work.

APPROACHES TO RESOLVING REALITY SHOCK

Kramer has suggested an anticipatory socialization program as one solution to reality shock. In brief, the intent is first to guide the student toward biculturalism while still in school through lectures, exposure to reality situations, discussion, and constant reinforcement and support in meeting and resolving reality shock issues.[19] A second aspect is to develop a postgraduate socialization process on the job as part of the orientation.[20]

Others, recognizing that some of the problems are related to the new graduate's need to have skills, have developed innovative orientation programs, internships or internship-type experiences planned cooperatively by school and service agency.*[21,22,23,24] One hospital created a nurses' ombudsman.[25] However, even beyond those early years, nurses find problems of professionalism-bureaucracy that must be met.

BURNOUT AND OTHER OCCUPATIONAL HAZARDS

Burnout, considered by some as an occupational hazard for those in service occupations, has been described as a debilitating psychological condition resulting from work-related frustrations. Maslack and her colleagues who have been studying the dynamics of burnout list some of the symptoms and effects: lack of motivation, cynicism, negativism, an overwhelming sense of hurt, rejection, failure, and severe loss of self-esteem.[26] Among the early symptoms is emotional and physical exhaustion—just not feeling "good," not sleeping well, reluctance to go to work, and being prone to all kinds of minor illnesses. Then the burned-out professional becomes negative and just wants to be left alone. A final phase, terminal burnout, would be "total disgust" with everyone and everything.

Burnout is caused by various situations. Sometimes it happens because of the emotionally charged, stressful environment found in clinical units where death and pain are constant companions, added to understaffing and interpersonal staff tensions. It has also been found that when there are personal or home problems, the situation is aggravated. Maslack suggests that prevention or cure starts with simply "being good to yourself," taking time for yourself and a break when necessary, and taking care of physical problems. A "decompression routine" is also helpful—perhaps some physical activity such as swimming, walking, jogging (not competitive sports), or even doing "meditative kinds of things." Sharing feelings and problems with others is also important. Sometimes a change of job is necessary, but lateral job transfers or a period in another type of unit often provide the necessary change.[27]

Whether or not burnout occurs, stress and frustration are certainly real problems. Obviously, these can occur in any job. The causes may overlap with burnout, and the cures may be somewhat similar. Gaining insight into one's own problems or concerns with the job is a first step and may be all that is necessary.[28,29] The feelings of role deprivation or alienation (powerlessness, meaninglessness, normlessness, isolation, self-estrangement), often felt by nurse professionals in a bureaucracy, have been described for some time.[30,31] As with any of these conditions, there is no pat answer, but self-efforts made by nurses (described later) are a key to overcoming them.

Job dissatisfaction is related to many aspects of the situations in which nurses find themselves. Surveys show that much dissatisfaction relates to lack of autonomy and unhappiness with the attitudes of administration, as well as understaffing, poor conditions of work,* and poor care for patients. Yet, most nurses still express reasonable satisfaction with their jobs; they like nursing. The question of what will keep nurses on the job varies with almost every survey. However, better staffing, opportunities for continuing education and a reward system for doing good nursing have been mentioned.[32]

For some nurses, succumbing to the Peter Principle, "every employee tends to rise to his level of incompetence,"[33] is a real threat. There is a tendency in nursing to promote a "good" nurse into administrative positions. If the person lacks the training, ability, or inclination to do so, but is tempted by the increased salary and perhaps better working conditions, the result can be disastrous.[34] The answer for upward mobility is in reward for clinical expertise—an approach that is

---

*See also Chapter 12.

*See Chapters 11 and 16.

being used by a number of health agencies and institutions.*

STRATEGIES FOR SURVIVAL AND SUCCESS

Students who have survived what might have been a reality shock in nursing education can adopt the strategies learned and used then to meet the new challenges of the work world.

Gortner makes some useful suggestions:

1. *Become competent in what you do.*
2. *Know well the organization in which you work.*
3. *Be a master of the art of the possible.*
4. *Recognize and seize the opportunity for doing more.*
5. *Consider few problems to be original. Hence, the solution is somewhere and that is the challenge.*
6. *Recognize the value of support systems. Build and use some for yourself.*
7. *Know yourself well.*[35]

Probably the first thing a new graduate must realize is that she/he may not have chosen or be able to choose an institution that wants to, or knows how to, help an entering employee to adjust. An early problem could arise from the graduate's belief in a printed job description. Too often, having one does not preclude the possibility of being asked (or assigned) to responsibilities not included in these job descriptions. The first consideration should be the safety of the patient, and nurses put in such positions must determine whether they are prepared and able to carry out such a function, and legally permitted to do so. If not, refusing to perform that function is necessary, although probably not pleasant. There is a tendency in some places of employment consistently to expect the nurse and others to carry out functions for which they are not prepared, or even licensed. Because nurses are responsible for

their own acts, this can become a serious legal situation, for eventually some patient will come to harm. The decision to refuse may cost a nurse the job, but it will also be only the first of many ethical decisions to be made. (Needless to say, this does not refer to the learning of new techniques of nursing care that evolve with advances in medical and nursing care.)

It is also not unusual for new graduates to be put temporarily in the position of charge nurse or team leader, for which they may not be prepared. This is especially likely to occur on the evening or night tour of duty. In a good orientation or in-service program, this possibility is foreseen and the nurse is given the appropriate learning experiences in such situations under supervision or guidance. When this kind of preparation is not included, the nurse should at least be assigned with a more experienced nurse to share the responsibilities. (In anticipation of such assignments, a new graduate might have inquired of the prospective employer as to the availability of such training and supervision and indicate willingness to learn and practice such responsibilities before assignments using them are made. The response of the employer could well be one means of judging the working environment.)

It may be necessary to learn new techniques to cope with unexpected assignments, such as learning to manage time and people,[36,37,38,39] and to activate beginning leadership skills. In some cases, assertiveness training and consciousness raising groups and internal support systems make the difference between disillusionment and challenge.[40,41,42] Other nurses have chosen to exercise their right to protest and seek help in collective bargaining.[43]*

Finally, knowing how to get along with others is often the keystone of success; there is little that a person can change alone.

---

*See Chapter 16.

*See also Chapters 16 and 22 for suggestions on gaining autonomy.

HARMONIOUS RELATIONSHIPS
WITH OTHERS

Nursing students are usually taught to respect the individuality of the patient/client and his family and to maintain therapeutically effective relationships with them. The importance of such relationships tend to increase when the student assumes the status of a professional registered nurse.

Not as much attention is given to human relationships with co-workers in the employment setting. If there are tensions among a student group, faculty often make an attempt to help the students resolve them through conferences, group sessions, and other accepted means. Yet the student may also be aware of tensions among the faculty or among the staff in the clinical setting. Perhaps the natural reaction of students is "to keep out of it" and hope that the problem does not affect them. However, lack of harmony in a work situation where the nurse must relate to everyone is not as easy to ignore. Anyone who has worked in an employment situation with tensions and pressures caused by personality conflicts and lack of respect for others knows the destructive nature of such an atmosphere. Whether it is caused by a sense of competition, disenchantment with the job, personal, mental, physical, or social problems; whether it emanates from authority groups or peer groups is irrelevant; the end result is not only an unhappy atmosphere, but often a poorer quality of nursing care.[44]

Harmonious interpersonal relationships are essential to one's growth in any profession. The stimulation of controversy is an added growth essential. Though the two may appear contradictory, ideally they should go hand in hand, provided, of course, that the controversies are not based on petty, personal disagreements, and stubborn behavior, but rather are the outgrowth of objective and constructive thought. Nurses can develop in their profession through healthy interpersonal relationships with their colleagues, or their paths can be obscured by personality limitations. Today's nurse is being educated to be a change agent; to be successful in this role requires the ability to relate well to others.[45]

The ability to live happily at home and in harmony with others at work and in the community is one of the principal constituents of successful living. This requires attention to the best use of one's personality assets and conscious control of one's liabilities, which can be particularly difficult for the nurse who works under trying circumstances. Married nurses who have family as well as professional responsibilities may find that both wife and husband will have to make many adjustments and be especially understanding and tolerant when the demands of their jobs interfere with their home life. Assuming too many responsibilities with fairness to all concerned is difficult even for older persons; young nurses may find it still more burdensome.

To study this problem and explore possible solutions are beyond the scope of this book; they might comprise the contents of several other books. However, the degree to which a nurse can cope with the situations mentioned might influence the nurse's entire attitude toward nursing, and the settings where nursing is done. Such stressful work situations are one major cause of employment turnover. Negative situations exist; the nurse, applying the principles of good mental health and understanding of human behavior, can at least maintain personal integrity, and perhaps help to improve the situation.

GROWTH THROUGH EDUCATION

As has been suggested several times in this book and in many other publications for nurses, the only way to advance, or keep abreast, in this fast-moving world is through continuing education that embraces general as well as professional subjects. This can partially be accomplished through selective reading, travel, community activities, and home study. The maintenance of professional competencies, however, takes a little more, and in terms of legal rights, responsibilities, and perhaps requirements, must not be neglected.*

Continuing Education

Continuing one's education after completion of a professional educational program is an inherent part of the responsibility of any professional person. One well-known nurse says:

> A commitment to lifelong learning is the mark of the truly professional person. To this individual, learning is as essential as breathing. Early in his career, he accepts a personal responsibility for his own continued education, seeing it as closely related to his own continued practice, and he pursues it with enthusiasm and zest. He is aware of and takes advantage of many different approaches to learning. He devotes time and attention to learning how to learn, and has identified those approaches that seem most useful to him. He has also learned how to be selective; he knows what activities will be beneficial to him, and which ones will not. He recognizes the value of concentrating on certain areas of interest, rather than dispersing his attention to a multiplicity of unrelated activities.
>
> The continuing learner identifies his learning goals and develops a plan for meeting those goals. He recognizes continuing education primarily as something that he does, rather than as something that is done to him.[46]

She concludes, "the involvement of nursing as a profession rests upon a commitment by nursing's practitioners to their own continued learning."[47]

The term *continuing education* has been interpreted many ways. Most agree that it includes any learning activity after the basic educational program. However, most often those programs leading to an academic degree are separated out. There is still much confusion among nurses who are sure that the renewed social and legal pressures for continuing education mean that they must enroll in a baccalaureate program. An ANA definition of *continuing education*, therefore is helpful:

> Continuing education in nursing consists of systematic learning experiences designed to enlarge the knowledge and skills of nurses. As distinct from education toward an academic degree or preparing as a beginning professional practitioner, continuing professional education activities have more specific content applicable to the individual's immediate goals; are generally of shorter duration; are sponsored by colleges, universities, health agencies and professional organizations; and may be conducted in a variety of settings.[48]

The basic and overriding purpose of continuing education in nursing is the maintenance of continued competence so that the care of the patient is safe and effective. The rapid changes in society, the emergence of new knowledge and technologies, make it impossible to function effectively with only the knowledge and skills gained in one's basic program, no matter how outstanding the program.

It has been noted that in the course of an individual's career, which might well cover a forty-year span, the knowledge needed to function effectively during the last years, or even earlier, would contain only a fraction of that available at the beginning of the professional's career.*

Although the tremendous advance of the sciences has provided an added impetus to the need for continuing education, the concept goes back to the beginning of modern nursing. In the writings of Florence Nightingale is found this statement:

> Nursing is a progressive art, in which to stand still is to go back. A woman who thinks to herself, "Now I am a full nurse, a skilled nurse, I have learnt all there is to be learnt" —take my word for it, she does not know

---

*See Chapter 20.

*See Chapter 13.

what a nurse is, and never will know; she is gone back already. Progress can never end but with a nurse's life.

Continuing education for nurses began early in modern nursing's history. Post-graduate courses were offered by hospitals and nursing alumnae associations beginning early in the 1900s, mainly to make up for the poor quality of education in many programs, where students were used almost entirely to meet service needs. At the same time some universities and colleges began to offer summer courses, often in the area of supervision. Institutes and workshops by the professional organization gained some momentum in the 1920s and are still a major source of continuing education. Refresher courses for inactive nurses were most prevalent in times of major nursing shortages, such as during World War II and the 1950s and 1960s. Federal funding under the Nurse Training Act in 1964 provided funding for short-term courses, and institutions of higher education took a renewed interest in providing continuing education, an interest that had dwindled through lack of funds and prepared faculty. Other federal funding for Regional Medical Programs also resulted in nursing workshops.[49] When these funds began to vanish during the Nixon administration, many colleges found it impossible to continue full programs. Others, seeing both the need and the trend, established institution-funded continuing education programs. Because these programs must generally be self-supporting it was expected that nurses or their employers would be willing to pay for the courses offered.

Who should bear the cost of the nurse's continuing education is a controversial issue. Formalized programs in continuing education are offered as in-service education in places of employment, through conferences, workshops, institutes, and other program meetings of professional or other health organizations, or in continuing education programs offered by colleges and universities. Only in-service education is always free. The other programs frequently charge at least a

token fee of some kind even for members because the cost of providing quality programs is high. Some courses, which may extend over a period of days or months, could run into hundreds of dollars; however, the average fee appears to be closer to $25.[50]

The professional nurse should expect to assume at least part of the cost. There are those who feel that because the employers ultimately benefit from the employee's improved performance they should provide such support as partial or full tuition payment, sabbaticals, or short-term leaves. On the other hand, hospitals and like institutions often maintain that these additional costs must be passed on unfairly to the patient, and that they have a right to expect competent practitioners.[51]

Of further concern is the measurement and recording of continuing education activities. The ANA, many state associations, some universities, and other groups have accepted the Continuing Education Unit developed by the National Task Force. The Continuing Education Unit, which emerged from a national planning conference attended by representatives of thirty-four national organizations and agencies, is defined as "ten contact hours of participation in an organized continuing education experience under responsible sponsorship, capable direction, and qualified instruction." The key word is "organized," but the CEU is *not* to be used for programs carrying academic credit or diplomas, in-service learning, orientation programs or short-term programs casually related to upgrading. The major benefit of the CEU is its acceptance as a standard unit not only in nursing but also in other disciplines.[52] The recording of an individual nurse's continuing education may be done through the agency offering the CE program. However, some state nursing organizations have begun to keep records for their members (or nonmembers, at a fee). Some approve CEU units for programs submitted to them by groups offering the program, using specific guidelines, as well as recognizing their own programs. If the number of nurses involved is large, this can become both expensive and unwieldy. The use of computers has been suggested, but the problem is not yet resolved.

Although there are no CEUs for informal study such as reading the professional literature, or such activities as research, teaching, writing a book, or other professional experiences, it is obvious that individuals do learn in these ways and some credit is given for them in certain states. Some nurses maintain that working in a patient setting is continuing education and, of course, it can be, depending on the setting, the opportunity for learning, and the nurse's inclination to use these opportunities. There are also nurses who merely repeat past experiences and do not recognize or choose to utilize available learning experiences.

Because the major stated purpose of continuing education is maintenance and improvement of professional skills (personal development aside), there is also concern as to the content of continuing education for nurses. Arguments range from the stand that anything which adds to the development of the nurse in any way is continuing education, to the equally firm stand that only clinical or directly related scientific studies should be acceptable. This argument may never be resolved for it is primarily philosophic. What benefits any specific nurse in improving practice is probably as individual as that nurse, and the conscientious nurse will seek out the educational experience needed whether it "counts" or not. Still, the matter must receive attention because programs must be planned to meet the needs of the learners. For accreditation of the programs, the objectives of the courses must pinpoint the expected changes in the behavior (learning) of the nurse. Possibly a significant message is relayed in a key governmental report, which states, "Continuing education in its present form—the bulk of which remains traditional —is destined for change; only those forms clearly related to continued competence should be maintained."[53] Eventually, it is

clear, there must be some type of peer review of practice.[54]

Little research has been done to determine the direct effects of continuing education on competency. Of the small studies done, the findings are sometimes contradictory, with improvement in practice either evidenced or absent. When nurses' participation is active and the program meets specific stated needs of the nurse, the result is likely to be more positive.[55,56] The majority of programs offered in the last few years stress updating skills, gaining new skills (particularly in preparation for the nurse practitioner role), and clinical knowledge, but it still is important to include nurses in the planning to assure meeting their needs. Because of the limited funds available for continuing education and the need for effective programs, further research is also strongly indicated.

One of the most controversial issues in continuing education is whether it should remain on a voluntary basis or whether, in order to ascertain that nurses (and others) do continue their education, it should be a requirement for relicensure.[57] This issue is discussed in Chapter 20. What is not controversial is the responsibility of the nurse, as a professional practitioner, to maintain competence in whatever area of practice is being engaged in: clinical, administrative, or other.

With continuing education programs proliferating, the nurse must give some thought to what is worth spending time and money on. One suggested plan for diagnosing one's continuing education needs is to develop a model of required competencies, assessing one's practice in relation to the model, and identifying the gaps between one's own knowledge and skills and those required. Some of this preliminary testing can be done by taking some of the tests in journals, but also by carefully evaluating one's own practice and getting feedback from peers and supervisors as well.[58]

Other methods of continuing education learning, besides formal classes or conferences, are well worth investigating, although, of course, there is often the added value of interaction with other nurses in group activities.[59] One expert in continuing education suggests some useful ways of weighing the choices offered, including figuring the costs (registration, travel, time off); looking at objectives, intent, and learning methods in relation to one's own specific needs; evaluating the quality of the program regarding speakers and sponsors; and finding programs that are suitable.[60]

Formal Higher Education

Besides participating in continuing education programs, the graduate of a diploma or associate degree program may want to give serious consideration to formal education leading to a baccalaureate degree, and the nurse with a baccalaureate degree may want to think about getting a master's. There is no question but that educational standards for all positions in nursing are growing steadily higher. The nurse who really wants to "move" professionally, to advance to positions of greater scope and challenge, will in the very near future, need at least a baccalaureate degree. The process of obtaining this and higher degrees not only will serve the nurse well professionally but will add considerably to the enrichment of his or her personal life and interests.

The problem of finances is undoubtedly the most common deterrent to advanced education for able professional nurses. There is good reason for viewing financial problems realistically before embarking on any new venture, but often a plan can be devised if the nurse is sincere in the desire to continue in higher education. Before enrolling in an educational program, it is advisable to estimate as accurately as possible expected income and expenses. Major educational expenses will include tuition, books, educational fees, and perhaps travel. Related personal expenses depend on where and how the nurse lives. Economizing may mean enrolling in a community college for the liberal arts and later transferring to a local or state

college. Economy should not include enrolling in a poor program. Graduating from a nonaccredited nursing program may create difficulties in advancing to the next higher degree. Not all nonaccredited programs are poor, but there is an additional risk that this might be so.

Although it would be difficult to denigrate the value to an individual of any good quality educational program, a nurse should give some thought to future goals. For many, the simple joy of exploring new fields and studying whatever one wishes to study without the pressure of time or the need to fulfill requirements for a program will take precedence. If these interests are in any of the liberal arts or social or physical sciences, which are also required or can be used as electives in most baccalaureate programs, a dual purpose will be accomplished in that the nurse is also started toward a degree. A conference with someone in the nursing program in which enrollment is planned, or at least a review of the catalog, might offer desirable courses that can be applied to the degree program.

If a nurse has definite plans for higher education and has specific time goals, it is essential to (1) select the most appropriate nursing program, (2) send for or get the catalog to ascertain requirements and review the program, (3) acquire and complete application blanks, (4) develop a plan of study and a time schedule.

Because baccalaureate courses with a nursing major are not always available (or affordable) to nurses in a particular geographic area, a number of programs have sprung up offering a degree in nursing or another field, giving credit for the lower-division nursing courses and offering no upper-division nursing courses. A nurse selecting such programs should evaluate them in relation to career goals. This program is *not* usually acceptable for future graduate studies in nursing, and the nurse may not be able to enroll in a graduate program without having taken upper-division nursing courses. With the crowded enrollments in most baccalaureate nursing programs, many will not accept students who wish to take only individual courses. Frequently, nurses have found it necessary to complete a second baccalaureate program, this time with a nursing major, in order to continue into a master's program.[61]

If a nurse is interested in a baccalaureate degree for personal development, any accredited baccalaureate program might, of course, meet these objectives. In some cases, individual courses would also enhance the nurse's understanding of nursing. The question remains as to whether a nurse wishes to enhance, deepen, and broaden the nursing knowledge already acquired and/or advance in newer nursing fields. If so, an accredited (or equivalent) nursing baccalaureate program is essential.

As noted in Chapter 12, registered nurses will find that they receive varying amounts of recognition or credit for their basic nursing courses, and may perhaps need to take challenging examinations. Nursing baccalaureate programs vary a great deal in this respect. The NLN *Directory of Career Mobility Opportunities in Nursing Education,* which is available from NLN or possibly found at the nurse's nursing school or place of employment, lists all those nursing programs offering some form of educational articulation, self-pacing, or other means of giving credit for previous knowledge, skill, and ability such as the external degree. There are also other NLN publications listing baccalaureate, master's, and doctoral programs.

Many of the same points apply to graduate education. There are still severe limitations in available nursing master's programs— limitations in their very existence, or in the major within nursing which is available. Therefore some nurses complete graduate programs in the various sciences or education, with or without any nursing input. Again, the nurse must consider the specific career goals selected. A nurse with a nursing major or at least minor may be given preference in a position requiring a graduate degree, particularly in educational positions.

Or if a nurse is hired now, there is no guarantee that later, when there are more nurses with graduate nursing degrees, he or she may not be bypassed for promotion or be required to take a second graduate degree in nursing, to hold the current position.

These are practical considerations presented here for information. Individual nurses must still make the educational decisions they wish which should not be made without as complete a knowledge of the pros and cons as possible. Some nurses simply do not want to acquire a degree. Other nurses may enroll in accredited nursing programs that seem to meet their needs financially and professionally, but then, in time, drop out. Sometimes the reason is lack of ability to perform at a particular academic level. There should be absolutely no negative attitude toward those nurses who do not want to, or cannot, earn a baccalaureate degree. These nurses can function perfectly well at their own level of competence and interest, maintaining and improving that competence through continuing education, and thereby make a valuable contribution to the profession and society. If, however, the nurse withdraws because of disappointment or lack of interest in that particular program, it may well be that the program is not congruent with that nurse's philosophy. Few nurses take the time, or recognize the wisdom of taking time, to determine whether a program's philosophy, objectives, approaches to teaching, and attitudes are what they want. Some of this information can be obtained from the catalog, the faculty or advisor interviews, informal contact with students or *recent* graduates (programs do change). Sometimes, if some courses may be taken without need for full matriculation, a sampling of courses will prove especially informative. It is time well spent for satisfaction gained and avoidance of negative experiences and wasted time.

Acquiring a degree takes time and effort, and is often expensive. It would be foolish to begin such an important venture without thought and careful investigation.

Sources of Financial Aid

The major sources of income for a self-supporting graduate nurse in an advanced educational program are savings or other personal resources, part-time work, scholarships, and loans.

The nurse who plans to do part-time work while attending college should make reasonably sure that the position is available at a satisfactory salary and that it seems to be professionally suitable, including enough flexibility to make the taking of courses possible. The nurse should also consider his or her mental and physical health under this double load. Overtaxing one's endurance over an extended period of time is always unwise; however, the motivated individual in good health can usually carry a heavy schedule of work and study—at least for a year or two—without untoward effects.

There are a number of scholarships, fellowships, and loans earmarked for educational purposes for which professional nurses are often eligible if they but seek them out and make application. Some sources of financial assistance are well known and used regularly; others are not used simply because people do not know about them. The financial-aid officer at the institution where the nurse plans to enroll is an excellent source of information.

In most instances educational scholarships, fellowships, and loans are defined as follows: (1) scholarship—a financial grant that does not involve repayment; (2) fellowship—a grant for graduate study not requiring reimbursement; (3) loan—a grant for educational purposes to be repaid by the recipient either with or without interest after completion of the course or education. Grants-in-aid are outright grants at both the undergraduate and graduate levels for accomplishment of a specific project. There may also be an outright grant to meet an immediate financial emergency or a grant to a student with a claim to a restricted scholarship fund. The term *traineeship* has also been used in recent years to denote federal grants with stipend and tuition costs, which need not be repaid, awarded to students in nursing programs, under the Nurse Training Act and its legislative successors.

Some funds are available to members of certain organizations or religious denominations or to students who meet other special requirements. Others are offered to any deserving person who has demonstrated such qualities as good character, leadership ability, and academic achievement. In general, scholarships, loans, and grants are available from both private and governmental sources and agencies.

The manner in which a person applies for financial assistance may have considerable bearing on whether or not he obtains it. Correspondence, personal interviews, application forms, references—all should show the same meticulous attention that is given to an application for a new position.

Professional nurses who wish financial assistance may find it at the local, state, regional, national, or international level. Where they should apply will depend upon how they plan to use the money. For example, some funds are available for advanced study in mental health and psychiatry only, or for other clinical specialties; others, to prepare nurses for teaching, supervisory, or administrative positions; still others have different stipulations; and many are unrestricted as long as the applicant meets the designated personal qualifications.

The National League for Nursing, 10 Columbus Circle, New York, N.Y. 10019, issues a pamphlet entitled *Scholarships, Fellowships, Educational Grants, and Loans for Registered Nurses*. Obtainable for one dollar, this pamphlet contains a great deal of specific information that may help a nurse decide where to apply first for financial assistance, thus saving valuable time in making applications.

The professional nursing journals frequently carry news items and articles about such funds, which can be found through the annual and cumulative indexes. Most college catalogs also list sources of student financial support. Given here, in more general terms, are some of the possible sources of scholarships, fellowships, and loans.

Local Sources. Local sources of funds include both professional and civic groups in the nursing school, community, district, and state. The alumni association of a school of nursing often has appropriations for scholarships and loans that are available to graduates of the school. The president of the association or the director of the school will have information about such sources of financial assistance. A few district and state nurses' associations may have funds for advanced study and other special purposes either as direct gifts or on a very reasonable interest and repayment basis. Some state legislatures have apportioned money to prepare selected professional nurses to work on state health problems and, more rarely, to provide loans and scholarships to nursing (and other) students. The state board of nursing and the operational institutions involved will have information about such appropriations.

Other local sources of funds include chapters of national sororities, fraternities, and clubs whose memberships are not restricted to nurses, but offer financial aid to anyone—whether a member or not—who meets their qualifications. There are church-affiliated groups, the Elks, Masons, Altrusa Club, American Legion Auxiliary, and other similar organizations; and private foundations and institutes. Other good sources of information are local or state colleges or universities and the hospital associations. The nurse's place of employment may also offer grants and loans, or pay part or all of the tuition fees.

In some instances, scholarships and loans are available to nurses in a region of the country comprising more than one state. Information about these is often carried in some of the previous sources mentioned.

National Sources. In recent years professional nurses interested in applying for a national scholarship, fellowship, or loan would, with the assistance of the advanced

nursing programs in which they were enrolled, have turned to the federal government. Both general scholarships and loans as well as some designated especially for registered nurses, grants, fellowships, and full-time nurse traineeships have been of increasing and invaluable aid to the RN. Although never enough to meet all needs, without them a large majority of RNs could not have completed advanced education. However, beginning in 1973 the administration became less interested in providing any financial aid to nurses and some loans and funds were cut back. Since 1975, funds for nurse traineeships have been progressively cut.* Loans and special scholarships for service in underserved areas continue to be available, but there are predictions that federal money for all health professions will gradually dry up. Much depends on the amount of pressure put on Congress to legislate funds. Such congressional action appears to fluctuate from year to year but has been leaning in the direction of fewer and more restricted funds.

The Nurses' Educational Funds, Inc., was established in 1954 to honor nursing pioneers. It was initiated largely through the efforts of the National League for Nursing, which saw the need for centralized administration of the three separate educational allocations for nurses that existed at that time: the Isabel Hampton Robb Memorial Fund, the Isabel McIsaac Loan Fund, and the Nurses' Scholarship and Fellowship Fund.[62] Since then, other funds have been initiated and turned over to NEF for administration. Many of the awards given are in the names of nurses who contributed greatly to the nursing profession. Nurses' Educational Funds, Inc., is an independent organization that grants and administers scholarships and fellowships to registered nurses for post-RN study. It is governed by a board of trustees, mainly leaders in nursing education, and supported by contributions from business corporations, foundations, nurses, and persons interested in nursing.

---

*See Chapter 19.

In 1973 the American Journal of Nursing Company assumed the administrative, accounting, and secretarial responsibilities for the Nurses' Educational Funds, Inc. Application forms and information about the necessary qualifications of applicants can be obtained from Nurses' Educational Funds, 10 Columbus Circle, New York, N.Y. 10019.

Financial aid is also available from the National Student Nurses' Association (see Chapter 24), miscellaneous private foundations, and some health organizations that may give financial assistance to nurses for advanced work in that organization's major area of interest. In addition, the armed services subsidize the advanced education of some of their nurses (see Chapter 15).

International Sources. The national nursing organizations may be able to supply information about scholarships, fellowships, and loans accessible to registered nurses who wish to study abroad. It would be well to contact these organizations first, although the International Council of Nurses, the World Health Organization, and the U.S. Public Health Service also are possible sources of information. As more and more professional nurses become interested in international nursing, governmental, professional, educational, and philanthropic groups may originate new scholarships, fellowships, and loans to assist them. The competition for available funds for international study is likely to be increasingly keen, however, because many other professional and occupational groups also are becoming more and more eager for education and experience in other countries.

The U.N.'s Educational, Scientific, and Cultural Organization publishes an annual catalog entitled *Study Abroad,* which gives information on approximately 75,000 opportunities for financial assistance for international education. The fellowships and scholarships are awarded by governments, foundations, universities, and other institutions in almost every country in the world. The subjects of study cover nearly all fields

of learning, including nursing. Complete data about the awards are given, such as the amount granted, qualifications, availability, length of study periods, and restrictions. Some funds are restricted; others are not. The common objective of the awards is to bring persons from different parts of the world into direct contact with each other and each other's cultures.

Although *Study Abroad* currently lists only a very limited number of sources of financial aid for U.S. nurses who wish to study abroad, it is hoped and anticipated that such opportunities will increase in the future. A large general library in a city or university might have a copy of the catalog or it can be purchased for a nominal sum directly from UNESCO at U.N. headquarters in New York City.

Conclusion

It should be realized that individuals and groups who contribute scholarships, fellowships, and loans want them to be used to the best possible advantage. If left unused for several years, the administering authority may decide to allocate the money elsewhere (if it is legally empowered to do so), or at least will be inclined to feel it unnecessary to try to increase the amounts or promote the establishment of new funds. Demands for and effective use of scholarships could increase the supply. Occasionally nursing and other journals list sources of educational funds, with guidelines for application and other useful information. These make good up-to-date references.[63]

PROFESSIONAL AND COMMUNITY ACTIVITIES

Active participation in community activities that allow the nurse to share and utilize the full dimensions of his or her professional background is also rewarding to the nurse. Some of the activities will be directly related to nursing, such as attending alumni and nurses' associations meetings and accepting appointments to committees and offices. Others will include volunteer work on a regular or special basis, such as participating in student nurse recruitment programs or career days, soliciting donations for various health organizations, helping with the Red Cross blood program, assisting with inoculation sessions for children, acting as adviser to a Future Nurse Club, or volunteering time at a free clinic.[64,65,66]

The importance of nursing input into the various community, state, and national joint provider-consumer groups which study means of improving the health care delivery system is obvious. Although participation at a state or national level may not be immediately feasible for a nurse who has not yet achieved professional recognition, just showing interest and volunteering one's services will often open doors at a local level. Nurses involved in direct patient care activities are particularly welcome, because there is the feeling that they can more specifically delineate some of the problems and suggest logical, down-to-earth solutions.

HSA's function in many major cities, but there are other variations in almost all communities. Participation of this kind is vital if nurses are to have a part in making policy decisions.*

Consumer activism has caused the formation of other groups concerned with health delivery, and nurses offering their expertise and understanding of health service problems can make valuable contributions. Sometimes nurses must sell themselves to these groups in the sense that they must assure the members of their sincere interest in improved health care services and their willingness to work cooperatively with the consumer to achieve that end. In some areas, ethnic and minority groups are especially suspicious of professional health workers outside of their own group, because unfortunate experiences have shown some of the workers to be more concerned with defending their own interests than the consumer's well-being, as the consumer sees it. In these

groups it is even more important to listen than to talk. Such participation can lead to development of free clinics, health fairs, health teaching classes, recruitment of minority students for nursing programs, tutoring sessions for students, liaison activities with health care institutions, programs for the aged, and legislative activities directed toward better health care.[67,68,69] The opportunities, challenges and satisfactions are unlimited.

Consumer health education is being stressed more and more today and where better can professional nurses offer their expertise? Such classes can be held under the auspices of health care institutions, public health organizations, and public and private community groups, and include teaching for wellness as well as teaching for those with chronic or long-term illnesses. Nurses who like to teach and are skilled and enthusiastic can participate in programs already set up, and, equally important, work toward developing other programs and involving others on the health team.

Keeping the public informed about nursing and the changes that have occurred in recent years in both education and practice is a contribution to the community. Offers to present programs about modern nursing are often welcome in the many community, social, business, professional and service groups that meet frequently and are interested in community service.

Activities such as these involve nurses in the community and are stimulating and satisfying. They also require time, effort, and often patience. But, besides the satisfaction of being of service, the nurse gains in self-development and growth as a professional and as an individual, a dual reward that cannot be bought.

A PHILOSOPHY OF LIFE AND OF NURSING

Early philosophers studied a wide range of subjects, including science and knowledge in general. Today philosophy usually is con-

---

*See Chapter 16.

fined to the study of the way man lives with himself, governs himself, thinks, learns, and views the world, and what he believes in. Philosophy does not create facts; it speculates about them—deeply, systematically, seriously.

An individual philosophizes when he/she thinks about his/her reasons for being and what she/he wants for the future. In addition to a personal philosophy of life, all successful career people develop a philosophy about their field of endeavor and their place in it. Nurses who can clearly state their beliefs in answer to the questions: What is professional nursing? What *should* it be? Why is it what it is today? What will its future be? have thoroughly explored the reasons and causes that determine their replies.

Undoubtedly, the kind of nursing education the nurse has had, the working experiences, relationships with other nurses and exposure to the ideas of nursing leaders and nursing organizations all influence the nurse's concept of nursing. Neither a personal philosophy nor a philosophy of nursing generally emerges fully developed, but evolves from the life experiences of the individual. To be able to think through one's philosophy and verbalize it is an important aspect of professional development.

Today, more than ever before in modern history, one's constructive talents and abilities are needed in full measure to help civilization advance on all fronts in every area of the globe, possibly of the universe. Nursing, with its unlimited frontiers and exciting future, also needs the full and unstinted output of its practitioners. The rewards promise to be many.

REFERENCES

1. Ida Simpson, "Patterns of Socialization into Professions: The Case of Student Nurses," *Soc. Inquiry*, 37:47 (Winter 1967).
2. Ada Sue Hinshaw, "Socialization and Resocialization of Nurses for Professional Nursing Practice," in *Socialization and Resocialization of Nurses for Professional Nursing Practice*, New York: NLN (1977), p. 2.
3. Ibid. pp. 5, 6.
4. Marlene Kramer. *Reality Shock* (St. Louis: C. V. Mosby Company, 1974), p. 15.
5. Ibid. pp. vii–viii, 3.
6. Ibid. pp. viii, 4–10.
7. Ibid. pp. 155–162.
8. Ibid. p. 162.
9. Margaret Treat and Marlene Kramer, "The Question Behind the Question," *J. Nurs. Admin.*, 2:20–27 (Jan.-Feb. 1972).
10. Marlene Kramer and Constance Baker, "The Exodus: Can We Prevent It?" *J. Nurs. Admin.*, 1:15–30 (May-June 1971).
11. Claudia Schmalenberg and Marlene Kramer, "Dreams and Reality: Where Do They Meet?" *J. Nurs. Admin.*, 6:35–43 (June 1976).
12. Marlene Kramer and Claudia Schmalenberg, "Conflict: The Cutting Edge of Growth," *J. Nurs. Admin.*, 6:19–25 (June 1976).
13. Linda Raker, "Treating Reality Shock," *Am. J. Nurs.*, 79:688 (Apr. 1979).
14. Ginger Alhadeff, "Anxiety in a New Graduate," *Am. J. Nurs.*, 79:687–688 (Apr. 1979).
15. Cynthia Schipani, "From the Ideal to the Real," *Am. J. Nurs.*, 78:1034–1035 (June 1978).
16. Sandra Miller, "Letter from a New Graduate," *Am. J. Nurs.*, 78:1688–1689 (Oct. 1978).
17. Sherril Santo, "A Beginning Nurse Reacts," *Am. J. Nurs.*, 78:1032–34 (June 1978).
18. Marlene Kramer, "The New Graduate Speaks," *Am. J. Nurs.*, 66:2420–2424 (Nov. 1966).
19. *Reality Shock*, op. cit., pp. 67–77.
20. Ibid. pp. 137–190.
21. Barbara Burrell et al., "Internships for AD Graduates," *Am. J. Nurs.*, 17:114–116 (Jan. 1977).
22. Barbara Fleming et al., "From Student to Staff Nurse: A Nurse Internship Program," *Am. J. Nurs.*, 75:595–599 (Apr. 1975).
23. Joan Goldsberry, "From Student to Professional," *J. of Nurs. Admin.*, 7:46–49 (Mar. 1977).
24. Dorothy del Bueno, "Special Orientation

Units Pay Off," *Am. J. Nurs.*, **76**:1629–1631 (Oct. 1976).

25. Regina Block, "The Nurses' Ombudsman," *Am. J. Nurs.*, **76**:1631–1633 (Oct. 1976).

26. Christina Maslack, "Burned Out" *Hum. Behavior*, **5**:16–22 (Sept. 1976).

27. Seymour Shubin, "Burnout, the Professional Hazard You Face in Nursing," *Nurs. 78*, **8**:22–27 (July 1978).

28. Kathleen Gunderson et al., "How To Control Professional Frustration," *Am. J. Nurs.*, **77**:1180–1183 (July 1977).

29. Seymour Shubin, "Rx for Stress, *Your* Stress," *Nurs. 79*, **9**:52–55 (Jan. 1979).

30. Eileen Zungolo, "A Study in Alienation: The Nurse Practitioner," *Nurs. Forum*, **7**(1) 38–48 (1968).

31. Mary Malone, "The Dilemma of a Professional in a Bureaucracy," *Nurs. Forum*, **3**(4) 36–60 (1964).

32. Joanne McCloskey, "What Rewards Will Keep Nurses on the Job?" *Am. J. Nurs.*, **75**:600–602 (Apr. 1975).

33. L. J. Peter and R. Hull. *The Peter Principle: Why Things Go Wrong* (New York: Bantam Books, Inc., 1969).

34. Michael Miller and Helen Bigles, "Nurses Beware: The Peter Principle May Be Upon You," *J. Nurs. Admin.*, **4**:32–33 (May-June 1974).

35. Susan Gortner, "Strategies for Survival in the Practice World," *Am. J. Nurs.*, **77**:618–619 (Apr. 1977).

36. Marlene Kramer and Claudia Schmalenberg, "Constructive Feedback," *Nurs. 77*, **7**:102–106 (Nov. 1977).

37. Loy Wiley, "The ABC's of Time Management," *Nurs. 78*, **8**:105–112 (Sept. 1978).

38. Edwina McConnell, "What Kind of a Delegator Are You?" *Nurs. 78*, **8**:105–110 (Oct. 1978).

39. Thora Kron, "How To Be A Better Leader," *Nurs. 76*, **6**:67–72 (Oct. 1976).

40. Loy Wiley, "Tips for the Timid or How Can One Little Nurse Hope to Change the Rules," *Nurs. 76*, **6**:CG1–CG6 (May 1976).

41. Gloria Donnelly, "The Assertive Nurse," *Nurs. 78*, **8**:65–69 (Jan. 1978).

42. Bonnie Randolph and Clydere Ross-Valliere, "Consciousness Raising Groups," *Am. J. Nurs.*, **79**:922–924 (May 1979).

43. Patricia Chaney, "Protest," *Nurs. 77*, **7**:20–33 (Feb. 1977).

44. Jeffrey Cooper, "Conflict: How To Avoid It and What To Do When You Can't," *Nurs. 79*, **9**:89–91 (Jan. 1979).

45. Jeffrey Cooper, "Actions Really Do Speak Louder Than Words," *Nurs. 79*, **79**:113–118 (Apr. 1979).

46. Signe Cooper, "This I Believe—About Continuing Education in Nursing," *Nurs. Outlook*, **20**:580 (Sept. 1972).

47. Ibid., p. 583.

48. American Nurses' Association, *Statement on Continuing Education in Nursing*. (Kansas City, Mo.: The Association, 1974).

49. Signe Cooper and May Hornback, *Continuing Nursing Education* (New York: McGraw-Hill Book Company, 1973), pp. 19–30.

50. Dorothy del Bueno, "How To Get Your Money's Worth Out of Continuing Education," *RN*, **41**:37–42 (April, 1978).

51. Maura Carroll, "Continuing Education as a Requirement for Relicensure: What Are the Issues?" *Critical Issues in Continuing Education in Nursing* (Madison: University of Wisconsin, 1971), pp. 84–85.

52. Betty Gwaltney, "The Continuing Education Unit," *Nurs. Outlook*, **21**:500–503 (Aug. 1973).

53. Harris Cohen and Lawrence Miike, *Developments in Health Manpower Licensure: A Follow-up Report to the 1971 Report on Licensure and Related Health Personnel Credentialling* (Washington, D.C.: Department of Health, Education, and Welfare, June, 1973), p. 42.

54. Ibid., pp. 39, 42.

55. Ruth Scheuer, "Coronary Care Nurse Training Program," *Nurs. Res.*, **21**:228 (May-June 1972).

56. Donald Sanborn, "Continuing Education for Nurses Via Interactive Closed Circuit Television; a Pilot Study," *Nurs. Res.*, **22**:448–451 (Sept.-Oct. 1973).

57. Gloria Hochman, "Mandatory Continuing Education: How Will It Affect You?" *Nurs. 78*, **8**:105–113 (Nov. 1978).

58. Andrea O'Connor, "Diagnosing Your Needs for Continuing Education," *Am. J. Nurs.*, **78**:405–406 (Mar. 1978).

59. Gloria Hochman, "Continuing Educa-

tion: How Can You Make the Most of It?'' *Nurs. 78,* **8**:81–89 (Dec. 1978).

60. del Bueno, op. cit.

61. Fay Carol Reed, ''Education or Exploitation,'' *Am. J. Nurs.,* **79**:1259–1261 (July 1979).

62. Eleanor A. Hall, ''A New Source of Educational Funds,'' *Am. J. Nurs.,* **54**:613 (May 1954).

63. ''Finding Funds For Further Education,'' *Nurs. 79,* **9**:49–56 (June 1979).

64. Kathleen Toms and Sister Frances Walker, ''A Free Clinic for the Working Poor,'' *Nurs. Outlook,* **21**:770–772 (Dec. 1973).

65. Madalon Amenta, ''Free Clinics Change the Scene,'' *Am. J. Nurs.,* **74**:284–288 (Feb. 1974).

66. Elizabeth Harding, Charles Harrington, and Gloria Manor, ''The Berkeley Free Clinic,'' *Nurs. Outlook,* **21**:40–43 (Jan. 1973).

67. Marion Moses, ''Viva La Causa,'' *Am. J. Nurs.,* **73**:842–848 (May 1973).

68. Mary Keaveney, ''A Community Health Fair,'' *Am. J. Nurs.,* **74**:270–271 (Feb. 1974).

69. Edna Anderson and Avery Andrew, ''Senior Citizens Health Conferences,'' *Nurs. Outlook,* **21**:580–582 (Sept. 1973).

BIBLIOGRAPHY

Armiger, Sister Bernadette. ''Scholarship in Nursing,'' *Nurs. Outlook,* **22** (Mar. 1974), 160–164. A thoughtful discussion of the importance of scholarship as a means to new experiences, knowledge, integrity, and the search for truth.

Buckholz, Linda. ''For the Self-Directed Professional Learner?'' *J. Cont. Ed.,* **10**(1):12–14. Interesting discussion of computer-assisted instruction (CAI).

Bushong, Nancy, and Susan Simms. ''Externship: A Way to Bridge the Gap,'' *Sup. Nurse,* **10** (June 1979), 14–16ff. Description of cost-effective training programs to improve clinical skills of new graduates, jointly developed by hospital and school.

Clemence, Sister Madeleine. ''Existentialism: A Philosophy of Commitment,'' *Am. J. Nurs.,* **66** (Mar. 1966), 500–505. Lucid, tightly reasoned explanation of the philosophy of existentialism and its special relevance for nursing. A nurse who lives this philosophy of commitment will care deeply about nursing, and it will be part of her life. Conversely, the ''uncommitted'' nurse is merely playing the nurse's role. This article demands thoughtful reading and careful reflection.

Cohn, Lucile. ''Coping With Your Anxieties: A Step-by-Step Guide,'' *Nurs. 79,* **9** (Dec. 1979), 34–39. Techniques for coping with on-the-job anxieties, including dealing with patients, families, doctors.

Cooper, Signe, and May Hornbach. *Continuing Nursing Education.* New York: McGraw-Hill Book Company, 1973. Within the framework of adult education and nursing, presents philosophy and rationale for continuing education, principles, trends, and issues.

Cooper, Signe, and Ella Allison. ''Mandatory Continuing Education?'' *Am. J. Nurs.,* **73** (Mar. 1973), 442–443. Two views on this controversial issue are presented.

Copp, Laurel. ''Professional Change: Which Trends Do Nurses Endorse?'' *Int. J. Nurs. Stud.,* **10** (Jan. 1973), 58–62. Purpose of this study was to determine if nurse administrators and educators, staff nurses, LPN's, and nursing assistants agreed on needed changes in nursing. Areas of agreement and disagreement are discussed.

Elsberry, Nancy. ''Power Relations in Hospital Nursing,'' *J. Nurs. Admin.,* **2** (Sept.-Oct. 1972), 75–77. Describes five types of power applicable to hospital nursing, the factors that limit power, and some methods to counter powerlessness.

Faulk, Paula. ''How I Boosted My Sagging Career,'' *RN,* **39** (June 1976), 44–46. A nurse quits her job to go to school.

''Finding Funds for Further Education,'' *Nurs. 79,* **9** (June 1979), 49–56. Guidelines for getting loans and some major sources.

Genn, Nancy. ''Where Can Nurses Practice as They're Taught?'' *Am. J. Nurs.,* **74** (Dec. 1974), 2212–2215. Committed new graduates struggle to innovate against rigid policies, staff resistance, and administrative inaction.

Harding, Elizabeth, et al. ''The Berkeley Free Clinic,'' *Nurs. Outlook,* **21** (Jan. 1973), 40–43. Description of non-traditional clinic, operated and staffed by volunteers and offering services to a community, with countercultural values and life-styles.

Keller, Nancy. ''The Nurse's Role: Is It Expanding or Shrinking?'' *Nurs. Outlook,* **21** (Apr. 1973), 236–240. A thoughtful discussion of the role of the nurse in today's society, with expressed concern that although nurses' capacity to serve increases, there are impediments to the delivery of these services.

Klasser, L. Kathryn, and Joanne White. "Health Career Day at Dodge City," *Nurs. Outlook,* **19** (Mar. 1971), 168–169. Description of a career day utilizing voluntary services of nurses.

Kramer, Marlene. *Reality Shock: Why Nurses Leave Nursing.* St. Louis: The C. V. Mosby Company, 1974. Reality shock describes the reactions of workers when they find themselves in a work situation for which they have been preparing themselves, and then find that they are not prepared. Based on the author's long-term study on baccalaureate students and graduates, this book reports the effect of reality shock and some possible solutions. The author indicates other graduates have similar reactions. Specific examples are given. Readable and interesting.

Kramer, Marlene, and Claudia Schmalenberg, eds. "Bicultural Training and New Graduate Role Transformation," entire issue, *Nurs. Dig.,* **5** (Winter 1978), 1–82. Reprint of some articles on topic as well as overview of the study. Short annotated bibliography.

Letellier, Marian. "*You* Can Change Nursing Practice," *Nurs. 77,* **7** (Mar. 1977), 59–65. Staff nurse identifies problem and decides to make a change.

Levin, Pamela, and Eric Berne. "Games Nurses Play," *Am. J. Nurs.,* **72** (Mar. 1972), 483–487. Instead of facing issues, nurses who work in hospitals play games, which are described in this article.

Lynch, Lillian. "Toward Appropriate Changes in Behavior Measuring Knowledge, Attitude, and Skills in Continuing Education," *J. Contin. Educ. Nurs.,* **3** (Sept.-Oct. 1972), 6–10. This study reports an attempt to measure these changes. The author concluded that a significant number of nurses tested changed in all three areas, with the greatest changes in knowledge and skills.

Matthews, Ann, and Sally Schumacher. "A Survey of Registered Nurses' Conception of and Participation Factors in Professional Continuing Education," *J. Cont. Ed.,* **10**(1) (1979), 21–27. Most nurses surveyed saw knowledge and skill benefits in continuing education but wanted CE credits, most preferred topics directly related to their job or interests.

Moses, Marion. "Viva la Causa," *Am. J. Nurs.,* **73** (May 1973), 842–848. A nurse who has worked with the National Farm Workers Union for five years without pay tells of the lack of care for migrants in health care facilities, and the care she and other volunteers give in free clinics. Extremely interesting.

Norris, Catherine. "Delusions that Trap Nurses," *Nurs. Outlook,* **21** (Jan. 1973), 18–21. A thought-provoking and controversial look at what the author feels moves nurses away from growth, relevance, and the ability to make an impact on health care.

Peplau, Hildegard. "An Open Letter to a New Graduate," *Nurs. Dig.,* **3** (Mar.-Apr. 1973), 36–37. A noted nurse gives her concept of the contribution new nurses can make to the profession.

Poole, Kathleen. "Things Our Instructors Never Told Us," *Nurs. 79,* **9** (Aug. 1979), 104. An amusing description by a new graduate of adjustments to her first job.

Reinkemeyer, Sister Mary Hubert. "An Inherited Pathology," *Nurs. Outlook,* **15** (Nov. 1967), 51–53. Based on the writer's research on attitudes of British nurses toward higher education. Comparisons are made to nurses in the United States.

Sandroff, Ronni. "Must Nursing Squeeze Out the Rest of Your Life?", *RN* **42** (Aug. 1979), 48–55. How a young OR supervisor balances job, husband and baby.

Schmalenberg, Claudia, and Marlene Kramer. "Bicultural Training: A Cost-Effective Program," *J. Nurs. Admin.,* **9** (Dec. 1979), 10–16. Data from study of a bicultural program shows savings, gives specific costs and analysis.

Skipper, James, and James King. "Continuing Education: Feedback from the Grass Roots," *Nurs. Outlook,* **22** (Apr. 1974), 252–253. A small study reveals how rank-and-file nurses feel about continuing education, the need for programs, and their impact.

Slalinka, Susan. "Baccalaureate Programs for RNs," *Am. J. Nurs.,* **79** (June 1979), 1095. Survey of 182 NLN-accredited BSN programs.

Socialization and Resocialization of Nurses for Professional Nursing Practice, New York: NLN, 1977. A collection of papers and group reports given at a workshop. Good presentation of theory. Panel and group discussion also brings out some interesting ideas.

Stevens, Barbara. "Improving Nurses' Managerial Skills," *Nurs. Outlook,* **27** (Dec. 1979), 774–777. Nurse manager must synthesize disciplines of both nursing and management. Good comparison of management's and nursing's work image.

Storlie, Frances. "Burnout: The Elaboration of a Concept," *Am. J. Nurs.*, **79** (Dec. 1979), 2108–2111. Describing burnout as professional autism, author gives some interesting examples of how nurses describe their feelings of frustration, particularly in the ICU.

Strauser, Carol. "An Internship With Academic Credit," *Am. J. Nurs.*, **79** (June 1979), 1070–1072. Describes program developed between VA hospital and a college of nursing.

Thomas, Barbara, and Merle Heick. "A Survey of Continuing Education Needs," *J. Contin. Educ. Nurs.*, **4** (May-June, 1973), 26–31. Study done in Iowa suggests need for a wide variety of continuing education programs, but also need to investigate what prevents RNs from utilizing CE opportunities.

Toms, Kathleen, and Sister Frances Walker. "A Free Clinic for the Working Poor," *Nurs. Out-look*, **4** (Dec. 1973), 770–772. Description of a clinic developed and staffed by volunteer nurses to assist the working poor.

Watson, Laurie. "Keeping Qualified Nurses," *Sup. Nurse*, **10** (Oct. 1979), 29, 32–34. Major reasons why nurses leave their positions are identified and discussed. Good bibliography.

Wiley, Loy. "Good Patient Care: Can You Give It in the Real World?" *Nurs. 77*, **77** (Sept. 1977), 105–109. Suggestions on what to do if care is incompetent.

See also references at end of Chapter 31, references and bibliography of Chapters 6, 10, 11, 12, 13, 15, 16, 19, 20, and 22. There are a number of journals with articles on assertiveness, such as *RN*, which had a series for most of 1979. *Nurs. 79* has published a guide, "Where to Get Your BSN Degree" in both the November and December, 1979 issues.

Appendix

Distinguished Nurses of the Past

Professional nursing, in its comparatively brief history of little more than one hundred years, has produced a great many outstanding men and women whose life stories are of interest to nurses. Detailed biographies of some of these can be found in books and journals in most nursing or health services libraries.

Here biographical material is presented in condensed, yet complete, form about some of the outstanding and representative nursing leaders of the past, realizing that others might well have been included had space not been so limited.[1] In gathering the data for these sketches, most of which was done by Mrs. Helen W. Munson, former associate editor of the *American Journal of Nursing* and, later, librarian at the Hartford (Conn.) Hospital School of Nursing, variations in dates were found; frequently dates and other information were not given in available sources. The material included here is as authentic and complete as possible.

_____

[1]This listing consists primarily of United States nurses, plus several whose names and contributions are internationally recognized. There were, undoubtedly, equally distinguished nurses in many other countries, but they are not included here.

Beard, Mary (1876–1946). As member of staff of Rockefeller Foundation, studied nursing conditions in Europe, Middle East, and Orient. Greatly interested in development of modern schools of nursing here and abroad. Instituted fellowship and travel grant programs under the Foundation to help nurses prepare for special service and to promote understanding between nurses and organizations in many countries. Persuaded Rockefeller Foundation to spend $4.25 million for nursing education and public health nursing (in which she was a recognized authority) in nearly twenty countries. As director of the nursing service of the American Red Cross, was responsible for promoting the enrollment of nurses in the ARC nursing reserve as the first reserve of nurses for military service during World War II; also for the great expansion of nursing services at home necessitated by war, especially the preparation of nurses' aides and teachers of home nursing.

BORN: Dover, N.H., 1876.

NSG. ED.: New York Hosp. Sch. of Nsg., New York City, 1903.

PRINCIPAL POSITIONS: dir., Instructive District Nsg. Assn., Boston; dir., Waterbury (Conn.) Visiting Nurse Assn.; mem., Rock. Found. staff, 1925–38; assoc. dir., Internat. Health Div., Rock. Found.; dir., nsg. serv., ARC, 1938–44.

PRINCIPAL OFFICES: pres., NOPHN, 1916–19; chm., Subcom. on Nsg., Health and Med. Com.,

Off. of Defense, Health and Welfare Serv., W. W. II; mem., many influential coms. inc. Com. for Study for Nsg. Ed.; Nat. Nsg. Council; Nat. Com. on Red Cross Nsg. Serv.; Gen. Med. Bd., Council of Nat. Defense.

AUTHOR: *The Nurse in Public Health,* Harper, New York, 1929; also numerous magazine articles.

HONORS: hon. L.H.D., Univ. of N.H., 1934; hon. LL.D. Smith College, 1945.

DIED: New York City, 1946.

Beck, Sister M. Berenice (c. 1893–1960). As chairman of the Ethical Standards Committee of the American Nurses' Association, led work on formulation of The Code for Professional Nurses. Promoter of collegiate programs for nurses. Organized Marquette University College of Nursing, Milwaukee, Wis., and helped develop the Nursing Education Department at Catholic University of America, Washington, D.C.

BORN: unknown, c. 1893.

NSG. ED.: St. Anthony's Hosp. Sch. of Nsg., St. Louis, 1915; B.A., M.A., Marquette Univ., Milwaukee; Ph.D., Cath. Univ. of Amer., Washington, D.C.

PRINCIPAL POSITIONS: instr. and asst. dir., St. Joseph's Hosp. Sch. of Nsg., Milwaukee; instr., Cath. Univ. of Amer.; asst. prof. and dean, Col. of Nsg., Marquette Univ., Milwaukee, 1936–43; asst. admin., St. Anthony's Hosp., St. Louis; prof. of nsg. ed. and chm., Dept. of Nsg. Ed., Graduate Sch., Marquette Univ., Milwaukee.

PRINCIPAL OFFICES: pres., vice-pres., and bd. mem., Wis. League of Nsg. Ed.; bd. mem., Dist. of Col. League of Nsg. Ed.; mem., Council of Nsg. Ed., Cath. Hosp. Assn.; secy., Cath. Fed. of Nurses; bd. mem., Wis. State Nurses Assn.; vice-pres., ANA Professional Counseling & Placement Serv.; mem., Bd. of Dir., ANA; mem., Bd. of Dir., Amer. J. Nurs. Co.; mem., Wis. Bd. of Nurse Examiners.

AUTHOR: *The Nurse, Handmaid of the Divine Physician,* Lippincott, Philadelphia, 1945; also several articles for professional journals.

DIED: Racine, Wis., 1960.

Breckinridge, Mary (1881–1965). Founded the Frontier Nursing Service of Kentucky in 1925, to offer maternal-child care to an estimated 10,000 people isolated in a 700-square mile area of the remote Cumberland mountains. During the forty years of Mrs. Breckinridge's stewardship, the service expanded from a staff of two to twenty-nine nurses, offered training in a nurse midwifery program, and provided a complete range of health services through six regional health centers and a twenty-seven-bed hospital.

Prior to establishing the Frontier Nursing Service, Mrs. Breckinridge worked for the American Commission for Devastated France, and in 1919 started France's first Child Hygiene and Visiting Nurse Service, now a permanent agency.

BORN: Memphis, Tenn., 1881.

NSG. ED.: St. Luke's Hospital Training School, New York, 1910. A.B., Keuka College, New York. CMB in nurse-midwifery from England, following her service in France.

PRINCIPAL POSITIONS: mem., Am. Comm. for Devastated France, c. 1919; founder and Director, Frontier Nursing Service of Kentucky, 1925–1965.

AUTHOR: *Wide Neighborhoods: A Story of the Frontier Nursing Service,* Harper, New York, 1952.

HONORS: (partial listing) Adelaide Nutting Award, 1961; Medaille Reconaissance, France; Governor's Medal for Distinguished and Meritorious Service to the Commonwealth of Kentucky.

DIED: Wendover, Kentucky, 1965.

Burgess, Elizabeth C. (1877–1949). An inspiring teacher, beloved by her many students at Teachers College, New York City, where she taught for twenty-four years. Authority on legal questions related to nursing. Credited with satisfactory development of NLNE accrediting program because of wide experience, good judgment, practical approach to problems, and leadership ability.

BORN: Bath, Me., 1877.

NSG. ED.: Roosevelt Hosp. Sch. of Nsg., New York City, 1904; B.S., 1923, M.A., 1925, Teachers Col., New York City.

PRINCIPAL POSITIONS: asst. supt. of nurses, Roosevelt Hosp., New York City, 1906–10; instr., Bellevue and St. Luke's Hosps., New York City, 1910–12; supt. of nurses, Michael Reese Hosp., Chicago, 1912–16; state inspector of nurses' training schs. of N.Y., 1916; asst. inspector of nsg. serv., Off. of Surg. Gen. of Army; secy., N.Y. State Bd. of Nurse Examiners, 1920–23; instr., asst. prof., assoc. prof., and prof., Div. Nsg. Ed., Teachers Col., New York City, 1923–47.

PRINCIPAL OFFICES: pres., NLNE, 1928–32; mem. and chm., many ANA and NLNE coms.; mem., Com. on Grading of Nsg. Schs.

AUTHOR: many articles in professional journals.

HONORS: endowed lectureship estab. in her name at Teachers Col., New York City, when she retired in 1948.

DIED: New York City, 1949.

Cavell, Edith (1865–1915). Best known in this country as the nurse who was executed by the Germans during World War I for assisting British and French soldiers and Belgians of military age to leave Belgium and "join their colors." Often referred to as a martyr. As director of first training school for nurses in Brussels, Belgium—l'Ecole belge d'Infirmières diplômeés—raised standards of nursing in Belgium remarkably. Began many innovations in nursing profession—started fourth year of nurses' training in maternity nursing; inaugurated practice of visiting children at home after their discharge.

BORN: Swardeston, Eng., 1865.

NSG. ED.: London Hosp. Sch. of Nsg., London, entered, 1896.

PRINCIPAL POSITIONS: night supt., Nor. St. Pancras Hosp., London, 1901–03; asst. matron, Shoreditch Infirmary, London, 1903–06; matron, l'Ecole belge d'Infirmières diplômeés, Brussels, 1907–15; matron, St. Gilles Hosp., Belg., 1912–15.

HONORS: sch. in Belg. of which she was first dir. now known as l'Ecole Edith Cavell-Marie Depage (Marie Depage was wife of sch's. founder, Dr. Antoine Depage); mountain peak in Alta., Can., named Mt. Edith Cavell; statue erected in St. Martin's Pl., London; Homes of Rest for Nurses estab. in Belg. in memory of her supreme sacrifice; Edith Cavell Ed., *Of the Imitation of Christ* —named in her honor because she carried copy of book while imprisoned in Belg. prior to her execution.

DIED: Brussels, 1915.

Davis, Mary E. (c. 1858–1924). Largely responsible, with Sophia Palmer, for planning the organization and financing of the *American Journal of Nursing* when it was launched in October, 1900. Evolved editorial plan. As business manager, instrumental in keeping *Journal* alive until it became self-supporting. Steadfastly maintained that the *Journal* must be "owned, edited, and controlled by nurses."

BORN: New Brusnwick, Can., c. 1858.

NSG. ED.: Mass. Gen. Hosp. Training Sch. for Nurses, Boston, 1878.

PRINCIPAL POSITIONS: supt. of hosp. and training sch., Hosp. of the Univ. of Penn., 1891–1900; bus. mgr., *Amer. J. Nurs.*, 1906–10; 1st registrar, Central Directory for Nurses, Washington, D.C., 1906; 1st registrar, Central Directory for Nurses, Boston, 1911; matron and supt. of nurses, Sch. for Nurses, Boston Insane Hosp., Dorchester, Mass.

PRINCIPAL OFFICES: mem., com. to organize the Amer. Soc. of Supts. of Training Schs. for Nurses of U.S. and Can. (now NLN), 1893; pres., Amer. Soc. of Supts. of Training Schs. for Nurses of U.S. and Can., 1895; chm., Com. on Periodicals, Nurses' Assoc. Alumnae of U.S. and Can. (now ANA), 1899–1902; pres., Bd. of Dir., Amer. J. Nurs. Co.

HONORS: nsg. sch. library at Mass. Gen. Hosp., Boston, named Palmer-Davis Library in honor of Mary Davis and Sophia Palmer, both grads. of the sch.; NLNE made Miss Davis a life mem. "in appreciation of her progressive work and sacrifices for the ideals of nsg. ed."

DIED: Norwood, Mass., 1924.

Delano, Jane A. (1862–1919). As director of Department of Nursing, American National Red Cross, perfected plan (with cooperation of ANA and a strong national committee) whereby more than 9,000 qualified professional nurses were enrolled and ready for military service when U.S. declared war against Germany in 1917; during the war, ARC nursing service supplied approximately 20,000 nurses to the Army, Navy, and USPHS nursing corps. Said to have rendered the greatest service of any woman in this country to the ultimate aim of winning World War I.

BORN: Montour Falls, N.Y., 1862.

NSG. ED.: Bellevue Training Sch. for Nurses, New York City, 1886.

PRINCIPAL POSITIONS: asst. supt. and instr. of nurses, Univ. of Penn. Hosp., 1891–96; dir., Sch. of Nsg., Bellevue Hosp., New York City, 1902–06; supt., ANC, 1909–12; volunteer in Red Cross Nsg. Serv., 1912–17; dir., Dept. of Nsg., 1917–19.

PRINCIPAL OFFICES: pres., Bd. of Dir., Amer. J. Nurs. Co., 1908–11; pres., Nurses Assoc. Alumnae of U.S. and Can. (now ANA), 1909–11; chm., Nat. Com., Red Cross Nsg. Serv., 1909–19; mem., Com. on Nsg., Gen. Med. Bd., Council of Nat. Defense.

AUTHOR: *ARC Textbook on Elementary Hygiene and Home Care of the Sick,* 1st ed. (in collaboration with Isabel McIsaac), Blakiston, Philadelphia, 1913.

HONORS: Distinguished Serv. Medal (U.S.) awarded posthumously; Distinguished Serv. Medal (ARC) awarded posthumously; Delano Memorial statue in Washington, D.C., residence at Army Med. Ctr., Washington, D.C., named for her; also many nurses' posts of Amer. Legion.

DIED: Savenay, France, 1919. Miss Delano's will provided for estab. of Delano Red Cross Nsg. Serv., financed by income from a bequest plus royalties from her textbook, which provides one or more visiting nurses for some of the communities unable to afford such services.

Dock, Lavinia L. (1858–1956). Very active in early development of nursing organizations in this country and of ICN. For twenty-three years edited "Foreign Department" of *Am. J. Nurs.* Wrote preamble to constitution of ICN. Encouraged among nurses concept of "one world" long before phrase became generally popular. Contributed to improvement of status of women and to social welfare. A militant woman suffragist and ardent crusader and benefactor. Leader in establishing sound foundations for nursing education.

BORN: Harrisburg, Pa., 1858.

NSG. ED.: Bellevue Training Sch. for Nurses, New York City, 1886.

PRINCIPAL POSITIONS: 1st visiting nurse employed by United Workers, a social org., Norwich, Conn., 1886; a pioneer nurse of New York City Mission; night supervisor, Bellevue Hosp., asst. supt. of nurses, Johns Hopkins Hosp., Baltimore, 1890–93; supt. of nurses, Illinois Training

Sch. for Nurses, Chicago, 1893–96; lived and worked with Lillian Wald at Henry St. Settlement, New York City, 1896–1916; editor "Foreign Dept.," *Am. J. Nurs.,* 1900–23.

PRINCIPAL OFFICES: secy., Am. Soc. of Supts. of Training Schs. for Nurses (now NLN), 1896–1902; secy., ICN, 1899–1922.

AUTHOR: *Textbook of Materia Medica for Nurses,* Putnam's, New York, 1890; *History of Nursing,* 4 vols. (in collaboration with Mary A. Nutting), Putnam's, New York, 1907–12; *Hygiene and Morality,* Putnam's, New York, 1910; *Short History of Nursing* (in collaboration with Isabel M. Stewart), Putnam's, New York, 1920; *History of American Red Cross Nursing* (in collaboration with Pickett and others), Macmillan, New York, 1922; also numerous articles for professional journals.

HONORS: chemistry lab. at Johns Hopkins Hosp. Sch. of Nsg., Baltimore, named in her honor, 1955; Lavinia L. Dock Fund estab. in ICN to help finance interchange and translation of educational materials; hon. mem., Johns Hopkins Nurses Alumnae Assn.

DIED: Fayetteville, Pa., 1956.

Fenwick, Ethel G. (Mrs. Bedford) (1856–1947). Proposed idea of an international organization of nurses at a meeting of Matron's Council of Great Britain in 1899. Enlisted support of nurses in United States, Canada, and other countries. Made first president of ICN following year. Influential in establishment of Florence Nightingale International Foundation in 1934. Leader in formation of British Nurses Association, first of its kind, which later was given royal charter and renamed Royal British Nurses Association.

BORN: Scot., 1856.

NSG. ED.: Children's Hosp., Nottingham, Eng., c. 1878.

PRINCIPAL POSITIONS: matron, St. Bartholomew's Hosp., London, 6 yrs.; editor, *Nurs. Rec.,* 1892, during which time she enlarged it to become *Brit. J. Nurs.*

PRINCIPAL OFFICES: first pres., ICN; pres., Brit. Nsg. Section, Chicago World's Fair, 1893; pres., Brit. Col. of Nurses, 1926; pres., Nat. Council of Nurses of Gr. Brit. and Ireland.

AUTHOR: *History of the International Council of Nurses, 1899–1925* (in collaboration with Margaret Breay), ICN, 1931.

HONORS: Greek Red Cross for effective serv. in Greece during war with Turkey; Belg. Order of Knights of St. Leopold, 1933; Silver Medal of the Ministry of Social Welfare of France.

DIED: London, Eng., 1947.

Foley, Edna L. (1879–1943). Leader in development of public health nursing all of professional life. Instrumental in organization of National Organization for Public Health Nursing, 1912. Helped organize public health nursing services in Italy after World War I. For many years edited "Department of Public Health Nursing" in *Am. J. Nurs.*

BORN: Hartford, Conn., 1879.

NSG. ED.: Hartford Hosp. Training Sch. for Nurses, Hartford, Conn., 1904; post grad. study at Boston Sch. of Social Work, 1908.

PRINCIPAL POSITIONS: supt., municipal tuberculosis nurses, Chicago, 3 yrs.; supt., Chicago Visiting Nurse Assn., 1912–37; asst. chief, Public Health Nsg., ARC Tuberculosis Commission to Italy, 1919–20.

PRINCIPAL OFFICES: vice-pres., acting pres., and pres., NOPHN; mem., Nat. Com. on Red Cross Nsg. Serv. for many yrs.; mem., com. to study standards of visiting nsg., which led to formation of NOPHN.

AUTHOR: *Visiting Nurse Manual*, published under auspices of NOPHN by Visiting Nurse Assn. of Chicago, c. 1914.

HONORS: hon. D.Sc., Smith Col., 1928; awarded first "citizen fellowship" conferred by Chicago Inst. of Med., 1934; Florence Nightingale medal, 1937; large substation of Chicago VNA named Edna L. Foley Substation in her honor.

DIED: New York City, 1943.

Gage, Nina D. (1883–1946). Primarily a nurse educator. Launched and developed nursing educational programs in China; influential in starting *Nurs. J. China;* did much work in organizing and developing School of Nursing, College of Yale, Changsha, China; instituted nursing school curricula, accreditation of schools, registration of nurses, and examinations. Kept Nursing Associa-

tion of China alive during critical times. Translated many English nursing textbooks into Chinese (China had no nursing texts before these translations). Helped organize Committee on Nursing Education in China.

BORN: Brooklyn, N.Y., 1883.

NSG. ED.: Sch. of Nsg., Roosevelt Hosp., New York City, 1908; A.B., Wellesley Col., Wellesley, Mass., 1905; M.A., Teachers Col., New York, 1925.

PRINCIPAL POSITIONS: instr. in anatomy and nsg. (in Chinese), Yale Hosp., Sch. of Nsg., Changsha, China, 1910–11; instr. (simultaneously), Yale Hosp. and Red Cross Hosp. Sch. of Nsg., Changsha, c. 1915–17; prof. of nsg. ed., Vassar Training Camp, ARC (summer), 1918; dean, Sch. of Nsg., Col. of Yale, Changsha, 1919; ed. dir. and dir. of nsg. serv., Willard Parker Hosp., New York, 1926–28; editor, "Nsg. Ed. Dept.," *Am. J. Nurs.*, 1929–31; dir., Sch. of Nsg., Hampton Inst., Hampton, Va., 1931–34; instr., Jersey City Med. Ctr. Sch. of Nsg., Jersey City, N.J., 1934–35; dir. of nsg. serv. and Sch. of Nsg., Newport Hosp., Newport, R.I., 1935–43; supt. of nurses, The Protestant Hosp., Nashville, Tenn., 1943–45.

PRINCIPAL OFFICES: pres., NAC, Shanghai, 1911–14; chm., Ed. Com., NAC, 1922–27; pres., ICN, 1925–29; exec. secy., NLNE, 1928–31; mem., Grand Council, ICN, 1929.

AUTHOR: *Communicable Diseases* (in collaboration with Landon), Davis Co., Philadelphia, 1939; also many articles in nsg. journals; translator of several Eng. nsg. textbooks into Chinese.

HONORS: Gage Hall, Sch. of Nsg., Newport Hosp., Newport, R.I., named in honor of Nina Gage, 1949.

DIED: Syracuse, N.Y., 1946.

Gardner, Mary S. (1871–1961). One of earliest directors and organizers of a visiting nurse association; much sought after for advice on organization and administration of public health nursing services. One of the founders of the National Organization for Public Health Nursing and its first secretary and second president. Her book, *Public Health Nursing,* published in 1916, is still considered an authority on the principles of public health nursing service administration.

BORN: Newton, Mass., 1871.

NSG. ED.: Newport Hosp. Sch. of Nsg., Newport, R.I., 1905.

PRINCIPAL POSITIONS: dir., Providence Dist. Nsg. Assn., Providence, R.I., 1905–31; while on leave from this position was dir., ARC Town and Country Nsg. Serv. (later ARC Bur. of Public Health Nsg.), 1917; dir., nsg. dept., ARC Commission for Tuberculosis to Italy, 1917–19; as special advisor to ARC on child health program, surveyed public health nsg. in Eastern Europe, 1920.

PRINCIPAL OFFICES: pres., NOPHN, 1913–15; chm., public health nsg. section, ICN; consultant, Henry St. Visiting Nurse Serv., New York City, 1923–24.

AUTHOR: *Public Health Nursing*, Macmillan, Toronto, 1916; *So Build We*, Macmillan, Toronto, 1942; *Katharine Kent* (a somewhat autobiographical novel), Macmillan, Toronto, 1946; also articles published in professional journals, particularly *Public Health Nursing*.

HONORS: hon. A.M., Brown Univ., 1918; made hon. pres., NOPHN, 1931; hon. dir., Providence Dist. Nsg. Assn., 1931; Walter Burns Saunders Medal for distinguished serv. in the cause of nsg., 1931.

DIED: Providence, R.I., 1961.

Goodrich, Annie W. (1866–1954). Distinguished educator and inspiring leader in professional nursing who aroused public to need for higher educational standards for nurses. First dean, Yale University School of Nursing. Had salutary influence on other members of nursing profession, her students, and co-workers. Contributed extensively to every position and office she held. Brilliant leader and crusader.

BORN: New Brunswick, N.J., 1866.

NSG. ED.: New York Hosp. Training Sch. for Nurses, New York City, 1892.

PRINCIPAL POSITIONS: supt. of nurses, Post-Graduate Hosp., New York City, 1893–1900, St. Luke's Hosp., New York City, 1900–02, New York Hosp., New York City, 1902–07, Bellevue and Allied Hosp., New York City, 1907–10; inspector of nurses training schs., N.Y. State Dept. of Ed., 1910–14; lecturer, Teachers Col., New York City, 1904–13; asst. prof., Dept. of Nsg. and Health, Teachers Col., New York City, 1914; dir. of nurses, Henry St. Settlement, New York City, 1917–23; dean, Army sch. of Nsg., 1918–19, "on

loan''; 1st dean, Yale Univ. Sch. of Nsg., New Haven, Conn., 1923–34.

PRINCIPAL OFFICES: pres., Amer. Soc. of Supts. of Training Schs. for Nurses (now NLN), 1905, 1st vice-pres., 1906; pres., Amer. Fed. of Nurses, 1909; pres., Assn. of Collegiate Schs. of Nsg., 1934; pres., ICN, 1912; vice-pres., Florence Nightingale Internat. Found., 1936; pres., ANA, 1915–18.

AUTHOR: *The Social and Ethical Significance of Nursing*, Macmillan, New York, 1932.

HONORS: hon. D.Sc., Mount Holyoke Col., 1912; Medal of the Inst. of Social Sciences, 1921; Distinguished Serv. Medal (U.S.), 1923; Médaille d'honneur de l'Hygiène Publique (France), 1928; Walter Burns Saunders Memorial Medal for distinguished serv. in the cause of nsg., 1932; Silver Medal of the Ministry of Social Welfare (France), 1933; hon. M.A., Yale Univ., 1923; hon. LL.D., Russell Sage Col., 1936; dean emeritus, Yale Univ. Sch. of Nsg., 1934; cited for distinguished serv. by ICN, 1947; citation and hon. fellowship, Amer. Col. of Hosp. Admin., 1948; Adelaide Nutting Award, 1949; Annie W. Goodrich Endowment Fund estab. by Yale Univ. Sch. of Nsg., 1942; Annie Goodrich Lectures estab. in her honor at Teachers Col., New York City.

DIED: Cobalt, Conn., 1954.

Gretter (Mrs.) Lystra E. (1858–1951). Leader in many forward trends in nursing in late nineteenth and early twentieth centuries. Established first eight-hour day for student nurses at Harper Hospital, Detroit, 1891. One of the first nursing directors to employ graduate nurses to supervise the work and instruction of students, which had been done formerly principally by physicians. Established one of the first preliminary courses for nursing students in this country in 1904. Was the "moving spirit" of group that wrote the Nightingale Pledge in 1893 which was taken that year for the first time by the graduating class of Farrand Training School (now Harper), Detroit.

BORN: Bayfield, Ontario, Can., 1858.

NSG. ED.: Buffalo Gen. Hosp. Training Sch. for Nurses, Buffalo, N.Y. 1888.

PRINCIPAL POSITIONS: prin., Farrand Training Sch. for Nurses, Harper Hosp., Detroit, 1889–1907; supt., Detroit Visiting Nurse Assn., 1907–23.

PRINCIPAL OFFICES: 1st pres., Mich. State Nurses Assn.; chm., Mich. State Com., Red Cross Nsg. Serv.; pres., Amer. Soc. of Supts. of Training Schs. for Nurses (now NLN), 1901; delegate to Internat. Conf. of Red Cross Soc. at which Florence Nightingale Medal was estab.; charter mem., NOPHN; bd. mem., Detroit Visiting Nurse Assn.

HONORS: Lystra Gretter Ed. Fund estab. in her honor by Farrand Training Sch. Alumnae Assn., 1920; hon. M.S., Wayne Univ., Detroit, 1937.

DIED: Detroit, Mich., 1951.

Hubbard, Ruth W. (1897–1955). Outstandingly effective interpreter of public health nursing to allied professions and the public through personal contacts, articles published in journals both within and outside the field of nursing, as an influential member of the National Health Council, and as president for two terms of the National Organization for Public Health Nursing.

BORN: Brooklyn, N.Y., 1897.

NSG. ED.: Army Sch. of Nsg., Washington, D.C., 1921; B.S., Teachers Col., New York City; graduate study, Yale Univ. and Univ. of Penn.

PRINCIPAL POSITIONS: head nurse and instr., Yale Univ. Sch. of Nsg., New Haven, Conn.; ed. dir., New Haven Visiting Nurse Assn., New Haven, Conn.; gen. dir., Visiting Nurse Soc. of Philadelphia, 1929–55.

PRINCIPAL OFFICES: pres., NOPHN; mem., nat. and internat. coms. in health field; bd. mem., Philadelphia Social Serv. Exchange; mem., ICN—Florence Nightingale Internat. Found. Com. on Nsg. Serv.

HONORS: bronze medal for dist. serv. in nsg., Pen. Nurses' Assn., 1949; Friendship Fete Award for outstanding serv. to humanity (sponsored by groups of professional women), 1955; Ruth Weaver Hubbard Found. estab. 1956 to enable nurses "to prepare for positions of leadership in nursing through advanced education, or to provide opportunities for selected nurses to pursue special studies in nursing."

DIED: Rush, N.Y., 1955.

Maass, Clara L. (1876–1901). Young Army nurse who was a martyr to medical science and humanity. During the investigation of yellow fever transmission in 1900–1901, in Cuba, she insisted on being allowed to volunteer for the experimental service; she was bitten by an infected mosquito, contracted yellow fever, and died. A dedicated nurse, she often worked in hospitals without compensation. Offered her services in Cuba, during the Spanish-American War, and during the insurrection in the Philippines.

BORN: East Orange, N.J., 1876.

NSG. ED.: Newark German (Memorial) Hosp., Newark, N.J., 1895.

PRINCIPAL POSITIONS: contract nurse, Field Hosps., 7th U.S. Army Corps, Jacksonville, Fla., Savannah, Ga., Santiago, Cuba, 1898–99; contract nurse, Field Reserve Hosp., Manila, P.I., 1899–1900; nurse for sanitary dept. of Havana, Las Animas Hosp., Havana, 1901 (until death in same yr.).

HONORS: buried with military honors in Fairmont Cem., Newark, at expense of U.S. Govt., 1902 (originally buried in Cuba; body returned to U.S. by U.S. Govt.); Lutheran Memorial Hosp. renamed the Clara Maass Memorial Hosp.; small Army stone on Clara Maass' grave replaced by a more fitting memorial, 1950; radio program, "Cavalcade of Amer.," dramatized story of Clara Maass, entitled, "No Greater Love," 1948; commemorative postage stamp honoring Clara Maass issued by Cuban Govt., 1951; unveiling of Clara Maass' portrait at commencement exercises of Lutheran Memorial Hosp., Newark, 1952; similar portrait presented to Republic of Cuba, 1952.

DIED: Cuba, 1901.

Mahoney, Mary E. (1845–1923). First professional Negro nurse in the U.S. Did much to inspire Negro nurses to strive for better working conditions and facilities in Negro nursing schools and to work towards combatting racial discrimination of nurses. Remains a symbol to the Negro nurse in the U.S.

BORN: Boston, Mass., 1845.

NSG. ED.: New England Hosp. for Women and Children, Boston, 1879.

PRINCIPAL POSITIONS: primarily private duty nurse, Boston.

PRINCIPAL OFFICES: chaplain, Nat. Assn. of Colored Grad. Nurses, 1909.

HONORS: Mary Mahoney Award (of the Nat. Assn. of Colored Grad. Nurses), awarded now by

ANA; recreation hall at Camp Livingstone, La., named in honor of Mary Mahoney in 1944; made life mem. of Nat. Assn. of Colored Grad. Nurses at 1st annual convention in Boston, 1909.

DIED: Boston, 1923.

Maxwell, Anna C. (1851–1929). Brilliant leader in all areas of nursing. Made nursing a more desirable and attractive occupation for women with high social standing. Interpreted nursing to her many acquaintances outside the profession and won support and interest for many causes. Instituted standardization of nursing techniques and procedures. Active in the American Society of Superintendents of Training Schools for Nurses (now NLN), the American Nurses' Association, *American Journal of Nursing,* the "nursing course" at Teachers College, the Robb Scholarship Fund, and the International Council of Nurses.

BORN: Bristol, N.Y., 1851.

NSG. ED.: Boston City Hosp. Training Sch. for Nurses, 1880.

PRINCIPAL POSITIONS: supt., Boston Training Sch. for Nurses, Mass. Gen. Hosp., Boston, 1882 –89; supt. of nurses, St. Luke's Hosp., New York City, 1889–91; supt. of nurses and prin. of Training Sch. for Nurses, Presbyterian Hosp., New York City, 1892–1921. In 1898, on leave from Presbyterian Hosp., in charge of nurses at Sternberg Hosp., Camp Thomas, Chicamauga Park, Ga., during Span.-Amer. War.

PRINCIPAL OFFICES: mem., com. for formulating plans for Red Cross Nsg. Serv. to become reserve of the ANC and NNC; mem., Bd. of Dir., ANA.

AUTHOR: *Practical Nursing* (in collaboration with Amy Pope), Putnam's, New York, 1907.

HONORS: hon. mem., Mass. Gen. Hosp. Training Sch. for Nurses Alumnae Assn., 1895; hon. M.A., Columbia Univ., 1917; nurses' residence at Presbyterian Hosp., New York City, named Anna C. Maxwell Hall; Médaille d'Honneur de l'Hygiene Publique (France), 1927, in recognition of her work in recruiting nurses and organizing the nsg. serv. of the Presbyterian Hosp. Unit (Base Hosp. 2).

DIED: New York City, 1929.

Nightingale, Florence (1820–1910). See Chapter 2.

Noyes, Clara D. (1869–1936). As president of the ANA and director of the American Red Cross Nursing Service simultaneously (in the post-World War I years), showed outstanding ability as organizer. Was instrumental in establishing ANA's national headquarters in 1921. Cited in *Am. J. Nurs.* obituary as "one of nursing's immortals."

BORN: Port Deposit, Md., 1869.

NSG. ED.: Johns Hopkins Hosp. Sch. of Nsg., Baltimore, 1896.

PRINCIPAL POSITIONS: supt. of nurses, New England Hosp. for Women and Children, Boston; supt. of hosp. and nurses, St. Luke's Hosp., New Bedford, Mass.; gen. supt. of nurses, Bellevue and Allied Hosp., New York City; dir., Bur. of Nsg., ARC, 1919; responsible for organizing staff of Red Cross nsg. units; dir. of nsg. serv., ARC, and chm., Nat. Com. on Red Cross Nsg. Serv., 1919–36.

PRINCIPAL OFFICES: 1st vice-pres., ICN, 1925 and 1929; pres., NLNE, 1913–15; pres., Bd. of Dir., Am. J. Nurs. Co., 1913–18; pres., ANA, 1918–22; chm., ANA Com. on Federal Legislation; chm., Com. on Mem., ICN; chm., Advisory Com. on Nsg., U.S. Veterans Admin.; editor, "Red Cross Nsg. Dept," *Am. J. Nurs.,* for many years.

HONORS: Nat. Inst. of Social Science Award; Florence Nightingale Medal; ARC Serv. Medal; decorated by Bulgarian Red Cross and Latvian Red Cross; Médaille d'Honneur d'Hygiene Publique (France); Médaille de la Reconnaissance (France); hon. mem., Polish and Costa Rican Red Cross Socs.; Walter Burns Saunders Memorial Medal, 1933; pin of the Florence Nightingale Sch. of Nsg., France, and hon. grad. of the sch., 1935; Clara D. Noyes Fund estab. following her death, for new wing at Nurses House, Babylon, N.Y.

DIED: Washington, D.C., 1936.

Nutting, Mary A. (1858–1948). As first head of Department of Institutional Administration at Teachers College, Columbia University (later the Department of Nursing and Health, and now, Department of Nursing Education), attracted nurses from all over the world who came to learn how to improve the preparation and status of nurses. Had tremendous vision and incalculable influence on the education of nurses, particularly in colleges and universities. Stressed importance of developing intellectual abilities and assuming professional and civic responsibilities. Was the first nurse to hold a professorship in a university.

BORN: Waterloo, Alta., Can., 1858.

NSG. ED.: Johns Hopkins Hosp. Sch. of Nsg., Baltimore, 1891.

PRINCIPAL POSITIONS: head nurse, asst. supt., and, in 1894, supt. of nurses, Johns Hopkins Hosp. Sch. of Nsg., Baltimore; adm. of dept. of nsg. (see above for exact names), Teachers Col., New York City, 1907–25.

PRINCIPAL OFFICES: hon. pres., Florence Nightingale Internat. Found., 1934–48; pres., Am. Soc. of Supts. of Training Schs. for Nurses (now NLN), 1896 and 1909, and secy., 1903 and 1905; one of founders of Am. Home Economics Assn. and its *Journal of Home Economics;* helped organize Nurses' Assoc. Alumnae of U.S. and Can. (now ANA); mem., Com. on Periodicals of the Nurses' Assoc. Alumnae of U.S. and Can. which estab. the *Am. J. Nurs.;* chm., Com. on Nsg. of the Council of Nat. Defense, W.W. I; pres., Amer. Fed. of Nurses; chm., Ed. Com., Am. Soc. of Supts. of Training Schs. for Nurses, for many years; mem., Com. for the Study of Nsg. Ed., which published the Winslow-Goldmark report: *Nursing and Nursing Education in the United States;* chm., Ed. Com., ICN; mem., group which persuaded Dean James E. Russell to introduce courses for professional nurses at Teachers Col., New York City.

AUTHOR: *History of Nursing,* 4 vols. (in collaboration with Lavinia L. Dock), Putnam's, New York, 1907; *Sound Economic Basis for Schools of Nursing,* Putnam's, New York, 1926; *Educational Status of Nursing* (research report), U.S. Off. of Ed., Washington, D.C., 1912.

HONORS: Mary Adelaide Nutting award estab. in her honor, 1943, to be awarded by NLNE, from time to time, in recognition of outstanding leadership in nsg. ed.; medal presented to Miss Nutting, herself, 1944; Liberty Serv. Medal—given by Council of Nat. Inst. of Social Sciences—for notable humanitarian and patriotic serv. furthering the nat. welfare; hon. M.A., Yale Univ., 1921; ed. unit at Johns Hopkins Sch. of Nsg. bears her name; Adelaide Nutting Historical Collection at Teachers Col. named in her honor—nucleus of collection contributed by her former students; 4 important funds estab. in her name: (1) for the historical collection at Teachers Col., (2) endow-

ment fund for the Johns Hopkins Hosp. Sch. of Nsg., (3) fund at NLN (associated with Adelaide Nutting Award) to make current and historical materials available for wider use, (4) Adelaide Nutting-Florence Nightingale Research Fund of the Florence Nightingale Internat. Found. to finance collection and preservation of Nightingaliana.

DIED: White Plains, N.Y., 1948.

Palmer, Sophia F. (1853–1920). Helped establish the *American Journal of Nursing* and was its editor from first issue, October, 1900, until her death in 1920. Pioneer work in journalism gave impetus to nursing profession. Leader in movement to secure state registration for nurses. Promoted in pages of *Am. J. Nurs.* legislation affecting nurse licensure. Helped organize both ANA and NLNE.

BORN: Milton, Mass., 1853.

NSG. ED.: Mass. Gen. Hosp. Training Sch. for Nurses, Boston, Mass., 1878.

PRINCIPAL POSITIONS: org. St. Luke's Hosp. Training Sch. for Nurses, New Bedford, Mass.; reorg. Garfield Memorial Hosp., Washington, D.C., and estab. training sch. for nurses; supt. Rochester City Hosp. (now Rochester Gen. Hosp.), Rochester, N.Y. and supt. of the training sch. for nurses; editor-in-chief, *Am. J. Nurs.,* 1900–20.

PRINCIPAL OFFICES: mem., com. to outline purposes of Amer. Soc. of Supts. of Training Schs. for Nurses (now NLN), qualifications of members, duties of officers, etc., 1893; mem., representing Nurses' Assoc. Alumnae of U.S. and Can. (now ANA), of the orig. com. on the Isabel Hampton Robb Ed. Fund, 1910; mem., Com. on Periodicals, Nurses' Assoc. Alumnae, which brought forth the *Am. J. Nurs.,* 1898; 1st pres., N.Y. State Bd. of Nurse Examiners; mem., local and nat. coms. on Red Cross nsg. serv.

HONORS: Palmer-Davis Library at Mass. Gen. Hosp. Sch. of Nsg., Boston, named for her and Miss Mary E. P. Davis; Sophia F. Palmer Memorial Library, Am. J. Nurs. Co., estab. in her honor, 1953.

DIED: Forest Lawn, N.Y., 1920.

Pope, Amy E. (1868–1949). Author and coauthor of numerous nursing texts translated into many languages and widely used in many countries. Served with Army in Cuba during Spanish-American War; in Cuba during yellow fever epidemic; went to the Philippines with Red Cross auxiliary unit. Appointed for service with Health Dept. of the Isthmian Canal Commission on Isthmus of Panama; appointed by governor of Puerto Rico as superintendent of the Government Insular Training School for Nurses, San Juan, P.R.

BORN: Quebec, Can., 1868.

NSG. ED.: Sch. of Nsg., Presbyterian Hosp., New York City, 1894.

PRINCIPAL POSITIONS: instr., Johns Hopkins Hosp., Sch. of Nsg., Baltimore, 1904; supt., Govt. Insular Training Sch. for Nurses, San Juan, P.R., 1907; instr., head nurse, and asst. supt., Sch. of Nsg., Presbyterian Hosp., New York City; instr., Sch. of Nsg., St. Luke's Hosp., San Francisco, 1914–28.

AUTHOR: *Practical Nursing* (coauthor), Putnam's New York, 1907; *Anatomy and Physiology for Nurses,* Putnam's, New York, 1913; *A Medical Dictionary for Nurses,* Putnam's, New York, 1914; *A Quiz Book of Nursing* (coauthor), Putnam's, New York, 1915; *Physics and Chemistry for Nurses,* Putnam's, New York, 1916; *Essentials of Dietetics in Health and Disease,* 2nd. ed. (coauthor), Putnam's, New York, 1917; *A Practical Dietary Computer,* Putnam's, New York, 1917; *Manual of Nursing Procedure,* Putnam's, New York, 1919; *Materia Medica, Pharmacology and Therapeutics for Nurses,* Saunders, Philadelphia, 1921; *A Textbook of Simple Nursing Procedure,* Putnam's, New York, 1921; *The Art and Principles of Nursing,* Putnam's, New York, 1934.

DIED: San Francisco, Calif., 1949.

Richards, Linda (1841–1930). Known as America's "first trained nurse." Primarily an organizer of training schools for nurses and nursing services. Organized or reorganized the schools in several hospitals: Massachusetts General (Boston), Boston City (Boston), Methodist Episcopal (Philadelphia), New England Hospital for Women and Children (Boston), Brooklyn Homeopathic Hosp. (Brooklyn, N.Y.), Hartford Hosp. (Hartford, Conn.), and University of Pennsylvania. Also a pioneer in establishing training schools for nurses in hospitals for the mentally ill. Comments in her *Reminiscenses:* "two years [was] my allotted time in an institution." Very

active in early work of organizing the national nursing organizations. Editor of "Hospital and Training School Items," *Am. J. Nurs.*

BORN: near Pottsdam, N.Y., 1841.

NSG. ED.: New England Hosp. for Women and Children, Boston, 1873.

PRINCIPAL POSITIONS: night supt., Bellevue Hosp., New York City, 1873–74; supt., Boston Training Sch., Mass. Gen. Hosp., Boston, 1874–77; supt., Training Sch. for Nurses, Boston City Hosp., Boston, 1878–85; org. 1st training sch. for nurses under missionary auspices in Japan, 1885–90; head, Philadelphia Visiting Nurses Society, 1891; between 1890 and 1909, supt. of Training Sch. for Nurses, Methodist Episcopal Hosp., Philadelphia; New England Hosp. for Women and Children, Boston; Brooklyn Homeopathic Hosp., Brooklyn, N.Y.; Hartford Hospital, Hartford, Conn.; and Univ. of Penn. Hosp., Philadelphia; supt. of nurses. Taunton Insane Hosp., Taunton, Mass.; Worcester Hosp. for the Insane, Worcester, Mass.; and Michigan Insane Hosp., Kalamazoo.

PRINCIPAL OFFICES: 1st pres., Amer. Soc. of Supts. of Training Schs. for Nurses (now NLN), 1894; mem., Supts. Soc. Com. on Ways and Means for the Teachers Course which approached Teachers Col. concerning courses there (later developed into what is now the Dept. of Nsg. Ed. at Teachers Col.); mem., 1st ed. com. of Amer. Soc. of Supts. of Training Schs. for Nurses (now NLN).

AUTHOR: *Reminiscences of Linda Richards: America's First Trained Nurse,* Whitcomb and Barrows, Boston, 1911.

HONORS: likeness engraved in corporate seal of ANA; hon. mem., Amer. Soc. of Supts. of Training Schs. for Nurses; Linda Richards Achievement Awards (medallion bearing likeness of Miss Richards on one side and letters ANA on the other) were presented to one nurse from each state by the ANA at the Diamond Jubilee of Nsg., 1948.

DIED: Boston, Mass., 1930.

Robb, Isabel H. (1860–1910). Brilliant leader who did much to improve and develop the curriculum in the early nursing schools. At Illinois Training School for Nurses, Chicago, extended theoretical instruction through two years; inaugurated a regular class schedule; provided for holidays for nurses; eliminated the monthly stipend. Has been credited with initiating proposal to establish nursing department at Teachers College, New York City. One of founders of American Society of Superintendents of Training Schools for Nurses, the Nurses' Associated Alumnae of the U.S. and Canada, the *American Journal of Nursing,* and the International Council of Nurses. One of earliest nurse authors.

BORN: Welland, Ont., Can., 1860.

NSG. ED.: Bellevue Training Sch. for Nurses, New York City, 1883; took nsg. course at St. Paul's House, Rome, Italy, 1883–85.

PRINCIPAL POSITIONS: supt., Illinois Training Sch. for Nurses, Chicago, 1886–89; org. Johns Hopkins Training Sch. for Nurses, Baltimore, and remained as supt., 1889–94.

PRINCIPAL OFFICES: 1st pres., Nurses Assoc. Alumnae, 1897; pres., Am. Soc. of Supts. of Training Schs. for Nurses, 1908; chm., Ed. Com., Am. Soc. of Supts. of Training Schs. for Nurses; mem., Com. on Periodicals of Assoc. Alumnae, which founded *Am. J. Nurs.;* mem., provisional com. to work out plan of org. for ICN; chm., Standing Com. on Ed. of the ICN.

AUTHOR: *Nursing, Its Principles and Practice,* E. C. Koeckert, Cleveland, 1893; *Nursing Ethics: for Hospital and Private Use,* J. B. Savage, Cleveland, 1901.

HONORS: Isabel Hampton Robb Fund estab. to provide scholarships for grad. nurses, 1910; Isabel Hampton Robb Fellowship awarded annually at Teachers Col., New York City, to advanced student specializing in nsg. ed.

DIED: Cleveland, O., 1910.

Roberts, Mary M. (1877–1959). As editor of *American Journal of Nursing* for twenty-eight years, was one of most influential figures in modern nursing. A great teacher and tireless worker and investigator with the intellectual ability, imagination, and insight to see the importance, significance, and relationships of various movements in nursing. Through the *Journal,* encouraged nurses to broaden concepts of service to patients and the community. A brilliant writer. Under her guidance the circulation of the *Journal* increased from approximately 20,000 subscribers to over 100,000.

BORN: Sheboygan, Mich., 1877.

NSG. ED.: Jewish Hosp. Sch. of Nsg., Cincinnati, O., 1899; B.S., Teachers Col., New York City, 1921.

PRINCIPAL POSITIONS: estab. Training Sch. for Nurses, Savannah Hosp., Savannah, Ga.; private duty in Chicago, 4 yrs.; asst. supt. and acting supt., Jewish Hosp., Cincinnati, 1904–1906; supt., Christian R. Holmes Hosp., Cincinnati 1908–17; dir., Bur. of Nsg., Lake Div., ARC, W.W. I; dir., Army Sch. of Nsg., Camp Sherman, O., 1918–19; editor, *Am. J. Nurs.,* 1921–49; editor emeritus, 1949–59.

PRINCIPAL OFFICES: mem. of innumerable coms. of ANA, NLNE, others; pres., Ohio State Nurses Assn.; mem., Ohio Nurse Examining Bd.; chm., ANA Com. on Florence Nightingale Internat. Found.; chm., Publications Com., ICN; mem., Ethics Com., ICN; mem., Nat. Com. on Red Cross Nsg. Serv., 1923–44; mem., Com. on Costs of Med. Care, 1929–33; consultant to Com. on the Grading of Nsg. Schs., 1926–34; nurse representative on New York Academy of Med. Com. on Med. in the Changing Order, 1944–47; consultant to the Procurement and Assignment Serv., War Manpower Commission, 1943–45; mem., Nsg. Council on Nat. Defense, W.W. II.

AUTHOR: *American Nursing: History and Interpretation,* Macmillan, New York, 1954; *The Army Nurse Corps—Yesterday and Today;* also many articles and guest editorials for professional journals.

HONORS: Florence Nightingale Medal; Army Certificate of Appreciation, 1949; citation by Bd. of Dir., Am. J. Nurs. Co., 1949; hon. fellowship, Am. Col. of Hosp. Admin.; Adelaide Nutting Award; Bronze Medal (France) for social serv. of outstanding merit; hospitality fund for nurses from other countries estab. at Nurses Home, Babylon, N.Y., in honor of Miss Roberts and Miss Florence M. Johnson; Mary M. Roberts Fellowship in Journalism (now Writing Awards) estab. by Am. J. Nurs. Co., 1950; Roberts Reading Room, *Am. J. Nurs.* Library, 1959.

DIED: New York City, 1959.

Shaw, Mrs. Clara Weeks (1857–1940). Credited with being first nurse to write a nursing textbook in the United States, 1885. Previously doctors had written most of the texts used in nursing schools.

BORN: Sanborton, N.H., 1857.

NSG. ED.: New York Hosp. Training Sch. for Nurses, New York City, 1880; had graduated from Rhode Island State Normal Sch. before entering nsg. sch.

PRINCIPAL POSITION: supt., Training Sch. for Nurses, Paterson Gen. Hosp., Paterson, N.J., 1883–88.

AUTHOR: *Textbook of Nursing for the Use of Training Schools, Families and Private Students*, Appleton, New York, 1885.

DIED: Mountainville, N.Y., 1940.

Stewart, Isabel Maitland (1878–1963). The influence of this great nursing leader and educator helped shape the development of twentieth century nursing education and practice. Miss Stewart was instrumental in developing the first program for preparing nurse faculty at Teachers College; aided in research which promoted the use of objective tests; and revived interest in the study of nursing schools by an outside group. The latter activity resulted in the 1926 study by the Committee on the Grading of Nursing Schools. As Chairman of the ICN Education Committee (1925–47) she wrote "Educational Program of the Schools of Nursing," published in four languages by the Nursing Bureau of the League of Red Cross Societies. During World War I, she wrote much nursing publicity and recruitment material which led to numbers of college women entering nursing through the Vassar Training Camp program. At the beginning of World War II, she suggested forming a National Nursing Council for National Defense; chaired its Committee on Educational Policies and Resources and prepared a brief that requested and helped to obtain federal funds for nursing education.

BORN: Fletcher, Ontario, Can., 1878.

NSG. ED.: Manitoba Normal School; Winnipeg General Hospital Training School (entered 1900; no graduation date available); Teachers College, Columbia Univ., B.S. 1910 to 1911, M.S. 1913. (First nurse in department to receive Master's degree.)

PRINCIPAL POSITIONS: Helen Hartley Foundation Professor of Nursing Education and Director of the Department, Teachers College, 1925–47; Professor Emeritus 1947–63.

PRINCIPAL OFFICES: sec., NLNE, 1914–19; Chm., Ed. Com. NLNE, 1920–37; mem., Bd. of

Dir. NLNE, 1925–43; FNIF mem., Com. on Management; mem., Foreign Policy Assn.; 2nd vice pres., Am. Council on Ed., 1944; one of founders and mem., Bd. of Dir. of Assn. of Coll. Schls. of Nsg. (pres. 1937–41); chm., NLN Com. on Early Nsg. Source Materials 1954; mem., Am. Soc. of Supts. of Trng. Schls. for Nurses; mem., Women's Board of Henry St. VNA; mem. and com. mem., ANA.

AUTHOR: *Short History of Nursing* (in collaboration with Lavinia Dock), Putnam's, New York, 1920; *Education of Nurses*, Macmillan, New York, 1943; and editor, AJN Dept. of Nursing Education, 1916–21.

HONORS: D. Hum. Col. Univ. 1954; LLD Western Res. Univ. 1948; Doctoral degree, Univ. of Manitoba; Adelaide Nutting Award, 1961; "Pro benignetate humana" medal of Finland; named one of twenty-three "Women of Achievement" by N.Y. League of Natl. Fed. Bus. and Prof. Women in 1936; hon. mem. Hist. of Nsg. Soc., McGill Univ.; Kappa Delta Pi; Pi Lambda Theta; honored by establishment of development fund at Teachers College in 1961 to endow Isabel Stewart Research Professorship in Nursing.

Stimson, Julia C. (1881–1948). First came to national notice through her spectacular work in organizing and administering the work of the nurses at General Hospital No. 12 in Rouen, France. First woman given rank of major in U.S. Army (promoted to colonel in 1945). Contributed greatly to nursing by her work in recruiting nurses for ANC and ARC; holds longest tenure in the history of ANC. Instrumental in forming the Nursing Council of National Defense (1940), later to become the National Nursing Council for War Service, Inc. (1942) and (in 1945) the National Council Inc.

BORN: Worcester, Mass., 1881.

NSG. ED.: New York Hosp. Sch. of Nsg., New York City, 1908; B.A., Vassar Col., Poughkeepsie, N.Y., 1901; M.A., Washington Univ., St. Louis, Mo., 1917.

PRINCIPAL POSITIONS: supt. of nurses, Harlem Hosp., New York City, 1908–11; dir. of hosp. social serv., Washington Univ., St. Louis, 1911; supt. of nurses, Barnes Hosp., Washington Univ., St. Louis, 1911–17; chief nurse, ANC, 1917; chief nurse, ARC, France, 1918; dir. of nsg. serv., Amer. Expeditionary Forces, 1918; dean,

Army Sch. of Nsg., 1919–33; supt., ANC, 1919–37.

PRINCIPAL OFFICES: pres., ANA, 1938–44; chm., Nsg. Council of Nat. Defense, 1940–42; secy.-treas., Isabel Hampton Robb Memorial Fund, Inc., 1945–47; mem., many Red Cross nsg. serv. coms. and military nsg. serv. coms.

AUTHOR: *Nurses' Handbook of Drugs and Solutions,* Whitcomb and Barrows, Boston, 1910; *Finding Themselves,* Macmillan, New York, 1918; also many articles and reports for nsg. and med. journals and Army med. bulls. and pamphs.

HONORS: First woman to become a major in U.S. Army, c. 1920; promoted to rank of colonel, 1945; Distinguished Serv. Medal for serv. overseas; cited by Gen. John J. Pershing for "exceptionally meritorious and efficient service"; received the Royal Red Cross, First Class Citation (Gr. Brit.); awarded Médaille de la Reconnaissance Francaise; given the silver Médaille d'Hygiene Publique (France); hon. Sc.D., Mount Holyoke Col., 1921; sch. library of Army Med. Field Serv. Sch., Fort Sam Houston, Tex., named in honor of Col. J. C. Stimson.

DIED: Poughkeepsie, N.Y., 1948.

Wald, Lillian D. (1867–1940). Founded Henry Street Visiting Nurse Service in New York City, the first nonsectarian public health nursing service in this country, now the Visiting Nurse Service of New York. Entire professional life spent in promoting public health and social welfare concepts and practices: was responsible for inauguration of school nursing in New York City; suggested that public health nurses visit ill persons insured by the Metropolitan Life Insurance Company; recommended that American Red Cross establish Town and Country Nursing Service, later ARC Public Health Nursing Service; fought for better housing in New York City slums; one of organizers of the National Child Labor Committee; establishing U.S. Children's Bureau was her idea.

BORN: Cincinnati, O., 1867.

NSG. ED.: New York Hosp. Training Sch. for Nurses, 1891; studied for a time at Women's Med. Col., New York City, after grad. from nsg. sch., but left col. to estab. program in Henry St. Settlement.

PRINCIPAL POSITIONS: head, Henry St. Settlement, New York City, 1893; founder, Henry St. Visiting Nurse Serv.

PRINCIPAL OFFICES: one of organizers and first pres., NOPHN; chm., Am. Union Against Militarism; mem., Com. on Nsg., Council of Nat. Defense, W.W. I; served on numerous local, nat., and internat. coms.

AUTHOR: *The House on Henry Street,* Henry Holt, New York, 1915; *Windows on Henry Street,* Little, Brown and Co., Boston, 1933.

HONORS: hon. LL.D., Mount Holyoke Col., 1912 and Smith Col., 1930; gold medal, Nat. Inst. of Sciences, 1912; gold medal, Rotary Club, 1923; "Better Times" medal for distinguished social serv., 1926; Abraham Lincoln High Sch. Award as "the citizen rendering the greatest service to the City of New York," 1936; cited by Mayor Fiorello LaGuardia of New York City, 1937; playground in New York City named for her.

DIED: Westport, Conn., 1940.

Of necessity, these sketches of distinguished nurses are brief. Although they contain basic information concerning the background and accomplishments of these nursing leaders, they contain none of the excitement of their lives, the spark each had that ignited the nursing of the time, the humanness, the force, the warmth. It is suggested that the reader review some of the early issues of the *American Journal of Nursing,* which contain information about, and often articles by, some of these individuals.

Index